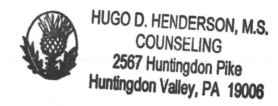

HUGO D. HENDERSON, M.S.
COUNSELING
2567 Huntingdon Pike
Huntingdon Valley, PA 19006

D0555901

# Late-Life Depression

# LATE-LIFE
# DEPRESSION

*Edited by*

STEVEN P. ROOSE
HAROLD A. SACKEIM

OXFORD
UNIVERSITY PRESS
2004

# OXFORD
UNIVERSITY PRESS

Oxford   New York
Auckland   Bangkok   Buenos Aires   Cape Town   Chennai
Dar es Salaam   Delhi   Hong Kong   Istanbul   Karachi   Kolkata
Kuala Lumpar   Madrid   Melbourne   Mexico City   Mumbai   Nairobi
São Paulo   Shanghai   Taipei   Tokyo   Toronto

Copyright © 2004 by Oxford University Press

Published by Oxford University Press, Inc.
198 Madison Avenue, New York, New York 10016
http://www.oup.org

Oxford is a registered trademark of Oxford University Press

Library of Congress Cataloging-in-Publication Data
Late-life depression / edited by Steven P. Roose, Harold A. Sackeim.
p. ; cm.   Includes bibliographical references and index.
ISBN 0-19-515274-3
1. Depression in old age.
2. Geriatric psychiatry.
I. Roose, Steven P., 1948– II. Sackeim, Harold A.
[DNLM: 1. Depressive Disorder—Aged.
2. Aged—psychology.
WM 171 L351 2004]
RC537.5.L38 2004   618.97'68527–dc22   2003069051

The science of medicine is a rapidly changing field. As new research and clinical experience broaden
our knowledge, changes in treatment and drug therapy do occur. The author and publisher of this work
have checked with sources believed to be reliable in their efforts to provide information that is accurate and complete, and in accordance with the standards accepted at the time of publication. However,
in light of the possibility of human error or changes in the practice of medicine, neither the author, nor
the publisher, nor any other party who has been involved in the preparation or publication of this work
warrants that the information contained herein is in every respect accurate or complete. Readers are
encouraged to confirm the information contained herein with other reliable sources, and are strongly
advised to check the product information sheet provided by the pharmaceutical company for each drug
they plan to administer.

9 8 7 6 5 4 3 2 1
Printed in the United States of America
on acid free paper

*For Liz,*
*Matthew and Katie Roose,*
*Alexander Sackeim,*
*and Judith Kiersky.*
*These are the people with whom we wish to grow old.*

# Preface

Detection and treatment of depression in the elderly are of paramount importance. The demographics are compelling: by the year 2030, over 70 million people in the United States will be over the age of 65 years. In fact, the most rapidly growing segment of the population is the group over the age of 85 years, whose numbers will double in the next decade. The remarkable growth of the segment of the population over the age of 65 is not restricted to the United States or Europe. Indeed, this rate of increase will be equaled, if not exceeded, in Africa, Asia, and South America. Thus, disorders that are prevalent and cause significant morbidity and mortality in older individuals will consume greater health care resources and require more intensive research.

Late-life depression is a public health problem of great concern. It is an illness that torments individuals and their families and can frequently frustrate the best attempts of the most caring and knowledgeable physicians. Given its significance, it is notable that until now there was no textbook specifically devoted to the comprehensive presentation of current knowledge about this disease. We felt that there was a compelling need for this book.

We sought out prominent scientists and clinicians expert in this field and asked them to write a fresh chapter, critically and comprehensively reviewing the state of knowledge about their topic. We also asked them to incorporate their own thinking about current theories of the illness, methodological problems endemic to the research area, and optimal treatment of their patients. Senior authors had to agree that they would write the chapter themselves and that it would constitute a new effort.

For whom is this book intended? Who should find this volume relevant to their work? Our first goal was to ensure that the volume be accessible, useful, and stimulating to the clinician who strives to understand the multiple dimensions of aging and the complexity of late-life depression and who aspires to practice evidence-based interventions. In addition, researchers wrote this book for other researchers, offering perspectives on where the field has been and where it should go. This is a volume that was also prepared for educators and students, including academic faculty, clinical and research fellows, residents, and graduate students. In addition to the review of current knowledge, each chapter illustrates how the author organizes an often methodologically disparate and large database, critically evaluates the findings, and distills justifiable conclusions.

It is our hope that the contents of this book will influence our judgment, empathy, and decision making as we struggle with the most complex and important task—the diagnosis, treatment, and understanding of the suffering patient.

*New York, NY*                                                                                 S. P. R.
*New York, NY*                                                                                 H. A. S.

# Acknowledgments

Throughout our careers, we have benefited from teachers, colleagues, students, and, most of all, patients who have taught, influenced, frustrated, and inspired us. To all of them, far too many to mention, we are grateful. We are also grateful to Fiona Stevens, our editor, who transformed our inchoate but strongly held opinions into the plan for this book, and to Judith Kiersky, who formatted and reformatted the chapters until the dawn.

# Contents

    Outcome, 150
Executive Dysfunction and Vascular
    Depression, 151
Cognitive Outcomes of Geriatric Depression, 151
Cognitive Outcomes of Vascular Depression, 151
Apolipoprotein E and Cognition, 151
Morbidity and Mortality Outcomes of Vascular
    Depression, 152
Leukoaraiosis and Lacunar Stroke: Apparently
    Different Outcomes, 152
Conceptual Framework, 152
Hippocampus and Geriatric Depression, 153

13. Hypothalamic-Pituitary-Adrenal Axis Activity
    in Mood and Cognition in the Elderly:
    Implications for Symptoms and Outcomes, 157
    Jennifer Keller, Theresa M. Buckley, and
    Alan F. Schatzberg

    Regulation and Function of the
        Hypothalamic-Pituitary-Adrenal Axis, 157
    Hypothalamic-Pituitary-Adrenal Axis and
        Depression, 158
    Geriatric Depression, Cognition, and
        Hypothalamic-Pituitary-Adrenal Activity, 159
    Aging and Hypothalamic-Pituitary-Adrenal
        Activity, 159
    Depression, Dementia, and Hypothalamic-Pituitary-
        Adrenal Activity, 160
    Brain Structures in Cognition and Depression, 160
    Frontal Lobe, 161
    Limbic and Fronto-Striatal Connections, 161
    Hippocampus and Amygdala, 161
    Depression, Aging, and Mortality, 162

14. The Neuroendocrinology of Aging, 167
    Stuart N. Seidman

    Hormones and Neuropsychiatry, 167
    Central Nervous System Mechanisms of Hormonal
        Action, 167
    Age-Related Changes in Hormone Axes, 168
    Carbohydrate Metabolism, 168
    Parathyroid, 168
    Hypothalamic-Pituitary-Thyroid Axis, 168
    Hypothalamic-Pituitary-Adrenal Axis, 169
    Dehydroepiandrosterone, 169
    Growth Hormone, 170
    Prolactin, 170
    Female Hypothalamic-Pituitary-Gonadal Axis, 171
    Male Hypothalamic-Pituitary-Gonadal Axis, 171
    Depression and Neuroendocrine Dysregulation in
        the Elderly, 172
    Hormonal Axis Dysregulation and Late-Life
        Depression, 173
    Hypothalamic-Pituitary-Adrenal Axis, Depression,
        and Age, 173

Dehydroepiandrosterone, Depression, and Age, 174
Hypothalamic-Pituitary-Thyroid Axis, Depression,
    and Age, 175
Hypothalamic-Pituitary-Gonadal Axis, Depression,
    and Age, 175
Testosterone and Male Neuropsychiatric
    Functioning, 175
Male Depressive Illness, Hypothalamic-Pituitary-
    Gonadal Axis Functioning, and Age, 177

## PART IV   TREATMENT

15. Pharmacokinetics and Pharmacodynamics in
    Late Life, 185
    Bruce G. Pollock

    Age-Associated Physiological Changes, 186
    Pharmacokinetics, 187
    Pharmacodynamics, 189

16. Antidepressant Medication for the Treatment of
    Late-Life Depression, 192
    Steven P. Roose and Harold A. Sackeim

    Moderators and Mediators of the Antidepressant
        Response, 192
    Antidepressant Medications, 195
    Tricyclic Antidepressants, 195
    Selective Serotonin Reuptake Inhibitors, 196
    Fluoxetine, 196
    Sertraline, 196
    Paroxetine, 197
    Citalopram, 197
    Selective Serotonin Reuptake Inhibitor Side Effect
        Profile in Geriatric Patients, 197
    Other Antidepressants, 197
    Placebo versus Comparator Controlled Trials, 198

17. Antidepressant Side Effects, 203
    Carl Salzman

    The Increased Likelihood of an Elderly Person
        Developing Side Effects, 203
    Receptor Mechanisms of Antidepressant Side
        Effects in the Elderly, 204
    Cardiovascular Side Effects, 206
    Vascular Side Effects, 207
    Falls, 207
    Inappropriate Antidiuretic Hormone Secretion, 207
    Weight Alterations, 208
    Medication Noncompliance as a Risk for
        Antidepressant Adverse Events, 208

18. Mood Stabilizers, 211
    Charles L. Bowden

    The Prevention of Depression in Elderly Bipolar
        Patients, 212
    Difficulties in Conducting Studies of Mood
        Stabilizers in Elderly Patients, 212
    Evidence of Spectrum of Efficacy, Tolerability,
        and Dosing, 213

# Contributors

GEORGE S. ALEXOPOULOS, MD
*Cornell Institute of Geriatric Psychiatry*
*Weill Medical College of Cornell University*
*White Plains, New York*

WILLIAM APFELDORF, MD, PhD
*Department of Psychiatry*
*University of New Mexico School of Medicine*
*Santa Fe, New Mexico*

PATRICIA A. AREAN, PhD
*Department of Psychiatry*
*University of California, San Francisco*
*San Francisco, California*

JOHN L. BEYER, MD
*Department of Psychiatry and Behavioral Sciences*
*Duke University Medical Center*
*Durham, North Carolina*

DAN G. BLAZER, MD, MPH, PhD
*Department of Psychiatry and Behavioral Sciences*
*Duke University Medical Center*
*Durham, North Carolina*

CHARLES L. BOWDEN, MD
*Department of Psychiatry*
*The University of Texas Health Science Center at*
  *San Antonio*
*San Antonio, Texas*

THERESA M. BUCKLEY, MD, MS
*Department of Psychiatry and Behavioral Sciences*
*Stanford University School of Medicine*
*Stanford, California*

ANJAN CHATTERJEE, MD
*The Gertrude H. Sergievsky Center, Columbia University*
*Department of Neurology*
*College of Physicians and Surgeons of Columbia University*
*New York, New York*

PAULA J. CLAYTON, MD
*Department of Psychiatry*
*University of New Mexico School of Medicine*
*Santa Fe, New Mexico*

YEATES CONWELL, MD
*Department of Psychiatry*
*University of Rochester School of Medicine*
*Rochester, New York*

D.P. DEVANAND, MD
*Departments of Psychiatry and Neurology*
*College of Physicians and Surgeons of Columbia University*
*New York State Psychiatric Institute*
*New York, New York*

CHRISTIAN R. DOLDER, PharmD
*Department of Psychiatry*
*University of California, San Diego*
*VA San Diego Healthcare System*
*San Diego, California*

P. MURALI DORAISWAMY, MD
*Department of Psychiatry and Behavioral Sciences*
*Duke University Medical Center*
*Durham, North Carolina*

VIRGINIA ELDERKIN-THOMPSON, PhD
*Department of Psychiatry and Bio-behavioral Sciences*
*David Geffen School of Medicine at UCLA*
*Los Angeles, California*

ELLEN FRANK, PhD
*Professor of Psychiatry and Psychology*
*University of Pittsburgh School of Medicine*
*Western Psychiatric Institute and Clinic*
*Pittsburgh, Pennsylvania*

ALEXANDER H. GLASSMAN, MD
*Department of Psychiatry*
*College of Physicians and Surgeons of Columbia University*
*New York State Psychiatric Institute*
*New York, New York*

DILIP V. JESTE, MD
*Department of Psychiatry*
*University of California, San Diego*
*VA San Diego Healthcare System*
*San Diego, California*

IRA R. KATZ, MD, PhD
*Section of Geriatric Psychiatry*
*Center for Interventions and Services Research*
*University of Pennsylvania*
*Mental Illness Research Education and Clinical Center*
*Philadelphia VA Medical Center*
*Philadelphia, Pennsylvania*

JENNIFER KELLER, PhD
*Department of Psychiatry and Behavioral Sciences*
*Stanford University School of Medicine*
*Stanford, California*

K. RANGA R. KRISHNAN, MD
*Department of Psychiatry and Behavioral Sciences*
*Duke University Medical Center*
*Durham, North Carolina*

ANAND KUMAR, MD
*Department of Psychiatry and Bio-behavioral Sciences*
*David Geffen School of Medicine at UCLA*
*Los Angeles, California*

JONATHAN P. LACRO, PharmD
*Department of Psychiatry*
*University of California, San Diego*
*VA San Diego Healthcare System*
*San Diego, California*

HELEN LAVRETSKY, MD
*Department of Psychiatry and Bio-behavioral Sciences*
*David Geffen School of Medicine at UCLA*
*Los Angeles, California*

BARRY D. LEBOWITZ, PhD
*Adult and Geriatric Treatment and*
  *Preventive Interventions Research Branch*
*National Institute of Mental Health*
*Bethesda, Maryland*

THOMAS R. LYNCH, PhD
*Department of Psychiatry and Behavioral Sciences*
*Duke University Medical Center*
*Durham, North Carolina*

KAREN MARDER, MD, MPH
*The Gertrude H. Sergievsky Center, Columbia University*
*Department of Neurology*
*College of Physicians and Surgeons of Columbia*
  *University*
*New York, New York*

J. CRAIG NELSON, MD
*Director of Geriatric Psychiatry*
*University of California, San Francisco*
*San Francisco, California*

JASON T. OLIN, PhD
*Clinical Development and Medical Affairs*
*Forest Research Institute*
*Jersey City, New Jersey*

DAVID W. OSLIN, MD
*Geriatric and Addiction Psychiatry*
*University of Pennsylvania*
*Philadelphia Veterans Affairs Medical Center*
*Philadelphia, Pennsylvania*

BRUCE G. POLLOCK, MD, PhD
*Academic Division of Geriatrics and Neuropsychiatry*
*University of Pittsburgh School of Medicine*
*Western Psychiatric Institute and Clinic*
*Pittsburgh, Pennsylvania*

CHARLES F. REYNOLDS III, MD
*Departments of Psychiatry, Neurology, and Neuroscience*
*University of Pittsburgh School of Medicine*
*Western Psychiatric Institute and Clinic*
*Pittsburgh, Pennsylvania*

ROBERT G. ROBINSON, MD
*Department of Psychiatry*
*The University of Iowa*
*Iowa City, Iowa*

STEVEN P. ROOSE, MD
*Department of Psychiatry*
*College of Physicians and Surgeons of Columbia*
  *University*
*New York State Psychiatric Institute*
*New York, New York*

JAMES C. ROOT, PhD
*Department of Psychiatry and Psychology*
*College of Physicians and Surgeons of Columbia*
  *University*
*New York State Psychiatric Institute*
*New York, New York*

HAROLD A. SACKEIM, PhD
*Departments of Psychiatry and Radiology*
*College of Physicians and Surgeons of Columbia*
  *University*
*New York State Psychiatric Institute*
*New York, New York*

CARL SALZMAN, MD
*Department of Psychiatry*
*Harvard Medical School*
*Massachusetts Mental Health Center*
*Boston, Massachusetts*

ALAN F. SCHATZBERG, MD
*Department of Psychiatry and Behavioral Sciences*
*Stanford University School of Medicine*
*Stanford, California*

STUART N. SEIDMAN, MD
*Department of Psychiatry*
*College of Physicians and Surgeons of Columbia*
  *University*
*New York State Psychiatric Institute*
*New York, New York*

GARY W. SMALL, MD
*Department of Psychiatry and Bio-behavioral Sciences and*
  *the Center on Aging*
*David Geffen School of Medicine at UCLA*
*Los Angeles, California*

JOEL STREIM, MD
*Section of Geriatric Psychiatry*
*Center for Interventions and Services Research*
*University of Pennsylvania*
*Mental Illness Research Education and Clinical Center*
*Philadelphia VA Medical Center*
*Philadelphia, Pennsylvania*

WILFRED G. VAN GORP, PhD
*Department of Psychiatry and Psychology*
*College of Physicians and Surgeons of Columbia University*
*New York State Psychiatric Institute*
*New York, New York*

ROBERT C. YOUNG, MD
*Cornell Institute of Geriatric Psychiatry*
*Weill Medical College of Cornell University*
*New York Presbyterian Hospital*
*White Plains, New York*

GEORGE S. ZUBENKO, MD, PhD
*Department of Psychiatry*
*University of Pittsburgh*
*Department of Biological Sciences*
*Carnegie-Mellon University*
*Pittsburgh, Pennsylvania*

# Introduction

STEVEN P. ROOSE AND HAROLD A. SACKEIM

Some medical specialties are dictated or bounded by the age of the patient—for example, pediatrics and geriatrics. What has not been appreciated is that age can sufficiently influence and modify the dimensions of an illness, including its etiology, pathophysiology, phenomenology, treatment response, and longitudinal course, that knowledge obtained about a disorder in one age group cannot necessarily be applied to patients substantially younger or older.

Though there have been many volumes, some excellent, devoted to various aspects of depressive disorders, their focus has been primarily on the illness as experienced by adults 18 to 60 years of age. The effect of aging on the brain, the physiological and behavioral consequences of recurrent depression, and the impact of other diseases common in the elderly make late-life depression a sufficiently distinct entity that it requires its own body of research, specialized treatment regimens, and its own book.

## LATE-LIFE DEPRESSION OR DEPRESSIONS?

Perhaps the title of this book should be *Late-Life Depressions*. Instead of a collection of chapters, it could be a series of case reports, each describing a unique life story, psychiatric and medical history, symptom presentation, course of treatment, and long-term outcome. The elderly are heterogeneous; their differences in health status, cognitive capacities, and personal relationships are often as extensive as the typical differences between the young and old.

It is often assumed that illnesses and people interact, and that the differences among people determine the differences in disease expression. For example, the course of pneumococcal pneumonia is often different in younger and older adults. In older adults, the course can be complicated by co-morbid medical conditions, such as congestive heart failure or emphysema, or by compromised immunological function, and is more commonly fatal. Thus, the same illness in different patients can vary considerably in signs and symptoms, treatment outcome, and long-term course. However,

these differences may not necessarily reflect an interaction between heterogeneous individuals and a homogeneous illness. Variability in illness expression and course may indicate that different people suffer from different disorders. For example, pneumonia in older individuals may result from diverse etiologies rarely seen in younger adults. Similarly, the differences in the presentation and course of late-life depression may not only result from a uniform disorder as expressed in the heterogeneous elderly. Rather, it may also or instead represent a heterogeneous group of disorders that differ in etiology, pathophysiology, and prognosis, some of which may be distinct for the depressive disorders experienced by younger adults.

One example of heterogeneity is the distinction between the older patient with recurrent depressive illness who had his or her first episode early in life and the older patient with onset of depressive illness during late life. The distinction between early- and late-onset depression is supported by epidemiological, imaging, treatment, and long-term outcome studies. Late-onset depression has been linked to a lower rate of family history of mood disorder, greater frequency of magnetic resonance imaging abnormalities compatible with ischemic cerebrovascular disease, and possibly the development of dementia. Another example concerns poststroke depression. Stroke, which occurs most commonly in late life, is frequently followed by a depressive syndrome. However, poststroke depression may present with a different phenomenology and response to antidepressant medications compared to late-life depressive syndromes unrelated to brain injury. Thus, as we evaluate the patients seeking treatment at our Late-Life Depression Research Center at Columbia University, we are faced with a collection of disorders that can present with a mosaic of symptoms. This is analogous to the patient with the syndrome of dementia that may result from Alzheimer's disease, multi-infarct dementia, acquired immune deficiency syndrome, and so on. Heterogeneity in the manifestations and course of late-life depression can interfere with accurate diagnosis and treatment selection.

## THE IMPORTANCE OF LATE-LIFE DEPRESSION: THE INDIVIDUAL AND SOCIETY

For patients and their families, late-life depression can have devastating effects on work, leisure time, personal relationships, and self-esteem. Late-life depression also takes a staggering toll through increased mortality. In the United States, suicide is the eighth leading cause of death, accounting for over 30,000 deaths a year. This is certainly an underestimation of the true rate of suicide since many suicide deaths are recorded as due to other causes because of concerns about stigma or the restrictions of insurance policies. There is a strong association between depression and suicide, especially in late life. People with depressive illness have a markedly increased risk of suicide, and there is a very high rate of current depressive illness, on the order of 80%, among people who commit suicide. In the United States and in virtually every country that reports suicide statistics, the rate is substantially greater for men than for women. One of the most striking statistics is the enormous increase in the suicide rate for men over 60.

## HEALTH CONSEQUENCES OF LATE-LIFE DEPRESSION

A less apparent, but no less devastating, impact of late-life depression on mortality results when late-life depression is co-morbid with other illness. This effect is best established for ischemic heart disease. Depression is an independent risk factor for the development of ischemic heart disease, and in patients with angina, congestive heart failure, or myocardial infarction, comorbid depression is associated with an increased risk of cardiovascular mortality. Thus, patients with depression are more likely to develop symptomatic vascular disease, and those with vascular disease are more likely to die if they are also depressed.

The brain is adversely impacted by depressive illness. These adverse effects may be reflected in disturbed cognitive function, sleep and appetite disturbance, other behavioral abnormalities, and, of course, mood alteration. It is also established that the physiology and structure of the brain are perturbed in late-life depression. Depression is accompanied by dysregulation of cerebral blood flow and metabolism, and patients with late-life depression often show marked deficits in functional brain activity. Abnormalities in brain structure have been reported in depressed patients across the life span. Especially in elderly patients, there is debate as to whether these abnormalities are a consequence or a cause of the depressive illness or both.

Although the causes and impact of depression are traditionally localized in the brain, the physiological consequences of depression for other organ systems have only recently been appreciated. For example, recent studies comparing platelet function and heart rate variability in healthy subjects, patients with depression, and patients with depression and ischemic heart disease have identified physiological mechanisms that may mediate the associations among depression, vascular disease, and sudden cardiac death. The pathophysiology of depressive illness involves dysregulation of neurotransmitter and hormonal systems that contribute to increased platelet activity and vascular injury. Depression is accompanied by autonomic nervous system imbalance that makes patients vulnerable to ventricular arrhythmia. These effects may underlie the association between depression and the development of vascular disease, as well as the increased mortality in patients with depression and symptomatic ischemic heart disease.

In addition to its physiological effects on multiple organ systems, depression is associated with poor compliance with medical regimens. This well-replicated phenomenon is observed across medical disciplines; comorbid depressive syndromes reduce compliance with the treatment of virtually all disorders. Thus, especially in late life, depression can exert a negative impact on health through multiple pathways. Not surprisingly, for almost every illness studied, such as, diabetes and cancer, individuals who are depressed have poorer outcomes.

The documentation that co-morbid depression adversely affects the course of other illnesses prevalent in the late-life population has stimulated research on the pathophysiological mechanisms and multiple studies of whether the treatment of depression reduces the risk of mortality. However, the most profound impact of the growing awareness of the relationship between depression and other illness has been a change in the concept of late-life depression from a psychiatric disorder that is diagnosed and treated in a psychiatrist's office to a disorder that is sufficiently common that it needs to be diagnosed and treated by all physicians who care for patients over the age of 60. Like hypertension, dementia, and diabetes, late-life depression is an illness that transcends traditional subspecialty boundaries, and every physician must be capable of providing at least an appropriate screening for the disorder.

## DIAGNOSIS AND TREATMENT

Traditionally, there have been a number of obstacles to the appropriate diagnosis and treatment of depression in late-life patients in both medical and psychiatric settings. First, older patients often present predominantly with somatic symptoms, such as sleep disturbance, appetite loss, fatigue, and pain, and may never complain of, or indeed may deny, the experience of depressed mood. Such presentations will cause the physician who thinks of depressed mood as the sine qua non of the illness to omit depression from the differential diagnosis. Furthermore, some of the symptoms that are criteria for a diagnosis of depression are also nonspecific symptoms of other medical conditions. Therefore, to make an accurate diagnosis of depression, the physician must be cognizant that the depressive syndrome can present with primarily somatic symptoms and should also take an inclusive approach to diagnosis in which all symptoms, if present, are counted toward the diagnosis of depression, regardless of whether they can be explained as due to co-morbid medical conditions or medication side effects.

Further complicating the issue of diagnosis are epidemiological studies indicating that among the elderly, milder subsyndromal depressive syndromes may be more common than major depression. Milder, chronic depressive disorders may be even harder for the clinician to recognize, especially if there is not a high index of suspicion for affective disorder. Moreover, even if a depressive syndrome is diagnosed, especially in the setting of serious medical illness, clinicians may often take a pseudoempathic approach in which the depression is considered a normal reaction to a serious or debilitating illness. In particular, younger clinicians may make a similar error by believing that depressive symptoms are normal in older patients, especially since the negative or stressful life events are common in late life, such as retirement, death of family members and lifelong friends, and medical illness and infirmity. The consequence of these beliefs is that, even when diagnosed, depression often goes untreated in this population.

## THE MIND AND THE AGING BODY: A LATE-LIFE DIALECTIC

Our organizing principle in creating this volume was to present what is known about the epidemiology, phenomenology, psychobiology, treatment, and consequences of late-life depression. The Table of Contents may prompt some readers to consider this book to be primarily biological, with too much emphasis on brain function and somatic therapies and not enough attention to social context, psychological theories, and psychotherapy. Indeed, the field of psychiatry is considered by many to be currently dominated by academic researchers and clinicians with a unidimensional biological perspective. However, we are not proponents of a restrictive biological model of the mind or illness, and that is not the point of view that determined the composition of this book. Rather, we felt that diagnosis and treatment should be evidence-based, and we sought to include comprehensively the established knowledge that

should inform clinical practice. In reviewing what had been learned, it became apparent that the psychobiology, brain function, and somatic treatments of late-life depression have been much more thoroughly researched than other areas. For example, psychological theories of depressive illness in the elderly are poorly developed, and the little theory that exists was generally developed in a younger population and exported wholesale to late life. The same is true for most psychotherapeutic treatments of depression, with some notable exceptions that are comprehensively and elegantly presented in the chapter devoted to psychotherapy (Chapter 23).

At every stage of life the interactions between the biology of the brain and experience are critical, but there are special circumstances in late life that make this process particularly important. During late life, losses in multiple domains are common, such as retirement, physical disability, and the death of family members and friends. These events are processed by a brain that has been transfigured by normal aging and/or illness. The aging brain may diminish a person's capacity to cope with painful life events, and the experience of stress may, in turn, accelerate depressive illness. This reality alone underscores the compelling need for a substantial program of rigorous research on the sociological and psychological dimensions of late-life depression and its treatment.

At its inception, the dominant concept that organized this book was that illness models and clinical treatment should be evidence-based. However, while as researchers and clinicians we embrace this perspective, we are also painfully aware that the available evidence is often strikingly limited. For example, there are only four placebo-controlled trials of selective serotonin reuptake inhibitor antidepressants in late-life depression, so the data on which to base conclusions about medication efficacy are scant. Moreover in some of these studies, sites differ markedly in rates of clinical response, regardless of the form of treatment, while differences between placebo and active medication across the sites are often of doubtful clinical importance, even if statistically significant. A reasonable and troubling conclusion is that recovery may depend more on where the patient is treated than on the prescribed medication. Determining why sites differ so widely in outcomes may help identify unrecognized dimensions that can contribute to recovery.

We must be cognizant of the limitations of research findings and recognize that the practice of evidence-based medicine is constrained by gaps in our knowledge. Nevertheless, we must continue to do research and treat patients, informed by our current, albeit inadequate, knowledge and eager for tomorrow's research and clinical contributions.

# I | EPIDEMIOLOGY AND THE BURDEN OF ILLNESS

EPIDEMIOLOGICAL studies have changed our view of the prevalence, etiology, and impact of psychiatric disorders. For example, the finding that schizophrenia is present in all societies at approximately the same rate strongly suggests that cultural influences are not a major contributor to its etiology. Nonetheless, the symptom presentation and course of schizophrenia are not invariant and may reflect cultural differences. For example, the World Health Organization studies reported that the long-term outcome of schizophrenia was superior in developing societies relative to developed industrial societies.

However, like all methodologies, the epidemiological approach has limitations that, if not appreciated, can lead to flawed conclusions. For example, it is reported that among the elderly there is a higher prevalence of subsyndromal depression relative to major depression. In younger adults the prevalence of these disorders is more similar. Do the relative rates of these illnesses simply change with age or are subsyndromal and/or major depression different illnesses in the young and old?

Despite a common set of symptoms, subsyndromal depression is a heterogeneous group of disorders in both younger and older adults, but is not necessarily the same heterogeneous disorder in both age groups. Only the late-life population includes men with an affective syndrome secondary to age-associated hypogonadism.

A devastating consequence of depression is suicide, and epidemiological studies have been crucial in identifying the population most at risk. At one time, suicide was considered a tragic event that occurred most often in young women. Though women attempt suicide more frequently than men, death from suicide occurs more frequently in men than in women. The suicide rate increases markedly among men once they reach the age of 60 years.

Though late-life depression causes suffering for individuals and their families, the broader impact of this disorder transcends the clinical case. Late-life depression has a marked effect on society, and particularly on the subculture of people over 60 years of age. The direct care of depression and the greater consumption of nonpsychiatric health-care services by the depressed elderly create substantial burdens on health-care systems. In particular, depression increases health care use and costs, as well as overall mortality, since depression worsens the prognosis for the co-morbid medical illnesses prevalent in the elderly, such as, ischemic heart disease. The impact of late-life depression on the individual, family, health-care system, and society is profound.

# 1 | The epidemiology of depressive disorders in late life

DAN G. BLAZER

Epidemiology provides the context for a comprehensive exploration of late-life depression. The importance of context in understanding disease was recognized as early as the time of the Hippocratic physicians.

Whoever wishes to investigate medicine properly should proceed thus: in the first place to consider the seasons of the year, and what effect each then produces. Then the winds . . . in the same manner, when one comes into a city to which he is a stranger, he should consider the situation, how it lies as to the wind and the rising of the sun . . . one should consider most attentively the water . . . and the mode in which the inhabitants live, and what are their pursuits, whether they are fond of drinking to excess, and given to indolence, or are fond of exercising and labor.

(Hippocrates, 1939; circa 400 BCE).

The study of context should attempt to inform the clinician and clinical investigator regarding the following questions (modified from Morris [1975]):

*Case identification.* What are the symptom patterns among the depressed elderly leading to the assignment as a "case" that is significant enough for attention by the mental health clinician?

*Prevalence, incidence, and distribution.* What is the frequency of various types of cases of late-life depression? How are they distributed across the population? How many new cases of depression evolve over time?

*Prognosis.* How is the outcome of a case of depression variously defined?

*Historical trends.* Has the frequency of late-life depression, variously defined, changed over the past century? If so, in what ways?

*Identification of causes of late-life depression.* What biological, psychological, and social risk factors have been identified as associated with and potentially causative of late-life depression? (This topic will not be addressed in this chapter, as it will be covered extensively in other chapters.)

*Use of psychiatric services.* What is the pattern of health service use among the depressed elderly, specif-

ically the use of medical and psychiatric services and the use of medications?

Other questions also might be appropriately addressed in the epidemiological study, such as the effectiveness (not efficacy) of an intervention study. Yet the questions posed above provide a reasonable framework for grasping the context of late-life depression. Given the veritable explosion of the literature addressing the epidemiology of late-life depression over the past few years, this review does not attempt to be comprehensive but rather representative, a view of the landscape. Data are presented primarily from community or large observational clinical epidemiological studies.

## CASE IDENTIFICATION

Most epidemiologists and clinicians agree on the core symptoms of clinically significant depression throughout the life cycle, yet the absolute distinction between a case and a noncase—that is, persons requiring psychiatric services versus those who do not—is not easily established (Blazer et al., in press). Many of the symptoms and signs of late-life depression are ubiquitous with aging. For example, 22% of elders in a community survey in North Carolina (Cornoni-Huntley et al., 1990; Hybels et al., 2001) reported feeling sad, and over 50% reported having at least two symptoms on the Center for Epidemiologic Studies Depression Scale most of the day every day for the past week. Over 50% also reported at least one complaint related to their sleep, thus blurring the distinction between cases and noncases. Though some have suggested that older adults are less likely to report depressive symptoms (or to somatize those symptoms), most community and institutional surveys do not substantiate that belief. Older persons may not be as forthcoming on their own regarding symptoms of depression, but there is little reason to believe that they are less likely to report those symptoms when asked.

When asked, "What is a case?", Copeland (1981) answered with the question, "A case for what?" The choice of criteria for a case depends upon the particular investigative or clinical inquiry. To determine the efficacy of a new antidepressant in older adults, the clinician may wish to identify cases of depression likely to respond to the antidepressant, such as cases of major depression. In another situation, an investigator may wish to identify older adults who have reacted with depressive symptoms to traumatic events, such as a tragic fire in a nursing home. The criteria for that study might be reaching a threshold of reported symptoms analogous to those of adjustment disorder with depressed mood.

How does the clinician determine whether a diagnostic category among older adults is appropriate? According to Goodwin and Guze (1979), diagnosis is prognosis. Consequently, diagnostic categories that approximate true disease processes have a number of characteristics, including the following (Weissman and Klerman, 1978):

1. A category should be distinguished on the basis of patterns of symptomatology; for example, a unique cluster of symptoms has been identified in vascular depression (Alexopoulos et al., 1997).

2. A category should predict the outcome of a disorder; for example, major depressive episodes in late life predict recurrence of depression over time (Murphy et al., 1987).

3. A category should reflect the underlying biological reality, confirmed by family members and genetic studies; for example, depression is found to be heritable in twin studies of older adults (Gatz et al., 1992).

4. Laboratory studies should eventually validate a diagnostic category; for example, sleep studies distinguish elders with major depression from normal controls (Reynolds et al., 1990).

5. The classification scheme should identify persons who may respond to a specific therapeutic intervention, such as a particular form of psychotherapy or a specific group of medications; for example, elders with major depression respond significantly better than controls to a combination of antidepressant therapy and interpersonal psychotherapy (Reynolds et al., 1999).

Diagnostic instruments (usually standardized interviews) have been developed that epidemiologists have used in community and clinic-based epidemiological studies to identify persons who meet these criteria. The Structured Clinical Interview for DSM Diagnoses (SCID) (Spitzer et al., 1990) and the Diagnostic Interview Schedule (DIS) (Robins et al., 1981) are examples of the most frequently used interview schedules in community and clinical epidemiological studies.

A second approach to case identification involves the use of a self-rating symptom scale. Frequently used scales in epidemiological surveys include the Center for Epidemiologic Studies Depression Scale (CES-D) (Radloff, 1977) and the Geriatric Depression Scale (Yesavage et al., 1983). The advantage of these scales is that, unlike diagnostic interviews, they do not subjectively assign patients to a particular diagnostic category; a disadvantage is the lack of diagnostic specificity that can be achieved with their use. Blazer et al. (1991), for example, estimated the prevalence of clinically significant depression symptoms among community-dwelling elders in North Carolina to be 9%, although most of these individuals would not be diagnosed with major depression.

Other authors define a case in part on the basis of the severity of physical, psychological, and social impairment secondary to the symptoms (Narrow et al., 2002). This approach to case identification is less popular among psychiatrists, who are more inclined to "treat major depression" than to "improve function." Improved function in theory should derive from remission of the disease. Nevertheless, function has special relevance in the care of older adults, especially the oldest old (Blazer, 2000). In fact, improving function as opposed to relieving symptoms may be the therapeutic goal (Hazzard, 1994). Nevertheless, introducing factors such as function clouds the clearer criteria based on the presence or absence of symptoms alone. A major debate in geriatric psychiatry revolves around the co-morbidity of depression and the dementing disorders, especially depression associated with lesions on magnetic resonance scanning. This has led one group to propose separate criteria for "depression of Alzheimer disease" (Olin et al., 2002), requiring, along with meeting criteria for Alzheimer's disease, at least three of the following symptoms: depressed mood, anhedonia, social isolation, poor appetite, a feeling of worthlessness, and suicidal thoughts.

## PREVALENCE, INCIDENCE, AND DISTRIBUTION

*Prevalence*—that is, the frequency of persons who meet criteria for the diagnosis of interest in a representative sample—is the most commonly used measure in psychiatric epidemiology. Examples include determining the prevalence of major depression or the prevalence of individuals with significant depressive symptoms, operationalized as exceeding a predetermined level as measured by the CES-D (Radloff, 1977) (see Tables 1.1 and 1.2).

Prevalence provides an estimate of the current burden of a disease, yet does not provide information about either the disease course or changing patterns in disease frequency through time (Blazer, 2002). *Lifetime prevalence* is the cumulative frequency of meeting criteria for a psychiatric disorder at any time during the past for all persons in the sample.

TABLE 1.1. *Prevalence Estimates of Depressive Symptoms and Minor Depression in Representative Samples of Older Adults*

| Author | Sample Site and Characteristics | N | Screening Instrument | Estimates |
|---|---|---|---|---|
| Blazer and Williams (1980) | Urban North Carolina | 997 | OARS Depression Scale (Fillenbaum, 1988) | 14.7% clinically significant depressive symptoms; no age or gender differences |
| Blazer et al. (1987) | Racially mixed sample, urban and rural North Carolina | 4163 | CES-D (Radloff, 1977) | 9% clinically significant depressive symptoms; more prevalent in the oldest old |
| Murrell et al. (1983) | Rural Kentucky | 2517 | CES-D | 16% significant depressive symptoms; more prevalent in the oldest old and in females |
| Copeland et al. (1987) | Liverpool | 1070 | GMS (Copeland et al., 1976) | 8.3% with minor depression |
| Beekman et al. (1995) | Netherlands | 3056 | CES-D | 12.9% with minor depression |
| Beekman et al. (1999) | EURODEP Consortium (combined estimates from varied European studies | Samples from multiple countries in Europe | Various instruments | 13.5% with clinically significant depressive symptoms, 9.8% with minor depression |
| Koenig et al., (1988) | VA inpatient sample | 171 | DIS | 23% with significant depressive symptoms |
| Parmelee, et al. (1989) | Nursing home and congregate apartments | 708 | DSM-III-R checklist (APA, 1987) | 35% with significant depressive symptoms |

CES-D, Center for Epidemiologic Studies Depression Scale; DIS, Diagnostic Interview Schedule; DSM-III-R, *Diagnostic and Statistical Manual of Mental Disorders*, 3rd rev. ed.; EURODEP Consortium, European Depression Study; GMS, Geriatric Mental State; OARS, Older Americans Resources and Services; VA, Veterans Administration.


TABLE 1.2. *Prevalence Estimates of Major Depression in Community and Clinical Samples of Older Adults*

| Author | Sample | N | Screening Method | Findings |
|---|---|---|---|---|
| Blazer et al., (1987) | Community sample in North Carolina | 1304 | DIS (Robins et al., 1981) | 0.8% with major depression |
| Beekman et al. (1995) | Community sample in the Netherlands | 3056 | DIS | 2.0 with major depression |
| Beekman et al. (1999) | EURODEP Consortium (combined estimates from varied European studies | Samples from multiple countries in Europe | Various instruments | 1.8% weighted average prevalence |
| Copeland et al. (1987) | Community sample in Liverpool | 1070 | GMS (Copeland et al., 1976) | 2.9% |
| Kessler et al. (2003) | National Community Sample in US | 5,554 (21% 60+) | CIDI (Robins et al. 1988) | Persons 30–44 years of age 1.8 times more likely to be diagnosed with major depression than persons 60+ years of age. |
| Koenig et al. (1988) | VA inpatient sample | 171 | DIS | 11.5% with major depression |
| Parmelee et al. (1989) | Nursing home and congregate apartments | 708 | DSM-III-R checklist (APA, 1987) | 12.4% with major depression |

DIS, Diagnostic Interview Schedule; DSM-III-R, *Diagnostic and Statistical Manual of Mental Disorders*, 3rd rev. ed.; EURODEP Consortium; GMS, Geriatric Mental State; VA, Veterans Administration.

*Incidence* complements prevalence and is the number of new cases of a disorder developing over a specified period of time (usually 1 year for psychiatric disorders) among persons free from the disorder at the beginning of the specified time. Incidence studies are much more difficult to perform in psychiatric epidemiology, and therefore the number of studies that report incidence is quite small.

Prevalence and incidence of depression are distributed unequally across older adults. For example, women, persons with functional impairment, and persons with cognitive impairment are more likely to be depressed (Blazer et al., 1991). In addition, depression is more prevalent among younger persons than older persons (Fig. 1.1). The lower prevalence of depression among the elderly, compared to younger persons, does not always hold in surveys of non-Western societies, such as Taiwan and Puerto Rico (Canino et al., 1987; Lin and Standley, 1962). When prevalence is compared across elders with and without cognitive impairment, one finds a relatively increased prevalence in the cognitively impaired. Therefore, the *odds* of being depressed are increased among the cognitively impaired. If, for example, the incidence of clinically significant depressive symptoms is compared across two samples of elders, one with and one without functional impairment, the incidence will be higher in the functionally impaired sample (Hays et al., 1997). Therefore, the *relative risk* of becoming depressed is higher in the functionally impaired than in the unimpaired.

Depression is also more frequent among the oldest old, women, persons in the lower socioeconomic strata, and persons with reduced social support (Blazer et al., 1991). The mechanisms by which these *risk factors* are associated with late-life depression cannot be determined via most epidemiological studies. Rather simple associations, usually reported as relative risk or odds ratios, in controlled and uncontrolled studies define the extant literature on risk. It is tempting to assume that longitudinal studies will correct this problem. Unfortunately, most risk factors are intermittent (such as a stressful event), and the time between the report of the event in community studies and the report of the depression (usually no less than 1 year) is too long to establish a meaningful association. Nevertheless, community studies do provide data that can be pursued in more detailed studies of clinical samples.

Risk factors that have been well established in clinical samples include family history, stressful life events, reduced social support (though the association varies across studies), lower socioeconomic status, and previous episodes of depression (as well as physical illness, functional impairment, and cognitive decline, which are discussed in more detail) (Alexopoulos et al., 1996b; Blazer et al., 1992; Bruce, 2001; George et al., 1989; Murphy, 1983). The higher prevalence of depression in urban dwellers compared to rural dwellers reported in a community sample from North Carolina (Blazer et al., 1985) is due to a difference in persons under the age of 45, not older adults (Blazer et al., 1986).

Prevalence estimates clearly depend upon case identification. Depression that is clinically significant is determined by preset criteria using various symptom scales or diagnostic criteria. For example, Beekman et al. (1995) defined minor depression as scoring 16+ on the CES-D (Radloff, 1977) but not meeting criteria for major depression. In contrast, DSM-IV (APA, 1994) provides a series of specific symptom criteria for minor depression in its Appendix. If these criteria had been used, the estimate would have been somewhat different.

Prevalence estimates for minor depression vary between 4% and 13% (Beekman et al., 1995; Blazer et al., 1987; Copeland et al., 1987). Most investigators estimate the prevalence of clinically significant depressive symptoms to be between 8% and 16% in community samples of older adults (Berkman et al., 1986; Blazer et al., 1991) (see Table 1.1), but it may reach higher levels in some subsamples, such as older Mexican Americans (Gonzalez et al., 2001). Case identification for minor depression and clinically significant depressive symptoms clearly overlaps due to criteria for case identification. In institutional settings, the estimated prevalence of clinically significant depressive symptoms ranges between 25% and 35% (Koenig et al., 1988; Parmelee et al., 1989).

Prevalence estimates for major depression are presented in Table 1.2. As can be seen, the estimates are quite low

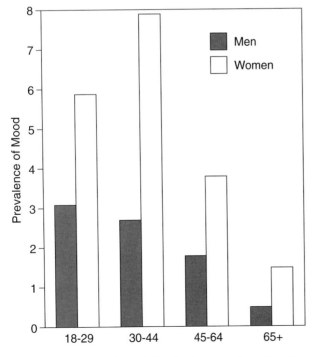

FIGURE 1.1 Prevalence of mood disorders by age and sex: Data from the Epidemiological Catchment Area study. (Weissman et al., 1991)

in community-based samples, ranging between 1% and 3%. Some have challenged these low estimates, yet the consistency of the estimates using various methodologies tends to substantiate them (Beekman et al., 1999; Blazer and Williams, 1980; Blazer et al., 1987). In contrast, estimates of major depression in clinical or institutional samples are much higher, ranging in institutional samples between 10% and 20% (Koenig et al., 1988; Parmelee et al., 1989). When samples of persons with Alzheimer's disease are surveyed for the prevalence of major depression, the estimates are similar to those for the institutional samples (Patterson et al., 1990; Reifler et al., 1982). Both depressive symptoms and cases of major depression are clearly more prevalent in the presence of co-morbid conditions such as physical illness, functional impairment, and cognitive decline. This association undoubtedly explains the higher prevalence among institutional samples compared to community samples.

The debate regarding the appropriate criteria across the life cycle for clinically significant depression has not ended, and is complicated (as noted above) in late life by the frequent co-morbidity of physical illness, functional impairment, and cognitive decline. In addition, whether minor depression, major depression, and the newly proposed depression in Alzheimer' disease actually represent different entities or different points along a continuum continues to be debatable. Regardless, how an individual investigator/clinician resolves this debate directly impacts the estimates of frequency and distribution of depression among the elderly.

As noted above, estimates of the incidence of late life depression are rare (and they suffer from the same problems in case identification found in prevalence studies). Rorsman et al. (1990) estimated the incidence of major depression in Lundby County, Sweden, to be 0.43 for men and 0.76 for women of all ages (with very little age variation). As would be expected, incidence estimates are lower than prevalence estimates. (Remember that if a subject is experiencing depression at the time of a study, that person will not qualify for an estimate of incidence because he or she is not at risk for developing depression over the follow-up period since he or she already has a diagnosis of depression.) Eaton et al. (1989) estimated the incidence of major depression in Baltimore. They found an overall annual incidence of 0.3, with a peak among 30-year-olds and a smaller peak among persons in their 50s. The incidence among older adults was much lower than that found earlier in the life cycle.

## PROGNOSIS

A number of naturalistic studies have been performed to track the course of depression in older adults, both in community and clinical samples. These studies, however, are not truly naturalistic because many of the subjects are treated with antidepressants or other medications as well as psychosocial therapies. In a long-term follow-up of community-dwelling older adults in the Netherlands, elders with clinically significant depression according to the CES-D experienced a chronically fluctuating course over time. Over 6 years, 25% of those with minor depression, 35% of those with major depression, and 52% of dysthymics experienced a chronic course. Overall, fewer than 50% recovered and remained well among all the subjects with CES-D scores in the clinically significant range.

Though the distribution varies across clinical studies, often due to different characteristics of the populations sampled, the *rule of thirds* usually applies. Namely, one-third of older persons diagnosed with major depression and followed for 1 year will recover and remain recovered, one-third will recover but will experience a relapse (or their recovery will be partial), and one-third will not recover (Alexopoulos et al., 1996a; Blazer et al., 1992; Murphy, 1983). The prognosis is considerably better for carefully selected samples that enter treatment trials, with approximately 80% recovering, and a lower relapse rate than found in naturalistic samples (Reynolds et al., 1999).

Nonsuicide mortality may be increased in elders who are depressed, but the data are mixed (Blazer et al., 2001; Fredman et al., 1989; Penninx et al., 2001; Schulz et al., 2000). In community samples, mortality appears to result from depressive symptoms through multiple pathways, such as decline in functional and cognitive status. For example, in data collected in North Carolina, when uncontrolled analyses were conducted, the risk of death over 3 years from depression was increased by twofold. However, when factors such as cognitive and functional status were controlled for, the association between depression and mortality disappeared (Blazer et al., 2001). Interpretation of an association (or lack of an association) depends upon which control variables are included in the study and the interpretation of the mechanisms by which depression and control variables interact over time. For example, depression predicts functional impairment over time (Bruce, 2001), yet functional impairment also predicts depression (Kennedy et al., 1990). Therefore, depression appears to lead to mortality through pathways such as increased functional decline and increased incidence of illness, yet both functional decline and physical illness may independently also lead to both depression and decreased life expectancy. In a recent controversial report, mild depressive symptoms actually protected against 3-year mortality in older women (Hybels et al., 2002). Therefore, the intricacies of the association of depression and mortality in the elderly remain to be established.

In contrast, when depressive symptoms are severe, such as when the diagnosis of major depression is made in community samples, mortality among elders is significantly increased (Bruce and Leaf, 1989). In clinical samples, elders with major depression are much more likely to die even when other factors are taken into account, such as physical illness (Murphy et al., 1988).

Depression is definitely related to increased mortality via suicide in the elderly (especially elderly white males). Suicide frequency in the 65+ age group in the United States was 16.9/100,000 per year in 1998 (Conwell et al., 2002; National Center for Health, 2001). The frequency among white males increased with age, being 623/100,000 in the 65+ age group. The association between depression and suicide in late life is well established (Conwell et al., 2000, 2002; Raern et al., 2002). Other risk factors for late-life suicide attempts include being a widow(er), living alone, perceived poor health, poor sleep quality, lack of a support network (especially a confidant), and the acute experience of a stressful event such as a change in financial status (Conwell et al., 2002; Turvey et al., 2002).

## HISTORICAL TRENDS

Klerman (1978) suggested that, in contrast to the "age of anxiety" that followed World War II, Western society has entered an "age of melancholy," precipitated in large part by social factors such as increasing secularization and societal instability. To support this finding, he and his colleagues analyzed family history data from the Psychobiology of Depression Study. They found an increased frequency of depression in successively younger birth cohorts through the twentieth century and an earlier age of onset of depression in each birth cohort (Klerman et al., 1985). A cross-national analysis of rates from nine community based epidemiological studies and 4000 relatives from three family studies confirmed that the most recent birth cohorts are at increased risk for major depression (Cross-National Collaborative Group, 1992). Analysis of data on suicide rates in the elderly tend to support these findings (Centers for Disease Control, 1995). Suicide rates among white males, after declining steadily from the mid-1940s to 1980, began to climb again during the 1980s. These rates plateaued during the 1990s (Conwell et al., 2002).

These findings must be considered within the context of historical trends, and these trends are best understood in terms of age, period, and cohort effects. For example, throughout the twentieth century, white males exhibited an increased frequency of suicide with age (an age effect: as a white male ages, he has an increased risk of suicide). Since about 1930, though, while the same age effect is noted, younger birth cohorts carry a higher risk of suicide (a cohort effect: white males born in 1930 are at lower risk for suicide throughout their lives than white males born in 1950) (Centers for Disease Control, 1995). Finally, suicide

rates may increase or decrease across the life cycle at different periods in history (a period effect: a particular historical period is associated with a change in rates). For example, Murphy and colleagues (1986) found that suicide rates in Britain declined dramatically from 1961 to 1975 and then leveled off. They speculated that a change in the cooking gas used in the British Isles (from a toxic to a nontoxic gas) eliminated one of the more common means of committing suicide.

We have very few data that can directly inform us of historical trends in depression, given that methods for identifying cases of depression have changed dramatically over the years and virtually no studies extend long enough in historical time and include adults of all ages such that age, period, and cohort effects can be sorted out. The suicide data, discussed elsewhere, provide a proxy, and some conclusions may be drawn.

First, the frequency of depression appears to increase with age only when other factors are not controlled for, such as functional status (Blazer et al., 1991). This does not diminish the simple fact that when these factors are not taken into account statistically, the frequency of depression may increase in older age groups. Second, the age of melancholy described by Klerman does not appear to have abated across society. Therefore, we appear to be carrying a greater burden of depression today than in past years. Third, younger birth cohorts are carrying a greater burden of depression (as well as many other psychiatric problems that are currently relatively rare among the elderly, such as drug and alcohol problems). As these cohorts age, there is no reason to believe that the frequency of depressive symptoms and major depression will decrease. Therefore, we can expect the burden of depression to increase among the elderly since a greater percentage of our population will be considered old.

Evidence from the twentieth century supports the prediction of progressively increasing rates of depression among the elderly (coupled with the presence of larger numbers of older persons). Nevertheless, public health initiatives or societywide changes could reduce this increase in rates. In the view of this author, the rates will increase. Though we may identify depression in younger cohorts earlier and treat the depression more effectively, such interventions may not compensate for other societal factors. For example, we will witness the probable decrease in financial stability of older adults as we progress into the twenty-first century, coupled with an increasingly secular and alienated society (Blazer, 2002; Putnam, 2000).

## USE OF PSYCHIATRIC SERVICES

In general, the elderly use fewer psychiatric services than younger persons. For example, German and colleagues (1985) reviewed data from the Baltimore Epidemiologic Catchment Area Study fielded in 1982 and found that among persons under the age of 65, 8.7% had made a visit to a specialty or primary care provider for mental health care during the 6 months before the survey. In contrast, for persons aged 65 to 74, the frequency of use was 4.2% and for those 75 years of age and above, the frequency was only 1.4%. Among those 75+ years of age, not one subject among the 292 surveyed had sought specialty mental health care for any reason. There is little reason to suspect that this overall pattern of use has changed dramatically during the past 20 years. Older persons are less likely to seek medical care for depression than younger persons. However, two caveats must be considered.

First, the use of antidepressant medications has increased dramatically among older adults since the introduction of the new generation of antidepressant medications (Blazer et al., 2000). In North Carolina, from 1986 to 1996, antidepressant use increased from 3.8% of a sample of persons 65 years of age and above to 11.0% over the 10 years of follow-up (subjects were 75 years of age and above at follow-up). This difference was most apparent among whites (an increase from 4.6% to 14.3%) compared to African Americans (an increase from 2.3% to 5.0%). Whites remained four times more likely to be taking antidepressant medications compared to African Americans even when income, health insurance, and reported mood were taken into account through controlled analysis. Though the elderly may use antidepressant medications for a number of reasons, it seems likely that most of them are used to treat depression. Therefore, the use of traditional mental health services remains low among older adults who experience depression, yet the use of antidepressant medications is quite high. Whether the rate of prescription of antidepressants to older adults is appropriate cannot be determined by epidemiological studies. The studies do not acquire information about the symptoms reported to the clinician (e.g., the primary care provider), the signs observed by the clinician, or the outcome of treatment. For example, many persons taking antidepressants at the time of community surveys may have been treated successfully and are therefore taking an appropriate maintenance dose. In older adults, most antidepressant therapy is prescribed by primary care providers. In one study, the effectiveness of antidepressant therapy prescribed by primary care physicians, even when the physicians were supplied with a report of depressive symptoms obtained by a checklist, was not demonstrated (Callahan et al., 1994).

Second, older adults who experience depression are much more likely to use general health services (Unutzer et al., 1997). In a cohort of older adults in primary care, depression was associated with increased use and cost of medical services. The increase was seen for every component of the health-care costs and was not ac-

counted for by an increase in specialty mental health care. The increase persisted even when age, sex, and chronic medical illnesses were controlled for. Therefore, though older adults experiencing depression may not use mental health services (or general health services for mental health treatment), they use general health services at a significantly higher rate and the cost to the health-care system for late-life depression is considerable. It should be noted that this cost remains significant even with the great increase in the use of antidepressant medications.

## CONCLUSION

The symptoms of depression are frequent among older adults, but they do not appear to increase with age except when accompanied by some of the common, though not inevitable, consequences of aging, such as functional impairment and cognitive impairment. The frequency of major depression in community surveys of older adults is low compared to the frequency at other ages. Nevertheless, if the current trend persists— namely, the trend for younger birth cohorts to carry a greater burden of depression—then we can expect the frequency of major depression to increase over the next few decades. Regardless, late-life depression is almost certainly undertreated except for the frequent use of antidepressant medications. Of course, many of the elderly with clinically significant depressive symptoms in the community are not taking antidepressant medications. The resultant undertreatment coupled with the inherent burden of depression in late life leads to an appreciable increase in the use of all health services by the depressed elderly.

ACKNOWLEDGMENTS
This work was supported in part by the Foundations Fund for Research in Psychiatry while Dr. Blazer was a Fellow at the Center for Advanced Studies in the Behavioral Sciences, Stanford, California.

REFERENCES

Alexopoulos, G., Meyers, B., Young, R., Campbell, S., Silbersweig, D., and Charlson, M. (1997) "Vascular depression" hypothesis. *Arch Gen Psychiatry* 54:915–922.
Alexopoulos, G., Meyers, B., Young, R., Kakuma, T., Feder, M., Einhorn, A., and Rosendahl, E. (1996a) Recovery in geriatric depression. *Arch Gen Psychiatry* 53:305–312.
Alexopoulos, G., Vrontou, C., Kakuma, T., Meyers, B., Young, R., Klausner, E., and Clarkin, J. (1996b) Disability in geriatric depression. *Am J Psychiatry* 153:877–885.
American Psychiatric Association. (1987) *DSM-III-R: Diagnostic and Statistical Manual of Mental Disorders*, 3rd rev. ed. Washington, D.C.: American Psychiatric Press.
American Psychiatric Association. (1994) *DSM-IV: Diagnostic and Statistical Manual of Mental Disorders*, 4th ed. Washington, D.C.: American Psychiatric Press.

Beekman, A., Copeland, J., and Prince, M. (1999) Review of community prevalence of depression in later life. *Br J Psychiatry* 174:307–311.

Beekman, A., Deeg, D., van Tilberg, T., Smit, J., Hooijer, C., and van Tilberg, W. (1995) Major and minor depression in later life: A study of prevalence and risk factors. *J Affect Disord* 36:65–75.

Berkman, L., Berkman, C., Kasl, S., Freeman, D., Leo, L., Ostfeld, A., Cornoni-Huntley, J., and Brody, J. (1986) Depressive symptoms in relation to physical health and functioning in the elderly. *Am J Epidemiol* 124:372–388.

Blazer, D. (2000) Psychiatry and the oldest old. *Am J Psychiatry* 157:1915–1924.

Blazer, D. (2002) *Depression in Late Life*, 3rd ed. New York: Springer.

Blazer, D., Burchett, B., Service, C., and George, L. (1991) The association of age and depression among the elderly: An epidemiologic exploration. *J Gerontol Med Sci* 46:M210–M215.

Blazer, D., Crowell, B., George, L., and Landerman, R. (1986) Urban-rural differences in depressive disorders: Does age make a difference? In: R.R. Barrett, J.E., ed. *Mental Disorders in the Community: Progress and Challenge*. New York: Guilford Press, pp. 233–255.

Blazer, D., Georg, L., Landerman, R., Pennybacker, M., Melville, M., Woodbury, M., Manton, K., Jordan, K., and Locke, B. (1985) Psychiatric disorders: A rural/urban comparison. *Arch Gen Psychiatry* 42:651–656.

Blazer, D., Hughes, D., and George, L. (1987) The epidemiology of depression in an elderly community population. *Gerontologist* 27:281–287.

Blazer, D., Hughes, D., and George, L. (1992) Age and impaired subjective support: Predictors of depressive symptoms at one-year follow-up. *J Nerv Ment Dis* 180:172–178.

Blazer, D., Hybels, C., and Hays, J. (in press) Epidemiology of psychiatric disorders in late life. In: Blazer, D., Steffens, D., and Busse, E., eds. *American Psychiatric Press Textbook of Geriatric Psychiatry*. Washington, DC: American Psychiatric Press.

Blazer, D., Hybels, C., and Pieper, C. (2001) The association of depression and mortality in elderly persons: A case for multiple independent pathways. *J Gerontol Med Sci* 56A:M505–M509.

Blazer, D., Hybels, C., Simonsick, E., and Hanlon, J. (2000) Marked differences in antidepressant use by race in an elderly community sample: 1986–1996. *Am J Psychiatry* 157:1089–1094.

Blazer, D., and Williams, C. (1980) The epidemiology of dysphoria and depression in an elderly population. *Am J Psychiatry* 137:439–444.

Bruce, M. (2001) Depression and disability in late life: Directions for future research. *Am J Geriatr Psychiatry* 9:102–112.

Bruce, M., and Leaf, P. (1989) Psychiatric disorders and 15-month mortality in a community sample of older adults. *Am J Public Health* 79:727–730.

Callahan, C., Hendrie, H., Dittus, R., Brater, D., Hui, S., and Tierney, W. (1994) Improving treatment of late-life depression in primary care: A randomized clinical trial. *J Am Geriatr Soc* 42:839–846.

Canino, G.L., Bird, H.R., Shrout, P.E., Rubio-Stipec, M.A., Bravo, M.R.M., Sesman, M., and Guevara, L.M. (1987) The prevalence of specific psychiatric disorders in Puerto Rico. *Arch Gen Psychiatry* 44:727–735.

Centers for Disease Control. (1995) *Suicide in the United States: 1980–1992. Violence Surveillance Summary Series, No. 1*. Atlanta: US Department of Heath and Human Services.

Conwell, Y., Duberstein, P., and Caine, E. (2002) Risk factors for suicide in later life. *Biol Psychiatry* 52:193–204.

Conwell, Y., Lyness, J., Duberstein, P., Cox, C., Seidlitz, L., and DiGiorgio, A. (2000) Completed suicide among older patients in primary care practices: A controlled study. *J Am Geriatr Soc* 48:23–29.

Copeland, J. (1981) What is a "case"? A case for what? In: Wing, J., Bebbington, P., and Robins, L., eds. *What Is a Case: The Problem of Definition in Psychiatric Community Surveys*. London: Grant McIntyre, pp. 1–14.

Copeland, J., Dewey, M., Wood, N., Searle, R., Davidson, I., and McWilliam, C. (1987) Range of mental illness among the elderly in the community: Prevalence in the Liverpool area using the GMS-AGECAT package. *Br J Psychiatry* 150:815–823.

Copeland, J., Kelleher, M., and Kellet, J. (1976) A semi-structured clinical interview for the assessment of diagnosis and mental state in the elderly. The Geriatric Mental State 1. Development and reliability. *Psychol Med* 6:439–449.

Cornoni-Huntley, J., Blazer, D., Lafferty, M., Everett, D., Brock, D., and Farmer, M. (eds.). (1990) *Established Populations for Epidemiologic Studies of the Elderly: Resource Data Book*, Vol. II. Bethesda, MD: National Institute on Aging.

Cross-National collaborative Group. (1992) The changing rate of major depression. *JAMA* 268:3098–3105.

Eaton, W., Kramer, M., Anthony, J., Dryman, A., Shapiro, S., and Locke, B. (1989) The incidence of specific DIS/DSM-III mental disorders: Data from the NIMH epidemiologic catchment area program. *Acta Psychiatr Scand* 79:109–125.

Fillenbaum, G. (1988). *Multidimensional Functional Assessment of Older Adults: The Duke Older Americans Resources and Services Procedures*. Hillsdale, NJ: Erlbaum.

Fredman, L., Schoenbach, V., Kaplan, B., Blazer, D., and James, S. (1989) The association between depressive symptoms and mortality among older participants in the Epidemiologic Catchment Area—Piedmont Health Survey. *J Gerontol Soc Sci* 44:S149–S156.

Gatz, M., Pedersen, N., Plomin, R., Nesselroade, J., and McClearn, G. (1992) Importance of shared genes and shared environments for symptoms of depression in older adults. *J Abnorm Psychol* 101:701–708.

George, L., Blazer, D., Hughes, D., and Fowler, N. (1989) Social support and the outcome of major depression. *Br J Psychiatry* 154:478–485.

German, P., Shapiro, S., and Skinner, E. (1985) Mental health of the elderly: Use of health and mental health services. *J Am Geriatr Soc* 33:246–252.

Gonzalez, H., Haan, M., and Hinton, L. (2001) Acculturation and the prevalence of depression in older Mexican Americans: Baseline results from the Sacramento Area Latino Study on Aging. *J Am Geriatr Soc* 49:948–953.

Goodwin, D., and Guze, S. (1979) *Psychiatric Diagnosis*, 2nd ed. New York: Oxford University Press.

Hays, J., Saunders, W., Flint, E., Kaplan, B., and Blazer, D. (1997) Depression and social support as risk factors for functional disability in late life. *Aging Ment Health* 3:209–220.

Hazzard, W. (1994) Introduction: The practice of geriatric medicine. In: Hazzard, W., Bierman, E., Blass, J., Ettinger, H., Jr., and Halter, J., eds. *Principles of Geriatric Medicine and Gerontology*, 3rd ed. New York: McGraw-Hill, pp. xxiii–xxiv.

Hippocrates (1938) On air, water, and places, circa 400 BC. Republished in *Medical Classics* 3:19.

Hybels, C., Blazer, D., and Pieper, C. (2001) Toward a threshold for subthreshold depression: An analysis of correlates of depression by severity of symptoms using data from an elderly community survey. *Gerontologist* 41:357–365.

Hybels, C., Pieper, C., and Blazer, D. (2002) Gender differences in the relationship between subthreshold depression and mortality in a community sample of older adults. *Am J Geriatr Psychiatry* 10:283–291.

Kennedy, G., Kelman, H., and Thomas, C. (1990) The emergence of depressive symptoms in late life: The importance of declining health and increasing disability. *J Community Health* 15:93–104.

Kessler, R., Bergland, P., Demler, O., Jin, R., Koretz, P., Merikangas, K., Rush, J., Waters, E., and Wans P. (2003). The epidemiology of major depression. *JAMA* 289:3095–3105.

Klerman, G. (1978) Affective disorders. In: Nicholi, A., ed. *Harvard Guide to Modern Psychiatry*. Cambridge, MA: Belknap Press, pp. 253–281.

Klerman, G.L., Lavori, P.W., Rice, J., Reich, T., Endicott, J., Andreasen, N.C., Keller, M.B., and Hirschfield, R.M. (1985) Birth-cohort trends in rates of major depressive disorder among relatives of patients with affective disorder. *Arch Gen Psychiatry* 42(7):689–693.

Koenig, H.G., Meador, K.G., Cohen, H.J., and Blazer, D.G. (1988) Depression in elderly hospitalized patients with medical illness. *Arch Intern Med* 148:1929–1936.

Lin, T.-Y., and Standley, C. (1962) *The Scope of Epidemiology in Psychiatry*. Geneva: World Health Organization.

Morris, J. (1975) *Uses of Epidemiology*, 3rd ed. Edinburgh: Churchill Livingstone.

Murphy, E. (1983) The prognosis of depression in old age. *Br J Psychiatry* 142:111–119.

Murphy, E., Lindesay, J., and Grundy, E. (1986) 60 years of suicide in England and Wales. A cohort study. *Arch Gen Psychiatry* 43(10):969–976.

Murphy, E., Smith, R., Lindsey, J., and Slattery, J. (1988) Increased mortality rates in late life depression. *Br J Psychiatry* **152**:347–353.

Murphy, J., Monson, R., Oliver, D., Sobol, A., and Mighton, A. (1987) Affective disorders and mortality: A general population study. *Arch Gen Psychiatry* 44:473–480.

Murrell, S., Himmelfarb, S., and Wright, K. (1983) Prevalence of depression and its correlates in older adults. *Am J Epidemiol* 117:173–185.

Narrow, W., Rae, D., Robins, L., and Regier, D. (2002) Revised prevalence estimates of mental disorders in the United States: Using a clinical significance criterion to reconcile 2 surveys' estimates. *Arch Gen Psychiatry* 59:115–123.

National Center for Health, S. (2001) *Death Rates for 72 Selected Causes by 5-Year Age Groups, Race, and Sex: United States, 1979–1998*. Washington, DC: National Center for Health Statistics.

Olin, J., Schneider, L., Katz, I., Meyers, B., Alexopoulos, G., Breitner, J., and Bruce, M. (2002) Provisional diagnostic criteria for depression of Alzheimer Disease. *Am J Geriatr Psychiatry* 10:125–128.

Parmelee, P., Katz, I., and Lawton, M. (1989) Depression among institutionalized aged: Assessment and prevalence estimation. *J Gerontol Med Sci* 44:M22–M29.

Patterson, M., Schnell, A., Martin, R., Mendez, M., and Smyth, K. (1990) Assessment of behavioral and affective symptoms in Alzheimer's disease. *J Geriatr Psychiatry Neurol* 3:21–30.

Penninx, B., Geerlings, S., Deeg, D., van Eijk, J., van Tilling, W., and Beekman, A. (2001) Minor and major depression and the risk of death in older persons. *Arch Gen Psychiatry* 56:889–895.

Putnam, R. (2000) *Bowling Alone*. New York: Simon and Schuster.

Radloff, L. (1977) The CES-D Scale: A self-report depression scale for research in the general population. *Appl Psychol Measures* 1:385–401.

Raern, M., Reneson, B., Allebeck, P., Beskow, J., Rubenowitz, E., Skoog, I., and Wilhelmsson, K. (2002) Mental disorder in elderly suicides: A case-control study. *Am J Psychiatry* 159:450–455.

Reifler, B., Larson, E., and Henley, R. (1982) Coexistence of cognitive impairment and depression in geriatric outpatients. *Am J Psychiatry* 139:623–626.

Reynolds, C., Busse, D., Kupfer, D., Hoch, C., and Houch, P. (1990) Rapid eye movements and sleep-deprivation as a probe in elderly subjects. *Arch Gen Psychiatry* 47:1128–1136.

Reynolds, C., Frank, E., Perel, J., Imber, S., Cornes, C., Miller, M., Mazumdar, S., Houck, R., Dew, M., Stac, J., Pollock, B., and Kupfer, D. (1999) Nortriptyline and interpersonal psychotherapy as maintenance therapies for recurrent major depression: A randomized controlled trial in patients older than 59 years. *JAMA* 281:39–45.

Robins, L., Helzer, J., and Croughan, J. (1981) Diagnostic Interview Schedule: Its history, characteristics and validity. *Arch Gen Psychiatry* 38:381–389.

Robins, L.N., Wing, J., and Wittchen, H.U., et al., (1988) The Composite International Diagnostic Interview. *Arch Gen Psychiatry* 45:1069–1077.

Rorsman, B., Grasbeck, A., Hagnell, O., Lanke, J., and Ohman, R. (1990) A prospective study of first-incidence of depression: The Lundby study, 1957–1972. *Br J Psychiatry* 156:336–342.

Schulz, R., Beach, S., and Ives, D. (2000) Association between depression and mortality in older adults: The Cardiovascular Health Study. *Arch Intern Med* 160:1761–1768.

Spitzer, R., Williams, J., Gibbon, M., and First, M. (1990) *Structured Clinical Interview for DSM-III-R*. New York: New York State Psychiatric Institute, Biometrics Research.

Turvey, C., Conwell, Y., Jones, M., Phillips, C., Simonsick, E., Pearson, J., and Wallace, R. (2002) Risk factors for late-life suicide: A prospective, community-based study. *Am J Geriatr Psychiatry* 10:398–406.

Unutzer, J., Patrick, D., Simon, G., Grembowski, D., Walker, E., Rutter, C., and Katon, W. (1997) Depressive symptoms and the cost of health services in HMO patients 65+ years and older. *JAMA* 277:1618–1623.

Weissman, M., and Klerman, G. (1978) Epidemiology of mental disorders. *Arch Gen Psychiatry* 25:705–715.

Weissman, M., Bruce, M., Leaf, P., Florio, L., and Holzer, C. (1991) Affective disorders. In: Regier, P. and Robins, L., eds. *Psychiatric Disorders in America*: New York, The Free Press, pp. 53–80.

Yesavage, J., Brink, T., and Rose, T. (1983) Development and validation of a geriatric depression screening scale: A preliminary report. *J Psychiatr Res* 17:37–49.

# 2 | The social and financial burden of late-life depression to society and individuals

BARRY D. LEBOWITZ AND JASON T. OLIN

Depression in late life is common, serious, and under-appreciated as a source of disability and suffering for older people and their families (Geriatric Psychiatry Alliance, 1997). Depression at any age is a matter of concern. In later life, depression is particularly important because of its widespread impact. Unrecognized and untreated depression in older persons is a significantly disabling condition in its own right. That clinical fact ought to be enough to merit significant attention. Beyond the suffering of depression, however, we have learned that depression is a source of considerable and unnecessary excess disability in older persons afflicted with a broad variety of chronic illnesses. Moreover, beyond even that, current studies have clearly shown that depression is a fatal illness in older people. Despite the compellingly solid and substantial body of research in this area, recognition of depression remains problematic and is often attributed to normal developmental changes in aging. Even when it is recognized, and despite the clear data on the efficacy and effectiveness of treatment, the adequacy and appropriateness of care are highly variable.

Two factors combine to make depression in late life a primary concern in worldwide public health. First, the global population is growing older, gaining nearly 30 years of life expectancy in the twenty-first century (Lebowitz et al., 1998). Second, our appreciation of the disabling consequences of depression has been underscored by the landmark report of the World Health Organization (WHO) on the "global burden of disease" (Murray and Lopez, 1996). Using a standard measure of disease burden (the DALY, or disability-adjusted life-year), the WHO shows that in the established market economies, depression is the second leading cause of lost years of healthy life, including those due to premature death or disability. Depression causes a greater burden than cardiovascular disease, alcohol use, or traffic accidents and is expected to overtake ischemic heart disease as the leading cause of disease burden.

The financial burden of depression across the entire life-course is enormous. The estimated cost in the U.S. alone is in the neighborhood of $50 billion per annum due to healthcare, suicide, and workplace costs (Greenberg et al., 1993). Depression doubles the number of absentee days for employed individuals (Kessler et al., 1999). In one study, 70% of workers with depression had an illness-related absence of at least six days (Birnbaum et al., 1999). Direct physical and psychiatric care and pharmaceutical costs are estimated to be $12.4 billion. Suicide, in addition, results in an equal amount ($12.4 billion) in lost productivity and wages (Kashner et al., 2000).

Depression in older people is acknowledged to be a significant public health problem (NIH, 1992). It is the cause of unnecessary suffering for those whose illness is unrecognized or inadequately treated, and it burdens families and institutions providing care for the elderly.

Because of the stereotypic notion that older people are necessarily beset by many physical illnesses and social and economic problems, clinicians, family members, and older people themselves often conclude that depression is a normal condition of late life. Clinically, the symptom of depressed mood may be less commonly reported than a variety of somatic complaints, sleep and appetite changes, and general loss of interest (Gallo et al., 1994). Finally, the stigma associated with mental illnesses, particularly among older people themselves, impairs accurate and timely recognition.

These factors combine to make diagnosis and treatment of depression highly variable and problematic (Lebowitz et al., 1997). The lack of treatment, as well as inadequate/inappropriate treatment, are general problems (U.S. Department of Health and Human Services, 1999) in depression care that are magnified in older persons (Unutzer et al., 1999, 2000).

## MORTALITY

There can be no doubt that depression increases the risk of mortality: over 60 studies have clearly documented its impact (Wulsin et al., 1999). Though questions remain about the mechanism, this is now becoming clearer (Musselman et al., 1998). Similarly, ongoing studies are clarifying the complex causal linkages and directionalities in the depression–mortality association.

In a recent study, for example, Schulz and colleagues (2000) found that high levels of depressive symptoms in the Cardiovascular Health Study sample increased the 6-year all-cause mortality rate by 24%. The number of depressive symptoms directly affected all–cause mortality in the Osteoporotic Fractures Research Group sample of older women: the 7-year all-cause mortality rate for those with six or more depressive symptoms at baseline (24%) was double that of those with five or fewer symptoms and more than triple the rate of those with no symptoms at baseline (7%) (Whooley and Browner, 1998). In this sample, depression was associated only with those deaths caused by diseases other than cancers. In a clinical sample of older persons with myocardial infarction, depression increased 6-month mortality by a factor of 5 (Frasure-Smith et al., 1993). The conclusion from this important line of research is that depression is as strong a factor in mortality as other, more established risk factors such as smoking, obesity, hypertension, and hyperlipidemia.

## CO-MORBIDITY AND DISABILITY

Depression coexisting with physical illness has been shown to increase levels of functional disability, increase the use of health-care resources, and reduce the effectiveness of rehabilitation in older patients with stroke, Parkinson's disease (PD), heart disease, pulmonary disease, and fractures (Katz, 1996). Depression has been shown to exert a strong and independent effect on functional disability. That effect is independent of the diagnosis or the overall medical burden. Functional disability itself predicts the development of depression; conversely, depressive symptomatology is a risk factor for the onset or progression of disability (Bruce, 1999; Bruce and Hoff, 1994; Bruce et al., 1994; Steffens et al., 1999). Studies have shown that treatment for depression is safe and effective in patients with complex patterns of co-morbidity, and they suggest that treatment for depression can reduce excessive levels of disability and result in improved levels of functioning (Borson et al., 1992).

Depression in PD appears common, with epidemiological studies suggesting prevalence rates between 24% and 42% (Slaughter et al., 2001), underscoring the need to determine its etiology and validate treatments. Although psychiatric problems can result secondarily from difficulties in adjusting to PD or its treatment, there is evidence that neuropsychiatric changes are intrinsic to the disease process, particularly depression (Slaughter et al., 2001). Whatever the cause, depression leads to significant morbidity and suffering in individuals with PD.

A small body of research has indicated, not surprisingly, that individuals with PD have lower levels of serotonin than nondepressed individuals (Mayeux et al., 1984). Other authors have hypothesized a role for dopaminergic function (Brown and Gershon, 1993; Mayberg and Solomon, 1995) and cortical changes (Rogers et al., 1987), but both have been little studied. Regarding treatment, there are no well-controlled trials. Despite the common use of selective serotonin reuptake inhibitors (SSRIs), there remains concern about the possibility of a *serotonin syndrome*, which can occur when an SSRI is coadministered with selegiline.

Depression commonly occurs in Alzheimer's disease (AD), sometimes preceding the dementia diagnosis. Converging evidence from neuropathologists, epidemiologists, clinicians, and trialists supports the existence of a specific depression that occurs in AD. Thus, a National Institute of Mental Health (NIMH) work group recently developed provisional diagnostic criteria for depression of Alzheimer's disease (dAD) (Olin et al., 2002a, 2002b). These proposed criteria were created to facilitate hypothesis-driven research that leads to a better understanding of the depression that co-occurs in AD and to generate more homogeneous cohorts for treatment studies.

Depression of Alzheimer's disease is similar to a major depressive episode, but the severity threshold of dAD is lower than that of a major depressive episode. Most individuals with AD do not develop major depressive episodes. Depression of Alzheimer's disease requires the presence of at least three symptoms for a period of 2 weeks, compared to five or more for a major depressive episode. In addition to the symptoms of major depressive episode, irritability and social isolation/withdrawal are included. Symptoms are not required to be present "nearly every day." Individuals must meet criteria for AD, and the symptoms should best be accounted for by dAD. Note that having dAD does not necessarily rule out the presence of other diagnoses, including psychosis of AD.

## HEALTH-CARE SERVICE AND RESOURCE USE

In mixed age samples, major depression leads to excessive use of medical services and greater health care costs (Henk et al., 1996; Johnson et al., 1992; Simon et al., 1995; von Korff et al., 1992). In nursing homes and among high users of medical services, patients with depression incur significant increases in direct costs for medical care (Fries et al., 1993). Longitudinal data demonstrate that depressive symptomatology in elderly primary care patients is associated with increases in physician visits, medication use, emergency room visits and outpatient charges (Callahan et al., 1994; Cooper-Patrick et al., 1994). Among medical inpatients, major depression has been associated with increased use of health-care resources, including longer hospital stays, and greater mortality, for example, in those undergoing elective coronary artery bypass grafting (Callahan and Wolinsky, 1995; Williams-Russo, 1996; Williams-Russo et al., 1996). After discharge, depression accounts for a substantial increase in ambulatory health care use (Koenig and Kuchibhatla, 1999).

It would seem logical, therefore, to expect that treatment of depression would result in reductions in general health-care costs. This cost-offset phenomenon has been difficult to document, however, with most studies being inconclusive or mixed in their conclusion. The most positive conclusion seems to be that there may be a relatively small offset for those using large amounts of specialty care, particularly for those individuals who receive the highest-quality care for depression (Katzelnick et al., 1997; Thompson et al., 1998; Zhang et al., 1999).

The general health-care sector is by far the principal source of treatment for older persons with depression. Data from the 1987 National Medical Expenditure Survey show that over 55% of older persons using mental health care received this care from general physicians. In contrast, less than 3% of individuals over age 65 report having received outpatient treatment from mental health professionals, a proportion lower than that for any other adult age group (Olfson and Pincus, 1996).

The scope and responsibility of primary care providers are being expanded and redefined in many health-care systems. Primary care providers are charged with greater responsibility for diagnosis, treatment, and long-term management in all areas of health care, including care of older patients with mental disorders. That being the case, older people may derive substantial benefit from increased sensitivity to identification of depression by their primary care physicians. Interventions directed to improved recognition and treatment, however, have not necessarily translated into added benefit when compared to practice as usual in the primary care setting (Callahan et al., 1994; Klinkman and Okkes, 1998; Lebowitz, 1998). Perhaps more troubling, even when the results of trials have been positive, there has been no durable effect on clinical practice patterns in the general health-care sector (Callahan, 2001). Trials directed to late-life depression

in primary care settings certainly offer the promise of improving approaches to treatment in this setting (Bruce and Pearson, 1999; Unutzer et al., 2001; Williams, et al., 2000), but they also raise the challenge of implementation in the postexperimental period.

## SUICIDE AND LATE-LIFE DEPRESSION

Suicide rates increase with age in most countries of the world, and men outnumber women suicide completers by a substantial percentage. Recent studies of completed suicide have reinforced the close association with major depressive illness, especially in the elderly (Conwell and Brent, 1995). With increased age, the relative importance of the contribution of depression to suicide risk is magnified. The typical clinical profile of the older suicide completer is one of late-onset, nonpsychotic, unipolar depression of moderate severity uncomplicated by substance abuse or personality disorder.

Tragically, the depression in these older people was rarely recognized or treated. The failure to recognize and treat depression was not due to restricted access to care. A majority of these depressed suicide victims had seen a health-care provider in the last month of life, 39% in the last week, and 20% on the day of suicide (Conwell et al., 2000).

## CONCLUSIONS

Depression remains a central concern to older people, their families, and the clinicians who take care of them. Even when it appears to be an understandable response to illness, the onset of depression should be viewed as a sentinel event that increases the risk of subsequent declines in health status and functional ability. Early recognition, diagnosis, and initiation of treatment of depression in older persons present opportunities for improvements in quality of life, the prevention of suffering or premature death, and the maintenance of optimal levels of function and independence for older people.

REFERENCES

Birnbaum, H.G., Greenberg, P.E., Barton, M., Kessler, R.C., et al. (1999) Workplace burden of depression: Case study in social functioning using employer claims data. *Drug Benefit Trends* 11:6–12.

Borson, S., McDonald, G.J., Gayle, T., et al. (1992) Improvement in mood, physical symptoms, and function with nortriptyline for depression in patients with chronic obstructive pulmonary disease. *Psychosomatics* 33:190–201.

Brown, A., and Gershon, S. (1993) Dopamine and depression. *J Neural Transm* 91:75–109.

Bruce, M.L. (1999) The association between depression and disability. *Am J Geriatr Psychiatry* 7:8–11.

Bruce, M.L., and Hoff, R.A. (1994) Social and physical health risk factors for first onset major depressive disorder in a community sample. *Soc Psychiatry Psychiatr Epidemiol* 29:165–171.

Bruce, M.L., and Pearson, J.L. (1999) Designing and intervention to prevent suicide: PROSPECT (Prevention of Suicide in Primary Care Elderly: Collaborative Trial). *Dialogues Clin Neurosci* 1:100–112.

Bruce, M.L., Seeman, T.E., Merrill, S.S., et al. (1994) The impact of depressive symptomatology on physical disability: MacArthur studies of successful aging. *Am J Public Health* 84:1796–1799.

Callahan, C. (2001) Quality improvement research on late-life depression in primary care. *Med Care* 39:772–784.

Callahan, C.M., Hendrie, H.C., Dittus, R.S., et al. (1994) Improving treatment of late-life depression in primary care: A randomized clinical trial. *J Am Geriatr Soc* 42:839–846.

Callahan, C.M., Hui, S.L., Nienaber, N.A., et al. (1994) Longitudinal study of depression and health services use among elderly primary care patients. *J Am Geriatr Soc* 42:833–838.

Callahan, C.M., and Wolinsky, F.D. (1995) Hospitalization for major depression among older Americans. *J Gerontol Med Sci* 50A:M196–M202.

Conwell, Y., and Brent, D. (1995) Suicide and aging. I: Patterns of psychiatric diagnosis. *Int Psychogeriatr* 7:149–164.

Conwell, Y., Lyness, J.M., Duberstein, P., Cox, C., et al. (2000) Completed suicide among older patients in primary care practices: A controlled study. *Am J Geriatr Psychiatry* 48:23–29.

Cooper-Patrick, L., Crum, R.M., and Ford, D.E. (1994) Characteristics of patients with major depression who received care in general medical and specialty health settings. *Med Care* 32:15–24.

Diagnosis and Treatment of Depression in Late Life. (1991) *NIH Consens Dev Conf Consens Statement* 9(3): Nov. 4–6.

Frasure-Smith, N., Lesperance, F., and Talajic, M. (1993) Depression following myocardial infarction: Impact on 6-month survival. *JAMA* 270:1819–1825.

Fries, B.E., Mehr, D.R., Schneider, D., et al. (1993) Mental dysfunction and resource use in nursing homes. *Med Care* 31:898–920.

Gallo, J.J., Anthony, J.C., and Muthen, B.G. (1994) Age differences in the symptoms of depression: A latent trait analysis. *J Gerontol Psychol Sci* 49:P251–P264.

Geriatric Psychiatry Alliance. (1997) *Depression in Late Life: Not a Natural Part of Aging.* Bethesda, MD: American Association for Geriatric Psychiatry.

Greenberg, P.E., Stiglin, L.E., Finkelstein, S.N., et al. (1993) The economic burden of depression in 1990. *J Clin Psychiatry* 54:405–419.

Henk, H.J., Katzelnick, D.J., Kobak, K.A., et al. (1996) Medical costs attributed to depression among patients with a history of high medical expenses in a health maintenance organization. *Arch Gen Psychiatry* 53:899–904.

Johnson, J., Weissman, M.M., and Klerman, G.L. (1992) Service utilization and social morbidity associated with depressive symptoms in the community. *JAMA* 267:1478–1483.

Kashner, T.M., Schoaf, T., and Rush, A.J. (2000) The economic burden of suicide in the United States in the year 2000. *TEN* 2:44–48.

Katz, I.R. (1996) On the inseparability of medical and physical health in aged persons: Lessons from depression and medical co-morbidity. *Am J Geriatr Psychiatry* 4:1–16.

Katzelnick, D.J., Kobak, K.A., Greist, J.H., et al. (1997) Effect of primary care treatment of depression on service use by patients with high medical expenditures. *Psychiatr Services* 48:59–64.

Kessler, R.C., Barber, C., Birnbaum, H.G., et al. (1999) Depression in the workplace: Effects of treatment on short-term disability. *Health Aff* 18:163–171.

Klinkman, M.S., and Okkes, I. (1998) Mental health problems in primary care: A research agenda. *J Fam Pract* 47:379–384.

Koenig, H.G., and Kuchibhatla, M. (1999) Use of health services by medically ill depressed elderly patients after hospital discharge. *Am J Geriatr Psychiatry* 7:48–56.

Lebowitz, B.D. (1998) Priorities for agenda building: Mental health and primary care. *J Fam Pract* 47:341.

Lebowitz, B.D., Pearson, J.L., and Cohen, G.D. (1998) Older Americans and their illnesses. In: Salzman, C., ed. *Clinical Geriatric Psychopharmacology*, 3rd ed. Baltimore: Williams & Wilkins, pp. 3–20.

Lebowitz, B.D., Pearson, J.L., Schneider, L.S., Reynolds, C.F., et al. (1997) Diagnosis and treatment of depression in late life: Consensus statement update. *JAMA* 278:1186–1190.

Mayberg, H., and Solomon, D. (1995) Depression in Parkinson's disease: A biochemical and organic viewpoint. In: Weiner, W.J., and Lang, A.E., eds. *Behavioral Neurology of Movement Disorders* (Advances in Neurology, vol. 65). New York, Raven Press, pp. 49–60.

Mayeux, R., Stern, Y., Cote, L., et al. (1984) Altered serotonin metabolism in depressed patients with Parkinson's disease. *Neurology* 34:642–646.

Murray, C.J.L., and Lopez, A.D., eds. (1996) *The Global Burden of Disease.* Cambridge, MA: Harvard University Press.

Musselman, D.L., Evans, D.L., and Nemeroff, C.B. (1998) The relationship of depression to cardiovascular disease: Epidemiology, biology, and treatment. *Arch Gen Psychiatry* 55:580–592.

NIH Consensus Development Panel on Depression in Late Life (1992) Diagnosis and treatment of depression in late life. *JAMA* 268:1018–1024.

Olfson, M., and Pincus, H.A. (1996) Outpatient mental health care in nonhospital settings: Distribution of patients across provider groups. *Am J Psychiatry* 153:1353–1356.

Olin, J.T., Katz, I.R., Meyers, B.S., Schneider, L.S., et al. (2002b) National Institute of Mental Health—Provisional Diagnostic Criteria for Depression of Alzheimer Disease: Rationale and Background. *Am J Geriatr Psychiatry* 10:125–128.

Olin, J.T., Schneider, L.S., Katz, I.R., Meyers, B.S., et al. (2002a) National Institute of Mental Health—Provisional Diagnostic Criteria for Depression of Alzheimer Disease. *Am J Geriatr Psychiatry* 10:129–141.

Rogers, D., Lees, A.J., Smith, E., et al. (1987) Bradyphrenia in Parkinson's disease and psychomotor retardation in depressive illness: An experimental study. *Brain* 110:761–776.

Schulz, R., Beach, S.R., Ives, D.G., et al. (2000) Association between depression and mortality in older adults: The Cardiovascular Health Study. *Arch Intern Med* 160:1761–1768.

Simon, G.E., Von Korff, M., and Barlow, W. (1995) Health care costs of primary care patients with recognized depression. *Arch Gen Psychiatry* 52:850–856.

Slaughter, J.R., Slaughter, K.A., Nichols, D., Holmes, S.E., and Martens, M.P. (2001). Prevalence, clinical manifestations, etiology, and treatment of depression in Parkinson's disease. *J Neuropsychiatry Clin Neurosci* 13(2):187–196.

Steffens, D.C., Hays, J.C., and Krishnan, R.R.K. (1999) Disability in geriatric depression. *Am J Geriatr Psychiatry* 7:34–40.

Thompson, D., Hylan, T.R., McMullen, W., et al. (1998) Predictors of a medical offset effect among patients receiving antidepressant therapy. *Am J Psychiatry* 155:824–826.

Unutzer, J., Katon, W., Russo, J., et al. (1999) Patterns of care for depressed older adults in a large staff model HMO. *Am J Geriatr Psychiatry* 7:235–243.

Unutzer, J., Katon, W., Williams, J.W., et al. (2001) Improving primary care for depression in late life: The design of a multicenter randomized trial. *Med Care* 39:785–799.

Unutzer, J., Simon, G., Belin, T.R., et al. (2000) Care for depression in HMO patients aged 65 and older. *J Am Geriatr Soc* 48:871–878.

U.S. Department of Health and Human Services. (1999) *Mental Health: A Report of the Surgeon General.* Rockville, MD: U.S. Department of Health and Human Services, Substance Abuse and Mental Health Services Administration, Center for Mental Health

Services, National Institutes of Health, National Institute of Mental Health.

Von Korff, M., Ormel, H., Katon, W., et al. (1992) Disability and depression among high utilizers of health care. *Arch Gen Psychiatry* 19:91–100.

Whooley, M.A., and Browner, W.S. (1998) Association between depressive symptoms and mortality in older women: Study of osteoporotic fractures research group. *Arch Intern Med* 158:2129–2135.

Williams-Russo, P. (1996) Barriers to diagnosis and treatment of depression in primary care settings. *Am J Geriatr Psychiatry* (Suppl 1) 4:S84–S90.

Williams-Russo, P., Petersen, J., Charlson, M.E., et al. (1996, July) Longitudinal course of depressive symptoms after bypass surgery. Presented at the NIMH Primary Care Conference, Rockville, MD.

Williams, J.W., Barrett, J., Oxman, T., et al. (2000) Treatment of dysthymia and minor depression in primary care: A randomized controlled trial in older adults. *JAMA* 284:1519–1526.

Wulsin, L.R., Vaillant, G.E., and Wells, V.W. (1999) A systematic review of the mortality of depression. *Psychosom Med* 61:6–17.

Zhang, M.L., Rost, K.G., and Fortney, J.C. (1999) Depression treatment and cost offset for rural community residents. *J Soc Service Res* 25:99–110.

# II | THE PHENOMENOLOGY AND DIFFERENTIAL DIAGNOSIS OF LATE-LIFE MOOD DISORDERS

## PHENOMENOLOGY: HISTORY OF THE TERM

The first use of the term *phenomenology* is attributed to a little-known German philosopher, Johann Heinrich Lambert, a contemporary of Kant. In *Neues Orqanon*, Lambert spoke of a discipline of phenomenology that focused on *phenomena*, which he took to be the illusory aspects of human experience. Thus, he defined phenomenology as the "theory of illusion."

Kant is given credit for generating wider interest in the concept of phenomenology, although he used the term only twice in his works. His view was that one must distinguish between the world (including ourselves) as we experience it and the world as it truly is. The former, our subjective experience of things, he termed *phenomena*, designating the latter *noumena* or *things-in-themselves*. To Kant, the only science we could have was phenomenological, as we could only know our experience of things, that is, phenomena, and not the things themselves.

During the nineteenth and twentieth centuries, the phenomenology movement in philosophy and psychiatry both embraced and rejected Kant. As espoused by Hegel, the notion was presented that phenomenology was our only valid method of attaining knowledge. However, especially with respect to knowledge of ourselves—that is, knowledge of the mind—ardent phenomenologists held that we could come to know the mind as it is—as a Kantian neumenon—with the method of the *science* relying on progressively deeper and more critical apprehension. Thus, in a curious twist of logic, and in many ways opposite to Kant's intent, there was and continues to be a deeply held view by some that disciplined analysis of subjective experience yields knowledge of reality. For decades, the ideological struggles between psychodynamic and biological approaches to mental illness have largely stemmed from the espousal or rejection of this view.

## PHENOMENOLOGY AND PSYCHIATRIC DIAGNOSIS

The most common current usage of the term *phenomenology* implies a less grand but perhaps more realistic vision. Phenomenology involves a descriptive investigation of what can be observed. In psychiatry, patients' thoughts, affects, and behaviors comprise the core of phenomenological study. Indeed, it may be unappreciated that the extraordinary progress made in recent decades in biological psychiatry and clinical neurosciences owes much to the reinstatement of a phenomenological approach as key to the diagnosis of disorders and the assessment of symptom severity.

Until DSM-III was published, diagnosis often mixed elements of phenomenology—that is, description and classification of the patient's mental states and behaviors—as reported or observed with psychodynamic and other speculations about causal processes. It was the return to more purely descriptive characterization ("of what was experienced") that led to consistency in the application of nosology and, often, impressive reliability in assessment and diagnosis. Reliability is no guarantee of accuracy. Our differential diagnoses may all be in agreement, and wrongfully so. However, reliability sets the upper limit for the validity of diagnosis. The concentration on phenomenologically based, criteria-driven assessment has not only ensured greater consistency in the diagnosis, but has also created the possibility of achieving greater accuracy.

## PHENOMENOLOGY: BOTH A BEGINNING AND AN END POINT

While phenomenology provides the substance of our assessment and diagnostic practices, it also is the end point of our investigations. Ultimately, the goal of our science is to be able to account for the phenomenological profiles of our patients. Whether on the basis of biological heritage, life events, somatic interventions, or other explanatory variables, we seek to explain how and why people are depressed, do or do not respond to treatments, or display cognitive decline. Presently, phenomenology defines the boundaries of psychiatric illness. Phenomenological differences determine nosological classification. Changes in phenomenology determine the success of treatments or characterize the course of illness. Explanations of phenomenological differences, whether age at onset, illness prevalence, or symptomatic profiles, speak to the factors that influence illness expression, and thus to etiology.

## STRENGTHS AND WEAKNESSES OF PHENOMENOLOGICAL METHODS

The ascendance and limitations of the phenomenological approach in psychiatry are readily apparent in mood disorders. Methods to assess variation among patients in severity of depressive symptoms have reached such an advanced stage of development, at least in studies of mid-life adults, that the reliability of symptom scores can rival that of any laboratory or radiological procedure. The subtypes of major depression—unipolar or bipolar, psychotic or nonpsychotic, typical or atypical, and melancholic and nonmelancholic—have each been validated by *pharmacological dissection* (different subtypes within a grouping preferentially benefit from different regimens), yet these subtypes were originally based on characterization of symptom clusters.

The limitations of a phenomenological approach are both practical and theoretical. Practically, there are intrinsic difficulties in relying on the reports of individuals as a prime source of information about their illness when the illness itself can distort memory or judgment. Particularly when the history is key to diagnosis or treatment decision making, elderly patients can present special difficulties. For example, the distinction between early- and late-onset depressive illness appears to be of growing significance. Yet, for elderly patients, prior episodes may have occurred so far in the past that they are forgotten, and the availability of other informants may be limited.

Theoretically, a purely phenomenological approach will prove unsatisfying as a system of classification. For example, late-life major depression is a syndrome that can result from many different etiologies, and can require different interventions and have different long-term courses. None of these distinctions, which are of key clinical concern, may necessarily be discerned at the phenomenological level. Progress in nosology will result from linking phenomenological observation with other realms of assessment, experimental manipulation, and treatment intervention.

## PHENOMENOLOGICAL DIFFERENCES IN DEPRESSION ACROSS THE AGE SPAN

There is a long-standing belief that there are important differences in phenomenology between late-life and mid-life depression. Two distinct, but not mutually exclusive, factors may alter the presentation of depressive illness in late life. One factor is the cumulative impact of recurrent depressive illness over a lifetime. In many patients, mood disorder begins early in life, and by the time they reach their 60s, they have had repeated episodes. There is evidence that the number of depressive episodes, as well as the cumulative time spent in a depressed state, are associated with a poorer response to treatment and the development of chronic symptoms. Furthermore, some studies suggest that the cumulative time spent in a depressed state is associated with atrophy in specific brain regions, which may affect the phenomenological presentation and the treatment outcome in future episodes. Thus, by the time a patient with recurrent depression reaches late life, the consequences of the disorder itself, and perhaps the treatments received, will influence the psychobiology, presentation, treatment response, and course of the illness.

The second factor that may independently influence the syndrome of late-life depression is a consequence of the psychosocial, behavioral, and physiological changes associated with aging. For example, functional impairment as a symptom of depression is often manifested differently throughout the life cycle. Depression-associated dysfunction in children can present as poor school performance or antisocial behavior, while in young adults it may manifest as dissatisfaction in work or love, and in older patients as hypochondriasis and increased use of medical services.

Imaging studies of normally aging individuals have revealed signficant age-associated changes in brain structure, cerebral blood flow, cerebral metabolism, and neurotransmitter function. These age-associated changes in brain structure and function can influence the phenomenology of depression in late life and may provide the basis for the increased frequency of the delusional and melancholic subtypes in older age groups. Furthermore, brain imaging studies in individuals with late-life depression have found a high rate of structural abnormalities compatible with cerebrovascular disease, especially among patients with late-onset illness. These abnormalities may predict a poorer treatment response and a deteriorating course of illness.

Changes in the brain may also affect how the individual reacts to the environment, increasing the vulnerability to stress and depression. Regional brain dysfunction, especially in the prefrontal areas, can produce changes in personality, temperament, vulnerability to distress, and coping mechanisms. Thus the effects of age and/or depression on neural systems may manifest as increased social isolation, loss of independence, cognitive impairment, and related behaviors that may precipitate, intensify, or prolong depressive episodes.

## DETECTION AND DIFFERENTIAL DIAGNOSIS OF LATE-LIFE DEPRESSIVE DISORDERS

It is widely recognized that a large percentage, perhaps the majority, of depressive disorders in the elderly goes undetected, let alone untreated. This lack of detection is not attributable to lack of contact with health-care providers. Instead, the elderly are especially likely to go undiagnosed with respect to mood disorder despite recent contact with medical professionals. Although the toll of depression in the elderly is so great, its detection in this age group seems particularly problematic. What are the barriers to detection and diagnosis?

### Symptom Profile Differences

As noted in Chapter 1, many elderly persons present with subsyndromal depressive symptoms that do not meet the threshold for a DSM-IV diagnosis of a depressive disorder. Nonetheless, these symptoms may result in functional deficits and suffering. The constellation of symptoms in older patients may not be typical of that seen in younger populations, with a greater incidence of somatic complaints, anhedonia, lack of interest, and cognitive deficits. Indeed, even in elderly patients with major depression, vegetative and somatic symptoms such as insomnia, lack of appetite, gastrointestinal disturbance, and so on may be incorrectly viewed as a consequence of medical co-morbidities or physiological effects of aging.

### Reporting Bias

Many of the key symptoms of depression refer to abnormal internal states, such as excessive sadness, fatigue, or a distinct quality of mood. Other symptoms of depression refer to the cognitive components of the self-schema—how we view ourselves and our place in the world. Although controversial, there is evidence that the elderly report fewer symptoms of depression than those found on formal evaluation. For example, scores on self-report measures of depressive symptoms tend to be lower in the elderly than scores on observer-rating instruments. In particular, it is thought that *cognitive symptoms*, such as thoughts of worthlessness or hopelessness and feelings of guilt, appear to be especially subject to this reporting bias, while this is less true of somatic symptoms.

This putative tendency to deny the cognitive symptoms of depression could reflect an aging or cohort effect regarding the stigma associated with receiving a psychiatric diagnosis. Specifically, older individuals may be more reluctant to accept a psychiatric diagnosis and may focus instead on the physical symptoms of their disorders. This view is far from validated. Nonetheless, there is clearly one subgroup that, at times, will actively deny that they have a psychiatric disorder. Patients with delusional (psychotic) depression are especially likely to deny that they are depressed or in any way in need of treatment. Almost invariably, marked discrepancies between self-report and observer ratings of depression occur in the assessment of patients with psychotic depression. This subgroup contains a large proportion of the elderly.

### Attributions of Depressive Symptoms

Across the adult age range, there is a powerful tendency to attribute the onset of depressive episodes to stressful life events. When patients are asked why they are depressed, they commonly state that the episode is triggered by some adverse life event. This phenomenon reflects a powerful bias for retrospective reconstruction of the genesis of depressive symptoms.

This bias is often shared by health-care providers. In this case, the attributional bias assumes that depressive symptoms are a *natural* or *expected* reaction to loss. Since the elderly are especially subject to frequent and profound negative life events, such as loss of spouse, relatives, and friends, loss of occupational and recreational roles, deteriorating physical health, and so on, there is a high frequency of depressive symptoms and syndromes in this age group. In essence, this bias assumes that negative life events and other types of loss (e.g., physical decline) play a primary etiological role in depressive syndromes in the elderly.

The elderly are not immune from this type of attributional bias. Both the patients and health-care providers may view depressive symptoms as simply emergent aspects of aging or a reaction to loss. Especially in the case of dysthymia or subsyndromal expression of depressive symptoms, some view insomnia, lack of interest in activities, reduced capacity to experience pleasure, loss of appetite, and so on as part of the aging process and not as an expression of a new disorder. The attribution to the aging process, as opposed to a reaction to loss, is especially nefarious. Depressive disorders in the elderly may become chronic conditions. By definition, this is the case in dysthymic disorder. When depressive symptomatology is viewed in this light, it is often further assumed that treatment is either unnecessary or would be ineffective. When depressive symptoms are an expected and normal expression of aging, little can be done to reverse or at least halt the march of aging.

Fundamentally, this bias may be characterized as stating that (1) "Anyone would be depressed if they were in their shoes" and (2) "Since the depressive symptoms reflect the aging process or are normal reactions to loss, treatment is unnecessary and, in any case, would not be successful."

This nihilistic view of the potential benefits of treatment can be easily challenged. In medicine, there is no certain relationship between etiological factors that lead to illness manifestation and responsiveness of the illness to treatment. Impaired vision may result from various etiological factors, including normative decline with aging, but various corrective procedures are still effective. The fact that, at times, negative life events may trigger illness has no clear-cut implications for the efficacy of psychological or biological interventions. Indeed, prolonged bereavement often responds to antidepressant treatment (Chapter 9).

One should also challenge the notions that depressive symptoms are an expected outgrowth of the aging process or that depressive syndromes are expected reactions to the losses and negative life events that accrue with aging. In practice, we often see individuals who have recurrent affective episodes of depression or mania with reliable periodicity (e.g., every spring). Many of these individuals retrospectively attribute syndromal onset to some life event, despite the regular emergence of symptoms regardless of overall life circumstances. In other words, there is a strong tendency to identify an environmental cause for the onset and expression of mood disorders. However, in many cases this would be akin to attributing the initial presentation or recurrence of cancer to a specific environmental event. Secondly, in medicine, often there is little relationship between the factors responsible for illness manifestation and the effectiveness of treatments. While some might argue that a trigger due to stressful life events should lead to use of a psychological treatment, our firmest evidence for efficacy in extended bereavement, poststoke depression, dysthymia, and major depression concerns biological interventions (Part III).

## Obscuring Effects of Comorbidity

Another key factor that inhibits the detection and differential diagnosis of depressive disorders in the elderly is the obscuring effect of co-morbid medical conditions. A variety of physical disorders (or their treatments) can produce some of the cardinal symptoms of depression, including insomnia or hypersomnia, fatigue, lack of interest, appetite loss, and so on. In this context, the depressive syndrome may not be detected due to attribution of the symptoms to the medical disorder. In dementing disorders, the cognitive decline may interfere with the detection and differential diagnosis of depressive disorders, since the patient is the primary informant but now has limited capacity to describe internal states.

Poststroke depression is a good example of how many of these biases can influence diagnosis and treatment. In the context of a recent stroke, many view depression as an expected psychological reaction for which treatment would be either unnecessary or unsuccessful. The behavioral effects of the stroke may mimic some of the symptoms of depression or reduce significantly the possibility of an informed self-report. The depressive syndrome following the stroke may not fully match the symptom profile in major depression, derailing the differential diagnosis. Depending largely on the location of the lesion and the time elapsed since the stroke, some patients will deny having depressive symptoms, complicating detection and diagnosis. Furthermore, the natural course of the depressive disorder may be distinct from that of major depression in patients without this neurological event. Indeed, there is some evidence that the treatments that are effective in poststroke depression have a more limited pharmacological profile than is the case for standard (idiopathic) major depression (Chapter 26).

In short, various biases impinge on the detection and differential diagnosis of depressive disorders in the elderly. It is probably fair to say that these biases stem from ideologies regarding the factors responsible for the emergence and maintenance of the depressed state and beliefs about the relationships between environmental triggers of depressive episodes and amenability to treatment and the choice of treatment. It should be kept in mind, however, that there is no necessary relationship between the efficacy of a treatment for a condition and the factors that influence its emergence or expression. We know of no one who has become depressed due to lack of a seizure, yet electroconvulsive therapy is our most effective antidepressant. Similarly, psychological interventions are often the most effective interventions in minimizing the behavioral deficits following a brain insult. Alternatively, pharmacological treatment may be the most effective strategy for treating the complications of bereavement.

Failure to detect and diagnose depressive disorders in the elderly can have dire consequences. Assuming that treatment is either unnecessary or of limited value can be especially damaging. As indicated repeatedly in the various chapters in this part, the depressive syndromes in the elderly are diverse in their phenomenology, course, and treatment response. Familiarity with these various presentations, and knowledge of the various factors that inhibit detection, diagnosis, and treatment, can only improve the provision of care for patients with late-life depression.

# 3 | Unipolar depression

GEORGE S. ALEXOPOULOS AND WILLIAM APFELDORF

Although depression affects a large number of elders, it is not an expected or a necessary consequence of aging. The Epidemiological Catchment Area study found that the prevalence of major depressive disorder in persons 65 years of age or older was 1.4% in women and 0.4% in men, with an overall combined prevalence of 1% (Weissman et al., 1988). The prevalence of depression changes with the setting. Some type of depressive disorder has been identified in 17%–30% of geriatric patients treated in primary care settings: approximately 30% of these patients meet criteria for major depressive disorder (Alexopoulos, 1996). Major depression has been found in 11% of patients hospitalized for treatment of medical illness (Blazer, 1994) and in 12% of patients confined to long-term care facilities (Parmelee et al., 1989). Depressive symptoms were documented in 50% of patients with dementia, and major depression was diagnosed in 17%–30% of demented patients (Alexopoulos and Abrams, 1991).

Despite its prevalence, late-life depression is under-recognized and undertreated, particularly in primary care practices, general hospitals, and nursing homes (Luber et al., 2001; Mulsant and Ganguli, 1999). The challenges unique to the diagnosis of late-life depression are the difficulties in differentiating it from the many other medical and neurological disorders of the elderly; the different presentation of depression in older patients, including the tendency of older people to deny feelings of depression; and the coexistence of depression and cognitive impairment. Depression in late life, more often than not, follows a relapsing or chronic course (Alexopoulos and Chester, 1992; Callahan et al., 1994; Cole and Bellavance, 1997). Hence, approaches to the care of depressed older adults must include efforts to minimize relapse, recurrence, and residual symptoms. Treating clinicians need to have a comprehensive knowledge of the illness and its management, and to educate their patients and their families about the necessity of long-term care.

In this chapter, we review the diagnoses, clinical assessment, course and consequences, and barriers to the recognition and treatment of late-life unipolar major depression. In this volume, separate chapters are devoted to bipolar disorder, dysthymia, subsyndromal depressions, mixed cognitive and affective syndromes, suicide, vascular depression, and complicated bereavement.

## DIAGNOSING LATE-LIFE DEPRESSION

The current diagnostic criteria for psychiatric disorders are codified in the *Diagnostic and Statistical Manual for Mental Disorders* (DSM), 4th edition—TR (American Psychiatric Association, 2000) and the *International Classification of Diseases*, 10th edition (2000). The DSM criteria for a major depressive episode include five or more symptoms during the same 2-week period (Table 3.1). The symptoms must represent a change from previous function.

The current DSM criteria are not modified to reflect the clinical features unique to the depressed elderly. Older depressed patients tend to report more somatic and cognitive symptoms than affective symptoms. Older patients who deny having a depressed mood may still report a lack of feeling/emotion or acknowledge a loss of interest and pleasure in activities (Gallo and Rabins, 1999; Gallo et al., 1994). The experience and expression of psychiatric symptoms are influenced by age, personal history, and culture. Furthermore, the presence of co-morbid conditions, which is the rule rather than the exception in a geriatric sample, can further complicate symptom assessment. Depression may intensify physical symptoms, lower self-rated health (Schulberg et al., 1998), and interfere with patient participation in treatment (diMatteo et al., 2000). Therefore, the ascertainment of symptoms, and perhaps the criteria for diagnosis, in the elderly should take these factors into consideration.

Approximately half of elders with depression have their first episode in late life. Therefore, accurate diagnosis cannot be helped by the past history, and many patients with late-onset depression have no family history of mood disorders (Mendlewicz and Baron, 1981). Older adults are often subject to losses and other stressors (e.g., bereavement, retirement, relocation, financial problems) that may contribute to diagnostic confusion, as behavioral changes following these events may mimic depressive symptoms. No biological tests can reliably aid the diagnostic assessment of depressed elders. To help make an accurate diagnosis, clinicians should use the reports of family informants or caregivers to supplement information provided by patient.

TABLE 3.1. *DSM IV-TR Criteria for Major Depressive Episode*

1. Depressed mood most of the day, nearly every day;
2. Markedly diminished interest or pleasure in all, or almost all activities;
3. Significant weight loss, or decrease or increase in appetite nearly every day;
4. Insomnia or hypersomnia;
5. Psychomotor agitation or retardation;
6. Fatigue or loss of energy;
7. Feelings of worthlessness or excessive or inappropriate guilt;
8. Diminished ability to think or concentrate, or indecisiveness;
9. Recurrent thoughts of death, suicidal ideation with or without a plan.

*Source:* American Psychiatric Association (2000).

The four major syndromes of late-life unipolar depression are unipolar major depression, psychotic major depression, depression due to a general medical condition, and adjustment disorder with depressed mood.

## Unipolar Major Depression/Major Depressive Disorder (296.2* or 296.3*)

The diagnosis of major depression requires at least five of the nine symptoms listed in Table 3.1 as criteria for a major depressive episode. Depressed mood or loss of interest or pleasure is necessary in order to meet criteria for major depression and must be one of the five required symptoms. Exclusion criteria include a history of mania or bipolar disorder.

Although not part of the diagnostic criteria, nondemented elderly individuals often have cognitive impairment, including disturbances in attention, speed of mental processing, and executive function (Boone et al., 1995; Kiosses et al., 2001; Lockwood et al., 2002). Processing speed and working memory deficits may lessen after remission of depression, but they are not normalized and may reflect a permanent underlying brain disturbance (Geerling et al., 2000; Kalayam and Alexopoulos, 1999).

The DSM-IV does not allow the diagnosis of unipolar major depression if it can be established that the symptoms of depression are a direct physiological effect of a medical disorder or substance. However, the usefulness of this rule in late-life depression is questionable. Co-morbidity of medical and cognitive disorders is the rule rather than the exception in patients with late-life depression, and the causal relationship between medical illness and depression cannot be easily ascertained.

However, the medical burden does not interfere with the response to antidepressant drugs (Gill and Hatcher, 2000). Depression occurring in the context of medical illnesses presumed to cause depression should be treated with antidepressants, while the coexisting medical condition is treated concurrently (Alexopoulos et al., 2001). Therefore, instead of emphasizing differences in etiology that cannot be reliably ascertained, it may be more fruitful to focus on differences in treatment approaches.

## Unipolar Major Depression with Psychotic Features/Major Depressive Disorder, Severe, with Psychotic Behavior (296.24 or 296.34)

Older patients with psychotic major depression have a severe depression and are experiencing delusions or hallucinations. The usual themes of depressive delusions are guilt, hypochondriasis, nihilism, persecution, and sometimes jealousy. Depressive delusions can be distinguished from delusions of demented patients in that the latter are less systematized and less congruent to the affective disturbance. Psychotic depression occurs in 20% to 45% of hospitalized elderly depressives and in 3.6% of elderly depressives living in the community (Linjakumpu et al., 2002).

## Depression due to a General Medical Condition/Organic Affective Syndrome (293.83)

The diagnosis of depression due to a general medical condition is limited to the medical illnesses with a known etiological link to depression. These include degenerative neurological diseases (e.g., parkinsonism, Huntington's disease), stroke, metabolic conditions (e.g., vitamin $B_{12}$ deficiency), thyroid, parathyroid, and adrenal diseases, autoimmune conditions (e.g., systemic lupus erythematosus), viral or other infections (e.g., hepatitis, infectious mononucleosis, human immunodeficiency virus), and malignancies (e.g., pancreatic cancer).

This syndrome is often misapplied to the large number of elderly patients in whom the overall medical burden contributes to their depression (Kukull et al., 1986; Mulsant et al., 1994; Schulberg et al., 1998; Zubenko et al., 1997). Physiological stress of an illness, functional disability, and life changes necessitated by chronic illness may precipitate demoralization and depression in susceptible individuals (Bruce et al., 1994; Kukull et al., 1986). Reciprocal patterns of causation are common in late-life depression associated with medical co-morbidity. Chronic pain is an example. Depression amplifies the perception of pain, and persistent pain worsens depression. Sleep disturbance, a symptom common in depression, is also linked to poor health, angina, limitations in activities of daily living, and chronic use of benzodiazepines (Newman et al., 1997).

## Adjustment Disorder with Depressed Mood/Depressive Reaction, prolonged (301.9)

Negative life events are associated with increased depressive symptoms in the elderly. Financial problems, socioeconomic deprivation, poor physical health, disability, and social isolation are significant contributors to depressive symptomatology in late life (Baumgarten et al., 1992). Other causes of adjustment disorders in the elderly are relocation to a long-term care facility and bereavement due to loss of a spouse. Marked increases in the risk of medical morbidity and mortality occur following involuntary relocation. However, when elderly persons have control over such decisions and when they move to a high-quality institution, relocation may have a neutral or even a beneficial effect.

## OTHER SYNDROMES OF LATE-LIFE DEPRESSION

Specific etiologies have been hypothesized for several syndromes related to late-life depression, and this has led to a line of research on brain mechanisms in late-life depression. While they are not included in the DSM-IV TR, these syndromes convey clinically and heuristically useful information.

### Late-Onset Depression

It has been suggested that depression with onset of the first episode in late life includes a large subgroup of patients with neurological brain disorders that may or may not be evident when the depression first appears (Alexopoulos et al., 1989). Compared to early-onset geriatric depressives, patients with late-onset depression appear to have a less frequent family history of mood disorders (Baldwin and Tomenson, 1995; Heun et al., 2001), a higher prevalence of dementing disorders (Jorm, 2000), more impairment on neuropsychological tests (Salloway et al., 1996), a higher rate of dementia development on follow-up (Baldwin et al., 2000), and greater enlargement of lateral brain ventricles and more white matter hyperintensities (Greenwald et al., 1996; Salloway et al., 1996).

The late-onset syndrome has served as the basis of pathogenetic hypotheses linking brain abnormalities to development of late-life depression. However, there are significant limitations in using age of onset as a distinguishing clinical characteristic. It can be difficult to identify the onset of depression, especially in patients whose early episodes are mild. On a theoretical level, an episode occurring in late life may receive a contribution from neurological brain changes, regardless of whether the patient did or did not have other depressive episodes in early life.

### Depression with Reversible Dementia

Some elderly depressed patients develop a reversible dementia syndrome that improves or completely subsides after remission of depression (Alexopoulos et al., 1993; Devanand et al., 1996). This syndrome has been termed *pseudodementia*, *depression with reversible dementia*, and *dementia of depression* and occurs mainly in patients with late-onset depression. Depressed elderly patients who still have some cognitive impairment even after improvement of depression are usually in the early stages of a dementing disorder whose cognitive manifestations are exaggerated when the depressive syndrome is superimposed. Though most of these patients do not meet criteria for dementia for 1–2 years after the initial episode of depression with reversible dementia, after 3 years even patients with more or less complete cognitive recovery have a 40% rate of irreversible dementia (Kral and Emery, 1989). Current pharmacological interventions for dementias allow stabilization of the cognitive status while not reversing any preexisting decline. Therefore, identification of a reversible dementia syndrome in elderly depressives is an indication for a thorough diagnostic workup aimed at the identification of treatable dementing disorders and frequent follow-up.

### Vascular Depression

It has been hypothesized that cerebrovascular disease may predispose to, precipitate, or perpetuate some geriatric depressive syndromes (Alexopoulos et al., 1997; Krishnan et al., 1997). The co-morbidity of depression and vascular risk factors and manifest vascular disease, as well as the association of ischemic lesions with distinct behavioral symptomatology, support the vascular depression hypothesis. Patients with late-onset depression and vascular risk factors have greater overall cognitive impairment, psychomotor retardation, and disability than elders with early-onset depression and no vascular risk factors (Alexopoulos et al., 1997). Fluency and naming are most impaired in vascular depression. Patients with vascular depression have more apathy and retardation and less agitation, as well as less guilt and greater lack of insight. Disruption of prefrontal systems or their modulating pathways, by single lesions or by an accumulation of lesions, is hypothesized to be the central mechanism underlying vascular depression. This topic is addressed elsewhere in this volume (Chapters 11, 12, 26).

### Depression-Executive Dysfunction Syndrome

Clinical, structural, and functional neuroimaging, as well as neuropathology studies, suggest that frontostriatal dysfunction contributes to the pathogenesis of at least some late-life depressive syndromes (Alex-opoulos, 2001; Beblo et al., 1999). Based on these findings, the *depression–executive dysfunction* syndrome has been described and conceptualized as an entity with pronounced frontostriatal dysfunction. The syndrome is characterized by psychomotor retardation, reduced interest in activities, impaired instrumental activities of daily living, and limited vegetative symptoms. Emerging evidence suggests that individuals with the depression–executive dysfunction syndrome have a poor and/or slow response to antidepressants (Kalayam and Alexopoulos, 1999), as well as frequent relapses and recurrences (Alexopoulos et al., 2000). There is some evidence that problem-solving therapy (PST) may be effective in patients with depression and executive dysfunction (Alexopoulos et al., 2003). However, the role of PST in preventing relapse and recurrence has not been investigated.

## ASSESSMENT

### Initial Evaluation

The most important symptoms in diagnosing depression in an older patient include a sad, downcast mood, frequent tearfulness, and recurrent thoughts of death and suicide (Alexopoulos et al., 2001). Other symptoms include diminished interest in pleasurable activities, feelings of hopelessness or helplessness, feelings of worthlessness, guilt or self-reproach, avoidance of social interactions or going out, psychomotor agitation or retardation, difficulty making decisions, and difficulty planning daily activities.

Elderly patients are most likely to report physical symptoms such as lack of sleep, energy, appetite, and weight rather than sadness, feelings of guilt, suicidal ideation, or feelings of hopelessness and worthlessness. Depressed elderly patients often have anhedonia rather than sadness. Thus, older depressed patients tend to report more somatic and cognitive symptoms than affective symptoms. The tendency of depressed older adults to report fewer affective symptoms is captured by the concept of *depression without sadness* (Gallo and Rabins, 1999). This variant has been described in elderly primary care populations and consists of apathy, loss of interest, fatigue, trouble sleeping, and other somatic symptoms but not a sad mood.

Given the medical and neurological disorders that often co-exist with late-life depression, the initial evaluation should include a psychiatric history and a mental status examination, a clinical examination of cognitive functions, a medical evaluation, and a focal neurological examination. Laboratory tests should include the thyroid stimulating hormone level, a chem-

### TABLE 3.2. *Drugs Associated with Depression*

| | | |
|---|---|---|
| Steroids | β-Interferon | Calcium channel blockers |
| Beta blockers | Clonidine | α-Methyldopa |
| Reserpine | Prazocin | Tetrabenazine |
| Amantadine | Bromocriptine | Baclofen |
| Metronidazole | Disulfiram | Stimulant withdrawal |

*Source:* Patten and Love (1994).

istry panel, complete blood count, and medication levels when appropriate. Often, electrocardiography and urinalysis are also performed, and serum vitamin $B_{12}$ and folate levels are measured. Although vitamin $B_{12}$ and folate deficiency-related depressions are rare, if identified they can be effectively treated. These recommendations (Alexopoulos et al., 2001) reflect the need to diagnose coexisting medical conditions that may contribute to depression or complicate its treatment.

Depressed elders typically receive multiple medications, some of which may contribute to depression. Chronic use of benzodiazepines is common among elders, who often resist discontinuation or dosage change. Alcohol use, although it declines with aging, may contribute to late-life depression. Patients who continue to use alcohol, substances of abuse, or medications known to cause depression (Table 3.2) frequently have an incomplete response to antidepressants. Moreover, the complicated medication regimens common in the elderly may lead to accidental medication misuse.

The elderly may also be subjected to physical, verbal, or emotional abuse by caregivers or relatives. Depression may both result from and exacerbate the consequences of elder abuse. It is important to evaluate the patient's level of functioning, environmental problems, and losses. The need to assume new functions after widowhood may result in chronic stress contributing to depression.

### Suicide Risk

Severe depression, psychotic depression, recent loss or bereavement, alcoholism, sedative-hypnotic abuse, or development of a disability increases the risk of suicide (Carney et al., 1994; Conwell et al., 1998; Dennis and Lindesay 1995). The majority of elderly suicide victims see their physicians within a few months of their death and over a third within the week of their suicide. Therefore, assessment of suicide risk is a necessary part of the assessment of late-life depression since protective measures and antidepressant treatment may avert suicide.

### Use of Rating Scales

Standardized clinical rating scales can be useful in the initial clinical assessment of depression and in monitoring depressive symptoms over time. Scales can be patient self-reports or interviews by trained staff of patients and/or informants. Different scales have been constructed to address specific clinical issues, such as screening for depression, rating depression severity, symptom profiling, and monitoring change. The choice of scale for an individual in a specific clinical setting requires knowledge of what a scale can and cannot assess.

The most widely used interviewer-rated scales in treatment studies are the Hamilton Depression Rating Scale (Ham-D) and the Montgomery-Asberg Depression Rating Scale (MADRS). The Ham-D was initially validated psychometrically in hospitalized patients (Hamilton, 1960). It is widely used in treatment studies of younger adults and in most of the available geriatric studies, although its psychometric properties have not been well established for elderly populations. Its emphasis on somatic symptoms may lead to higher scores and overestimates of depression severity in medically ill elderly subjects. The MADRS (Montgomery and Asberg, 1979) assesses 10 symptoms of depression and has been shown to be sensitive to change. Both of these assessments require a trained interviewer.

A widely used self-report in geriatric psychiatry is the Geriatric Depression Scale (Yesavage et al., 1983), a symptom inventory with a yes/no format that is available in versions of different length (30 items and 15 items). The Beck Depression Inventory (BDI) is a self-report inventory not specifically designed for administration to elderly subjects, but is widely used and includes a severity rating and a suicide item (Beck and Steer, 1987). The Center for Epidemiological Studies—Depression Scale (Radloff, 1977) has been used as a screen for depression principally in community-based samples (Foelker and Shewchuk, 1992). Other self-reports include The Mood Scales—Elderly (Raskin and Crook, 1988) and the SELFCARE (D) (Bird et al., 1987).

## Distinguishing Depression from Dementia

The assessment of depression in the presence of cognitive impairment is a critical clinical issue. Communication difficulties in patients with severe dementia can force diagnostic decisions to be made on the basis of behavior alone. Moreover, many symptoms of depression overlap with symptoms of dementing disorders, such as, psychomotor slowing, emotional lability, crying spells, insomnia, weight loss, inability to describe mood states, and pessimism (McGuire and Rabins 1994). Nonetheless, depressed Alzheimer's disease patients display more self-pity, rejection sensitivity, and anhedonia and fewer neurovegetative signs than nondemented, depressed older patients (Greenwald et al., 1989). There is a consensus that as the severity of dementia increases, assessment of depressive symptoms directly from the patient becomes less reliable and proxy measures become necessary.

Instruments developed for the quantification of depressive symptomatology in geriatric patients have used one or more of the following approaches:

1. Avoidance of items in areas where the symptoms and signs of depression overlap with those of medical illness (Yesavage et al., 1983) or of dementia (Alexopoulos et al., 1988a, 1988b; Sunderland et al., 1988).
2. Exclusive rating of depressive signs, since symptoms may be unreliably reported by demented-depressed patients (Katona and Aldridge, 1985).
3. Reliance on informants' reports as well as patient evaluation (Alexopoulos et al., 1988a, 1988b).
4. Use of rather long periods of observation.

A limitation of these approaches is that they may fail to identify a significant part of the depressive syndrome, such as disturbances in concentration, guilt, or somatic complaints, and thus may result in erroneously low scores. A second limitation is that the validity of some of these scales may be compromised if unreliable informants are used. It should be emphasized, however, that caregivers as a group appear to be more sensitive than trained raters in identifying depressive symptoms and signs in demented patients (Alexopoulos and Abrams, 1991).

## Distinguishing Medical from Depressive Symptoms

Most older adults have one or more chronic medical illnesses leading to somatic complaints and in some cases contributing to depression. Nonetheless, depressed older patients have a wide range of depressive manifestations rather than just increased somatic complaints or another restricted subset of depressive symptoms (Chemerinski et al., 2001; von Ammon Cavanough, 1986). The existing diagnostic criteria appear applicable even in the presence of specific medical disorders (Paradiso and Robinson 1999). Medical acuity and the complexity of the individual patient may be more of an obstacle to the diagnosis of depression than the inadequacy of the diagnostic system (Goldman et al., 1999). Some depression severity scales can perform reliably in medically ill patients (Borson et al., 1992; Zubenko et al., 1994).

Medical disorders may mimic depression. Apathetic delirium is a rather common condition (Camus et al., 2000). It may present with withdrawal and reduced speech and causes nonspecific dysphoria (Armstrong et al., 1997). Some depressive symptoms are often misattributed to medical illnesses (Hendrie et al., 1995; Knauper and Wittchen, 1994; Mulsant et al., 1994). These include loss of interest, low energy, changes in appetite and sleep, weight loss, or difficulty with concentration (Alexopoulos et al., 1988b; Mulsant et al., 1994; Silverstone, 1991). In elderly community-dwelling persons, internists attributed these symptoms to a physical illness or medication in more than 50%

of patients in whom psychiatrists had identified depressive symptoms (Linden et al., 1995).

Several approaches have been used to identify depressive symptoms in the elderly. The *exclusive approach* does not consider symptoms that can result from medical illnesses in diagnosing depression (e.g., changes in sleep, energy, appetite, and weight). The *substitutive approach* substitutes somatic symptoms with nonsomatic cognitive symptoms (e.g., hopelessness) in the definition of a major depressive episode. The *best-estimate approach* requires a clinical judgment to be made concerning whether each depressive symptom is caused by a physical disorder or is part of a depressive syndrome. Finally, the *inclusive approach* assumes that all depressive symptoms contribute to the syndrome, regardless of their cause (Cohen-Cole and Stoudemire, 1987; Endicott, 1984; Kathol et al., 1990; Mulsant et al., 1994; Rapp and Vrana, 1989).

In a study of cognitively unimpaired elderly medical inpatients, the prevalence of major depression varied from 10% to 20%, depending on the diagnostic approach (Koenig et al., 1997). Similarly, the prevalence of minor depression varied from 14% to 25%. Depressed patients classified with different diagnostic approaches had similar psychological and health characteristics (predictive validity) and similar severity of depression (concurrent validity). The diagnostic approach that best distinguished severe and persistent depression was the exclusive/best-estimate approach. However this approach missed 49% of patients identified with the inclusive approach, of whom 60% continued to experience persistent symptoms of depression many weeks after discharge.

The diagnostic strategy chosen should be based on the specific goals and purposes of the examiner. While the exclusive/best-estimate approach identifies the most severe and persistent depressions, the inclusive approach is the most sensitive and reliable approach and is an intermediate predictor of persistent depression. The inclusive approach to diagnosis may be preferable in settings in which older, medically ill patients may be misdiagnosed, such as primary care settings, general hospitals, or nursing homes (Borson et al., 1992, 1998; Cohen-Cole and Stoudemire, 1987; Endicott, 1984; Kathol et al., 1990; Mulsant et al., 1994; Rapp and Vrana, 1989). Conversely, in specialized clinical services with advanced psychiatric expertise, the contributors to depressive symptoms (e.g. medical causes) need to be considered in order to avoid unnecessary treatment.

## COURSE AND CONSEQUENCES OF LATE-LIFE DEPRESSION

Depression is a relapsing and remitting illness; 50% to 80% of patients who have had one depressive episode can expect a recurrence. The recurrence rate increases with each successive episode. In mixed-age unipolar depressives, 34% of patients have a depressive episode during the year after recovery (Keller et al., 1983, 1984), with the relapse rate being higher during the first 6 months immediately after recovery. The figures for relapse/recurrence in major depression in geriatric patients (Alexopoulos et al., 1989) are comparable to those of mixed-age populations (21% in Keller et al., 1983:4). For the elderly, the time between episodes is shorter, with most relapses and recurrences occurring within 2 years (Georgotas and McCue, 1989; Reynolds et al., 1999a).

In mixed-age populations, a history of three or more previous depressive episodes and late age of depression onset are the strongest predictors of relapse/recurrence (Keller et al., 1983:4). In geriatric populations, most studies suggest that the likelihood of relapse is increased in patients with a history of frequent episodes, intercurrent medical illnesses, and possibly high severity of depression (Alexopoulos et al., 1989; Georgotas and McCue, 1989; Georgotas et al., 1988). Chronic medical illness represents a risk factor for both chronicity and relapse. Disability sets the stage for demoralization and depression and worsens its course (Bruce, 2001). Increases in disability over time predict the emergence of depressive symptoms (Bruce et al., 1994; Kennedy et al., 1990). Being confined to a bed or chair for a 2-week period predicts the first onset of depression (OR: 5.03) after controlling for potential covariates. Further, cerebrovascular disease and neurodegenerative disorders like Alzheimer's disease and Parkinson's disease (Alexopoulos et al., 1996), chronic insomnia (Ford and Kamerow, 1989), multiple personal losses and bereavement (Reynolds et al., 1999b), and progressive depletion of psychosocial resources (Dew et al., 1997) often accompany late-life depression and may contribute to a chronic and/or relapsing course. Finally, patients with prolonged index episodes, those who take longer to respond, and those who have residual symptoms of anxiety are all at high risk for recurrence (Flint and Rifat, 2000).

These observations highlight the importance of keeping patients well following the acute treatment of a depressive episode via continuation and maintenance therapy. The primary goal of continuation therapy is to prevent relapse; the primary goals of maintenance therapy are to prevent recurrence and to prolong recovery.

Once recovery is achieved, continuation treatment should be administered to all patients for at least 6 months with the same dosage of the antidepressant that was used during the acute treatment (Alexopoulos et al., 2001). Failure to provide continuation treatment results in relapse in 30%–35% of cases (Bump et al., 2001).

The indications for and duration of maintenance treatment for late-life depression are less well established than the indication for continuation treatment.

The Expert Consensus Guideline (Alexopoulos et al., 2001) recommends long-term treatment of elderly patients with a history of frequent and/or multiple episodes of major depression, those who have had a major depressive episode plus preexisting dysthymia, those with onset of major depression after the age of 60, those with a long duration of individual episodes, severe index episodes, and poor symptom control during continuation therapy, and those with co-morbid anxiety disorders or substance abuse.

The most conservative approach is to offer longer rather than shorter maintenance treatment, as most frequently used antidepressants (selective serotonin reuptake inhibitors, nonselective reuptake inhibitors) have side effects that do not endanger the health of elderly patients. Avoiding recurrences has clinical advantages. A proportion of patients with recurrence may fail to respond to reinitiation of treatment with the agent that induced remission; 10% of patients with a recurrence of major depression failed to respond to nortriptyline even though their index episodes had remitted with this agent (Reynolds et al., 1994). With each succeeding episode, there appears to be an increased risk of nonresponse and chronicity.

## MEDICAL CO-MORBIDITY

Depression increases mortality in a variety of elderly populations. Epidemiological studies have shown that depression increases the mortality of patient without a significant medical burden (Gurialnik et al., 1991; Philibert et al., 1997). There is evidence that depression increases mortality in hospitalized patients even when the severity of medical illnesses and disability is controlled (Arfken et al., 1999; Covinsky et al., 1999). Depression has been associated with increased mortality in residents of nursing homes and congregate apartments. It has been reported that the presence of major depression on admission to a nursing home increases the likelihood of death by 59% 1 year later (Rovner, 1993) the effect of depression on mortality was independent of other medical health parameters.

Depression may increase medical morbidity. Depressive symptoms, especially chronic symptoms, are associated with more medical morbidity than other psychiatric disorders of late life. In older community residents, long-term, but not short-term, depressive symptoms had an adverse impact on health (Meeks et al., 2000). In contrast, the medical burden contributed only to short-lived depressive symptoms. In elderly medical inpatients, those with six depressive symptoms had greater co-morbid illness, cognitive impairment, and functional impairment.

Depression may adversely affect the prognosis of individuals with co-morbid disease, as suggested by evidence of prolonged recovery from illness, long hospital stays, increased medical complications, and earlier mortality in depressed patients (Koenig et al., 1997). Increased mortality risk has been reported in depressed compared to nondepressed medical (Frasure-Smith et al., 1993, 1995) and psychiatric patients (Lyness et al., 1993). Depression after surgery has been associated with poorer recovery of both functional and psychosocial status. Among patients hospitalized after hip fractures, those with chronic or acute cognitive and depressive symptoms had poorer functional recovery 1 year after discharge than those who did not (Magaziner et al., 1990). Depressed medical patients report a reduced health-related quality of life and increased medical costs (Creed et al., 2002). Depressed medical patients stay in bed more days than do patients with chronic diseases such as chronic lung disease, diabetes, arthritis, and hypertension (Callahan and Wolinsky, 1995; Unutzer et al., 1996, 1997).

Depression increases the perception of poor health and use of medical services. Depressed primary care patients had almost twice as many medical appointments per year as nondepressed patients (5.3 vs. 2.9: Luber et al., 2001). Depressed patients had more than twice as many hospital days over the expected length of stay as nondepressed patients (Callahan et al., 1994). Finally, 65% of depressed patients received more than five medications compared to 35.6% of nondepressed patients (Luber et al., 2001).

## COGNITIVE IMPAIRMENT DISORDERS

Depression is often a prodrome to dementing disorders. Individuals with late-life depression and dementia that subsides after remission of depression (pseudodementia) frequently develop dementia within a few years after the onset of depression (Alexopoulos et al., 1993). A history of depression is associated with an increased incidence of Alzheimer's disease. Depressive symptoms are associated with poorer cognitive function at baseline and with cognitive decline during follow-up (Bassuk et al., 1998). Depressive symptoms are common in elderly individuals who later develop dementia (Devanand et al., 1996; Geerling et al., 2000). Patients with Alzheimer's dementia showed reduced perfusion when studied by perfusion single photon emission computed tomography (SPECT) imaging in the left temporoparietal cortex (Ebmeier et al., 1997). In these regions of interest, patients with late-onset depression tended to have perfusion values intermediate between those of patients with early-onset depression and demented patients (Ebmeier et al., 1997). Among elderly individuals with subclinical cognitive dysfunction, those who developed dementia 3 years later had more depressive symptoms (Ritchie et al., 1999) as subjects were progressing to dementia, they exhibited fewer affective symptoms and more agitation and psychomotor slowing. These changes paralleled reduction of cerebral blood flow in the left temporal region.

A lifetime history of depression may increase the risk of Alzheimer's disease, regardless of the presence or absence of a family history of dementing disorders. In elderly twins, depression was one of the risk factors for development of dementia, regardless of the presence or absence of an ApoE4 allele (Steffens et al., 1997). Depressive symptoms and diagnoses were found to be associated with cognitive decline and a high risk of Alzheimer's disease (Devanand et al., 1996). In a meta-analytic study, a history of depression was associated with the onset of Alzheimer's disease after the age of 70 years only when depressive symptoms had appeared within 10 years before the onset of dementia (Zubenko, 2000). However, depression with onset more than 10 years before the diagnosis of dementia was associated with the onset of Alzheimer's disease at any age, suggesting that previous depression can sometimes represent a risk factor in some patients and a prodromal expression of dementing illness in others (Zubenko et al., 1996).

## DISABILITY

The World Health Organization defines *functional disability* as problems with self-care, household activities, getting around, understanding and communicating, getting along with others, and participating in society (Murray and Lopez, 1996). While disability has a reciprocal relationship with psychiatric and medical disorders, it constitutes a distinct functional dimension of health status (Ferrucci et al., 1991). Disability compromises the quality of life and has various negative outcomes such as a high rate of hospital admissions, nursing home placement, mortality, and even morbidity for specific medical conditions.

The Global Burden of Disease Initiative identified unipolar depression as the leading cause of disability worldwide (Murray and Lopez, 1996). Depression accounts for 10.7% of disability and is responsible for more than 1 in 10 years lived with disability. Depression ranked among the strongest contributors to disability in a review of 78 studies of community-residing elders. In a 12-year follow-up study, individuals with major depression at baseline were four times more likely to report incident disability after controlling for medical illness (Bruce et al., 1994). Depression may lead to disability in medically healthy elderly individuals directly and by contributing to and increasing the impact of the medical burden (Bruce, 2001). Moreover, disability resulting from medical or neurological illnesses has been found to be a risk factor for depressive

disorders in late life. Therefore, depression and disability interact with each other in a variety of ways with potentially detrimental consequences.

The course of disability parallels the course of depression. In community-residing individuals, residual depressive symptoms covary with disability over time (Lenze et al., 2001). Reduction in the level of depression was shown to result in an approximately 50% reduction in disability days 1 year later. In patients with chronic obstructive pulmonary disease, nortriptyline was superior to placebo in improving both depression and day-to-day function, although it did not influence the physiological measures of pulmonary insufficiency (Borson et al., 1992).

Several studies have examined the relationship of specific clinical characteristics of depressed elderly patients to disability. In elderly populations, disability often has been classified as impairment in self-maintenance functions (ability to eat, dress, groom, bathe, use the toilet, and ambulate) and impairment in instrumental activities of daily living (IADLs), including the ability to go to places beyond walking distance, shop for groceries, prepare meals, do housework, launder clothes, use the telephone, take medications, and manage money.

Self-maintenance is predicted by different demographic and clinical factors than IADLs in depressed elderly patients (Spector et al., 1987). Among older depressed adults, impairment in self-maintenance competence is associated with increasing age, more severe chronic medical illness, psychomotor retardation, and lower subjective social support, while depressed mood had a lower impact (Steffens et al., 1999).

Clinical findings ascertained during a comprehensive clinical examination of depressed elderly patients—that is, severity of depression, cognitive impairment, medical burden—appear to predict approximately 40% of the variance in IADLs. Unlike self-maintenance skills, IADLs are significantly influenced by depressive symptoms and signs (Bruce, 2001). Specific depressive symptoms can contribute uniquely to IADL impairment (Lawton and Brody, 1969). In depressed elderly psychiatric patients, IADL impairment was found to be associated with high severity of depression and more specifically with anxiety, depressive ideation, apathy, psychomotor retardation, and weight loss but with less pathological guilt (Alexopoulos et al., 1996). Similar findings have been reported in community-residing elders, in whom IADL impairment was associated with dysphoria, sleep disturbance, appetite disturbance, feelings of guilt, death wishes and suicidal thoughts, loss of interest, concentration difficulties, psychomotor change, and loss of energy (Forsell et al., 1994; Ormel et al., 2002).

Executive dysfunction is strongly related to IADL impairment in depressed elderly patients (Kiosses et al., 2000). A similar association between executive dysfunction and disability was reported in nondepressed patients with Alzheimer's disease of mild to moderate severity. Since both geriatric depression and executive dysfunction often occur in patients with frontostriatal impairment, these observations raise the question of whether disability is an early indicator of impairment of the frontal and prefrontal areas.

## SUICIDE

Suicide is more frequent in elderly individuals than in any other population (Hoyert et al., 1999). Depression is the most common psychiatric diagnosis in elderly suicide victims, unlike younger adults, in whom substance abuse alone or with co-morbid mood disorders is the most frequent diagnosis. Major depression was identified in 80% of suicide victims older than 74 years of age, while its frequency ranged from 3.1% to 29.4% in younger victims (Conwell et al., 1996). These findings indicate that depression is the psychiatric disorder most likely to increase the risk of successful suicide in the elderly. Despite the high frequency of suicide in late life, suicidal attempts and suicidal ideation decrease with aging. Older adults commit more carefully planned and lethal self-destructive acts and give fewer indications of suicidal intent. Therefore, while suicide attempts are more rare in old than young age, their lethality is increased.

## BARRIERS TO EFFECTIVE RECOGNITION AND TREATMENT OF GERIATRIC UNIPOLAR DEPRESSION

Depression in older adults not only causes distress and suffering but also leads to impairments in physical, mental, and social functioning. Despite being associated with excess morbidity and mortality, depression often goes undiagnosed and untreated (NIH, 1992; USDHHS, 1999; Young et al., 2001). A substantial proportion of older patients receive no treatment or inadequate treatment in primary care settings (Lebowitz et al., 1997; Unutzer et al., 1997) or psychiatric settings (Sirey et al., 1999). Barriers to translating our advances in the identification, characterization, and treatment of geriatric depression exist at the patient level, the provider level, the health-care system level, and the societal level.

Depressed elderly patients often misattribute symptoms of depression to aging or medical illness (Gallo et al., 1994). It is often misattribution shared by patients, families, and providers that reduces the chances for effective treatment. Psychosocial antecedents such as loss, combined with decrements in physical health and sensory impairment, can also divert attention from clinical depression. Being poor or old significantly decreases

the likelihood of receiving treatment for depression (Brown et al., 1995). Men are less likely to report mood-related symptoms than women (Brown et al., 1995), and primary care physicians are less able to recognize depression in men than in women (Potts et al., 1991). Depression can and frequently does amplify physical symptoms, distracting attention from the underlying depression. Elderly patients may attach a stigma to depression, disagree with physicians when informed of their diagnosis, and be concerned about the impression they make on their families (Sirey et al., 2001). They often fear that antidepressants will be addictive or interfere with treatment of their medical disorders (Goldman, 1997). These attitudes lead to underreporting of depressive complaints.

At the provider level, inadequate awareness and skills contribute to underrecognition of depression (Shah and Harris, 1997). In a study of primary care physicians, only 55% of internists felt confident in diagnosing depression, and only 35% felt confident in prescribing antidepressants to older persons (Callahan et al., 1992). Coexisting medical disorders often make physicians focus on medical causes and disregard depression. Symptom overlap of depression and dementia adds to diagnostic difficulties (Rabins, 1996). Clinicians may not recognize that patients with coexisting depression and dementia can benefit from treatment of depression. Physicians may disregard depression when the patient has reasons to be depressed (Cole and Bellavance, 1997). Cognitive decline, both normal and pathological, may interfere with the reporting of depressive symptoms. The time required for interviewing and offering treatment interventions to a depressed patient competes with the treatment of other medical disorders during a short visit (Glasser and Gravdal, 1997).

At the health-care system level, limited availability of mental health services and inadequate reimbursement are barriers to care. Appropriate reimbursement for counseling, availability of support staff, and training in mental health are critical for improving the care of depressed patients (Glasser and Gravdal, 1997). Primary care providers are four times more likely to report difficulties in making a mental health referral for their patients than making a referral for other specialty services (Center for Studying Health Systems Change, 1997). Moreover, there are clear limits to the distance that patients are willing to travel in order to receive mental health care (Marcus et al., 1997). In many health plans, mental health is *carved out* and introduces fragmentation of care that elderly patients cannot deal with easily (NIH, 1992; Unutzer et al. 1999). Medicare continues to require a 50% copayment for most outpatient mental health services compared to 20% for medical services. This policy discourages patients and physicians from using mental health services (Unutzer et al., 1999).

Finally, stereotypes about normal aging make the diagnosis and treatment of geriatric depression more difficult. Many patients and their families may believe that depression and hopelessness are natural conditions of older age, especially with prolonged bereavement (Bartels et al., 1997). The underdiagnosis and undertreatment of geriatric depression and other psychiatric disorders in the elderly represent a serious public health problem (USDHHS, 1999).

REFERENCES

Alexopoulos, G.S. (1996) Geriatric depression in primary care. *Int J Geriatr Psychiatry* 11:397–400.

Alexopoulos, G.S. (2001) The depression-executive dysfunction syndrome of late life: A target for D3 receptor agonists. *Am J Geriatr Psychiatry* 9:1–8.

Alexopoulos, G.S., and Abrams, R.C. (1991) Depression in Alzheimer's disease. *Psychiatr Clin North Am* 14:327–340.

Alexopoulos, G.S., Abrams, R.C., Young, R.C., et al. (1988a) Cornell scale for depression in dementia. Biol Psychiatry 23:271–284.

Alexopoulos, G.S., Abrams, R.C., Young, R.C., et al. (1988b) Use of the Cornell scale in nondemented patients. *J Am Geriatr Soc* 36:230–236.

Alexopoulos, G.S., Bruce, M.L., Hull, J., and Kakuma, T. (1999) Clinical determinants of suicidal ideation and behavior in geriatric depression. *Arch Gen Psychiatry* 56:1048–1053.

Alexopoulos, G.S., and Chester, J.G. (1992) Outcomes of geriatric depression. *Clin Geriatr Med* 8:363–376.

Alexopoulos, G.S., Katz, I.R., Reynolds, C.F., Carpenter, D., and Docherty, J.P. (2001, October) The Expert Consensus Guideline Series. Pharmacotherapy of Geriatric Depression. *Postgrad Med* (Special Report).

Alexopoulos, G.S., Meyers, B.S., Young, R.C., Campbell, S., Silberswig, D., and Charlson, M. (1997) The "vascular depression" hypothesis. *Arch Gen Psychiatry* 54:915–922.

Alexopoulos, G.S., Meyers, B.S., Young, R.C., Hull, J., Sirey, J.A., and Kakuma, T. (2000) Executive dysfunction and risk for relapse and recurrence of geriatric depression. *Arch Gen Psychiatry* 57:285–290.

Alexopoulos, G.S., Meyers, B.S., Young, R.C., Matiis, S., and Kakuma, T. (1993) The course of geriatric depression with "reversible dementia": A controlled study. *Am J Psychiatry* 150:1693–1699.

Alexopoulos, G.S., Raue, P., and Arean, P. (2003) Problem solving therapy versus supportive psychotherapy in geriatric major depression with executive dysfunction. *Am J Geriatr Psychiatry* 11:46–52.

Alexopoulos, G.S., Vrontou, C., Kakuma, T., Meyers, B.S., Young, R.C., Klausner, E., and Clarkin, J. (1996) Disability in geriatric depression. *Am J Psychiatry* 153:877–885.

Alexopoulos, G.S., Young, R.C., Abrams, R.C., Meyers, B., and Shamoian, C.A. (1989) Chronicity and relapse in geriatric depression. *Biol Psychiatry* 26:551–564.

American Psychiatric Association. (2000) *Diagnostic and Statistical Manual of Mental Disorders, Fourth Edition, Text Revision.* Washington, DC: American Psychiatric Association.

Arfken, C.L., Lichtenberg, P.A., and Tancer, M.E. (1999) Cognitive impairment and depression predict mortality in medically ill older adults. *J Gerontol A Biol Sci Med Sci* 54:152–156.

Armstrong, S.C., Cozza, K.L., and Watanabe, K.S. (1997) The misdiagnosis of delirium. *Psychosomatics* 38(5):433–439.

Baldwin, R.C., and Tomenson, B. (1995) Depression in later life. A comparison of symptoms and risk factors in early and late onset cases. *Br J Psychiatry* 167:649–652.

Baldwin, R.C., Walker, S., Simpson, S.W., et al. (2000) The prognostic significance of abnormalities seen on magnetic resonance imaging in late-life depression. *Int J Geriatr Psychiatry* 15:1097–1104.

Bartels, S.J., Horn, S., Sharkey, P., and Levine, K. (1997) Treatment of depression in older primary care patients in Health Maintenance Organizations. *Int J Psychiatry Med* 3:215–231.

Bassuk, S.S., Berkman, L.F., and Wypiy, D. (1998) Depressive symptomatology and incident cognitive decline in an elderly community sample. *Arch Gen Psychiatry* 55:1073–1081.

Baumgarten, M., Bartista, R., Infante-Rivard, C., et al. (1992) The psychological and physical health of family members caring for an elderly person with dementia. *J Clin Epidemiol* 45:61–70.

Beblo, T., Wallesch, C.W., and Herrmann, M. (1999) The crucial role of frontostriatal circuits for depressive disorders in the postacute stage after stroke. *Neuropsychiatry, Neuropsychol Behav Neurol* 12(4):236–246.

Beck, A.T., and Steer, R. (1987) *The Beck Depression Inventory Manual.* San Antonio: Psychological Corporation, Harcourt Brace Jovanovich.

Bird, A.S., MacDonald, A.J.D., Mann, A.H., and Philpot, M.P. (1987) Preliminary experience with the SELFCARE (D): A self-rating depression questionnaire for use in elderly, non-institutionalized subjects. *Int J Geriatr Psychiatry* 2:31–38.

Blazer, D.G. (1994) Depression in the elderly. *Hosp Pract* 29:37–41.

Boone, K.B., Lesser, I.M., Miller, B.L., et al. (1995) Cognitive functioning in older depressed outpatients: Relationship of presence and severity of depression to neuropsychological test scores. *Neuropsychology* 9:390–398.

Borson, S., Claypoole, K., and McDonald, G.J. (1998) Depression and chronic obstructive pulmonary disease: Treatment trials. *Semin Clin Neuropsychiatry* 3(2):151–130.

Borson, S., McDonald, G.J., Gayle, T., et al. (1992) Improvement in mood, physical symptoms, and function with nortriptyline for depression in patients with chronic obstructive pulmonary disease. *Psychosomatics* 33:190–201.

Brown, S.L., Salive, M.E., Guralnik, J.M., Pahor, M., Chapman, D.P., and Blazer, D. (1995) Antidepressant use in the elderly: Association with demographic characteristics, health related factors, and health care utilization. *J Clin Epidemiol* 48:445–452.

Bruce, M.L. (2001) Depression and disability in late life. *Am J Geriatr Psychiatry* 9:102–112.

Bruce, M.L., Seeman, T.E., Merrill, S.S., et al. (1994) The impact of depressive symptomatology on physical disability: MacArthur Studies of Successful Aging. *Am J Public Health* 84:1796–1799.

Bump, G.M., Mulsant, B.H., Pollack, B.G., et al. (2001) Paroxetine versus nortriptyline in the continuation and maintenance treatment of depression in the elderly. *Depress Anxiety* 13:38–44.

Callahan, C.M., Hui, S.L., Nienaber, N.A., et al. (1994) Longitudinal study of depression and health services use among elderly primary care patients. *J Am Geriatr Soc* 42:833–838.

Callahan, C.M., Nienaber, N.A., Hendrie, H.C., et al. (1992) Depression of elderly outpatients: Primary care physicians' attitudes and practice patterns. *J Gen Int Med* 7:26–31.

Callahan, C.M., and Wolinsky, F.D. (1995) Hospitalization for major depression among older Americans. *J Gerontol Ser A, Biol Sci Med Sci* 50:M196–M202.

Camus, V., Gonthier, R., Dubos, G., Schwed, P., and Simeone, I. (2000) Etiologic and outcome profiles in hypoactive and hyperactive subtypes of delirium. *J Geriatr Psychiatry Neurol* 13(1):38–42.

Carney, S.S., Rich, C.L., Burke, P.A., and Fowler, R.C. (1994) Suicide over 60: The San Diego Study. *JAGS* 42:174–180.

Center for Studying Health System Change (1997, Fall) *Newsletter.* Washington, DC.

Chemerinski, E., Petracca, G., Sabe, L., Kremer, J., and Starkstein, S.E. (2000) The specificity of depressive symptoms in patients with Alzheimer's disease. *Am J Psychiatry* 158(1):68–72.

Cohen-Cole, S.A., and Stoudemire, A. (1987) Major depression and physical illness. *Psychiatr Clin North Am* 10:1–17.

Cole, M.G., and Bellavance, F. (1997) Depression in elderly medical inpatients: A meta-analysis of outcomes. *CMAJ* 157:1055–1060.

Conwell, Y., Ouberstein, P.R., Cox, C., Herrmann, J., Forbes, N.T., and Caine, E.D. (1996) Relationships of age and axis I diagnoses in victims of completed suicide: a psychological autopsy study. *Am J Psychiatry* 153:1001–1008.

Conwell, Y., Duberstein, P.R., Herrmann, J., Forbes, N., and Caine, E.D. (1998) Age differences in behaviors leading to completed suicide. *Am J Geriatr Psychiatry* 6:122–126.

Covinsky, K.E., Kahana, E., Chin, M.H., Palmer, R.M., Fortinsky, R.H., and Landefeld, C.S. (1999) Depressive symptoms and 3-year mortality in older hospitalized medical patients. *Ann Intern Med* 130:563–569.

Coyne, J., Thompson, R., Palmer, S., et al. (2000) Should we screen for depression? Caveats and potential pitfalls. *Appl Prev Psychol* 9:101–121.

Creed, F., Morgan, R., Fiddler, M., et al. (2002) Depression and anxiety impair health-related quality of life and are associated with increased costs in general medical inpatients. *Psychosomatics* 43:302–309.

Dennis, M.S., and Lindesay, J. (1995) Suicide in the elderly: The United Kingdom perspective. *Int Psychogeriatr* 7:263–274.

Devanand, D.P., Sano, M., Tang, M.X., et al. (1996) Depressed mood and the incidence of Alzheimer's disease in the elderly living in the community. *Arch Gen Psychiatry* 53:175–182.

Dew, M.A., Reynolds, C.F., III, Houck, P.R., et al. (1997) Temporal profiles of the course of depression during treatment. Predictors of pathways toward recovery in the elderly. *Arch Gen Psychiatry* 54:1016–1024.

DiMatteo, M.R., Lepper, H.S., and Croghan, T.W. (2000) Depression is a risk factor for non-compliance with medical treatment. Meta-analysis of the effects of anxiety and depression on patient adherence. *Arch Intern Med* 160:2101–2107.

Ebmeier, K.P., Prentice, N., and Ryman, A., et al. (1997) Temporal lobe abnormalities in dementia and depression. *J Neurol Neurosurg Psychiatry* 63:597–604.

Endicott, J. (1984) Measurement of depression in patients with cancer. *Cancer* 53:2243–2249.

Ferrucci, L., Guralnik, J.M., Baroni, A., Tesi, G., Antonini, E., and Marchionni, N. (1991) Value of combined assessment of physical health and functional status in community-dwelling aged: A prospective study in Florence, Italy. *J Gerontol* 46:M52–M56.

Flint, A.J., and Rifat, S.L. (2000) Maintenance treatment for recurrent depression in late life. A four-year outcome study. *Am J Geriatr Psychiatry* 8:112–116.

Foelker, G.A., and Shewchuk, R.M. (1992) Somatic complaints and the CES-D. *J Am Geriatr Soc* 40:259–262.

Ford, D.E., and Kamerow, D.B. (1989) Epidemiologic study of sleep disturbances in the elderly. *Am J Psychiatry* 262:1479–1484.

Forsell, Y., Jorm, A.F., and Winblad, B. (1994) Association of age, sex, cognitive dysfunction, and disability with major depressive symptoms in an elderly sample. *Am J Psychiatry* 151:1600–1604.

Frasure-Smith, N., Lesperance, F., and Talajic, M. (1993) Depression following myocardial infarction. Impact on 6-month survival. *JAMA* 270:1819–1825.

Frasure-Smith, N., Lesperance, F., and Talajic, M. (1995) Depression and 18-month prognosis after myocardial infarction. *Circulation* 91:999–1005.

Gallo, J.J., Anthony, J.C., and Muthen, B.O. (1994) Age differences in the symptoms of depression: A latent trait analysis. *J Gerontol* 49:251–264.

Gallo, J.J., and Rabins, P.V. (1999) Depression without sadness: Alternative presentations of depression in late life. *Am Fam Physician* 60(3):820–826.

Geerling, M., Schoevers, R.A., Beekman, A.T., Jonker, C., Deer, D.J.,

Schmand, B., Ader, H.J., Bouter, L.M., and van Tilburg, W. (2000) Depression and risk of cognitive decline and Alzheimer's disease. Results of two prospective studies. *Br J Psychiatry* 176:568–575.

Georgotas, A., and McCue, R.E. (1989) Relapse of depressed patients after effective continuation therapy. *J Affect Disord* 17:159–164.

Georgotas, A., McCue, R.E., Cooper, T.B., et al. (1988) How effective and safe is continuation therapy in elderly depressed patients? Factors affecting relapse rate. *Arch Gen Psychiatry* 45:929–932.

Gill, D., and Hatcher, S. (2000) Antidepressants for depression in medical illness. *Cochrane Database Syst Rev* (4):CD001312.

Glasser, M., and Gravdal, J.A. (1997) Assessment and treatment of geriatric depression in primary care settings. *Arch Fam Med* 6:433–438.

Goldman, L.S. (1997) Psychiatry in primary care: Possible roles for organized medicine. *Psychiatr Ann* 27:1–5.

Goldman, L.S., Nielsen, N.H., and Champion, H.C. (1999) Awareness, diagnosis, and treatment of depression. *J Gen Intern Med* 14:569–580.

Greenwald, B.S., Kramer-Ginsberg, E., Krishnan, R.R., et al. (1996) MRI signal hyperintensities in late-life depression. *Am J Psychiatry* 53:1212–1215.

Greenwald, B.S., Kramer-Ginsberg, E., Marin, D.B., et al. (1989) Dementia with coexistent major depression. *Am J Psychiatry* 146:1472–1478.

Gurialnik, J.M., LaCroix, A.Z., Branch, L.G., Kasl, S.V., and Wallace, R.B. (1991) Morbidity and disability in older persons in the years prior to death. *Am J Public Health* 82:443–447.

Gurland, B.J., Cross, P.S., and Katz, S. (1996) Epidemiological perspectives on opportunities for treatment of depression. *Am J Geriatr Psychiatry* 4(Suppl 1):S7–S13.

Hamilton, M. (1960) A rating scale for depression. *J Neurol Neurosurg Psychiatry* 23:56–62.

Hendrie, H.C., Callahan, C.M., Levitt, E.E., et al. (1995) Prevalence rates of major depressive disorders: The effects of varying the diagnostic criteria in an older primary care population. *Am J Geriatr Psychiatry* 3:119–131.

Heun, R., Papassotiropoulos, A., Jessen, F., et al. (2001) A family study of Alzheimer's disease and early- and late-onset depression in elderly patients. *Arch Gen Psychiatry* 58:190–196.

Hoyert, D.L., Kochanek, K.D., Murphy, S.L. (1999) Deaths: Final data for 1997. *National Vital Statistics Reports* 47. Hyattsville, MD: National Center for Health Statistics.

Jorm, A.F. (2000) Is depression a risk factor for dementia or cognitive decline? A review. *Gerontology* 46:219–227.

Kalayam, B., and Alexopoulos, G. (1999) Prefrontal dysfunction and treatment response in geriatric depression. *Arch Gen Psychiatry* 56:713–718.

Kathol, R.G., Mutgi, A., Williams, J., et al. (1990) Diagnosis of major depression in cancer patients according to four sets of criteria. *Am J Psychiatry* 147:1021–1024.

Katona, C.L.E., and Aldridge, C.R. (1985) The dexamethasone suppression test and depressive signs in dementia. *J Affect Disord* 8:83–89.

Keller, M.B., Klerman, G.L., Lavori, P.W., Coryell, W., Endicott, J., and Taylor, J. (1984) Long-term outcome of episodes of major depression. *JAMA* 252:788–792.

Keller, M.B., Lavori, P.W., Lewis, C.E., and Klerman, G.L. (1983) Predictors of relapse in major depressive disorder. *JAMA* 250:3299–3304.

Kennedy, G.J., Kelman, H.R., and Thomas, C. (1990) The emergence of depressive symptoms in late life: The importance of declining health and increasing disability. *J Community Health* 15:93–104.

Kiosses, D.N., Klimstra, S., and Murphy, C. (2001) Executive dysfunction and disability in elderly patients with major depression. *Am J Geriatr Psychiatry* 9:269–274.

Knauper, B., and Wittchen, H.U. (1994) Diagnosing major depression in the elderly: Evidence for response bias in standardized diagnostic interviews? *J Psychiatr Res* 28:147–164.

Koenig, H.G., George, L.K., Peterson, B.L., and Pieper, C.F. (1997) Depression in medically ill hospitalized older adults: Prevalence, characteristics, and course of symptoms according to six diagnostic schemes. *Am J Psychiatry* 154:1376–1383.

Kral, V.A., and Emery, V.O.B. (1989) Long term follow-up of depressive pseudodementia of the aged. *Can J Psychiatry* 34:445–447.

Krishnan, K.R.R., Hays, J.C., and Blazer, D.G. (1997) MRI-defined vascular depression. *Am J Psychiatry* 154:497–500.

Kukull, W.A., Koepsell, T.D., Inui, T.S., et al. (1986) Depression and physical illness among elderly general medical clinic patients. *J Affect Disord* 10:153–162.

Lawton, M.P., and Brody, E.M. (1969) Assessment of older people: Self-maintaining and instrumental activities of daily living. *Gerontologist* 9:179–186.

Lebowtiz, B.D., Pearson, J.L., Schneider, L.S., Reynolds, C.F., III, et al. (1997) Diagnosis and treatment of depression in late life. Consensus statement update. *JAMA* 278:1186–1190.

Lenze, E.J., Rogers, J.C., Martire, L.M., Mulsant, B.H., Rollman, B.L., Dew, M.A., Schulz, R., and Reynolds, C.F. (2001) The association of late-life depression and anxiety with physical disability: A review of the literature and prospectus for future research. *Am J Geriatr Psychiatry* 9:113–135.

Linden, M., Borcheil, M., Barnow, S., and Geiselmann, B. (1995) The impact of somatic morbidity on the Hamilton Depression Rating Scale in the very old. *Acta Psychiatr Scand* 92:150–154.

Linjakumpu, T., Hartikainen, S., Klaukka, T., et al. (2002) Psychotropics among the home-dwelling elderly. *Int J Geriatr Psychiatry* 9:874–883.

Lockwood, K.A., Alexopoulos, G.S., and van Gorp, W.G. (2002) Executive dysfunction in geriatric depression. *Am J Psychiatry* 159:1119–1126.

Luber, M.P., Meyers, B.S., Williams-Russo, P.G., et al. (2001) Depression and service utilization in elderly primary care patients. *Am J Geriatr Psychiatry* 9:169–176.

Lyness, J.M., Caine, E.D., Conwell, Y., et al. (1993a) Depressive symptoms, medical illness, and functional status in depressed psychiatric inpatients. *Am J Psychiatry* 50:910–915.

Magaziner, J., Simonsick, E.M., Kashner, T.M., et al. (1990) Predictors of functional recovery one year following hospital discharge for hip fracture: A prospective study. *J Gerontol* 45:M101–M107.

Manton, K.G. (1988) A longitudinal study of functional change and mortality in the United States. *J Gerontol* 43:S153–S161.

Marcus, S.C., Fortney, J.C., Olfson, M., and Ryan, N.E. (1997) Travel distance to outpatient treatment for depression. *Psychiatr Services* 48:1005.

McGuire MH, and Rabins PV (1994) Mood disorders, In: Coffey, C.E., and Cummings, J.L., eds. *Textbook of Geriatric Neuropsychiatry*. Washington, DC: American Psychiatric Press, pp. 246–260.

Meeks, S., Murrell, S.A., and Mehl, R.C. (2000) Longitudinal relationship between depressive symptoms and health in normal older and middle-aged adults. *Psychol Aging* 15:100–109.

Mendlewicz, J., and Baron, M. (1981) Morbidity risks in subtypes of unipolar depressive illness: Differences between early and late onset forms. *Br J Psychiatry* 139:464–466.

Montgomery, S.A., and Asberg, M. (1979) A new depression scale designed to be sensitivie to change. *Br J Psychiatry* 134:383–389.

Mulsant, B.H., and Ganguli, M. (1999) Epidemiology and diagnosis of depression in late-life. *J Clin Psychiatry* 60(suppl 20):9–15.

Mulsant, B.H., Ganguli, M., and Seaberg, E.C. (1997) The relationship between self-rated health and depressive symptoms in an epidemiological sample of community-dwelling older adults. *J Am Geriatr Soc* 45:954–958.

Mulsant, B.H., Sweet, R.A., Rifai, A.H., et al. (1994) The use of the Hamilton rating scale for depression in elderly patients with cognitive impairment and physical illness. *Am J Geriatr Psychiatry* 2:220–229.

Murray, C.J.L., and Lopez, A.D., eds. (1996) *The Global Burden of Disease*. Cambridge, MA: Harvard University Press.

National Institutes of Health. (1992) NIH Consensus Conference. Diagnosis and Treatment of Depression in Late Life. *JAMA* 268:1018–1024.

Newman, A.B., Enrigt, P.L., Manolio, T.A., Haponik, E., and Wahl, P.W. (1997) Sleep disturbance, psychosocial correlates, and cardiovascular disease in 5201 older adults. *J Am Geriatr Soc* 45:1–7.

Ormel, J., Rijsdijk, F.V., Sullivan, M., et al. (2002) Temporal and reciprocal relationship between IADL/ADL disability and depressive symptoms in late life. *J Gerontol B Psychol Sci Soc Sci* 57:P338–P347.

Paradiso, S., and Robinson, R.G. (1999) Minor depression after stroke: An initial validation of the DSM-IV construct. *Am J Geriatr Psychiatry* 7(3):244–251.

Parmelee, P.A., Katz, I.R., and Lawton, M.P. (1989) Depression among institutionalized aged: Assessment and prevalence estimation. *J Gerontol* 44:22–29.

Patten, S.B., and Love, E.J. (1994) Drug-induced depression. Incidence, avoidance and management. *Drug Saf* 10(3):203–219.

Philibert, P.A., Richards, L., Lynch, C.F., and Winokur, G. (1997) The effect of gender and age at onset of depression on mortality. *J Clin Psychiatry* 58:355–360.

Potts, M., Burnam, M., and Wells, K.B. (1991) Gender differences in depression detection: A comparison of clinical diagnosis and standardized assessment. *Psychol Assess* 3:609–615.

Rabins, P. (1996) Barriers to diagnosis and treatment of depression in elderly patients. *Am J Geriatr Psychiatry* 4(4):79–84.

Radloff, L. (1977) The CES-D Scale: A self-report depression scale for research in the general population. *Appl Psychol Measure* 1:385–401.

Rapp, S.R., and Vrana, S. (1989) Substituting nonsomatic for somatic symptoms in the diagnosis of depression in elderly male medical patients. *Am J Psychiatry* 146:1197–1200.

Raskin, A., and Crook, T. (1988) Mood Scales—Elderly (MS-E). *Psychopharmacol Bull* 24:727–732.

Reynolds, C.F., III, Frank, E., Dew, M.A., et al. (1999a) Treatment of 70(+)-year-olds with recurrent major depression. Excellent short-term but brittle long-term response. *Am J Geriatr Psychiatry* 7:64–69.

Reynolds, C.F., III, Frank, E., Perel, J.M., Miller, M.D., Cornes, C., et al. (1994) Treatment of consecutive episodes of major depression in the elderly. *Am J Psychiatry* 151:1740–1743.

Reynolds, C.F., III, Miller, M.D., Pasternak, R.E., et al. (1999b) Treatment of bereavement-related major depressive episodes in later life: A controlled study of acute and continuation treatment with nortriptyline and interpersonal psychotherapy. *Am J Psychiatry* 156:202–208.

Ritchie, K., Gilham, C., Ledesert, B., Touchon, J., and Kotzki, P.O. (1999) Depressive illness, depressive symptomatology and regional cerebral blood flow in elderly people with sub-clinical cognitive impairment. *Age Ageing* 28:385–391.

Rovner, B.W. (1993) Depression and increased risk of mortality in the nursing home patient. *Am J Med* 94:19S–22S.

Rovner, B.W., and Ganguli, M. (1998) Depression and disability associated with impaired vision: The MoVies Project. *J Am Geriatr Soc* 46(5):617–619.

Salloway, S., Malloy, P., Kohn, R., Gillard, E., et al. (1996) MRI and neuropsychological differences in early- and late-life-onset geriatric depression. *Neurology* 46:1567–1574.

Schulberg, H.C., Mulsant, B.H., Schulz, R., Rollman, B.L., Houck, P.R., and Reynolds, C.F. (1998) Characteristics and course of major depression in older primary care patients. *Int J Psychiatr Med* 28(4):421–436.

Shah, S., and Harris, M. (1997) A survey of general practitioners' confidence in their management of elderly patients. *Aust Fam Physician* 26(suppl 1):S12–S17.

Silverstone, P.H. (1991) Measuring depression in the physically ill. *Int J Methods Psychiatr Res* 1:3–12.

Sirey, J.A., Bruce, M.L., Alexopoulos, G.S., et al. (2001) Perceived stigma as a predictor of treatment discontinuation in young and older outpatients with depression. *Am J Psychiatry* 158(3):479–481.

Sirey, J.A., Meyers, B.S., Bruce, M.L., Alexopoulos, G.S., Perlick, D.A., and Raue, P. (1999) Predictors of antidepressant prescription and early use among depressed outpatients. *Am J Psychiatry* 156:690–696.

Spector, W.D., Katz, S., Murphy, J.B., and Fulton, J.P. (1987) The hierarchical relationship between activities of daily living and instrumental activities of daily living. *J Chronic Dis* 40:481–489.

Steffens, D.C., Hays, J.C., and Krishnan, K.R. (1999) Disability in geriatric depression. *Am J Geriatr Psychiatry* 7:34–40.

Steffens, D.C., Plassman, B.L., Helms, M.J., et al. (1997) A twin study of late-onset depression and apolipoprotein E epsilon 4 as risk factors for Alzheimer's disease. *Biol Psychiatry* 41:851–856.

Sunderland, T., Alterman, I.S., Yount, D., et al. (1988) A new scale for the assessment of depressed mood in demented patients. *Am J Psychiatry* 145:955–959.

U.S. Department of Health and Human Services (1999) *Mental Health: A Report of the Surgeon General—Older Adults and Mental Health*. Rockville, MD: U.S. Department of Health and Human Services, Substance Abuse and Mental Health Services Administration, Center for Mental Health Services, National Institutes of Health, National Institute of Mental Health.

Unutzer, J., Katon, W.J., Simon, G., et al. (1996) Depression, quality of life, and use of health services in primary care patients over 65: A 4-year prospective study. *Psychosomatics* 37:35.

Unutzer, J., Katon, W., Sullivan, M., and Miranda, J. (1999) Treating depressed older adults in primary care: Narrowing the gap between efficacy and effectiveness. *Milbank Q* 77:225–256.

Unutzer, J., Patrick, D.L., Simon, G., et al. (1997) Depressive symptoms and the cost of health services in HMO patients aged 65 years and older. A 4-year prospective study. *JAMA* 277:1618–1623.

Weissman, M.M., Leaf, P.J., Tischler, B.L., et al. (1988) Affective disorders in five United States communities. *Psychol Med* 18:141–153.

Yesavage, J.A., Brink, T.L., Rose, T.L., et al. (1983) Development and validation of a geriatric depression scale. *J Psychiatr Res* 17:31–49.

Young, A.S., Klap, R., Sherbourne, C.D., and Wells, K.B. (2001) The quality of care for depressive and anxiety disorders in the United States. *Arch Gen Psychiatry* 58:55–61.

Zubenko, G.S. (2000) Neurobiology of major depression in Alzheimer's disease. *Int Psychogeriatr* 12(Suppl 1):217–230.

Zubenko, G.S., Marino, L.J., Sweet, R.A., Rifai, A.H., Mulsant, B.H., and Pasternak, R.E. (1997) Medical co-morbidity in elderly psychiatric inpatients. *Biol Psychiatry* 41:724–736.

Zubenko, G.S., Mulsant, B.H., Rifai, A.H., Sweet, R.A., Pasternak, R.E., Marino, L.J. Jr., and Tu, X.M. (1994) Impact of acute psychiatric inpatient treatment on major depression in late life and prediction of response. *Am J Psychiatry* 151(7):987–994.

Zubenko, G.S., Rifai, A.H., Mulsant, B.H., Sweet, R.A., and Pasternak, R.E. (1996) Association of premorbid history of major depression with the depressive syndrome of Alzheimer's disease. *Am J Geriatr Psychiatry* 4:85–90.

# 4 | Bipolar disorders

ROBERT C. YOUNG

Elderly patients with mania and bipolar (BP) disorders constitute a substantial subgroup among elderly patients presenting for psychiatric treatment, and they often have severe illness that requires high use of services. These patients have diverse clinical characteristics, co-morbidities, and presumed etiologies and pathophysiologies. Their illness courses and outcomes differ widely among individuals, and their response to interventions is difficult to predict. Age-associated factors contribute to these dimensions of heterogeneity and this discussion is organized around age and age-at-onset of illness.

## HISTORICAL PERSPECTIVE

Kraepelin, who distinguished mood disorder (*manic depressive insanity*) from schizophrenia, discussed the incidence of first-episode mania, depression, and mixed states across the age span (Kraepelin, 1921). In a sample of 903 cases, he observed that mania as a first episode of illness was less frequent with increased age, although it tends to increase between ages 45 and 50 years. He also observed that, in contrast to depressive first episodes, the incidence of mixed first episodes declined consistently with age. Yet, he noted that affective episodes could appear first in old age—for example, at age 80 years. Kraepelin, however, did not differentiate unipolar depression from BP disorder.

Roth and colleagues (Slater and Roth, 1977) suggested that although the manic syndrome in elders is qualitatively similar to that in younger patients, older patients demonstrate attenuation or exaggeration of particular features. Post (1965) suggested that elderly manic patients less often have a typical flight of ideas, and that they more often have persecutory delusions that are not mood-congruent compared to younger patients. In the experience of Slater and Roth (1977), many cases of mania in old age are "relatively mild." They observed that euphoria in older manic patients is often not "infectious," and speech and thought lack the usual "sparkle and versatility" and are commonly "threadbare and repetitious." These clinicians suggested, however, that "hostility and resentment" are often marked.

These psychiatrists also pointed out that cognitive impairments frequently accompany manic syndromes, and impairments are particularly apparent in aged manic patients. They described disorientation and delirium in manic patients (Kraepelin, 1921; Post, 1965; Slater et al., 1977). However, Kraepelin observed that dementia was not a necessary outcome of late-onset affective episodes.

Early literature also commented on manic psychopathology in the context of brain lesions and mental disorders (Shulman, 1997). Welt (1888) described disinhibited behavior in the context of lesions of the orbital surface of the frontal lobes. This was referred to as *Witzelsucht* by European psychiatrists (Oppenheim, 1890) and as *pseudopsychopathic syndrome* by neurologists (Blumer and Benson, 1975). These set the stage for more recent investigations of neuroanatomical specificity in brain lesions associated with mania and depression (see below). Early writing also mentions the association between vascular disease and mood disorder in late life (Kraepelin, 1921). Kay et al. (1955) and Post (1965) proposed that mood disorder with onset in late life reflects, in part, age-associated brain changes.

In the mid-twentieth century, investigation of mood disorders in late life was advanced by validation of the distinction between unipolar depression and BP disorder (Marneros and Angst, 2000). The introduction of lithium salts (Cade, 1949) and other mood stabilizers reinforced the utility of the BP category across the age spectrum. It also encouraged testing, in younger patients, distinctions within BP disorder such as atypical or type II patients, and broadening the concept of BP disorder.

## DIAGNOSIS

Diagnostic categories (e.g., American Psychiatric Association, 1994) used in younger patients are broadly applicable to aged BP patients. The knowledge base concerning geriatric BP disorders is too preliminary to warrant modification of existing nosologies. However, differential diagnosis and co-morbidity warrant discussion.

## DIFFERENTIAL DIAGNOSIS OF MANIA IN LATE LIFE

### Type I Bipolar Disorders (DSM-IV)

These disorders are defined by idiopathic manic states. Manic states have thus far been the main focus of clinical description and investigation of bipolarity in late life. Type I BP disorders in the elderly can be recurrent from a young age or they may begin in late life. Manic states can also occur in patients with a prior history of recurrent major depression, representing a change in polarity. Idiopathic, recurrent manic states in the absence of depressive episodes, referred to as *unipolar* mania, can occur in aged patients, although relatively infrequently (Shulman and Tohen, 1994).

### Type II Bipolar Disorders (DSM-IV)

These disorders are characterized by hypomanic states and major depressive episodes. Benazzi (2000) reported that the ratio of type II BP depression to unipolar depression in an ambulatory private practice sample was less in aged patients than in younger patients.

### Manic States and Mood Disorders Associated with Medical Conditions or Drug Treatments (DSM-IV)

In elderly BP patients, medical and neurological disorders are prevalent, and they may have significance for psychiatric management. Particular conditions and treatments are implicated in the etiology of manic syndromes (see below). These syndromes have been referred to as *symptomatic* (Slavney et al., 1977), *secondary* mania (Krauthammer and Klerman, 1978), or *complicated* mania (Black et al., 1988).

### Organic Mental Disorders

Delirious patients can present with manic features. Delirium has also been described as a manifestation of manic episodes of BP disorder (Kraepelin, 1921; Slater and Roth, 1977).

Patients with dementing illness can present with either manic features or manic syndromes (Burns et al., 1990; Lyketsos et al., 1995). Manic psychopathology and manic syndromes in patients with dementia may not be correctly identified by caregivers and clinicians and may be treated as agitation (Folstein, 1999). Manic patients with dementia may or may not have had affective episodes prior to the onset of the dementia. This group of patients has received little investigation, except as a focus of preliminary pharmacological study (Mega et al., 2000; Tariot et al., 2001).

### Chronic Psychoses

Bipolar schizoaffective disorders can present with manic syndromes in late life. Schizoaffective disorders have presented challenges for classification and have not been well described in the elderly. In an early study by Post (1971), BP and depressive subtypes were not distinguished. Bipolar-type schizoaffective disorders may constitute a substantial proportion of geriatric schizoaffective inpatients (Yu and Young, 2001). Paranoid schizophrenic patients can have manic features such as grandiose delusions. The clinical differentiation of chronic psychosis from primary BP disorder depends on longitudinal history.

### Substance Abuse

Active substance abuse/dependence and intoxication can contribute to manic-like signs and symptoms. Alcohol, anxiolytic, and analgesic dependence in particular must be considered in the differential diagnosis of mania in the elderly. In a sample of 81 manic patients aged >55 years, one-third had a history of substance abuse (Himmelhoch et al., 1980). More information on patterns of drug and alcohol abuse in BP elders is needed.

### Psychiatric Co-morbidity

Anxiety disorders in elderly BP patients have not been characterized. Data regarding personality traits in geriatric BP patients are also lacking.

Clinicians need to consider a broad range of possibilities in the assessment and differential diagnosis of mania and BP disorders in old age. An adequate history is central to management, and longitudinal assessment can help clarify the diagnosis. Manic states can reflect underlying medical and neurological disorders and treatments, and this highlights the need for thorough medical evaluation of these patients.

## EPIDEMIOLOGY

Epidemiological issues related to BP disorders in late life are reviewed in Chapter 1. A few points are highlighted here. In this review, the definition of *aged*, *elderly*, or *geriatric* is 60 years of age and older, since this is one commonly used convention. In some studies, older adults have been defined by a younger index age, and this will be indicated.

### Age and Prevalence

The lifetime and 1-year prevalence rates for mania in the elderly community detected in the Epidemiological Catchment Area Study were only 0.1% (Weissman et al., 1990). On the other hand, the prevalence of mania at age 60 years and older in patients presenting to psychiatric services for treatment ranges from 5% to 19% (Dunn and Rabins, 1996; Yassa et al., 1988). The sex distribution favors women. Comparisons in racial and ethnic groups are lacking.

## Age and Incidence

Wertham (1929) observed a decline in first psychiatric admissions of manic patients over the age of 50. Clayton (1986a, 1986b) concluded that the risk of new-onset mania declines, or at least does not increase, with aging. This is consistent with findings of a retrospective study of psychiatric inpatients by Loranger and Levine (1978), although these investigators excluded an unspecified number of elderly patients with medical illnesses. In contrast to this experience, the geropsychiatry literature indicates that age-at-onset of mania tends to be late, often in the fifth or sixth decade (Broadhead and Jacoby, 1990; Charron et al., 2001; Glasser and Rabins, 1984; Shulman and Post, 1980; Stone, 1989). Angst (1978) suggested a bimodal distribution for age-at-onset of BP disorder based on findings in a sample of 95 mixed-age patients. Spicer et al. (1973) found that first admissions of male manic patients increased above 60 years of age, and Eagles and Whalley (1985) observed a gradual increase with age in first hospital admissions of manic patients—especially males, an increase that was sustained past the age of 70. These findings are similar to the later age-at-onset in males noted by Snowdon (1991); however, Shulman and Post (1980) reported later age-at-onset in females.

Episodes of depression often predate the onset of mania in late life, and this interval can be more than a decade (Broadhead and Jacoby, 1990; Glasser and Rabins, 1984; Shulman and Post, 1980; Snowdon, 1991; Stone, 1989; Yassa et al., 1988). There has also been speculation that the availability of antidepressant pharmacotherapies may be increasing the rate of BP disorder in late life. One report suggests that a pattern of unipolar mania in late life may be linked to a history of early-onset illness (Shulman et al., 1994).

Ascertainment of age-at-onset can be difficult in late-life mood disorder. The definition of late onset differs among studies (Young and Klerman, 1992). Definitions have included use of conventional age values, and values derived from distribution of age-at-onset in particular samples.

## PATHOPHYSIOLOGY AND ETIOLOGY

### Overview

Age-associated factors may modify the pathophysiology of early-onset illness. They may modify the clinical features and course of BP disorders. Potential mechanisms could include both physical/physiological changes with-in the range of normal aging that interact with the pathophysiology of early-onset illnesses and other disorders or illnesses. Age-associated brain changes have been proposed as mediators of change from unipolar depression to BP disorder (Shulman, 1997). Other potential mechanisms include learning and adaptation, as well as changes in social context, environment, and resources. An optimal strategy for studying age effects on illness would be to compare elderly patients with early-onset BP disorder with younger BP disorder patients, but the limited available data generally involve index age alone.

Patients who develop BP disorder in late life can be conceptualized as manifesting age-associated pathogenic factors for the disorder and/or loss of protective factors. Whether these patients are different from elders with early-onset BP disorder has received limited investigation. To examine age-at-onset effects requires comparison of aged patients with either early- or late-onset illness.

### Vascular Risk Factors

Elderly manic patients as a group may have increased risk factors for stroke (Nadeem et al., 2000). Berrios and Bakshi (1991) recorded high Hachinski scores in patients with manic symptoms compared to those with depressive symptoms. Broadhead and Jacoby (1990) and Snowdon (1991) indicated that some of the patients in their samples had onset of mania soon after a central neurological event.

### Age-at-onset

Excess risk factors for stroke may be particularly associated with late onset of BP disorder (Cassidy et al., 2001; Wylie et al., 1999). Steffens and Krishnan (1998) proposed a vascular subtype of mania similar to the concept of vascular depression (Alexopoulos et al., 1997).

### Brain Lesions and Mania

Studies of patients with focal brain pathology have implicated specific neural circuits in manic psychopathology. Right hemisphere lesions have been linked to mania. Sackeim et al. (1982) reported that pathological laughing was associated with destructive lesions of the right brain and that right hemispherectomy often produces a euphoric mood. Further, Starkstein et al. (1988, 1990) reported a preponderance of right-sided or bilateral hemispheric localization of heterogeneous brain lesions including tumors, strokes, and head injuries in patients with mania. However, some left-sided lesions, including basal ganglia lesions, have also been associated with mania (Liu et al., 1996; Turecki et al., 1993).

A number of reports have linked mania and *disinhibition syndrome* with pathology of the medial orbitofrontal cortex (OFC)—subcortical circuits, including the thalamus and caudate (Cummings, 1993; Starkstein et al., 1991). The behavioral abnormalities encompassed by disinhibition overlap with the psychopathology of mania, for example in some forms of *secondary* mania (Cummings, 1993; Shulman, 1997; Starkstein and Robinson, 1997). Involvement of OFC dysfunction in mania is supported by functional imaging studies in mixed-age manic patients (Blumberg et al., 2002). Frontal lobe dementia can present with disinhibition (Miller et al., 1991). Primate studies also link OFC lesions to disruption of social behavior (Kling and Steklis, 1976).

Basotemporal cortical lesions also have been implicated in mania (Starkstein, 1997; Starkstein et al., 1991). A study of head injury found predominantly basotemporal injury in the 9% of patients in this sample who developed mania (Jorge et al., 1993).

## Abnormalities Found on Structural Neuroimaging in Psychiatric Patients

Brain morphological abnormalities found on neuroimaging may be prominent in elderly manic and BP disorder patients treated at psychiatric services. A limited number of studies have been conducted, but investigators have described both excess signal hyperintensities (SH) on magnetic resonance imaging and loss of tissue volume. They describe prominent deep frontal white matter and periventricular SH (deAsis et al., 1998; McDonald et al., 1991, 1999) and subcortical gray matter SH (McDonald et al., 1999). SH in aged patients with BP disorder may reflect different processes than those seen in unipolar depressed elders. However, a greater rate of silent strokes have also been described in aged BP disorder patients (Fujikawa et al., 1995).

Aged patients with mania have excess cortical sulcal widening on computed tomography (Broadhead and Jacoby, 1990; Young et al., 1999) and magnetic resonance imaging scans (Rabins et al., 2000). In one report, aged BP disorder patients also had greater left sylvian fissure and greater left and right temporal sulcal widening than aged controls (Rabins et al., 2000). One study found a larger lateral ventricle/brain ratio in aged manic patients than in controls (Young et al., 1999), while another study did not (Broadhead and Jacoby, 1990).

## Age

SH scores were higher in both older and younger BP disorder patients compared to controls in a mixed-age sample (McDonald et al., 1999), although there was a trend toward more confluent SH in the younger pa-

tients. In this study, subcortical gray nuclei SH scores were also higher than in controls, which has not been reported in studies of young BP patients. Caudate volume was inversely associated with age in a study of mixed-age BP disorder patients (Brambilla et al., 2001).

## Age-at-onset

Some abnormalities seen on structural neuroimaging may be particularly prominent in those BP elders with late age-at-onset, and these include small strokes (Fujikawa et al., 1995; McDonald et al., 1991; Young et al., 1999). A study of SH in older patients with late-onset illness revealed greater SH than in aged controls (McDonald et al., 1991); however, a study of a mixed-age sample did not support an association with age-at-onset (McDonald et al., 1999).

Greater cortical sulcal widening was associated with later age-at-onset of illness in one study (Young et al., 1999) but not in another (Broadhead and Jacoby, 1990).

## Other Neurological Disorders and Treatments

Kay et al. (Kay et al., 1955) and Post (1965) proposed that mood disorder with onset in late life reflects in part degenerative brain changes. Shulman and Post (1980) reported that the onset of manic states in the geriatric age range was associated with clinical evidence of coarse brain diseases. Stone (1989) reported evidence of *organic cerebral impairment* in 24% of 92 elderly manic inpatients studied retrospectively, and found that these patients had later onset of illness. Tohen et al. (1994) observed neurological co-morbidity in 74% of late-onset cases.

Geriatric manic patients also have a higher prevalence of heterogeneous neurological disorders compared to age- and sex-matched unipolar depressives (Shulman et al., 1993). In addition to cerebrovascular disease, degenerative brain disorders linked to BP disorders include multiple sclerosis (Joffe et al., 1987) and Huntington's disease (Folstein, 1989).

There has been only preliminary study of manic psychopathology in Alzheimer's disease. Burns et al. (1990) recorded manic features in 3.5% of Alzheimer's disease patients. Lyketsos et al. (1995) found that 2.2% of Alzheimer patients had a manic syndrome and that two-thirds of this subgroup had had manic episodes prior to the onset of dementia.

## Other Medical Disorders and Treatments

Krauthammer and Klerman (1978) demonstrated that a range of medical disorders can be associated with late-onset mania. Black et al. (1988) observed that older age was a characteristic of patients with mania complicated by medical disorders including endocrinopathies, nutrient deficiencies, and infections. The breadth of this list has been underscored by recent reviews (Strakowski et al., 1994; Verdoux and Bourgeois, 1995). Drugs used to treat medical disorders, for example corticosteroids, also have been implicated in manic states. Roose et al. (1979) cautioned that psychiatrists may be the only physicians involved with elderly BP disorder patients despite their prevalent medical co-morbidities.

## Familial and Genetic Factors

Bipolar disorder is strongly associated with hereditary factors. The relatives of late-onset BP probands have a lower rate of affective disorder than do the relatives of probands with early-onset illness. This is true in mixed-age patient samples (Hays, 1976; Mendlewics et al., 1972; Rice et al., 1987; Taylor and Abrams, 1981) and is also observed in elderly BP patients (Glasser and Robins, 1984; Shulman and Post, 1980; Snowdon, 1991; Stone, 1989). However, genetic factors may contribute to late age-at-onset (McMahon and DePaulo, 1996).

## Life Events

There is limited information concerning life events in geriatric manic or BP disorder patients (Walter-Ryan, 1983). Yassa et al. (1988) reported a history of stressful events in 70% of elderly manic patients studied.

### Age

In a mixed-age sample, negative life events preceding a manic episode were associated with an older index age (Ambelas, 1987). Controlled studies of this methodologically difficult issue are needed.

Late age-at-onset manic syndromes and BP disorders represent models for studying age-associated constitutional and psychosocial factors in relationship to pathogenesis. Thus, familial and genetic contributions may be different and may include different balances between protective factors and causal vulnerabilities. Brain changes may play an important role, particularly those arising from cerebrovascular or degenerative changes at a microscopic or clinical level. Manic and BP disorders arising out of brain lesions have implicated particular neuronal circuits in these disorders, including dysfunction of cortico-striatal circuits, and these may be relevant to the pathophysiology of idiopathic disorders. Dementing disorders and subcortical neurological diseases present additional opportunities for investigation. Models of late-life illness may be relevant to mechanisms of early-life illness.

## FEATURES OF EPISODES: PSYCHOPATHOLOGY AND ITS ASSESSMENT

### Mania

In this syndrome, the predominant affective signs and symptoms represent acceleration and/or excesses of behavior, mental activity, or emotion. These characteristics can result in harm to the patient and to others. For example, Petrie et al. (1982) observed that 9%–16% of aggressive or violent geriatric inpatients are manic.

### Age

Few studies have used rating scales to compare manic psychopathology in elderly patients to that in younger patients. In symptomatic inpatients of mixed age studied prospectively (Young and Falk, 1989) age was negatively associated with scores on the "activity-energy" item of the Mania Rating Scale (Young et al., 1978). There was a low negative correlation between age and scores on the "language-thought disorder" item and a trend toward decreased "sexual interest" scores with age. In aged manic patients, Broadhead and Jacoby (1990) found that total scores on the Modified Manic Rating Scale (Blackburn et al., 1977) on hospital admission were lower than those of a young patient comparison group. While older patients had lower scores on the "religiosity" item of the scale, other items did not differentiate old from young patients.

### Age-at-onset

Broadhead and Jacoby (1990) found higher average item ratings for "happiness" and "cheerfulness" on the Modified Manic Rating Scale in late-compared to early-onset cases. However, a retrospective report (Glasser and Robins, 1984) detected no differences in psychopathology between aged patients with late-onset and early-onset illness.

### Mixed States

A mixture of depressive features in mania occurs in young adult patients, that is, mixed states (e.g., DSM-IV) or dysphoric mania (Swann, 1995). Post (1965) suggested that older manic patients exhibit concomitant depressive features more often than do younger patients based on clinical impressions.

### Age

In the study by Broadhead and Jacoby (1990), there were equivalent mixed features in elderly and young manic patients.

## Age-at-onset

The authors found no difference in depressive features during the manic episode between late-onset and early-onset elderly patients.

## Bipolar Depression

Bipolar depressed states in elderly patients have received minimal study. This group was included in the sample studied by Wylie et al. (1999).

## Age

In the study by Broadhead and Jacoby (1990), a greater proportion of elderly compared to young manic patients cycled into a depressive episode during their hospitalization. Rapid cycling has apparently not been studied in aged BP patients.

## Psychosis

Psychotic symptoms, that is, delusions and hallucinations, can occur in manic and BP depressed elders. For example, 58% of the symptomatic geriatric BP patients studied by Wylie et al. (1999) were psychotic. The distinction between mood-congruent and mood-incongruent psychotic features awaits study in these patients. Benazzi (1999) observed, in his private practice, that among aged depressed patients, those who were psychotic had BP disorder more often than those who were not psychotic.

## Age

A prospective assessment of mixed-age manic inpatients did not find an association between age and the presence of hallucinations and/or delusions (Young et al., 1983). Evaluation of geriatric manic patients did not reveal differences in rate of psychosis compared to younger adults (Broadhead and Jacoby, 1990). Benazzi (1999) did not detect an age effect on BP preponderance among depressed patients with psychotic features.

## Age-at-onset

Wylie et al. (1999) found an association between late age-at-onset and psychosis in a sample of aged BP disorder patients with manic and depressed states. Tohen et al. (1994) reported delusions in 45% of their late-onset manic sample. Broadhead and Jacoby (1990) did not detect a difference in rate of delusions between early- and late-onset manic elders. There have been conflicting reports concerning age-at-onset and psychosis in the mixed-age BP literature (Angst et al., 1973; Rosen et al., 1984).

## Assessment

Rating scales for manic psychopathology (Bech et al., 1978; Blackburn et al., 1977; Young et al., 1978) have been applied in elderly patients and can be used to monitor change. They are likely to be most useful in cognitively intact and mildly impaired patients. Instruments need to be developed for use in demented patients.

## COGNITIVE IMPAIRMENT

Consistent with early clinical descriptions, symptomatic states in BP disorders can be associated with impaired performance on cognitive tests. In mixed-age BP patients, deficits in attention and memory have been documented using neurocognitive tests during manic states (Bearden et al., 2001; Kerry et al., 1983; Strauss et al., 1984). Cognitive dysfunction has also been reported in remitted mixed-age BP patients (Coffman et al., 1990; Rubinsztein et al., 2000; Chowdry et al., 2000).

## Age

Recent clinical investigation in BP elders has supported the presence of cognitive impairment. In one study of symptomatic elderly psychiatric inpatients, those with manic syndromes had lower performance on the Blessed cognitive scale than those with depression or those lacking predominant affective features (Berrios and Bakshi, 1991). Stone (1989) reported that more than 14% of elderly manic patients had memory impairment. Burt et al. (2000) found greater memory impairment in BP depressed elders compared to younger BP depressed patients; this difference was greater than in unipolar depressed patients. Broadhead and Jacoby (1990) found that a greater proportion of elderly patients successfully treated for mania performed in the demented range on subtests of the Kendrick neuropsychological battery compared to young patients; however, they observed a large discrepancy between verbal and performance IQ in both age groups.

While cognitive performance may improve with treatment of BP episodes in elders (Wylie et al., 1999), impairment may persist. Savard et al. (1980) reported that neuropsychological task performance was poorer in remitted BP patients aged 40 years or older than in controls. Stone (1989) indicated that memory impairment, when it was noted, was persistent in elderly manic patients; this may be consistent with the experience of Broadhead and Jacoby (1990). The potential effects of psychotropics, as well as of residual psychopathology on cognition, must be taken into account in ongoing studies of these issues in elders.

Beyond global impairment, preliminary interest has focused on whether particular cognitive functions are impaired in late-life BP disorders. Some evidence suggests that executive functions can be impaired (Bearden et al., 2001; Young et al., 2001; Murphy et al., 2001).

### Age-at-Onset

In Stone's study (1989), cerebral organic impairment was associated with late age-at-onset. Broadhead and Jacoby (1990) did not detect an effect of age-at-onset on their cognitive measures.

### Assessment

Assessment with standardized instruments during symptomatic states may be feasible if limitations of cooperation are taken into account. The Minimental State Examination (MMSE) (Folstein et al., 1975) has been used widely in this population, although it is rather insensitive compared to more extensive instruments. The strategy of testing cognitive function both during episodes of illness and on follow-up, when patients are in affective remission, is important to clinical work and investigation.

### Other Issues

Exacerbation of cognitive impairment can be minimized by identifying treatments that are best tolerated. On the other hand, some psychotropic treatments such as mood stabilizers may have neuroprotective/neurotropic effects (Moore et al., 2000a, 2000b; Manji et al., 1999). Cognitive rehabilitation has not been studied in impaired BP disorder patients.

## FUNCTION/BEHAVIORAL DISABILITY

Functional impairment is described in young BP disorder patients (Arnold et al., 2000) during illness episodes. Behavioral disability has received almost no investigation in elders with BP disorder (Bartels et al., 1997).

## COURSE OF ILLNESS: CHRONICITY

### Age

There is little information on whether the rates of recovery from mania are different in elderly and younger patients. Several investigators (Lundquist, 1945; Mac-

Donald, 1918; Wertham, 1929) have reported a positive association between age and duration of the acute manic episode in mixed-age samples. Wertham's 2000 patients ranged in age up to the eighth decade. In Mac-Donald's sample, 12 of 451 patients were 60 years of age or older, and in Lundquist's sample, 11 of 103 manic patients were older than 50 years. Chronic mania has been associated with increased age (Henderson and Gillespie, 1956; Wertham, 1929). Wertham observed that seven patients with manic episodes lasting for at least 5 years ranged in age from 31 to 60 years. Henderson and Gillespie (1956) reported that patients with chronic mania were frequently more than 40 years old. Among Lundquist's patients, fewer of those more than 40 years of age recovered (84%) compared to younger patients (95%).

Roth (1955) suggested a relatively poor outcome for elderly patients with mania. He reported that among 28 geriatric inpatients with mania, 65% of those still living at the 2-year follow-up had remained in the hospital; this was a poorer outcome than that of geriatric depressed patients.

Van der Velde (1970) observed worse acute outcomes with increased age in patients receiving naturalistic lithium treatment. In a mixed-age sample of manic patients examined prospectively, older age was associated with a longer duration of acute psychiatric hospitalization (Young and Falk, 1989). In that sample, consistent with clinical observation by Post (1965), older age was also associated with greater residual impairment of insight after 2 weeks of naturalistic lithium treatment. Berrios and Bakshi (1991) observed worse acute outcomes in geriatric mania than in geriatric depression. However, Himmelhoch et al. (1980) did not find an effect of age on recovery from mania in 81 patients studied retrospectively, although all were aged 55 years or more. In the prospective study by Broadhead and Jacoby (1990), there was no difference in duration of the index manic episode between elderly and younger patients. Stone (1989) reported episodes lasting for 2–13 years in 5 of 92 geriatric manic patients, but only 8% of patients remained in the hospital at 6 months. Glasser and Rabins (1984) found that 79% of manic elderly inpatients were discharged home after acute treatment, which supports an improved short-term prognosis since the era of Roth's investigations.

### Age-at-Onset

In mixed-age patient groups, some reports have suggested an association between older age-at-onset and a greater duration of the episode and/or chronicity. Mac-Donald's (1918) and Lundquist's (1945) patients were selected on the basis of first psychiatric hospitalization. In Wertham's (1929) study, four of seven chronic patients were age 38–60 years at the onset of illness.

In the geriatric literature, neither the report of Broadhead and Jacoby (1990) nor that of Stone (1989) indicated differences in duration of episode between late-onset and early-onset geriatric manic patients. Dhingra and Rabins (1991) and Shulman et al. (1993) did not comment on this issue.

## COURSE OF ILLNESS: RELAPSE AND RECURRENCE

### Age

In BP patients of mixed ages, MacDonald (1918) reported an association between older age and shorter intervals between episodes. Studies of geriatric manic patients found further episodes in a high proportion but suggested a better prognosis than that observed by Roth. Their designs have differed in measures and duration of assessment. Shulman and Post (1980) observed further episodes in 76% of the patients in their sample. Stone (1989) reported a 52% readmission rate on 1 month to 10 year follow-up. Dhingra and Rabins (1991) recorded relapse requiring hospitalization in 32% of patients followed up over 5–7 years.

### Age-at-Onset

In mixed-age BP disorder patients, investigators (Angst et al., 1973; Swift HM, 1907) have reported an association between shorter interepisode intervals and later age-at-onset.

Among geriatric patients, Stone (1989) found an increased frequency of readmission in those with a history of previous affective episodes compared to those without such a history. On the other hand, Shulman et al. (1993) found that an age-at-onset above 55 years predicted decreased time to psychiatric rehospitalization at 3- to 10-year follow-up. Dhingra and Rabins (1991) reported no difference in this regard between early- and late-onset patients.

## COURSE OF ILLNESS: SUICIDE

Suicidal ideation, suicide attempt, or completed suicide, are not well characterized in geriatric BP disorders. Shulman et al. (1993) did not detect suicide as a cause of mortality in their follow-up study. Given the associations of suicide with age and with mood disorder in mixed-age populations, investigation of elderly BP patients is warranted.

## COURSE OF ILLNESS: PSYCHIATRIC SERVICES USE AND CAREGIVER BURDEN

The public health importance of BP disorders in the elderly stems not only from their clinical characteristics

and the burden that they impose on patients themselves, but also from their impact on caregivers, families, and care systems. Elderly BP disorder patients use psychiatric services frequently (Sajetovic et al., 1997). Bartels et al. (1997) reported that they use these services almost four times more often than aged unipolar depressed patients. The burden on families and caregivers in late-life with BP disorders has not been explored.

## MODIFICATION OF THE COURSE BY OTHER AGE-ASSOCIATED FACTORS

### Psychiatric Co-morbidity

Substance abuse was associated with a poor acute therapeutic outcome in older patients with mania in one study (Himmelhoch et al., 1980).

### Medical/Neurological Co-morbidity

In the study of Shulman et al. (1993), neurological disorders were associated with higher rates of subsequent psychiatric hospitalization. Berrios and Bakshi (1991) reported that high Hatchinski scores predicted a worse acute outcome in mania. In another study, patients more than 55 years old with mania accompanied by dementia had a poorer acute response to antimanic treatment (Himmelhoch et al., 1980). Other medical disorders may also contribute to poor acute outcomes in mania (Black et al., 1988).

### Lack of Social Support

O'Connell et al. (1991) observed that low levels of social support were associated with poor function in a sample of BP patients ranging in age up to the tenth decade. Among geriatric BP disorder patients (Bartels et al., 1997), lack of a spouse was associated with residence in a nursing facility rather than residence in the community. Geriatric BP disorder patients report low perceived social support (Beyer et al., 2002). Lack of social support in geriatric depression is associated with poor outcomes, and it may contribute to poor adherence to medication regimens.

### Disability

In young BP disorder patients, disability can worsen the symptom course (Gitlin et al., 1995). This has not been studied in elderly BP patients.

In summary, the course of illness in late-life mania and BP disorders is heterogeneous and may be more malignant than that of unipolar depression. Neurological disorders may predict poor outcomes.

## NONAFFECTIVE OUTCOMES

### Nonsuicide Mortality

Mortality rates are relatively high in aged patients with BP disorder. Roth (1955) observed a mortality rate over 2 years of 11%; this was lower than that for elderly demented patients but was higher than that for elderly depressed patients. There were two deaths among nine patients followed for 2 years by Yassa et al. (1988). Stone (1989) observed a mortality rate over 2 years of 16% in geriatric mania. In the study by Dhingra and Rabins (1991), mortality at 5- to 7-year follow-up was 34%; these authors commented that the survival rate was significantly lower than the expected rate calculated from census data. Similarly, Shulman et al. (1993) found that the mortality rate of geriatric manic patients, 50% at an average interval of 6 years, exceeded the 20% mortality rate in geriatric depressed patients.

The mechanisms for this increased nonsuicide mortality are not clear, but they include effects of cerebrovascular disease (Tohen et al., 1994). Mortality was not increased by neurological disorder in the sample of Shulman et al. (1993).

Affective episodes themselves may be lethal, and manic episodes have in the past been linked to mortality through *exhaustion.* Decreased sleep, impaired nutritional status through overactivity and distraction, and decreased compliance with medical regimens all pose a threat to health. These issues carry added weight in the frail elderly patient. Although deaths from *manic exhaustion* were reported to occur most often among young patients (Derby, 1933), the age distribution of the total samples was not clear. The incidence of manic exhaustion has apparently been reduced dramatically in the psychopharmacological era (Wendkos, 1979).

### Age

Mortality among elderly patients has apparently not been compared to that among younger BP disorder patients in the same study. There is evidence for greater mortality among BP disorder patients of mixed ages—at least among those with a medical illness (Jamison and Goodwin, 1990)—than among the general population.

### Age-at-Onset

Late-onset mania has a high mortality rate (Tohen et al., 1994). Male patients had higher mortality than female patients in that sample. Neither the study of Dhingra and Rabins (1991) nor that of Shulman et al. (1993) detected differences in mortality between patients with late-onset and early-onset disorder.

### Emergent Dementia

A proportion of elderly manic patients have cognitive impairment and/or dementia on follow-up. Stone (1989) reported that 3% of 92 geriatric patients with mania went on to develop moderate to severe dementia over an average of 3 years of follow-up. Dhingra and Rabins (1991) found that at 5- to 7-year follow-up, 32% of elderly manic patients, who had been cognitively intact at index episode, had MMSE scores in the cognitively impaired range (less than 24). However, these authors commented that this was greater than the incidence of all forms of dementia expected in this age group in the community; the rate was not greater than that of geriatric depressed patients.

### Age

Emergent dementia occurs relatively infrequently in BP disorder patients of mixed ages and has received only limited study as an outcome measure (Coffman et al., 1990). In the study of Astrup et al. (1959), less than 5% of patients with affective disorders were clinically demented on 7- to 19-year follow-up.

### Age-at-onset

It is not known whether late-onset manic patients are at particularly high risk for development of cognitive dysfunction/dementia. Dhingra and Rabins (1991) did not detect a difference in MMSE scores between late-onset and geriatric early-onset patients at 5- to 7-year follow-up. Charron et al. (2001) did not observe dementia on 2-year follow-up in their six late-onset patients.

### Function/Behavioral Disability

While a substantial proportion of young BP disorder patients have impaired function, when in remission, i.e., behavioral disability (Coryell et al., 1993), the course of disability has not been studied in geriatric BP disorder patients. Nursing home/chronic institutional placement is reported in 20%–30% in recent follow-up studies of elderly manic patients (Dhingra and Rabins, 1991; Shulman et al., 1993). In young BP disorder patients, disability may be worsened by symptomatic states (Gitlin et al., 1995).

Function in patients with geriatric BP disorder is likely to be impaired. Behavioral disability needs to be assessed as an outcome in treatment studies; particular interventions may have different effects on psychopathology and function.

## Modification of Nonaffective Outcomes by Other Age-Associated Factors

### Cognitive impairment

In a cross-sectional study of geriatric BP disorder patients (Bartels et al., 1997), global cognitive performance (MMSE) accounted for a substantial proportion of interindividual differences (46% of the variance) function in contrast to psychopathology ratings, which accounted for little (3%–7% of the variance).

## RESPONSE TO ANTIMANIC TREATMENT

The treatment literature related to aged BP disorder patients understandably deals almost entirely with pharmacotherapy. However, there has been little information about the role of electroconvulsive therapy (Chapter 21). There has also been essentially no investigation of nonsomatic components of management of BP disorder in the elderly, such as education and supportive psychotherapy for patients, and for families and caregivers, or rehabilitative interventions for patients. In what follows, limited evidence is reviewed regarding potential modifier of outcomes of interventions that are particularly important in BP elders. Related issues including pharmacokinetic distortions with advanced age and tolerability are discussed in Chapters 15, 16, 18, and 20.

### Age

There is limited information regarding the influence of age on acute outcomes in BP disorders. Van der Velde (1970) noted poorer acute therapeutic benefits of lithium in older manic patients compared to a sample of younger (aged <60 years) patients. In fact, only 3 of 12 elderly manic patients responded to lithium compared to 51 of 63 younger patients. A prospective study of naturalistic lithium treatment in mixed-age manic patients suggested that the benefit was attenuated by increased age (Young and Falk, 1989). There are no analyses of age effects on divalproex (DVP) efficacy in mania. Okuma et al. (1990) did not analyze separately the response to carbamazepine or lithium in aged patients. Cycling immediately into a depressive episode may occur more often after inpatient management of mania in elders than in younger patients (Broadhead and Jacoby, 1990).

### Age-at-Onset

Little attention has been paid to the relationship, if any, of age-at-onset to treatment outcome in geriat-

ric BP disorder patients (Young and Klerman, 1992b). There was no effect of age-at-onset on the outcome at the end point in one naturalistic study of BP elderly (Wylie et al., 1999) or in a preliminary retrospective report (Lehman and Rabins, 2001). In BP disorder patients, two chronological events related to age-at-onset are pertinent in the examination of illness: the first affective episode and the first manic episode. The reliability of retrospective course assessment in geriatric patients is a limiting factor in research; multiple sources of information clearly must be used.

### Other Factors

Cognitive impairments may be associated with limitation of acute therapeutic outcomes in older BP disorder patients. Impairments of executive function, for example, are prevalent in BP disorders, particularly in late life (Bearden et al., 2001); these are often associated with frontostriatal pathology. Executive dysfunction was associated with an attenuated acute response to pharmacotherapy in a preliminary study of elderly manic patients (Young et al., 2001). This observation may be similar to that concerning the effects of executive impairment on outcomes described in geriatric unipolar depression (Kalayam and Alexopoulos, 1999). Co-morbid dementia may also be associated with worse antimanic outcomes of lithium treatment (Himmelhoch et al., 1980). In one report, DVP benefited BP disorder patients with dementia (Niedermier and Nasrallah, 1998). However, in a placebo-controlled trial involving demented patients with manic symptoms, DVP reduced agitation but not mania ratings (Tariot et al., 2001). Carbamazepine has been reported to reduce agitation in dementia, but these patients were not manic (Leibovici et al., 1988). Mechanisms through which cognitive impairments may be associated with differences in response to antimanic agents await elucidation.

Acute treatment can improve cognitive performance in geriatric BP disorder patients (Wylie et al., 1999). Alleviation of affective psychopathology can be associated with improvement of cognitive performance, a phenomenon referred to as *reversible dementia*. In addition, mood stabilizers may have neuroprotective effects (Manji et al., 1999; Moore et al., 2000b) and, in fact, may promote regeneration of cortical gray matter (Moore et al., 2000a). Systemic effects of behavioral improvement may also be relevant to cognitive improvement. However, cognitive impairments may also persist in euthymic mixed-age BP disorder patients (van Gorp et al., 1998; Thompson et al., 2000).

Elderly manic patients with neurological compromise may have worse therapeutic outcomes than those without compromise. Berrios and Bakshi (1991) reported an association between higher Hachinski scores, indicating cerebrovascular disease, and worse acute treatment outcomes. Himmelhoch et al. (1980) observed that extrapyramidal impairment predicted a poorer antimanic effect of lithium treatment. On the other hand, in one case series, mixed-age patients with brain disease responded well to DVP (Stoll et al., 1994).

Other co-morbid conditions may have negative influences on treatment outcomes in mania. Substance abuse was associated with a poor antimanic response to lithium in elderly manic patients in one report (Himmelhoch et al., 1980). Co-morbid medical conditions (Black et al., 1988) also can predict a poor acute response to lithium. In the mixed-age sample of Black et al., patients with medical co-morbidity had a mean age of 51 years, higher than that of patients without such co-morbidity.

The potential relationship of psychopathological features to treatment outcomes in geriatric mania has received little study. In a retrospective study, Chen et al. (1999) observed that lithium had a better therapeutic effect than DVP in patients with classic mania compared to those with mixed mania; drug levels were not provided in this comparison. Elderly patients with rapidly cycling states are another subgroup who await study from this perspective.

## RESPONSE TO ANTIDEPRESSANT TREATMENT IN BIPOLAR DEPRESSION

There has been minimal investigation of the treatment of BP disorder in late life (Chapter 16). For example, the effect of age on outcome was not examined in a recent study of mixed-age patients (Nemeroff et al., 2001).

The nature of the "switch" to mania or the change to a rapidly cycling course during antidepressant treatment has long been of clinical concern, though primarily in younger patients. Antidepressant-associated mania has been reported in aged patients and may be a particular issue in patients who have their first episode of mania late in life (van Scheyen and van Kammen, 1979; Young et al., 2003).

## RELAPSE AND RECURRENCE IN MAINTENANCE TREATMENT

Since aged BP disorder patients are at risk for repeated episodes requiring treatment, continuation and maintenance pharmacotherapy and other long-term management is central to their care. There is even less literature regarding their long-term treatment than there is on acute management. Efficacy data are summarized in Chapter 18.

## Age

Abou-Saleh and Coppen (1983) observed no age effect on affective morbidity in mixed-aged unipolar and BP disorder patients; however, there were few BP elders in the sample. In a naturalistic study of patients aged 25 to 90 years, the affective outcome of BP disorder patients receiving lithium treatment was independent of age (O'Connell et al., 1991). On the other hand, Van der Velde (1970) found that, over 3 years of observation, 52% of the younger patients and 8% of the older patients remained free of affective episodes during lithium treatment. Murray et al. (1983) observed only trends toward greater manic psychopathology, although no more frequent hospitalizations, among older compared to younger patients treated with lithium. Interpretation of another report (Hewick et al., 1977) is confounded by differing plasma concentrations with age.

## Age-at-Onset

This factor was not evaluated as a predictor in existing reports. However, Stone (1989) found that a history of prior episodes predicted a higher rate of recurrence in geriatric mania on naturalistic follow-up.

## Other Factors

Cognitive impairments or neurologic compromise may have adverse implications for long-term treatment outcomes in elderly BP disease patients. Bartels et al. (1997) observed that cognitive deficits were associated with poor community living skills, with deficits in activities of daily living, and with nursing home placement. In a naturalistic prospective study, however, elderly manic patients with or without global cognitive impairment had an equal risk of relapse with hospitalization (Dhingra and Rabins, 1991). Shulman et al. (1993) found that patients with neurological co-morbidity had a higher risk of psychiatric rehospitalization and institutionalization. Data from controlled treatment trials are needed.

## CONCLUSIONS

Manic syndromes in late life have a broad differential diagnosis. Affective psychopathology in mania in old age is qualitatively similar to that in younger patients, although quantitative changes have been suggested. Cognitive impairments are prominent, and these may have both state- and trait-related components. The antecedent course includes early recurrence, change in polarity, and late-onset illness. Co-morbidities are prevalent. Vascular pathology and other brain lesions may be linked to pathogenesis in late-onset patients. The course of illness in elderly manic and BP disorder patients appears to be characterized by excess mortality and by vulnerability to further episodes. Age-associated modifiers of treatment outcomes have been suggested, but these associations await validation in controlled treatment trials. Investigation of late-life BP illness, in addition, can provide models that may be relevant to the pathophysiology and pathogenesis of early-life BP illness.

ACKNOWLEDGMENTS
This work was supported by NIMH Grants K02 MH01192, K02 MH067028, and R01 MH52763, and by Grant P20 MH49762 (P.I.: G.S. Alexopoulos). The author thanks C.F. Murphy.

REFERENCES

Abou-Saleh, M.T., and Coppen, A. (1983) Prognosis of depression in old age. The case for lithium therapy. *Br J Psychiatry* 143: 527–528.

Alexopoulos, G., Meyers, B.S., Young, R.C., Kakuma, T., Silbersweig, D., and Charlson, M. (1997) Clinically defined vascular depression. *Am J Psychiatry* 154:562–565.

Ambelas, A. (1987) Life events and mania. A special relationship? *Br J Psychiatry* 150:235–240.

American Psychiatric Association. (1994) *Diagnostic and Statistical Manual*, 4th ed. Washington, DC: American Psychiatric Press.

Angst, J. (1978) The course of affective disorders. II. Typology of bipolar manic-depressive illness. *Arch Psychiatr Nervenkr* 226: 65–73.

Angst, J., Baastrup, P., Grof, P., Hippius, H., Poldinger, W., and Weis, P. (1973) The course of monopolar and bipolar depression and bipolar psychosis. *Psychiatr Neurol Neurochir* 76:489–500.

Arnold, L.M., Witzeman, K.A., Swank, M.L., McElroy, S.L., and Keck, P.E., Jr. (2000) Health-related quality of life using the SF-36 in patients with bipolar disorder compared with patients with chronic back pain and the general population. *J Affect Disord* 57(1–3):235–239.

Astrup, C., Fossum, A., and Holmboe, R. (1959) A follow-up study of 270 patients with acute affective psychoses. *Acta Psychiatr Scand* Suppl 135:1–65.

Bartels, S.J., Meuser, K.T., and Miles, K.M. (1997) A comparative study of elderly patients with schizophrenia and bipolar disorder in nursing homes and the community. *Schizophr Res* 27(2–3): 181–190.

Bearden, C.E., Hoffman, K.M., and Kannon, T.D. (2001) The neuropsychology of neuroanatomy of bipolar affective disorder. *Bipolar Dis* 3:106–150.

Bech, P., Rafaelsen, O.J., Kramp, P., and Bolwig, T.G. (1978) The Mania Rating Scale. Scale construction and interobserver agreement. *Neuropsychopharmacology* 17:430–431.

Benazzi, F. (1999) Psychotic late-life depression. A 376-case study. *Int Psychogeriatr* 11(3):325–332.

Benazzi, F. (2000) Late-life chronic depression. A 339-case study in private practice. *Int J Geriatr Psychiatry* 15:1–6.

Berrios, G.E., and Bakshi, N. (1991) Manic and depressive symptoms in the elderly. Their relationships to treatment outcome, cognition and motor symptoms. *Psychopathology* 24:31–38.

Beyer, J.L., Kuchibhatala, M., Cassidy, F., Looney, C., and Krishnan, K.R.R. (2003) Social support in elderly patients with bipolar disorder. *Bipolar Disord* 5:22–27.

Black, D.W., Winokur, G., Bell, S., Nasrallah, A., and Hulbert, J. (1988) Complicated mania. *Arch Gen Psychiatry* 45:232–236.

Blackburn, J., Loudon, J., and Ashworth, C. (1977) A new scale for measuring mania. *Psychol Med* 7:453–458.

Blumberg, H.P., Charney, D.S., and Krystal, J.H. (2002) Frontotemporal neural systems in bipolar disorder. *Semin Clin Neuropsychiatry* 7:243–254.

Blumer, D., and Benson, D.F. (1975) Personality changes with frontal and temporal lobe lesions. In: Benson, D.F., and Blumer, D. (eds.) *Psychiatric Aspects of Neurologic Disease*. New York: Grune and Stratton, pp. 151–170.

Brambilla, P., Harensi, K., Nicoletti, M.A., Mallinger, A.G., Frank, E., Kupfer, D., et al. (2001) Anatomical MRI study of basal ganglia in bipolar disorder patients. *Psychiatry Res Neuroimag Sect* 106:65–80.

Broadhead, J., and Jacoby, R. (1990) Mania in old age. A first prospective study. *Int J Geriatr Psychiatry* 5:215–222.

Burns, A., Jacoby, R., and Levy, R. (1990) Psychiatric phenomena in Alzheimer's disease. III. Disorders of mood. *Br J Psychol* 157: 81–86.

Burt, T., Prudic, J., Peyser, S., Clark, J., and Sackeim, H.A. (2000) Learning and memory in bipolar and unipolar major depression. Effects of aging. *Neuropsychiatr Neuropsychol Behav Neurol* 13:246–253.

Cade, J.F.J. (1949) Lithium salts in the treatment of psychotic excitement. *Med J Aust* 36:349–352.

Cassidy, F., and Carroll, B.J. (2001) Vascular risk factors in late-onset mania. *Psychol Med* 32(2):359–362.

Charron, M., Fortin, L., and Paquette, I. (2001) De novo mania among elderly people. *Acta Psychiatr Scand* 84:503–507.

Chen, S.T., Altshuler, L.L., Melnyk, K.A., Erhart, S.M., Miller, E., and Mintz, J. (1999) Efficacy of lithium vs. valproate in the treatment of mania in the elderly. A retrospective study. *J Clin Psychiatry* 60:181–185.

Chowdry, R., Ferrier, I.N., and Thompson, J.M. (2003) Cognitive dysfunction in bipolar disorder. *Curr Opin Psychiatry* 16:7–12.

Clayton, P.J. (1986a) Manic symptoms in the elderly. In: Busse, E., ed. *Aspects of Aging*. III. Disturbed Behavior in the Elderly. Report no. 3. Philadelphia: Smith Kline and French, pp. 3–13.

Clayton, P.J. (1986b) The epidemiology of bipolar affective disorder. *Compr Psychiatry* 22:31–43.

Coffman, J.A., Bornstein, R.A., Olson, S.C., Schwarzkopf, S.B., and Nasrallah, H.A. (1990) Cognitive impairment and cerebral structure by MRI in bipolar disorder. *Biol Psychiatry* 27:1188–1196.

Coryell, W., Scheffner, W., Keller, M., Endicott, J., Maser, J., and Klerman, G.L. (1993) The enduring psychosocial consequences of mania and depression. *Am J Psychiatry* 150(5):720–727.

Cummings, J.L. (1993) Fronto-subcortical circuits and human behavior. *Arch Neurol* 50:873–880.

De Asis, J., Young, R.C., Alexopoulos, G.S., Greenwald, B., Kakuma, T., and Ashtari, M. (1998) Signal hyperintensities in geriatric mania. Abstract, annual meeting, American Psychiatric Association, Chicago, Ill.

Derby, I.M. (1933) Manic depressive "exhaustion" deaths. *Psychiatr Q* 7:436–449.

Dhingra, U., and Rabins, P.V. (1991) Mania in the elderly. A five-to-seven year follow-up. *J Am Geriatr Soc* 39:581–583.

Dunn, K.L., and Rabins, P.V. (1996) Mania in old age. In: Shulman, K.I., Tohen, M., and Kutcher, S.P., eds. *Mood Disorders Across the Life Span*. New York: John Wiley and Sons, pp. 399–406.

Eagles, J.M., and Whalley, L.J. (1985) Ageing and affective disorders. The age at first onset of affective disorders in Scotland 1966–1978. *Br J Psychiatry* 147:180–187.

Folstein, M. (February 1999) Mania, agitation and Alzheimer's disease. Abstract, annual meeting, American Association of Geriatric Psychiatry,

Folstein, M.F., Folstein, S.E., and McHugh, P.R. (1975) Mini-Mental State. A practical method for grading the cognitive state of patients for the clinician. *J Psychiatr Res* 12:189–198.

Folstein, S.E. (1989) *Huntington's Disease. A Disorder of Families.* Baltimore: Johns Hopkins University Press.

Fujikawa, T., Yamawaki, S., and Touhouda, Y. (1995) Silent cerebral infarctions in patients with late-onset mania. *Stroke* 26:946–949.

Gitlin, M.H., Swendsen, J., and Heller, T.L. (1995) Relapse and impairment in bipolar disorder. *Am J Psychiatry* 152:1635–1640.

Glasser, M., and Rabins, P.V. (1984) Mania in the elderly. *Age Aging* 13:210–213.

Hays, P. (1976) Etiological factors in manic depressive psychosis. *Arch Gen Psychiatry* 33:1187–1188.

Henderson, D., and Gillespie, R.D. (1956) *A Textbook of Psychiatry for Students and Practitioners*, 8th ed. London: Oxford University Press.

Hewick, D.S., Newburg, P., Hopwood, S., Naylor, G., and Moody, J. (1977) Age as a factor affecting lithium therapy. *Br J Clin Pharmacol* 4:201–205.

Himmelhoch, J., Neil, J.R., May, S.J., Fuchs, S., and Licata, S.M. (1980) Age, dementia, dyskinesias, and lithium response. *Am J Psychiatry* 137:941–945.

Jamison, K.R., and Goodwin, F.K. (1990) In: Jamison, K.R., and Goodwin, F.K. (eds.) Medical treatment of acute bipolar depression. *Manic Depressive Illness* New York: Oxford University Press, 631–664.

Joffe, R.T., Lippert, G.P., Gray, T.A., Sawa, G., and Horrath, Z. (1987) Mood disorder and multiple sclerosis. *Arch Neurol* 44:376–378.

Jorge, R.E., Robinson, R.G., Starkstein, S.E., Arndt, S.V., Forrester, A.W., and Geisler, F.H. (1993) Secondary mania following traumatic brain injury. *Am J Psychiatry* 150:916–921.

Kalayam, B., and Alexopoulos, G.S. (1999) Prefrontal dysfunction and treatment response in geriatric depression. *Arch Gen Psychiatry* 56:713–718.

Kay, D.W.K., Roth, M., and Hopkins, B. (1955) Affective disorders arising in the senium, I. Their association with organic cerebral degeneration. *J Ment Sci* 101:302–316.

Kerry, R.J., McDermott, C.M., and Orme, J.E. (1983) Affective disorders and cognitive performance. *J Affect Disord* 5:345–352.

Kling, A., and Steklis, H.D. (1976) A neural substrate for affiliative behavior in nonhuman primates. *Brain Behav Evol* 13:216–238.

Kraepelin, E. (1921) *Manic-Depressive Insanity and Paranoia* (Barclay, R.M., trans. and ed.). Edinburgh: E. and S. Livingstone.

Krauthammer, C., and Klerman, G. (1978) Secondary mania. *Arch Gen Psychiatry* 35:1333–1339.

Lehman, S., and Rabins, P.V. (2001) Factors influencing treatment outcomes in geriatric mania. Abstract, Annual Meeting Soc. of *Biol Psychiatry* New Orleans, LA.

Leibovici, A., and Tariot, P.N. (1988) Carbamazepine treatment of agitation associated with dementia. *J Geriatr Psychiatry Neurol* 1:110–112.

Liu, C.-Y., Wang, S.-J., Fuh, J.-L., Yang, Y.-Y., and Liu, H.-C. (1996) Bipolar disorder following a stroke involving the left hemisphere. *Aust NZ J Psychiatry* 30:688–691.

Loranger, A.W., and Levine, P.M. (1978) Age-at-onset of bipolar affective illness. *Arch Gen Psychiatry* 35:345.

Lundquist, G. (1945) Prognosis and course in manic depressive psychoses. A follow-up study of 319 first admissions. *Acta Psychiatr Scand* Suppl 1:1–96.

Lyketsos, C.G., Corazzini, K., and Steele, C. (1995) Mania in Alzheimer's disease. *J Neuropsychiatry Clin Neurosci* 7:350–352.

MacDonald, J.B. (1918) Prognosis in manic-depressive insanity. *J Nerv Ment Dis* 47:20–30.

Manji, H.K., Moore, G.J., and Chen, G. (1999) Lithium at 50. Have the neuroprotective effects of this unique cation been overlooked? *Biol Psychiatry* 46:929–940.

Marneros, A., and Angst. J. (2000) Bipolar disorders. Roots and evolution. In: Marneros, A., and Angst. J., eds. *Bipolar Disorders.* Dordrecht, the Netherlands: pp. 1–35.

McDonald, W.M., Krishnan, K.R., Doraiswamy, P.M., and Blazer, D.G. (1991) Occurrence of subcortical hyperintensities in elderly subjects with mania. *Psychol Res* 40(4):211–220.

McDonald, W.M., Tupler, L.A., Marsteller, F.A., Figiel, G.S., DeSouza, S., Nemeroff, C.B., and Krishnan, K.R.R. (1999) Hyperintense lesions on magnetic resonance images in bipolar disorder. *Biol Psychiatry* 45:965–971.

McDonald, W.M., Krishnan, K.R., Doraiswamy, P.M., and Blazer, D.G. (1991) Occurrence of subcortical hyperintensities in elderly subjects with mania. *Psychol Res* 40:211–220.

McMahon, F.J., and DePaulo, J.R. (1996) Genetics and age-at-onset. In: Shulman, T.K., ed. *Mood Disorders Across the Life Span.* New York: Wiley-Liss, pp. 35–48.

Mega, M.S., Dinov, I.D., Lee, L., O'Connor, S.M., Masterman, D.M., Wilen, N., Mishkin, F., Toga, A.W., and Cummings, J.L. (2000) Orbital and dorsolateral perfusion defect associated with behavioral response to cholinesterase inhibitor therapy in Alzheimer disease. *Neuroscience* 12:209–218.

Mendlewics, J., Fieve, R.R., Rainer, J.D., and Fleiss, J.L. (1972) Manic depressive illness. A comparative study of patients with and without a family history. *Br J Psychiatry* 120:523–530.

Miller, B.L., Cummings, J.L., Villanueva-Meyer, J., Boone, K., Mehringer, C.M., Lesser, I.M., et al. (1991) Frontal lobe degeneration. Clinical, neuropsychological, and SPECT characteristics. *Neurology* 41:1374–1382.

Moore, G.J., Bebchuk, J.M., Hasanat, K., et al. (2000a) In vivo evidence in support of bcl-2's neurotrophic effects? *Biol Psychiatry* 48(1):1–8.

Moore, G.J., Bebchuk, J.M., Wilds, I.B., Chen, G., and Manji, H.K. (2000b) Lithium-induced increase in human brain grey matter. *Lancet* 356(9237):1241–1242.

Murphy, C., Klimstra, S., Alexopoulos, G.S., and Young, R.C. (2001) Perseveration in geriatric manic disorder vs. unipolar depression. AAGP Annual Meeting, December, 2001.

Murray, E., Hopwood, S., and Balfour, J. (1983) The influence of age on lithium efficacy and side-effects in outpatients. *Psychol Med* 13:53–60.

Nadeem, A., Young, R.C., deAsis, J., and Alexopoulos, G.S. (2000) Stroke risk factors in geriatric mania. In:

Nemeroff, C.B., Evans, D.L., Gyulai, L., Sachs, G.S., Bowden, C.L., Gergel, I.P., and Oakes, R. (2001) Double-blind, placebo-controlled comparison of imipramine and paroxetine in the treatment of bipolar depression. *Am J Psychiatry* 158(6):906–912.

Niedermier, J.A., and Nasrallah, H.A. (1998) Clinical correlates of response to valproate in geriatric inpatients. *Ann Clin Psychiatry* 10:165–168.

O'Connell, R.A., Mayo, J.A., Flatow, L., et al. (1991) Outcome of bipolar disorder on long-term treatment with lithium. *Br J Psychiatry* 159:123–129.

Okuma, T., et al. (1990) Comparison of the antimanic efficacy of carbamazepine and lithium carbonate by double-blind controlled study. *Pharmacopsychiatry* 23(3):143–150.

Oppenheim, J. (1890) Zur pathologie der grosshirngeschwulste. *Arch Psychiatr Nervenkr* 21:560–587.

Petrie, W.M., et al. (1982) Violence in geriatric patients. *JAMA* 248:443–444.

Post, F. (1965) The clinical psychiatry of late life. In: Oxford: Pergamon Press, pp. 79–82.

Post, F. (1971) Schizo-affective symptomatology in late life. *Br J Psychiatry* 118:437–445.

Rabins, P.V., Aylward, E., Holroyd, S., and Pearlson, G. (2000) MRI findings differentiate between late-onset schizophrenia and mood disorder. *Int J Geriatr Psychiatry* 15:954–960.

Rice, J.P., and Reich, T., et al. (1987) The familial transmission of bipolar illness. *Arch Gen Psychiatry* 44:441–447.

Roose, S.P., Nurnberger, J., Dunner, D., et al. (1979) Cardiac sinus node dysfunction during lithium treatment. *Am J Psychiatry* 136: 804–806.

Rosen, L.N., Rosenthal, N.E., Van Dusen, P.H., Dunner, D.L., and Fieve, R.R. (1984) Age-at-onset and number of psychotic symptoms in bipolar I and schizoaffective disorder. *Am J Psychiatry* 140:1523–1524.

Roth, M. (1955) The natural history of mental disorder in old age. *J Ment Sci* 101:281–301.

Rubinsztein, J.S., Michael, A., Paykel, E.S., and Sahakian, B.J. (2000) Cognitive impairment in remission in bipolar affective disorder. *Psychol Med* 30:1025–1036.

Sackeim, H.A., Greenberg, M.S., Weiman, A.L., Gur, R.C., Hungerbuhler, J.P., and Geschwind, N. (1982) Hemispheric asymmetry in the expression of positive and negative emotions. *Arch Neurol* 39:210–218.

Sajatovic, M., Vernon, L., and Semple, W. (1997) Clinical characteristics and health resource use of men and women veterans with serious mental illness. *Psych Serv* 48(11):1461–1463.

Savard, R.J., Rey, C., and Post, R.M. (1980) Halstead-Reitan Category Test in bipolar and unipolar affective disorders. Relationship to age and phase of illness. *J Nerv Ment Dis* 168:297–304.

Shulman, K.I. (1997) Disinhibition syndromes, secondary mania and bipolar disorder in old age. *J Affect Disord* 46:175–182.

Shulman, K., and Post, F. (1980) Bipolar affective disorders in old age. *Br J Psychiatry* 136:26–32.

Shulman, K.I., and Tohen, M. (1994) Unipolar mania reconsidered. Evidence from an elderly cohort. *Br J Psychiatry* 164:547–549.

Shulman, K.I., Tohen, M., Satlin, A., Gopinath, M., and Kalunian, D. (1993) Mania compared with unipolar depression in old age. *Am J Psychiatry* 149:341–345.

Slater, E., and Roth, M. (1977) *Mayer-Gross, Slater, and Roth's Clinical Psychiatry*, 3rd ed. London: Bailliere, Tindall and Cassell.

Slavney, P.R., Rich, G.B., Pearlson, G.D., and McHugh, P.R. (1977) Phencyclidine abuse and symptomatic mania. *Biol Psychiatry* 12:697–700.

Snowdon, J. (1991) A retrospective case-note study of bipolar disorder in old age. *Br J Psychiatry* 158:485–490.

Spicer, C.C., Hare, E.H., and Slater, E. (1973) Neurotic and psychotic forms of depressive illness. Evidence from age incidence in a national sample. *Br J Psychiatry* 123:535–541.

Starkstein, S.E., Boston, J.D., and Robinson, R.G. (1988) Mechanisms of mania after brain injury. Twelve case reports and review of the literature. *J Nerv Ment Dis* 176:87–100.

Starkstein, S.E., Mayberg, H.S., Berthier, M.L., Fedoroff, P., Price, T.R., Dannals, R.F., Wagner, H.N., Leiguarda, R., and Robinson, R.G. (1997) Mechanism of disinhibition after brain lesions. *J Nerv Ment Dis* 185:108–114.

Starkstein, S.E., et al. (1990) Mania after brain injury. Neuroradiological and metabolic findings. *Ann Neurol* 27:652–659.

Starkstein, S.E., Federoff, P., Berthier, M.L., and Robinson, R.G. (1991) Manic depressive and pure manic states after brain lesions. *Biol Psychiatry* 29:773–782.

Steffens, D.C., and Krishnan, K.R.R. (1998) Structural neuroimaging and mood disorders. Recent findings, implications for classification, and future directions. *Biol Psychiatry* 43:705–712.

Stoll, A.L., Banov, M., Kolbrener, M., Mayer, P.V., Tohen, M., Strakowski, S.M., et al. (1994) Neurologic factors predict a favorable valproate response in bipolar and schizoaffective disorders. *J Clin Psychopharm* 14:311–313.

Stone, K. (1989) Mania in the elderly. *Br J Psychiatry* 155:220–224.

Strakowski, S.M., McElroy, S.L., Keck, P., and West, S. (1994) The co-occurrence of mania with medical and other psychiatric disorders. *Int J Psychiatry Med* 24:305–328.

Strauss, M.E., Bohannon, W.E., Stephens, J.H., and Paulker, N.E.

(1984) Perceptual span in schizophrenia and affective disorders. *J Nerv Ment Dis* 172:431–435.

Swann, A.C. (1995) Mixed or dysphoric manic states. Psychopathology and treatment. *J Clin Psychiatry* 56:6–10.

Swift, H.M. (1907) The prognosis of recurrent insanity of the manic depressive type. *Am J Insanity* 64:311–326.

Tariot, P.N., Schneider, L.S., Mintzer, J.E., Cutler, A.J., Cunningham, M.R., Thomas, J.W., et al. (2001) Safety and tolerability of divalproex sodium in the treatment of signs and symptoms of mania in elderly patients with dementia. Results of a double-blind, placebo-controlled trial. *Curr Ther Res* 62:51–67.

Taylor, M.A., and Abrams, R. (1981) Prediction of treatment response in mania. *Arch Gen Psychiatry* 38:800–803.

Thompson, J.M., Ferrier, I.N., Hughes, J.H., Gray, J.M., and Young, A.H. (2000) Neuropsychological function in a cohort of bipolar patients prospectively verified as euthymic. *Acta Neuropsychiatrica* 12:170.

Tohen, M., Shulman, K.I., and Satlin, A. (1994) First-episode mania in late life. *Am J Psychiatry* 151:30–132.

Turecki, G., Mari, J.D.J., and Porto, J.A.D. (1993) Bipolar disorder following left basal ganglia stroke. *Br J Psychiatry* 163:690.

van der Velde, C.D. (1970) Effectiveness of lithium carbonate in the treatment of manic-depressive illness. *Am J Psychiatry* 123:345–351.

van Gorp, W., Altshuler, L., Theverg, D.C., Wilkins, J., and Dixon, W. (1998) Cognitive impairment in euthymic bipolar patients with and without prior alcohol dependence. *Arch Gen Psychiatry* 55: 41–46.

van Scheyen, J.D., and van Kammen, D.P. (1979) Clomipramine-induced mania in unipolar depression. *Arch Gen Psychiatry* 36: 560–565.

Verdoux, H., and Bourgeois. M. (1995) Manies secondaires a des pathologies organiques cerebrales. *Ann Med Psychol* 153:161–168.

Walter-Ryan, W.G. (1983) Mania with onset in the ninth decade. *J Clin Psychiatry* 44:430–431.

Weissman, M.M., Bruce, M.L., Leak, P.J., Leak, P.J., Florio, L.P., and Holzer, C., III. (1990) Affective disorders. In: Robins, L.N., and Regier, D.A., eds. *Psychiatric Disorders in America. The Epidemiologic Catchment Area Study.* New York: Free Press, pp. 53–80.

Welt, L. (1888) Uber characterveranderungen der menschen infolge von lasionen des stirnhirn. *Arch Klin Med* 42:339–390.

Wendkos, M.H. (1979) Acute Exhaustive mania. In: *Sudden Death in Psychiatric Illness.* New York: SP Medical and Scientific Books, pp. 165–176.

Wertham, F.I. (1929) A group of benign chronic psychoses. Prolonged manic excitements with a statistical study of age, duration and frequency in 2,000 manic attacks. *Am J Psychiatry* 86:17–78.

Wylie, M.E., Mulsant, B.H., Pollock, B., Sweet, R.A., Zubenko, G. S., Begley, A.E., et al. (1999) Age-at-onset in geriatric bipolar disorder. *Am J Geriatr Psychiatry* 7:77–83.

Yassa, R., Nair, N.P.V., and Iskandar, H. (1988) Late onset bipolar disorder in psychosis and depression in the elderly. *Psychiatr Clin North Am* 11:117–131.

Yassa, R., Nair, V., and Nastase, C. (1988) Prevalence of bipolar disorder in a psychogeriatric population. *J Affect Disord* 14:197.

Young, R.C., Jain, J., Kiosses, D., and Meyers, B.S. (2003) Antidepressant-associated mania in late life. *Int J Geriatr Psychiatry* 18:421–424.

Young, R.C., Biggs, J.T., Ziegler, V.E., and Meyer, D.A. (1978) A rating scale for mania. Reliability, validity, and sensitivity. *Br J Psychiatry* 133:429–435.

Young, R.C., Gyulai, L., Mulsant, B., Flint, A., Beyer, J., Shulman, K.I., and Reynolds, C.F. Pharmacotherapy of bipolar disorder in old age. *Am J Geriatric Psychiatry* (in press).

Young, R.C., Murphy, C.F., DeAsis, J.M., Apfeldorf, W.J., and Alexopoulos, G.S. (2001) Executive dysfunction and treatment outcome in geriatric mania. New Research Abstract, Annual Meeting, American Psychiatric Associates, New Orleans, LA.

Young, R.C., Murphy, C.F., Stern, Y., and Alexopoulos, G.S. (2001) Response inhibition in geriatric mania. Abstract, annual meeting of the American College of Neuropsychopharmacology, Hawaii.

Young, R.C., Nambudiri, D., Jain, H., DeAsis, J., and Alexopoulos, G. (1999) Brain computed tomography in geriatric manic disorder. *Biol Psychiatry* 45:1063–1065.

Young, R.C., and Falk, J.R. (1989) Age, manic psychopathology and treatment response. *Int J Geriatr Psychiatry* 4:73–78.

Young, R.C., and Klerman, G.L. (1992) Mania in late life. Focus on age-at-onset. *Am J Psychiatry* 149:867–876.

Young, R.C., Schreiber, M.T., and Nysewander, R.W. (1983) Psychotic mania. *Biol Psychiatry* 18:1167–1173.

Yu, X.L., and Young, R.C. (2001) Geriatric schizoaffective disorder: Subtypes. Abstract. Annual Meeting, American Association of Geriatric Psychiatry San Francisco, CA.

# 5 | Dysthymic disorder in the elderly

D.P. DEVANAND

Several terms have been used for chronic mild to moderate depressive illness: *chronic minor depression, depressive neurosis, depressive personality, chronic dysphoria*, and *intermittent depression*. *Dysthymic disorder* denotes chronic depression with fewer symptoms than in major depressive disorder, and it affects 2%–4% of adults (Gwirtsman et al., 1997).

## PREVALENCE

In the Epidemiological Catchment Area (ECA) study of five U.S. communities, the prevalence of DSM-III dysthymic disorder was 3.1% in the adult population (Weissman et al., 1988). In the age range of 18–44 years, the rate of dysthymic disorder was higher in people of lower socioeconomic status. More than 75% of adults with dysthymia had other psychiatric disorders, particularly major depression, anxiety disorders, and substance abuse. In the elderly subsample in the ECA study, the prevalence of dysthymic disorder was only 1.5%, a rate lower than that reported in most other epidemiological studies. The decline in prevalence after age 65 was difficult to interpret because the sample size of elderly subjects was relatively small, age at onset of dysthymic disorder was not determined, and subjects in assisted living and nursing home facilities were not evaluated.

Other epidemiological studies conducted in elderly community samples indicate that dysthymic disorder ranges in prevalence from 2% to 5%. In a population study in North Carolina, Blazer et al. (1987) reported that 27% of community-residing elderly individuals reported depressive symptoms: 19% mild dysphoria, 4% symptomatic depression, 1.2% mixed depression/anxiety, 0.8% major depression, and 2% dysthymia. In European studies, the prevalence of dysthymia in the elderly has been somewhat higher, ranging from 4% to 7% (Carta et al., 1995; Fichter et al., 1995; Stefansson et al., 1991). Ernst and Angst (1995) suggested that severe depressive disorders decrease in old age and are replaced by milder forms of depressive illness, including dysthymia.

In the Cache County epidemiological study in Utah, nursing homes and other assisted living facilities were included in the survey (Steffens et al., 2000). Among 4559 elderly subjects, 25.1% endorsed depressed mood, 12.4% endorsed anhedonia, and 7.9% endorsed irritability. Women endorsed these items more often than men, and the prevalence of major depression was 2.7% in men and 4.4% in women, with no effect of age across the age range studied. The prevalence of major depression was higher than that reported in other epidemiological studies (Blazer et al., 1988; Carta et al., 1995). Among depressed patients, 35.7% were taking antidepressants and 27.4% were taking a sedative/hypnotic. Using a narrow definition of dysthymic disorder (requiring two of four symptoms that were arbitrarily selected from the list of six symptoms in the DSM-III criteria), the prevalence of dysthymia in the elderly was less than 1%. The selection of the four symptoms to make the diagnosis was problematic because two of them were vegetative symptoms that are not commonly endorsed by elderly patients (Devanand et al., 1994; Oxman et al., 2000). Another limitation was the homogeneity of the almost exclusively Mormon sample, and the results obtained may not generalize well to other populations.

In a community screening study, 40 elderly subjects with dysthymic disorder were compared to 630 non-depressed elderly subjects (Kirby et al., 1999). Dysthymic disorder was of late onset in 93% and was associated with a major stressor in 65%. Co-morbid Axis I disorders were present in 15% and Axis II disorders in 10%. Greater physical impairment was present in the dysthymic subjects than in the nondepressed subjects, and 83% presented to their general practitioner with anxiety/depressive symptoms at some stage during the course of their dysthymic disorder. These results indicate that dysthymic disorder in elderly subjects is predominantly of the late-onset type with few co-morbid Axis I or II disorders.

Clinical studies also show that elderly dysthymic subjects typically have late onset (in middle age or later) and are not merely young dysthymic subjects who simply grew older (Devanand et al., 1994; 2004). This finding raises the intriguing question of what happens to young adults with dysthymic disorder as they grow older. There are several possible explanations: progression to recurrent or chronic major depression, remission from depressive illness, or death due to suicide. The long-term studies needed to clarify these issues—for example, following up dysthymic patients from young adulthood to old age—have not yet been conducted. Data on young adults with dysthymic disorder followed for a few years suggest that the majority have a persistent, chronic illness (Klein et al., 2000). In community samples, chronicity appears to be characteristic of elderly dysthymic subjects as well (Pulska et al., 1998).

## DIAGNOSIS

The diagnosis of dysthymic disorder was introduced in DSM-III to describe a chronic depressive disorder less severe (defined as fewer symptoms) than major depressive disorder. There has been a long-standing debate about whether the diagnosis of patients with chronic mild to moderate depressive symptoms should be classified under personality disorder or affective disorder. The evidence from a variety of studies of phenomenology, clinical course, family history, and response to treatment has led to the classification of dysthymic disorder as an affective disorder. However, within the framework of affective disorder, it remains unclear if dysthymic disorder is indeed separate or is on a continuum with chronic major depressive disorder (Gwirtsman et al., 1997; Hirschfeld, 1994). There is some evidence that major depression and panic disorder are better differentiated by specific symptoms than are dysthymia and generalized anxiety disorder (Clark et al., 1994), suggesting that the latter two diagnostic entities need further validation studies.

Akiskal's (1983) subtyping of mild to moderate chronic depressive syndromes provides a useful conceptual approach to understand the main subtypes among these conditions. One limitation to using this approach is that a large enough body of research is not available to validate this subtyping in young adults, and there has been no research on this classification in the elderly. Akiskal's classification was developed partly to address the problem of separating trait (personality) from state (depression). In this classification, *subaffective dysthymia* resembles dysthymic disorder in the DSM-III system. The other diagnostic categories are primary depression with residual chronicity (resembles major depression in partial remission), chronic secondary dysphoria secondary (occurring later in time) to a medical or other psychiatric condition, and character-spectrum disorder (depressive personality) unresponsive to antidepressants.

The classification of subthreshold (defined as less severe than major depression) depression in the elderly remains the subject of ongoing debate. Geiselmann and Bauer (2000) classified subthreshold depression in the elderly as a quantitatively minor variant of depression or a depression-like state with fewer symptoms or with less continuity, and as a qualitatively different condition from major depression with fewer suicidal thoughts or feelings of guilt or worthlessness, but accompanied by prominent worries about health and weariness of living. However, empirical data and validation studies to back up these clinical assertions are still lacking.

In DSM-III, the types of symptoms selected to make the diagnosis of dysthymic disorder were arbitrary, as was the minimum 2-year duration criterion (Kocsis and Francis, 1987). Subsequently, a field trial for DSM-IV was conducted in 524 depressed adults evaluated at several clinical sites. Double depression (dysthymia plus major depression) was common: 62% of dysthymic patients had concurrent major depression, and 79% had lifetime major depressive disorder (Keller et al., 1995). The results of this field trial showed that chronic major depression, double depression (major depression plus dysthymic disorder), and dysthymic disorder were all common conditions in psychiatric outpatient clinics. Evaluation of the frequency of symptom presentation suggested that the neurovegetative symptoms of appetite disturbance and decreased libido were uncommon in dysthymic patients, and insomnia was less common in dysthymic patients than in patients with major depression. The cognitive symptoms of hopelessness and worthlessness, and other symptoms indicating demoralization, were common in dysthymic disorder. In this study, content validity of the symptom criteria for dysthymia suggested emphasizing cognitive and social/motivational symptoms rather than neurovegetative symptoms (Keller et al., 1995). However, the results of this field trial did not impact materially on the DSM-IV symptom criteria for dysthymic disorder, which remained essentially unchanged from DSM-III (and DSM-III-R). As a compromise, the most frequent symptoms reported by dysthymic patients in the field trial were listed under the Alternative Research Criterion B for dysthymia in the DSM-IV Appendix. A minimum 2-year duration criterion continues to be required to make this diagnosis, but empirical research to support this duration cutoff is still lacking. In the DSM-IV field trial, there was moderate 6-month test-retest reliability for the diagnosis of dysthymia (Keller et al., 1995).

Studies of elderly patients with dysthymic disorder have shown that the majority of these patients have a mid- to late-life age of onset and that loss of appetite, weight loss, and decreased libido are uncommon (Devanand et al., 1994). In elderly patients with dysthymic disorder who participated in a double-blind trial comparing fluoxetine to placebo, sleep changes were common (80.5%) but appetite changes were less frequent (20.7%). Feelings of hopelessness (53.2%) and worthlessness (67.5%) were common symptoms, both usually mild in severity (Devanand et al., in press). The few published studies on the symptom profile of elderly dysthymic patients indicate predominant amotivational (e.g., loss of interest, lack of energy) and cognitive (e.g., feelings of hopelessness and worthlessness) symptoms, with neurovegetative symptoms being less frequent (Devanand et al., 2004; Oxman et al., 2000). Therefore, for both young adult and elderly patients, the symptom criteria listed under the Alternative Research Criterion B for dysthymia in the DSM-IV Appendix may be more valid than the symptom criteria listed under the main DSM-IV diagnostic criteria for dysthymic disorder.

## AGE-AT-ONSET

In 84 consecutive adult outpatients with dysthymic disorder, a history of major depressive disorder, social phobia, panic disorder, and conversion disorder was more common in early-onset compared to late-onset patients (Barzega et al., 2001). These findings replicated those of earlier systematic studies that demonstrated that co-morbid major depression, anxiety disorders, substance abuse, and personality disorders are common in patients with early-onset dysthymic disorder (Klein et al., 1988a, 1998).

These studies used the DSM-IV specifier for early onset in the diagnosis of dysthymic disorder. DSM-IV defines early onset as age of onset of less than 21 years and late onset as age of onset after 21 years. However, recent studies indicate that 85%–95% of elderly patients with dysthymic disorder have an onset after 21 years of age (Devanand et al., 1994, 2004; Oxman et al., 2000) and that an age cutoff of 50 or 60 years may be more appropriate in defining early- versus late-onset dysthymia in elderly subjects. More important, the findings on age of onset and co-morbidity suggest that dysthymia is typically a different disorder in the elderly than in young adults.

In the first clinical study of elderly (≥60 years) patients with dysthymic disorder, the mean age of onset was 55.2 ± 15.4 years, and the vast majority had late age-at-onset. There was an equal gender distribution and limited co-morbid Axis I and II pathology (Devanand et al., 1994). These results stand in contrast to those concerning dysthymic disorder in young adults, where patients are predominantly female and early onset and co-morbid Axis I and II disorders are common (Klein et al., 1988b; Kocsis et al., 1988a). Double depression appears to be much less common in elderly dysthymic patients compared to young adults with this disorder (Devanand et al., 1994, 2004). Of note, in a sample of 416 adults with primary dysthymia who participated in a clinical trial (Thase et al., 1997), those

with onset in middle age had few co-morbid mental disorders compared to young adults, a finding similar to that in elderly dysthymic patients with onset in old age. These reports indicate some similarities between dysthymic patients with onset in middle age and old age.

Oxman et al. (2000) evaluated 216 patients with dysthymic disorder in the age groups 18–59 years and above 60 years in primary care settings. Younger patients were more likely to have symptoms of worthlessness, guilt, feeling trapped, feeling blue, feeling lonely, blaming the self, decreased sexual interest, and overeating. However, age-at-onset was not systematically evaluated, and it is possible that elderly dysthymic patients with early onset were more similar to young dysthymic patients than to patients with late-onset dysthymia. In another study of 106 patients, age was related positively to concomitant medical illnesses and to the number of recent life events but was negatively related to the presence of avoidant or dependent personality disorder. In young adults, dysthymic disorder was associated with abnormalities of personality and in the elderly with health problems and life losses (Bellino et al., 2001).

The high prevalence of co-morbid Axis I and II disorders in young adults with dysthymic disorder is particularly prominent in patients with DSM-IV early-onset disorder, that is, before 21 years of age. In fact, the average age-at-onset among adults with early onset varies from 5 to 12 years across studies (Klein et al., 1995, 2000; Markowitz et al., 1992), suggesting that many of these patients report having felt depressed from early childhood or as long as they could remember. In contrast, less than 10%–20% of elderly dysthymic patients present with such a long-standing history (Devanand et al., 1994, 2004).

In a series of 211 patients with major depression and 159 patients with dysthymic disorder who presented to a late-life depression clinic, late-onset (≥60 years) patients had a higher rate of cardiovascular disease, a lower rate of anxiety disorder, and a lower rate of family history of affective disorder compared to early-onset patients (Devanand et al., 2004). Late-onset dysthymic patients were more likely to have cardiovascular disease than early-onset dysthymic patients, but the rate of cardiovascular disease did not differ between late- and early-onset patients with major depression. Late-onset patients with major depression were less likely to have a family history of affective disorder than early-onset patients with major depression. Prevalence of anxiety disorders did not differ between the early- and late-onset patients with major depression, but was more common in the early-onset compared to the late-onset dysthymic patients. Late-onset dysthymic disorder did not differ from late-onset major depression in the rates of cardiovascular disease, anxiety disorders, and family history of affective disorder.

These results support the view that in the elderly, late-onset dysthymic disorder is typically different from early-onset dysthymic disorder. Cerebrovascular disease may play a role in the etiology of late-onset dysthymic disorder. The similarities between late-onset dysthymic disorder and late-onset major depressive disorder suggest that many elderly depressed patients have a single condition along a continuum.

In summary, it appears that in the vast majority of elderly dysthymic patients, their disorder begins in middle to old age, and that these late-onset patients typically do not have double depression or co-morbid Axis I or Axis II psychiatric disorders. It has also been suggested that there is an equal sex distribution in elderly patients with dysthymic disorder (Devanand et al., 2004; Oxman et al., 2000). This finding stands in striking contrast to that obtained in young adults with early age of onset, who are typically female with frequent co-morbid Axis I and II pathology.

## CO-MORBIDITY

Antecedent adverse life events are commonly reported by depressed patients in all age groups. In the elderly, as in young adults, the characteristic feature of depressed patients is that they perceive life events as having a much greater impact on them than do healthy controls (Devanand et al., 2002). This difference from healthy controls applies to both patients with major depression and patients with dysthymic disorder.

Dysthymic disorder usually predates co-morbid psychiatric disorders and is associated with specific comorbid Axis I and II diagnoses (Klein et al., 1998; Markowitz et al., 1992). Compared to patients with onset of dysthymic disorder after age 21, patients with early-onset dysthymic disorder have higher lifetime rates of co-morbid major depression (double depression) and anxiety disorders, seek treatment more frequently, have a higher rate of major affective disorders in first-degree relatives, and exhibit more severe depressive symptoms (Klein et al., 1995, 1998).

Studies in young adults consistently show that the vast majority of patients with the diagnosis of dysthymic disorder have a history of major depression or will develop a superimposed major depressive episode within the first 5 years of onset of dysthymia (Keller and Shapiro, 1982; Klein et al., 1998; Markowtiz et al., 1992). This finding raises the question of whether these patients with double depression indeed have a unique syndrome, dysthymic disorder, or whether they have chronic major depression with partial, sustained improvement (spontaneous or treatment-related) leading to the diagnosis of dysthymic disorder (primary depression with residual

chronicity in Akiskal's classification). In contrast to these findings in young adults, double depression appears to be infrequent in elderly patients with dysthymic disorder, suggesting a relatively *pure* syndrome.

When adults with double depression are treated with antidepressants, one-third of them improve to the extent that diagnostic criteria for major depression are no longer met, but dysthymia often persists. This also appears to be true of adults with double depression who are treated with electroconvulsive therapy (ECT) (Prudic et al., 1993). It remains unclear if similar results will be obtained in studies of double depression in the elderly, in whom this diagnosis is not common (Devanand et al., 1994; in 2004).

Co-morbid anxiety disorder is common in young adults with dysthymic disorder (Pini et al., 1997) but is uncommon in elderly patients with dysthymic disorder (Devanand et al., 1994, 2004). Alcohol/substance abuse is also common in young adults with dysthymic disorder (Klein et al., 2000). As is the case with major depressive disorder, it remains unclear which of the two disorders came first. Alcohol abuse does occur in a small proportion of elderly patients with dysthymic disorder, but other forms of substance abuse are rare (Devanand et al., 2004).

In young adults, personality disorders are frequent co-morbid diagnoses in patients with dysthymic disorder, particularly those with double depression. The most common Axis II disorders in young adults with dsythymic disorder are in Cluster B according to the DSM classification: borderline, narcissistic, and histrionic, with avoidant and obsessive-compulsive being the most common Cluster C diagnoses (Klein et al., 1988b; Pepper et al., 1995; Riso et al., 1996; Sansone et al., 1998). Elderly patients with dysthymic disorder have a different profile with respect to personality disorders. In a series of 76 elderly patients with dysthymic disorder, 31% met criteria for at least one personality disorder (Devanand et al., 2000). Obsessive-compulsive (17.1%) and avoidant (11.8%) personality disorders were the most common types of personality disorder, while borderline (5.3%), narcissistic (2.6%), histrionic (0%), and antisocial (0%) subtypes were rare or nonexistent. These data suggest that elderly patients with dysthymic disorder are different from young adults with dysthymic disorder but similar to elderly patients with major depressive disorder, in whom obsessive-compulsive and avoidant personality disorders are not infrequent (Abrams et al., 1994, 1998).

## FAMILY HISTORY

A strong familial relationship between dysthymia and major depression has been reported in patients with early-onset dysthymic disorder. Across subtypes of dysthymic disorder, there is limited evidence that dysthymia may run "true" in the families of these patients (Klein et al., 1995). In these early-onset patients, dysthymia may have a stronger familial association with personality disorders than with major depression (Klein et al., 1995). A family history of affective disorder is not uncommon in elderly patients with dysthymic disorder, with a somewhat higher rate in early-onset compared to late-onset patients (Devanand et al., 2004). As is the case with major depressive disorder, elderly patients with late-onset (in middle to old age) dysthymic disorder typically do not have high familial loading for affective disorder, indicating that genetic etiology is not a likely explanation for late-onset depressive illness.

## SOCIAL ADJUSTMENT, QUALITY OF LIFE, AND DISABILITY

Increased service use and social morbidity are associated with depressive symptoms in the community (Johnson et al., 1992). There are well-established associations among dysthymic disorder, poor social adjustment, and poor functioning in young adults (Leader and Klein, 1996). Subsyndromal depressive symptoms and disorders, including dysthymic disorder, are associated with functional impairment across many areas of daily living (Judd et al., 1996). In 416 young adult patients with primary dysthymia who were randomized to treatment with sertraline, imipramine, and placebo, the outcome on social adjustment was superior in the two medication groups compared to the placebo group (Kocsis et al., 1997), consistent with the findings of prior studies (Kocsis et al., 1988b; Stewart et al., 1988). Similar findings have been obtained in studies of elderly depressed patients. Elderly patients with major depressive disorder who responded to treatment with nortriptyline and/or interpersonal therapy improved on the General Life Functioning scale (Mazumdar et al., 1996). In a study comparing fluoxetine to placebo in elderly patients with dysthymic disorder, a treatment response was associated with improvement in measures related to quality of life, despite the fact that the response to fluoxetine was limited (Devanand et al., in press).

Lack of social support, loneliness, and handicap are common in depressed patients in old age (Prince et al., 1997). In a sample of 113 elderly subjects with unipolar major depression followed for 1 year, instrumental support was protective against worsening performance on instrumental activities of daily living (Hays et al., 2001). Subjective and structural dimensions of social support protected the more severely depressed patients against the loss of basic maintenance abilities.

The Global Burden of Disease Report of the World Health Organization identified unipolar depression as the world's leading cause of disability, accounting for 10.7% of disability and responsible for more than 1 in 10 years lived with disability (WHO, 1996). In a study involving 11,242 medical outpatients, depression was associated with physical, social, and role impairment, poor perceived current health, and greater bodily pain (Wells et al., 1989). In a Finnish survey with 6 to 12 years of follow-up, dysthymic disorder in the elderly was associated with higher mortality, mainly due to physical illness and disability (Pulska et al., 1998).

From these reports, it is clear that depressive disorders, including dysthymic disorder, across the life span are associated with poor social adjustment and poor general functioning. In addition, the elderly demonstrate considerable disability as a result of depressive illness, and interventions directed at improving depressive symptoms should also aim at improving function and quality of life.

## PROGNOSIS

The intervening confound of treatment, or lack of it, makes it difficult to develop an accurate model to describe the likely prognosis for patients with dysthymic disorder. Nonetheless, several studies in young adults, and a few reports in the elderly, provide useful information on this issue. Overall, the data in young adults suggest a chronic illness with a low likelihood of sustained remission, but comparable long-term clinical data are not yet available in elderly patients with dysthymic disorder.

In a 12-year follow-up study of adults with depressive disorders, diagnostic criteria for minor depression and dysthymia were met frequently during the course of recurrent major depressive disorder, suggesting that diagnoses shifted over time during long-term follow-up (Judd et al., 1996). The confound of antidepressant treatment was analyzed but not fully controlled in this study. In 86 young adults with dysthymic disorder who presented for clinical evaluation, the diagnosis of dysthymic disorder was stable over 30 months of follow-up in the majority of these outpatients (Klein et al., 1998). Only 39% of patients with early-onset (<21 years) dysthymic disorder recovered during the follow-up period. In a young adult outpatient study, half of the patients with dysthymic disorder did not recover during 5-year follow-up, and dysthymic disorder was typically a chronic condition with a protracted course and a high risk of relapse (Klein et al., 2000). In adults with dysthymic disorder, Hayden and Klein (2001) reported that the presence of co-morbid anxiety disorder, personality disorders, and chronic stress was associated with a lower rate of recovery from dysthymic disorder during follow-up. A family history of bipolar disorder was associated with a higher probability of recovery, suggesting that the presentation of dysthymic disorder in some patients was a forme fruste of bipolar depression. Double depression may have a worse long-term prognosis than dysthymia alone and major depression alone (Chen et al., 2000). The relatively low rate of double depression in elderly dysthymic patients indirectly suggests that the prognosis may not be as poor as in young adults (Devanand et al., 1994, 2004), but systematic studies are needed to address this issue directly.

In a long-term follow-up study of healthy elderly men, the presence of affective spectrum disorder, broadly defined, before age 53 predicted a poor psychosocial outcome and poor physical health at age 65 (Vaillant et al., 1996). In a European epidemiological study of elderly subjects, both men and women with dysthymic disorder in old age had a poor prognosis (Pulska et al., 1998). In 1920 adults followed long-term in the Baltimore Longitudinal Study on Aging, the lifetime prevalence of major depression was 9.8%, that of dysthymia was 7.3%, and that of depressive syndrome (broadly defined, including minor depression) was 16%. Double depression had the earliest onset and the worst course (Chen et al., 2000). Dysthymia, unlike the other disorders, was not associated with a family history of depression or stressful life events. In a separate report from the same cohort, a history of depressive disorder was associated with an increased risk (relative risk 2.6) of stroke during a 13-year follow-up period. In another study, dysthymia was also associated with an increased risk of stroke but the relationship was not statistically significant (Larson et al., 2001).

In an epidemiological study of elderly Finns, there was lower survival of both elderly men and women with dysthymic disorder, but this association was largely explained by the frequent occurrence of somatic diseases and disabilities in these subjects (Pulska et al., 1998). In a 6-year follow-up study of Dutch community subjects with late-life depression, symptoms generally persisted and the majority of patients had either a chronic course or an unfavorable but fluctuating course (Beekman et al., 2002). In another study of 489 community subjects averaging 63 years of age with repeat evaluation up to 4 years after the initial assessment, the average annual incidence of a major depressive episode in the subset with baseline dysthymic disorder was 210 per 1000 but only 21 per 1000 for those with minor depression and 13 per 1000 for those with subsyndromal depression (Murphy et al., 2002). This suggests an overlap between dysthymic disorder and major depressive disorder but not between the other subthreshold depressive syndromes and major depressive disorder in the elderly. In subjects without a diagnosis of a depressive disorder at baseline evaluation, the symptoms of wanting to die and feeling worthless were the most predictive of future depression in the cohort interviewed 4 years later. Therefore, psycholog-

ical symptoms of self-disparagement appeared to be important indicators of future depressive illness in the elderly. In that study, sleep disturbance, especially insomnia, was not specific for diagnosis or prognosis. In a psychological autopsy study of 85 completed suicides in Sweden, recurrent major depression and substance use disorder were found to be very strong risk factors for suicide (Waern et al., 2002). Dysthymic disorder also posed an increased risk of suicide, but this risk was lower than that posed by major depression.

Most studies have focused primarily on elderly community samples. Less is known about the long-term prognosis of elderly patients with dysthymic disorder who present for clinical evaluation and treatment. Nonetheless, the evidence to date strongly suggests that dysthymic disorder, which is chronic by definition, usually persists and may worsen over time to reach the level of major depression in the elderly, particularly in the absence of effective treatment.

## DYSTHYMIC DISORDER IN PRIMARY CARE

Most elderly patients with dysthymic disorder present to a primary care physician rather than to a mental health professional (Williams et al., 2000). In a recent study that used the mental component summary of the SF-36 rating form in an elderly Medicare fee-for-service sample, the prevalence of either major depression or dysthymia was 25% (McCall et al., 2002).

The ability of primary care physicians to identify dysthymic disorder and other depressive disorders is known to be less than optimal, and treatment for these patients is often lacking or inadequate (Sherbourne et al., 1994). The low-grade chronicity of dysthymic disorder may contribute to the problems of inaccurate diagnosis and undertreatment. Wells et al. (2000) conducted a large-scale study in primary care and established that it is cost-effective to treat depression in the primary health care setting. Quality improvement in the standard of care is crucial, and the usual primary care model may need to be modified to be cost-effective. A collaborative care model has been shown to be effective in the treatment of depression in primary care (Unutzer et al., 2002). In an ongoing multicenter study, there is initial evidence that using a case manager to identify and arrange for treatment of depressed patients helps to improve the clinical outcome in the primary care setting (Mulsant et al., 2001a).

## RATING SCALES

As discussed earlier, the DSM-IV symptom criteria for major depression maintain an emphasis on neurovegetative symptoms, even though the DSM-IV field trial indicated that cognitive/behavioral symptoms are more common in adults with dysthymic disorder. The most frequent symptoms reported by patients with dysthymic disorder in the DSM-IV field trial are the nine items in the Alternative Criterion B for Dysthymic Disorder in the DSM-IV Appendix. Studies in elderly dysthymic patients also show that cognitive/behavioral symptoms such as poor self-esteem and social withdrawal are more common than neurovegetative symptoms (Devanand et al., 2004; Oxman et al., 2000). These findings suggest that traditional rating scales that have been used to evaluate major depression may need to be modified for use in dysthymic disorder. The Cornell Dysthymia Rating Scale was developed precisely for this purpose, and has been used both in studies of phenomenology and in clinical trials.

In contrast to the Hamilton Rating Scale for Depression, which has a restricted range of scoring for many items, the Cornell Dysthymia Rating Scale has a wide 5-point range for all the items in the scale (Mason et al., 1993). The scale's anchor points relate to current and recent frequency and severity of symptoms, rather than referring to normal premorbid periods, thereby making it more suitable for use in a chronic illness like dysthymic disorder. The Cornell Dysthymia Rating Scale has been shown to have good convergent validity with the Hamilton Rating Scale for Depression, the Beck Depression Inventory, and the Clinical Global Impression Scale (Mason et al., 1993). In young adults, a Cornell Dysthymia Rating Scale score of 20 showed the best sensitivity and specificity to clinical response (Hellerstein et al., 2002). The scale has a greater severity range and better content validity than the Hamilton Rating Scale for Depression in the evaluation of patients with dysthymic disorder (Mason et al., 1993). The scale has also been shown to be sensitive to response in a clinical trial comparing fluoxetine and placebo in elderly patients with dysthymic disorder (Devanand et al., in press).

While administration of this rating scale is not necessary for routine clinical practice, it can prove useful in the evaluation and monitoring of patients with dysthymic disorder who have unclear/ambiguous presentations or are difficult to treat effectively.

## NEUROBIOLOGY

Most neurobiological studies, particularly biochemical and neurophysiological studies, have been conducted in young adults. Some neurobiological abnormalities in dysthymic disorder are similar to those observed in major depressive disorder, but other findings suggest a similarity to healthy controls. Heterogeneity among patients diagnosed with dysthymic disorder may contribute to the inconsistent findings across studies.

Subgroups of patients with dysthymic disorder have been shown to have abnormalities in plasma and urinary metabolites of catecholamines, and lower platelet monoamine oxidase (MAO) activity, but no consistent abnormalities have been reported (Ravindran et al., 1994a, 1994b). Immunological abnormalities have been reported in some studies. Interleukin-1B levels in patients with dysthymic disorder were elevated before and after sertraline treatment, suggesting that this abnormality is a trait and not a state phenomenon (Anisman et al., 1999). Dysthymic disorder has been shown to be associated with elevated levels of circulating natural killer cells, but with no increase in adrenocorticotropic hormone or norepinephrine (Ravindran et al., 1996).

Seidman et al. (2002) reported that testosterone levels were lower in elderly men with dysthymic disorder compared to healthy male controls, with no significant differences between elderly men with major depression and healthy controls. The issue of whether testosterone deficiency is related to dysthymic disorder in elderly men clearly merits further investigation. There is indirect evidence that women with major depression who are receiving estrogen may show a superior response to antidepressants (Schneider et al., 1997), but this issue has not been studied in elderly patients with dysthymic disorder.

In recent years, the putative association between late-life depression and cerebrovascular disease has been the subject of intense investigation. Hyperintensities on magnetic resonance imaging (MRI) scans are two- to fivefold greater in patients with late-life major depression than in normal controls (Boone et al., 1992; Christiansen et al., 1994) and are more frequent in late- versus early-onset patients with major depression (Dahabra et al., 1998; Fujikawa et al., 1994; Krishnan et al., 1993, 1997; Lesser et al., 1996; O'Brien et al., 1998), with a few contradictory reports (Greenwald et al., 1996; Iidaka et al., 1996). In most MRI studies in late-life major depression, hyperintensities have been found across a wide spectrum of severity, suggesting that they may also occur frequently in elderly late-onset patients with dysthymic disorder. In a series of 159 elderly patients with dysthymic disorder, cardiac disease was more common in late-onset than early-onset patients, indirectly suggesting that cerebrovascular pathology may be more common in late-onset than early-onset dysthymic disorder (Devanand et al., 2004).

Most MRI hyperintensities appear to be caused by microvascular pathology, as they are associated with age, hypertension, coronary heart disease, or other vascular risk factors. Functional brain imaging studies show decreased blood flow or metabolism globally and regionally, as well as in and around MRI hyperintensities (Bench et al., 1993; Curran et al., 1993; Herholz et al., 1990; Kobayashi et al., 1991; Kumar et al., 1993, 1998; Sackeim et al., 1990). The pathophysiology of late-onset depression may be similar to that of the cortical deafferentation syndrome in Binswanger's disease, resulting from subcortical lesions due to hypoperfusion in watershed areas (limited collateral supply, vulnerability to vascular insult) supplied by small arterioles that branch off long, penetrating medullary and lenticulostriate arteries. Early clinical signs of Binswanger's disease are blunted affect, slowness, and decreased concentration and learning, features similar to those seen in elderly patients with major depression and, to some extent, dysthymic disorder. Reflecting this vulnerability, elderly patients with major depression who have basal ganglia hyperintensities are prone to develop delirium when treated with antidepressants or ECT (Figiel et al., 1989, 1990).

Elderly patients with major depression have high rates of basal ganglia, thalamic, and frontal hyperintensities (Greenwald et al., 1998). The *vascular depression hypothesis* postulates that cerebrovascular disease predisposes to, precipitates, and perpetuates late-life depression (Alexopoulos et al., 1997; Steffens and Krishnan, 1998). Dysthymic disorder is a condition mainly of late-onset patients. Therefore, a large number of elderly patients with dysthymic disorder are likely to have cerebrovascular disease and hyperintensities, as commonly occur in late-onset major depression. However, empirical data are not yet available to support this assertion.

There is some evidence that hyperintensities predict a poor response to antidepressants in geriatric major depression (Hickie et al., 1997). Moreover, hyperintensities have been associated with executive dysfunction, which may be related to a poor response to antidepressants (Alexopoulos et al., 2000; Kalayam and Alexopoulos, 1999). In a study of 60 patients (>55 years old) with major depression followed for a mean period of 32 months, those with severe hyperintensities had a two- to threefold shorter time to relapse or cognitive decline (O'Brien et al., 1998). In geriatric major depression, several studies show that MRI hyperintensities are associated with a poor short-term response to antidepressants and ECT (Figiel et al., 1990; Fujikawa et al., 1996; Hickie et al., 1995). Given the commonalities between dysthymic disorder and major depression in the elderly, hyperintensities are also likely to predict a poor response to antidepressants in geriatric dysthymic disorder. However, published data on this issue are lacking in elderly patients with dysthymic disorder.

Abnormalities other than hyperintensities, such as degenerative changes, may lead to executive dysfunction and medication resistance. The finding of increased cerebral atrophy in elderly patients with major depression suggests that degenerative changes have taken place. A structural MRI study in geriatric patients found that the degree of atrophy in patients with minor depression was intermediate between those of patients with major depression and controls (Kumar et al., 1998). Hippocampal atrophy may also characterize late-onset major depression (Sheline et al., 1999; 2000), and this may explain the memory loss that sometimes accompanies depression in the elderly. One possibility is that persistently high levels of corticosteroids in major depression (exemplified by an abnormal dexamethasone suppression test) lead to hippocampal damage and atrophy (Sheline et al., 1999; Sheline, 2000).

Recent studies suggest that late-life major depressive disorder is associated with cortical deafferentation contributing to striatofrontal dysfunction, clinically expressed as executive dysfunction, a pathophysiological defect associated with a reduced response to antidepressants (Alexopoulos, 2001). Cognitive deficits occur in geriatric major depression and may be more common in late- compared to early-onset patients. The cognitive deficits in patients with late-onset major depression who have hyperintensities are mainly in executive functions and processing speed, as well as in nonverbal intelligence, nonverbal memory, and constructional ability. Many elderly patients with dysthymic disorder may have executive deficits because they often have late age of onset and vascular risk factors or disease, and there is evidence of frontal lobe atrophy in geriatric nonmajor depression (Kumar et al., 1998). Executive dysfunction, psychomotor retardation, and prolonged latency of the P300 auditory evoked potential predicted a poor or slow response to antidepressants in a series of elderly patients with major depressive disorder, indicating that striatofrontal dysfunction may contribute to antidepressant resistance (Kalayam et al., 1999). In contrast, memory dysfunction was not associated with the treatment outcome, suggesting that the relationship of executive dysfunction to medication resistance is rather specific. This assertion is supported by data showing that executive dysfunction, but not memory deficits, predicted early relapse and recurrence of geriatric major depression, further demonstrating specificity (Alexopoulos et al., 2000). There is also evidence that depressive symptoms in general, and psychomotor retardation and diminished interest in activities in particular, interact significantly with executive dysfunction in contributing to disability.

In summary, there is considerable evidence that cerebrovascular disease, cerebral atrophy (global and regionally specific), and executive function deficits characterize geriatric major depression, particularly in late-onset patients. These features appear to be associated with a poor treatment response and prognosis. A similar profile may occur in elderly late-onset patients with dysthymic disorder, but more research is needed to establish if this is indeed the case.

## TREATMENT

The increase in antidepressant prescribing in the 1990s in the United States was greatest for patients with psychiatric disorders of mild to moderate severity like dysthymic disorder (Olfson et al., 1998). However, dysthymic disorder continues to be commonly under-treated in young adults (Shelton et al., 1997), and this also appears to be true in the elderly (Devanand et al., in press; Williams et al., 2000).

Several studies in young adults have demonstrated that antidepressant medications are efficacious in the treatment of dysthymic disorder, both in patients with primary dysthymic disorder (no antecedent Axis I or II diagnoses) and in patients with double depression (de Lima et al., 1999). Kocsis et al. (1988a) reported a 59% response rate to imipramine compared to 13% for placebo in 96 patients with chronic, mainly double, depression. Other studies suggest moderate efficacy of antidepressants in young adults with dysthymic disorder (Boyer et al., 1999; Hellerstein et al., 1993; Lecrubier et al., 1997; Smeraldi, 1998; Versiani et al., 1997). In a double-blind study of 416 (310 completers) young adult outpatients with primary dysthymic disorder, Thase et al. (1996) reported intent-to-treat response rates of 64% to imipramine, 59% to sertraline, and 44% to placebo. Although significant, the 15% advantage of sertraline over placebo was not robust. Both sertraline and imipramine were superior to placebo in psychosocial outcomes (Kocsis et al., 1997), and another study found better extended family adjustment in responders compared to nonresponders (Friedman et al., 1995b).

In patients with double depression, antidepressant response rates to acute treatment appear to be similar to those of patients with primary dysthymia (Keller et al., 1998). One report suggested that patients whose dysthymia began after major depression may have a poorer response to antidepressant treatment than patients who had dysthymia before the first major depressive episode (Levitt et al., 1998).

Studies comparing a selective serotonin reuptake inhibitor (SSRI) to placebo in adults with dysthymic disorder have generally shown a small advantage for the SSRI (Hellerstein et al., 1993; Ravindran et al., 2000; Vanelle et al., 1997). Venlafaxine may also be an effective treatment in dysthymic disorder in young adults, but placebo-controlled trials are lacking (Ballus et al., 2000; Dunner et al., 1997; Ravindran et al., 1998). Moclobemide (an MAO inhibitor available in Europe but not in the United States) and imipramine have been shown to be superior to placebo in a trial of dysthymic disorder (two-thirds primary dysthymia and one-third double depression) (Versiani et al., 1997). An earlier study found superior efficacy for phenelzine up to 75 mg/day compared to imipramine up to 250 mg/day in

32 patients with dysthymic disorder (Vallejo et al., 1987).

In contrast, there is a paucity of controlled data on the treatment of elderly patients with dysthymic disorder. The only published, randomized, double-blind, placebo-controlled treatment study in elderly dysthymic patients was conducted in primary care, and it found a small but significant advantage for paroxetine over problem-solving therapy or placebo on the Hopkins Symptom Checklist, with similar response rates (40% to 51%) among the three conditions (Williams et al., 2000). In that study, patients with lower education, higher scores on the personality dimension of neuroticism, and severe medical illness were less likely to respond to active treatment or placebo (Katon et al., 2002). Perceived social support was associated with improvement in the placebo plus clinical management group, and impairment in activities of daily living was associated with subsequent increases in depression (Oxman and Hull, 2001).

An initial open pilot trial of fluoxetine in elderly dysthymic patients found moderate efficacy with relatively few side effects (Nobler et al., 1996), but a subsequent double-blind, placebo-controlled study has found minimal superiority for fluoxetine over placebo, with response rates of 27.3% for fluoxetine and 19.6% for placebo in intent-to-treat analyses, and response rates of 37.5% for fluoxetine and 23.1% for placebo in completer analyses (Devanand et al., in press). Interestingly, placebo-controlled trials of SSRIs in elderly patients with major depression have also found small to no advantages for active medication over placebo (Gottfries, 1996; Nyth et al., 1992; Schatzberg and Cantillon, 2000; Schneider et al., 2003; Tollefson and Holman, 1993). However, in geriatric major depression, response rates in studies not including a placebo and evaluating drug–drug comparisons (Finkel et al., 1999; Mulsant et al., 2001b; Oslin et al., 2000) have been higher than those reported in placebo-controlled trials.

In a large-scale study of adults with chronic depression, half of the patients who did not respond to sertraline responded to imipramine, and half of the patients who did not respond to imipramine responded to sertraline (Thase et al., 2002). In elderly patients with major depression, those who do not respond to one antidepressant usually respond to subsequent trials of alternative antidepressants (Flint and Rifat, 1996). It is possible that in elderly patients with dysthymic disorder, treating nonresponders to one class of medication with another class of medication may be an effective strategy. Clinically, the choice of medication should be based more on potential side effects than on putative differences in efficacy that have been small in magnitude across studies.

## LONG-TERM RESPONSE AND RELAPSE

After an acute response to antidepressant treatment, adults with dysthymic disorder invariably maintain their improvement if continued on medication for extended periods of time (Hellerstein et al., 1996; Koran et al., 2001). Conversely, adults with dysthymic disorder commonly relapse if the antidepressant medication is discontinued (Bogetto et al., 2002; Kocsis et al., 1995), but recover if the antidepressant medication is reinstituted (Friedman et al., 1995a). In a small sample of elderly patients with dysthymic disorder, 6 of 12 patients relapsed within 6 months of discontinuation of fluoxetine after a clinical response was achieved (Devanand et al., 1997). These initial findings in elderly patients, taken together with the literature on long-term antidepressant treatment of dysthymic disorder in adults, suggests that antidepressant medications should be continued for at least a year, and perhaps longer, after a clinical response is achieved in elderly patients with dysthymic disorder.

## ANTIPSYCHOTIC MEDICATIONS

In European studies, atypical antipsychotic medications have been shown to be efficacious in treating adults with dysthymic disorder. Amisulpiride, which is available in Europe, is a presynaptic dopamine-blocking antipsychotic at low doses and a postsynaptic blocker at higher doses, and it does not act in the striatum. Both amisulpiride and amineptine (approved as an antidepressant in some European countries) were superior to placebo in a trial of 323 patients with dysthymic disorder (Boyer et al., 1999). In a study of 313 outpatients with dysthymic disorder, including double depression, amisulpride 50 mg/day was compared to sertraline 50–100 mg/day (Amore and Jori, 2001). Response rates after 8 weeks of treatment were 82% with amisulpride and 69% with sertraline. Patients on amisulpride showed a shorter time to response and good tolerability. There are no data on the use of atypical antipsychotics in elderly patients with dysthymic disorder, but these results suggest that this class of medication merits investigation in the elderly.

## PSYCHOTHERAPY

A few uncontrolled and controlled studies of psychotherapy in dysthymic disorder have been conducted in young adults. In a small series of depressed outpatients, half of whom had dysthymic disorder, nonresponders to cognitive therapy responded to imipramine but not to placebo (Stewart et al., 1993). There is evidence that cognitive behavior therapy is effective in milder forms of major depression, indirectly suggesting that this approach may also work in dysthymic disorder. A recent study reported that combining a cognitive behavioral analysis system of psychotherapy with the antidepressant nefazodone was superior to treatment with nefazodone alone or to this type of psychotherapy alone in treating adults with chronic, nonpsychotic, major depression (Keller et al., 2000). The differences between the groups were larger than those in prior studies of antidepressant medication and psychotherapy in major depression, and further studies are clearly required using these treatment approaches. Nonetheless, these results suggest that this form of psychotherapy may have some utility in dysthymic disorder, and studies of this type in dysthymic disorder are clearly needed.

Group therapy may have some utility in adults with dysthymic disorder, particularly when used in conjunction with antidepressant medication treatment (Hellerstein et al., 2001; Ravindran et al., 1999). In a study of 26 married women who received doxepin, marital therapy, placebo, and minimal contact, both active treatments appeared to reduce depressive symptoms but marital therapy had a superior effect on marital intimacy (Waring et al., 1988). In a nonblind study that compared sertraline 50–200 mg/day plus 10 sessions of interpersonal therapy (IPT) to sertraline plus IPT in a primary care sample, response rates (40% improvement in symptoms) were 60.2% for sertraline, 46.6% for IPT, and 57.5% for combined treatment (Browne et al., 2002). The response rates would have been lower if the standard response criterion of 50% rather than 40% improvement in symptoms were used. There was a small economic advantage for the combined treatment group with respect to lower health-care costs.

In the only study that compared an antidepressant, placebo, and psychotherapy in elderly patients with dysthymic disorder, problem-solving therapy was not superior to placebo or paroxetine treatment (Williams et al., 2000). Of note, there were large intersite differences in response rates to problem-solving therapy, emphasizing the difficulty in standardizing psychotherapy in treatment trials in elderly patients.

Overall, while psychotherapy of several types has shown limited efficacy in depressed patients, this remains to be demonstrated in controlled studies of elderly patients with dysthymic disorder.

## CONCLUSIONS

Dysthymic disorder affects 2%–4% of the elderly population and leads to disability and a poor quality of life. Both epidemiological and clinical studies show that dysthymic disorder in the elderly is different from dysthymic disorder in young adults. Dysthymic disorder in the elderly is predominantly of the late-onset type, with onset typically above 40 years of age, and it is associated with few co-morbid Axis I or II disorders. This suggests that most elderly patients with dysthymic disorder are not young patients with dysthymic disorder who simply grew older.

For both young adult and elderly patients, the symptom criteria listed under the Alternative Research Criterion B for dysthymia in the DSM-IV Appendix, which emphasizes motivational and cognitive/ideational symptoms, may be more valid than the symptom criteria listed under the main DSM-IV diagnostic criteria for dysthymic disorder, which emphasize neurovegetative symptoms. In elderly patients with dysthymic disorder, obsessive-compulsive and avoidant personality disorders are the most common personality disorders; these findings are similar to those in elderly patients with major depressive disorder. In elderly patients with dysthymic disorder, the co-morbid Cluster B diagnoses of borderline, antisocial, narcissistic, and histrionic personality disorder are rare. Patients with onset of dysthymia in middle to old age typically do not have high familial loading for affective disorder, indicating that genetic etiology is not a likely explanation for late-onset dysthymia.

Depressive disorders, including dysthymic disorder, across the life span are associated with poor social adjustment and poor general functioning. In addition, the elderly demonstrate considerable disability as a result of depressive illness, and interventions directed at improving depressive symptoms should also aim at improving function and quality of life. A collaborative care model has been shown to be effective in the treatment of depression in primary care, and ongoing research is likely to define the optimal model needed to improve the management of patients in the primary care setting.

There is considerable evidence that cerebrovascular disease, cerebral atrophy (global and regionally specific), and executive function deficits characterize geriatric major depression, particularly in late-onset patients. These features appear to be associated with a poor treatment response and a poor prognosis. A similar profile may occur in elderly late-onset patients with dysthymic disorder, but more research is needed to establish if this is indeed the case.

There is a lack of data on the treatment of elderly patients with dysthymic disorder. The only published, randomized, double-blind, placebo-controlled treatment study in elderly patients with dysthymic disorder was conducted in primary care, and it found a small but significant advantage for paroxetine over problem-solving therapy or placebo on one rating scale. However, response rates were similar (40% to 51%) among the three conditions. Results of a recent study comparing fluoxetine to placebo also suggest that SSRIs have minimal advantages over placebo in the treatment of this disorder (Devanand et al., in press). Therefore, despite general progress in antidepressant therapeutics, no treatment with proven efficacy exists for geriatric dysthymic disorder.

There is preliminary evidence that a treatment response in elderly patients with dysthymic disorder should be followed by continued treatment for an extended period of time. A few European studies suggest that atypical antipsychotics may have some value in the treatment of this condition, and further research in this area is clearly needed. While psychotherapy of different types has shown limited efficacy in elderly patients with major depression, this remains to be demonstrated in controlled studies of elderly patients with dysthymic disorder.

REFERENCES

Abrams, R.C., Spielman, L.A., Alexopoulos, G.S., and Klausner, E. (1998) Personality disorder symptoms and functioning in elderly depressed patients. *Am J Geriatr Psychiatry* 6:24–30.

Akiskal, H.S. (1983) Dysthymic disorder: Psychopathology of proposed chronic depressive subtypes. *Am J Psychiatry* 140:11–20.

Alexopoulos, G.S. (2001) The "depression-executive dysfunction syndrome" of late life. A target for D3 agonists. *Am J Geriatr Psychiatry* 9:22–29.

Alexopoulos, G.S., Meyers, B.S., Young, R.C., Campbell, S., Silbersweig, D., and Charlson. M. (1997) "Vascular depression" hypothesis. *Arch Gen Psychiatry* 54:915–922.

Alexopoulos, G.S., Meyers, B.S., Young, R.C., Hull, J., Sirey, J.A., and Kakuma, T. (2000) Executive dysfunction and risk for relapse and recurrence of geriatric depression. *Arch Gen Psychiatry* 57:285–290.

Amore, M., and Jori, M.C. (2001) Faster response on amisulpride 50 mg versus sertraline 50–100 mg in patients with dysthymia or double depression: A randomized, double-blind, parallel group study. *Int Clin Psychopharmacol* 16(6):317–324.

Anisman, H., Ravindran, A.V., Griffiths, J., and Merali, Z. (1999) Interleukin-1 beta production in dysthymia before and after pharmacotherapy. *Biol Psychiatry* 46(12):1649–1655.

Ballus, C., Quiros, G., De Flores, T., de la Torre, J., Palao, D., Rojo, L., Gutierrez, M., Casais, L., and Riesgo, Y. (2000) The efficacy and tolerability of venlafaxine and paroxetine in outpatients with depressive disorder or dysthymia. *Int Clin Psychopharmacol* 15(1):43–48.

Barzega, G., Maina, G., Venturello, S., and Bogetto, F. (2001) Dysthymic disorder: Clinical characteristics in relation to age at onset. *J Affect Disord* 66(1):39–46.

Bellino, S., Patria, L., Ziero, S., Rocca, G., and Bogetto, F. (2001) Clinical features of dysthymia and age: A clinical investigation. *Psychiatry Res* 103(2–3):219–228.

Bench, C.J., Friston, K.J., Brown, R.G., Frackowiak, R.S., and Dolan, R.J. (1993) Regional cerebral blood flow in depression measured by positron emission tomography: The relationship with clinical dimensions. *Psychol Med* 23:579–590.

Blazer, D., Hughes, D.C., and George, L.K. (1987) The epidemiology of depression in an elderly community population. *Gerontologist* 27:281–287.

Blazer, D., Swartz, M., Woodbury, M., Manton, K.G., Hughes, D., and George, L.K. (1988) Depressive symptoms and depressive diagnoses in a community population. *Arch Gen Psychiatry* 45:1078–1084.

Bogetto, F., Bellino, S., Revello, R.B., and Patria, L. (2002) Discontinuation syndrome in dysthymic patients treated with selective serotonin reuptake inhibitors: A clinical investigation. *CNS Drugs* 16(4):273–283.

Boone, K.B., Miller, B.L., Lesser, I.M., Mehringer, C.M., Hill-Gutierrez, E., Goldberg, M.A., and Berman, N.G. (1992) Neuropsychological correlates of white-matter lesions in healthy elderly subjects. *Arch Neurol* 49:549–554.

Boyer, P., Lecrubier, Y., Stalla-Bourdillon, A., and Fleurot, O. (1999) Amisulpride versus amineptine and placebo for the treatment of dysthymia. *Neuropsychobiology* 39:25–32.

Browne, G., Steiner, M., Roberts, J., Gafni, A., Byrne, C., Dunn, E., Bell, B., Mills, M., Chalklin, L., Wallik, D., and Kraemer, J. (2002) Sertraline and/or interpersonal psychotherapy for patients with dysthymic disorder in primary care: 6-month comparison with longitudinal 2-year follow-up of effectiveness and costs. *J Affect Disord* 68(2–3):317–330.

Carta, M.G., Carpiniello, B., Kovess, V., Porcedda, R., Zedda, A., and Rudas, N. (1995) Lifetime prevalence of major depression and dysthymia: Results of a community survey in Sardinia. *Eur Neuropsychopharmacol* 5(suppl):103–107.

Chen, L., Eaton, W.W., Gallo, J.J., and Nestadt, G. (2000) Understanding the heterogeneity of depression through the triad of symptoms, course and risk factors: A longitudinal, population-based study. *J Affect Disord* 59(1):1–11.

Christiansen, P., Larsson, H.B., Thomsen, C., Wieslander, S.B., and Henriksen, O. (1994) Age dependent white matter lesions and brain volume changes in healthy volunteers. *Acta Radiol* 35:117–122.

Clark, D.A., Beck, A.T., and Beck, J.S. (1994) Symptom differences in major depression, dysthymia, panic disorder, and generalized anxiety disorder. *Am J Psychiatry* 151(2):205–209.

Curran, S.M., Murray, C.M., Van Beck, M., Dougall, N., O'Carroll, R.E., Austin, M.P., Ebmeier, K.P., and Goodwin, G.M. (1993) A single photon emission computerised tomography study of regional brain function in elderly patients with major depression and with Alzheimer-type dementia. *Br J Psychiatry* 163:155–165.

Dahabra, S., Ashton, C.H., Bahrainian, M., Britton, P.G., Ferrier, I.N., McAllister, V.A., Marsh, V.R., et al. (1998) Structural and functional abnormalities in elderly patients clinically recovered from early- and late-onset depression. *Biol Psychiatry* 44:34–46.

de Lima, M.S., Hotoph, M., and Wessely, S. (1999) The efficacy of drug treatments for dysthymia: A systematic review and meta-analysis. *Psychol Med* 29:1273–1289.

Devanand, D.P., Adorno, E., Cheng, J., Burt, T., Pelton, G.H., Roose, S.P., and Sackeim, H.A. (2004) Late onset dysthymic disorder and major depression differ from early onset dysthymic disorder and major depression in elderly outpatients, *J Affect Disord* 78:259–267.

Devanand, D.P., Kim, M.K., and Nobler, M.S. (1997) Fluoxetine discontinuation in elderly dysthymic patients. *Am J Geriatr Psychiatry* 5:83–87.

Devanand, D.P., Kim, M.K., Paykina, N., and Sackeim, H.A. (2002) Adverse life events in elderly patients with major depression or dysthymic disorder and in healthy control subjects. *Am J Geriatr Psychiatry* 10(3):265–274.

Devanand, D.P., Nobler, M.S., Cheng, J., Turret, N., Pelton, G.H., Roose, S.P., and Sackeim, H.A. (in press) A randomized, double-blind, placebo-controlled trial of fluoxetine treatment for elderly patients with dysthymic disorder.

Devanand, D.P., Nobler, M.S., Singer, T., Kiersky, J.E., Turret, N., Roose, S.P., and Sackeim, H.A. (1994) Is dysthymia a different disorder in the elderly? *Am J Psychiatry* 151:1592–1599.

Devanand, D.P., Turret, N., Moody, B.J., Fitzsimons, L., Peyser, S., Mickle, K., Nobler, M.S., and Roose, S.P. (2000) Personality disorders in elderly patients with dysthymic disorder. *Am J Geriatr Psychiatry* 8:188–195.

Dunner, D.L., Hendrickson, H.E., Bea, C., and Budech, C.B. (1997) Venlafaxine in dysthymic disorder. *J Clin Psychiatry* 58:528–531.

Ernst, C., and Angst, J. (1995) Depression in old age. Is there a real decrease in prevalence? A review. *Eur Arch Psychiatry Clin Neurosci* 245:272–287.

Fichter, M.M., Bruce, M.L., Schroppel, H., Meller, I., and Merikangas, K. (1995) Cognitive impairment and depression in the oldest old in a German and in U.S. communities. *Eur Arch Psychiatry Clin Neurosci* 245:319–325.

Figiel, G.S., Krishnan, K.R., Breitner, J.C., and Nemeroff, C.B. (1989) Radiologic correlates of antidepressant-induced delirium: The possible significance of basal-ganglia lesions. *J Neuropsychiatry Clin Neurosci* 1:188–190.

Figiel, G.S., Krishnan, K.R., and Doraiswamy, P.M. (1990) Subcortical structural changes in ECT-induced delirium. *J Geriatr Psychiatry Neurol* 3:172–176.

Finkel, S.I., Richter, E.M., and Clary, C.M. (1999) Comparative efficacy and safety of sertraline versus nortriptyline in major depression in patients 70 and older. *Int Psychogeriatr* 11:85–99.

Flint, A.J., and Rifat, S.L. (1996) The effect of sequential antidepressant treatment on geriatric depression. *J Affect Disord* 36:95–105.

Friedman, R.A., Mitchell, J., and Kocsis, J.H. (1995a) Retreatment for relapse following desipramine discontinuation in dysthymia. *Am J Psychiatry* 152:926–928.

Friedman, R.A., Parides, M., Baff, R., Moran, M., and Kocsis, J.H. (1995b) Predictors of response to desipramine in dysthymia. *J Clin Psychopharmacol* 4:280–283.

Fujikawa, T., Yamawaki, S., and Touhouda, Y. (1994) Background factors and clinical symptoms of major depression with silent cerebral infarction. *Stroke* 25:798–801.

Fujikawa, T., Yokota, N., Muraoka, M., and Yamawaki, S. (1996) Response of patients with major depression and silent cerebral infarction to antidepressant drug therapy, with emphasis on central nervous system adverse reactions. *Stroke* 27:2020–2042.

Geiselmann, B., and Bauer, M. (2000) Subthreshold depression in the elderly: Qualitative or quantitative distinction? *Compr Psychiatry* 41(2 suppl 1):32–38.

Gottfries, C.G. (1996) Scandinavian experience with citalopram in the elderly. *Int Clin Psychopharmacol* 11:41–44.

Greenwald, B.S., Kramer-Ginsberg, E., Krishnan, K.R., Ashtari, M., Auerbach, C., and Patel, M. (1998) Neuroanatomic localization of magnetic resonance imaging signal hyperintensities in geriatric depression. *Stroke* 29:613–617.

Greenwald, B.S., Kramer-Ginsberg, E., Krishnan, R.R., Ashtari, M., Aupperle, P.M., and Patel, M. (1996) MRI signal hyperintensities in geriatric depression. *Am J Psychiatry* 153:1212–1215.

Gwirtsman, H.E., Blehar, M.C., McCullough, J.P., Kocsis, J.H., and Prien, R.F. (1997) Standardized assessment of dysthymia: Report of a National Institute of Mental Health conference. *Psychopharmacol Bull* 33:3–11.

Hayden, E.P., and Klein, D.N. (2001) Outcome of dysthymic disorder at 5-year follow-up: The effect of familial psychopathology, early adversity, personality, comorbidity, and chronic stress. *Am J Psychiatry* 158(11):1864–1870.

Hays, J.C., Steffens, D.C., Flint, E.P., Bosworth, H.B., and George, L.K. (2001) Does social support buffer functional decline in elderly patients with unipolar depression? *Am J Psychiatry* 158(11):1850–1855.

Hellerstein, D.J., Batchelder, S.T., Lee, A., and Borisovskaya, M. (2002) Rating dysthymia: An assessment of the construct and content validity of the Cornell dysthymia rating scale. *J Affect Disord* 71:85–96.

Hellerstein, D.J., Little, S.A., Samstag, L.W., Batchelder, S., Muran, J.C., Fedak, M., Kreditor, D., Rosenthal, R.N., and Winston, A. (2001) Adding group psychotherapy to medication treatment in dysthymia: A randomized prospective pilot study. *J Psychother Pract Res* 10(2):93–103.

Hellerstein, D.J., Samstag, L.W., Cantillon, M., Maurer, M., Rosenthal, J., Yanowitch, P., and Winston, A. (1996) Follow-up assessment of medication-treated Dysthymia. *Biol Psychiatry* 20:427–442.

Hellerstein, D.J., Yanowitch, P., Rosenthal, J., et al. (1993) A randomized double-blind study of fluoxetine versus placebo in the treatment of dysthymia. *Am J Psychiatry* 150:1169–1175.

Herholz, K., Heindel, W., Rackl, A., Neubauer, I., Steinbrich, W., Pietrzyk, U., Erasmi-Körber, H., and Heiss, W.-D. (1990) Regional cerebral blood flow in patients with leukoaraiosis and atherosclerotic carotid artery disease. *Arch Neurol* 47:392–396.

Hickie, I., Scott, E., Mitchell, P., Wilhelm, K., Austin, M.P., and Bennett, B. (1995) Subcortical hyperintensities on magnetic resonance imaging: Clinical correlates and prognostic significance in patients with severe depression. *Biol Psychiatry* 37:151–160.

Hickie, I., Scott, E., Wilhelm, K., and Brodaty, H. (1997) Subcortical hyperintensities on magnetic resonance imaging in patients with severe depression—a longitudinal evaluation. *Biol Psychiatry* 42:367–374.

Hirschfeld, R.M. (1994) Major depression, dysthymia and depressive personality disorder. *Br J Psychiatry Suppl.* (26):23–30.

Iidaka, T., Nakajima, T., Kawamoto, K., Fukuda, H., Suzuki, Y., Maehara, T., and Shiraishi, H. (1996) Signal hyperintensities on brain magnetic resonance imaging in elderly depressed patients. *Eur Neurol* 36:293–299.

Johnson, J., and Weissman, M.M., and Klerman, G.L. (1992) Service utilization and social morbidity associated with depressive symptoms in the community. *JAMA* 267:1478–1483.

Judd, L.L., Paulus, M.P., Wells, K.B., and Rapaport, M.H. (1996) Socioeconomic burden of subsyndromal depressive symptoms and major depression in a sample of the general population. *Am J Psychiatry* 153(11):1411–1417.

Kalayam, B., and Alexopoulos, G. (1999) Prefrontal dysfunction and treatment response in geriatric depression. *Arch Gen Psychiatry* 56:713–718.

Katon, W., Russo, J., Frank, E., Barrett, J., Williams, J.W., Jr., Oxman, T., Sullivan, M., and Cornell, J. (2002) Predictors of nonresponse to treatment in primary care patients with dysthymia. *Gen Hosp Psychiatry* 24(1):20–27.

Keller, M.B., Gelenberg, A.J., Hirschfeld, R.M.A., Rush, A.J., Thase, M.E., Kocsis, J.H., Markowitz, J.C., et al. (1998) The treatment of chronic depression, part 2: A double-blind, randomized trial of sertraline and imipramine. *J Clin Psychiatry* 59:598–607.

Keller, M.B., Klein, D.N., Hirschfeld, R.M.A., Kocsis, J.H., McCullough, J.P., Miller, I., First, M.B., et al. (1995) Results of the DSM-IV mood disorders field trial. *Am J Psychiatry* 152:843–849.

Keller, M.B., McCullough, J.P., Klein, D.N., Arnow, B., Dunner, D.L., Gelenberg, A.J., Markowitz, J.C., Nemeroff, C.B., Russell, J.M., Thase, M.E., Trivedi, M.H., and Zajecka, J. (2000) A comparison of nefazodone, the cognitive behavioral-analysis system of psychotherapy, and their combination for the treatment of chronic depression. *N Engl J Med* 342(20):1462–1470.

Keller, M.B., and Shapiro, R.W. (1982) "Double depression": Superimposition of acute depressive episodes on chronic depresssive disorders. *Am J Psychiatry* 139:438–442.

Kirby, M., Bruce, I., Coakley, D., and Lawlor, B.A. (1999) Dysthymia among the community-dwelling elderly. *Int J Geriatr Psychiatry* 14(6):440–445.

Klein, D.N., Norden, K.A., Ferro, T., Leader, J.B., Kasch, K.L., Klein, L.M., Schwartz, J.E., Aronson, T.A. Thirty-month naturalistic follow-up study of early-onset dysthymic disorder: Course, diagnostic stability, and prediction of outcome. *J Abnorm Psychol* 1998; 107, 338–348.

Klein, D.N., Riso, L.P., Donaldson, S.K., Schwartz, J.E., Anderson, R.L., Ouimette, P.C., Lizardi, H., et al. (1995) Family study of early-onset dysthymia. *Arch Gen Psychiatry* 52:487–496.

Klein, D.N., Schwartz, J.E., Rose, S., and Leader, J.B. (2000) Five-year course and outcome of dysthymic disorder: A prospective, naturalistic follow-up study. *Am J Psychiatry* 157(6):931–939.

Klein, D.N., Taylor, E.B., Dickstein, S., and Harding. K. (1988a) The early–late onset distinction in DSM-III-R dysthymia. *J Affect Disord* 14:25–33.

Klein, D.N., Taylor, E.B., Harding, K., and Dickstein, S. (1988b) Double depression and episodic major depression: Demographic, clinical, familial, personality, and socioenvironmental characteristics and short-term outcome. *Am J Psychiatry* 145:1226–1231.

Kobayashi, S., Okada, K., and Yamashita, K. (1991) Incidence of silent lacunar lesion in normal adults and its relation to cerebral blood flow and risk factors. *Stroke* 22:1379–1383.

Kocsis, J.H., and Frances, A.J. (1987) A critical discussion of DSM-III dysthymic disorder. *Am J Psychiatry* 144:1534–1542.

Kocsis, J.H., Frances, A.J., Voss, C., Mann, J.J., Mason, B.J., and Sweeney, J. (1988a) Imipramine treatment for chronic depression. *Arch Gen Psychiatry* 45:253–257.

Kocsis, J.H., Frances, A.J., Voss, C., Mason, B.J., Mann, J.J., and Sweeney, J. (1988b) Imipramine and social-vocational adjustment in chronic depression. *Am J Psychiatry* 145:997–999.

Kocsis, J.H., Friedman, R.A., Markowitz, J.C., et al. (1995) Stability of remission during tricyclic antidepressant continuation therapy for dysthymia. *Psychopharmacol Bull* 31:2:213–216.

Kocsis, J.H., Zisook, S., Davidson, J., Shelton, R., Yonkers, K., Hellerstein, D.J., Rosenbaum, J., et al. (1997) Double-blind comparison of sertraline, imipramine, and placebo in the treatment of dysthymia: Psychosocial outcomes. *Am J Psychiatry* 154:390–395.

Koran, L.M., Gelenberg, A.J., Kornstein, S.G., Howland, R.H., Friedman, R.A., DeBattista, C., Klein, D., Kocsis, J.H., Schatzberg, A.F., Thase, M.E., Rush, A.J., Hirschfeld, R.M., LaVange, L.M., and Keller, M.B. (2001) Sertraline versus imipramine to prevent relapse in chronic depression. *J Affect Disord* 65:27–36.

Krishnan, K.R., Hays, J.C., and Blazer, D.G. (1997) MRI-defined vascular depression. *Am J Psychiatry* 154:497–501.

Krishnan, K.R., McDonald, W.M., Doraiswamy, P.M., Tupler, L.A., Husain, M., Boyko, O.B., Figiel, G.S., and Ellinwood, E.H., Jr. (1993) Neuroanatomical substrates of depression in the elderly. *Eur Arch Psychiatry Clin Neurosci* 243:41–46.

Kumar, A., Jin, Z., Bilker, W., Udupa, J., and Gottlieb, G. (1998) Late-onset minor and major depression: Early evidence for common neuroanatomical substrates detected by using MRI. *Proc Natl Acad Sci USA* 95:7654–7658.

Kumar, A., Newberg, A., Alavi, A., Berlin, J., Smith, R., and Reivich, M. (1993) Regional cerebral glucose metabolism in late-life depression and Alzheimer disease: A preliminary positron emission tomography study. *Proc Natl Acad Sci USA* 90:7019–7023.

Larson, S.L., Owens, P.L., Ford, D., and Eaton, W. (2001) Depressive disorder, dysthymia, and risk of stroke: thirteen-year follow-up from the Baltimore epidemiologic catchment area study. *Stroke* 32(9):1979–1983.

Leader, J.B., and Klein, D.N. (1996) Social adjustment in dysthymia, double depression and episodic major depression. *J Affect Disord* 37:91–101.

Lecrubier, Y., Boyer, P., Turjanski, S., and Rein, W. (1997) Amisulpride versus imipramine and placebo in dysthymia and major depression. *J Affect Disord* 43:95–103.

Lesser, I.M., Boone, K.B., Mehringer, C.M., Wohl, M.A., Miller, B.L., and Berman, N.G. (1996) Cognition and white matter hyperintensities in older depressed patients. *Am J Psychiatry* 153:1280–1287.

Lesser, I.M., Miller, B.L., Boone, K.B., Hill-Gutierrez, E., Mehringer, C.M., Wong, K., and Mena, I. (1991) Brain injury and cognitive function in late-onset psychotic depression. *J Neuropsychiatry Clin Neurosci* 3:33–40.

Levitt, A.J., Joffe, R.T., and Sokolov, S.T. (1998) Does the chronological relationship between the onset of dysthymia and major depression influence subsequent response to antidepressants? *J Affect Disord* 47(1–3):169–175.

Markowitz, J.C., Moran, M.E., Kocsis, J.H., and Frances, A.J. (1992) Prevalence and co-morbidity of dysthymic disorder among psychiatric outpatients. *J Affect Disord* 24:63–71.

Mason, B.J., Kocsis, J.H., Leon, A.C., Thompson, S., Frances, A.J., Morgan, R.O., and Parides, M.K. (1993) Measurement of severity and treatment response in dysthymia may have been limited by the structure and format of existing rating instruments. *Psychiatr Ann* 23:625–631.

Mazumdar, S., Reynolds, C.F., Houck, P.R., Frank, E., Dew, M.A., and Kupfer, D.J. (1996) Quality of life in elderly patients with recurrent major depression: A factor analysis of the General Life Functioning Scale. *Psychiatry Res* 63:183–190.

McCall, N.T., Parks, P., Smith, K., Pope, G., and Griggs, M. (2002) The prevalence of major depression or dysthymia among aged Medicare fee-for-service beneficiaries. *Int J Geriatr Psychiatry* 17(6):557–565.

Mulsant, B.H., Alexopoulos, G.S., Reynolds, C.F., 3rd, Katz, I.R., Abrams, R., Oslin, D., and Schulberg, H.C. (2001a) Pharmacological treatment of depression in older primary care patients: The PROSPECT algorithm. *Int J Geriatr Psychiatry* 16(6):585–592.

Mulsant, B.H., Pollock, B.G., Nebes, R., Miller, M.D., Sweet, R.A., Stack, J., Houck, P.R., Bensasi, S., Mazumdar, S., and Reynolds, C.F., 3rd. (2001b) A twelve-week, double-blind, randomized comparison of nortriptyline and paroxetine in older depressed inpatients and outpatients. *Am J Geriatr Psychiatry* 9:406–414.

Murphy, J.M., Nierenberg, A.A., Laird, N.M., Monson, R.R., Sobol, A.M., and Leighton, A.H. (2002) Incidence of major depression: Prediction from subthreshold categories in the Stirling County Study. *J Affect Disord* 68(2–3):251–259.

Nobler, M.S., Devanand, D.P., Kim, M.K., Fitzsimons, L.M., Singer, T.M., Turret, N., Sackeim, H.A., et al. (1996) Fluoxetine treatment of dysthymia in the elderly. *J Clin Psychiatry* 57:254–256.

Nyth, A.L., Gottfries, C.G., Lyby, K., Smedegaard-Andersen, L., Gylding-Sabroe, J., Kristensen, M., Refsum, H.E., Ofsti, E., Eriksson, S., and Syversen, S. (1992) A controlled multicenter clinical study of citalopram and placebo in elderly depressed patients with and without concomitant dementia. *Acta Psychiatr Scand* 86(2):138–145.

O'Brien, J., Ames, D., Chiu, E., Schweitzer, I., Desmond, P., and Tress, B. (1998) Severe deep white matter lesions and outcome in elderly patients with major depressive disorder: Follow-up study. *BMJ* 317:982–984.

Olfson, M., Marcus, S.C., Pincus, H.A., Zito, J.M., Thompson, J.W., and Zarin, D.A. (1998) Antidepressant prescribing practices of outpatient psychiatrists. *Arch Gen Psychiatry* 55(4):310–316.

Oslin, D.W., Streim, J.E., Katz, I.R., Smith, B.D., DiFilippo, S.D., Ten Have, T.R., and Cooper, T. (2000) Heuristic comparison of sertraline with nortriptyline for the treatment of depression in frail elderly patients. *Am J Geriatr Psychiatry* 8:141–149.

Oxman, T.E., Barrett, J.E., Sengupta, A., and Williams, J.W., Jr. (2000) The relationship of aging and dysthymia in primary care. *Am J Geriatr Psychiatry* 8(4):318–326.

Oxman, T.E., and Hull, J.G. (2001) Social support and treatment response in older depressed primary care patients. *J Gerontol B Psychol Sci Soc Sci* 56(1):P35–P45.

Pepper, C.M., Klein, D.N., Anderson, R.L., Riso, L.P., Ouimette, P.C., and Lizardi, H. (1995) DSM-III-R axis II co-morbidity in dysthymia and major depression. *Am J Psychiatry* 152:239–247.

Pini, S., Cassano, G.B., Simonini, E., Savino, M., Russo, A., and Montgomery, S.A. (1997) Prevalence of anxiety disorders co-morbidity in bipolar depression, unipolar depression and dysthymia. *J Affect Disord* 42(2–3):145–153.

Prince, M.J., Harwood, R.H., Blizard, R.A., Thomas, A., and Mann, A.H. (1997) Impairment, disability and handicap as risk factors for depression in old age. The Gospel Oak Project V. *Psychol Med* 27(2):311–321.

Prudic, J., Sackeim, H.A., Devanand, D.P., and Kiersky, J.E. (1993) The efficacy of ECT in double depression. *Depression* 1:38–44.

Pulska, T., Pahkala, K., Laippala, P., and Kivela, S. (1998) Survival of elderly Finns suffering from dysthymic disorder: A community study. *Soc Psychiatry Psychiatr Epidemiol* 33:319–325.

Ravindran, A.V., Anisman, H., Merali, Z., Charbonneau, Y., Telner, J., Bialik, R.J., Wiens, A., Ellis, J., and Griffiths, J. (1999) Treatment of primary dysthymia with group cognitive therapy and pharmacotherapy: clinical symptoms and functional impairments. *Am J Psychiatry* 156(10):1608–1617.

Ravindran, A.V., Bialik, R.J., Brown, G.M., and Lapierre, Y.D. (1994a) Primary onset dysthymia, biochemical correlates of the therapeutic response to fluoxetine: II. Urinary metabolites of serotonin, norepinephrine, epinephrine, and melatonin. *J Affect Disord* 31:119–123.

Ravindran, A.V., Bialik, R.J., and Lapierre, Y.D. (1994b) Primary early onset dysthymia, biochemical correlates of the therapeutic response to fluoxetine: I. Platelet monoamine oxidase and the dexamethasone suppression test. *J Affect Disord* 31:111–117.

Ravindran, A.V., Charbonneau, Y., Zaharia, M.D., Al-Zaid, K., Wiens, A., and Anisman, H. (1998) Efficacy and tolerability of venlafaxine in the treatment of primary dysthymia. *J Psychiatry Neurosci* 23:288–292.

Ravindran, A.V., Griffiths, J., Merali, Z., and Anisman, H. (1996) Primary dysthymia: A study of several psychosocial, endocrine and immune correlates. *J Affect Disord* 40:73–84.

Ravindran, A.V., Guelfi, J.D., Lane, R.M., and Cassano, G.B. (2000) Treatment of dysthymia with sertraline: A double-blind, placebo-controlled trial in dysthymic patients without major depression. *J Clin Psychiatry* 61(11):821–827.

Riso, L.P., Klein, D.N., Ferro, T., Kasch, K.L., Pepper, C.M., Schwartz, J.E., and Aronson, T.A. (1996) Understanding the comorbidity between early-onset dysthymia and cluster B personality disorders: A family study. *Am J Psychiatry* 153:900–906.

Sackeim, H.A. (2001) Brain structure and function in late-life depression. In: Morihisa, J.M., ed. *Review of Psychiatry*, vol. 20, *Advances in Brain Imaging*. Washington, DC: American Psychiatric Press, pp. 83–121.

Sackeim, H.A., Prohovnik, I., Moeller, J.R., Brown, R.P., Apter, S., Prudic, J., Devanand, D.P., and Mukherjee, S. (1990) Regional cerebral blood flow in mood disorders. I. Comparison of major depressives and normal controls at rest. *Arch Gen Psychiatry* 47:60–70.

Sansone, R.A., Wiederman, M.W., Sansone, L.A., and Touchet, B. (1998) Early-onset dysthymia and personality disturbance among patients in a primary care setting. *J Nerv Ment Dis* 186:57–59.

Schatzberg, A., and Cantillon, M. (2000) Antidepressant early response and remission with venlafaxine or fluoxetine in depressed geriatric outpatients. Presented at the European College of Neuropsychopharmacology meeting, Nice. July 2000.

Schneider, L.S., Small, G.W., Hamilton, S.H., Bystritsky, A., Nemeroff, C.B., and Meyers, B.S. (1997) Estrogen replacement and response to fluoxetine in a multicenter geriatric depression trial. Fluoxetine Collaborative Study Group. *Am J Geriatr Psychiatry* 5(2):97–106.

Schneider, L.S., Nelson J.C., Clary C.M., Newhouse P., Krishnan K.R. Shiovitz T., and Weihs K. (2003) Sertraline Elderly Depression Study Group. An 8-week multicenter parallel-group, double-blind, placebo-controlled study of sertraline in elderly out-patients with major depression. *Am J Psychiatry* 160:1277–1285.

Seidman, S.N., Araujo, A.B., Roose, S.P., Devanand, D.P., Xie, S., Cooper, T.B., and McKinlay, J.B. (2002) Low testosterone levels in elderly men with dysthymic disorder. *Am J Psychiatry* 159:456–459.

Sheline, Y.I. (2000) 3D MRI studies of neuroanatomic changes in unipolar major depression: The role of stress and medical comorbidity. *Biol Psychiatry* 48(8):791–800.

Sheline, Y.I., Sanghavi, M., Mintun, M.A., and Gado, M.H. (1999) Depression duration but not age predicts hippocampal volume loss in medically healthy women with recurrent major depression. *J Neurosci* 19:5034–5043.

Shelton, R.C., Davidson, J., Yonkers, K.A., Koran, L., Thase, M.E., Pearlstein, T., and Halbreich, U. (1997) The undertreatment of dysthymia. *J Clin Psychiatry* 58(2):59–65.

Sherbourne, C.D., Wells, K.B., Hays, R.D., Rogers, W., Burnam, M.A., and Judd, L.L. (1994) Subthreshold depression and depressive disorder: Clinical characteristics of general medical and mental health specialty outpatients. *Am J Psychiatry* 151(12):1777–1784.

Smeraldi, E. (1998) Amisulpride versus fluoxetine in patients with dysthymia or major depression in partial remission: A double-blind, comparative study. *J Affect Disord* 48:47–56.

Stefansson, J.G., Lindal, E., Bjornsson, J.K., and Guomundsdottir, A. (1991) Lifetime prevalence of specific mental disorders among people born in Iceland in 1931. *Acta Psychiatr Scand* 84:142–149.

Steffens, D.C., and Krishnan, K.R. (1998) Structural neuroimaging and mood disorders: Recent findings, implications for classification, and future directions. *Biol Psychiatry* 43:705–712.

Steffens, D.C., Skoog, I., Norton, M.C., Hart, A.D., Tschanz, J.T., Plassman, B.L., Wyse, B.W., Welsh-Bohmer, K.A., and Breitner, J.C. (2000) Prevalence of depression and its treatment in an elderly population: The Cache County study. *Arch Gen Psychiatry* 57(6):601–607.

Stewart, J.W., McGrath, P.J., Quitkin, F.M., Rabkin, J.G., Harrison, W., Wager, S., Nunes, E., Ocepek-Welikson, K., and Tricamo, E. (1993) Chronic depression: Response to placebo, imipramine, and phenelzine. *J Clin Psychopharmacol* 13(6):391–396.

Stewart, J.W., Quitkin, F.M., McGrath, P.J., Rabkin, J.G., Markowitz, J.S., Tricamo, E., and Klein, D.F. (1988) Social functioning in chronic depression: Effect of 6 weeks of antidepressant treatment. *Psychiatry Res* 25:213–222.

Thase, M.E., Fava, M., Halbreich, U., Kocsis, J.H., Koran, L., Daidson, J., Rosenbaum, J., and Harrison, W. (1996) A placebo-controlled, randomized clinical trial comparing sertraline and imipramine for the treatment of dysthymia. *Arch Gen Psychiatry* 53:777–784.

Thase, M.E., Greenhouse, J.B., Frank, E., Reynolds, C.F., Pilonis, P.A., Hurley, K., and Grochinski, V., et al. (1997) Treatment of major depression with psychotherapy or psychotherapy-pharmacotherapy combinations. *Arch Gen Psychiatry* 54:1009–1015.

Thase, M.E., Rush, A.J., Howland, R.H., Kornstein, S.G., Kocsis, J.H., Gelenberg, A.J., Schatzberg, A.F., Koran, L.M., Keller, M.B., Russell, J.M., Hirschfeld, R.M., LaVange, L.M., Klein, D.N., Fawcett, J., and Harrison, W. (2002) Double-blind switch study of imipramine or sertraline treatment of antidepressant-resistant chronic depression. *Arch Gen Psychiatry* 59(3):233–239.

Tollefson, G.D., and Holman, S.L. (1993) Analysis of the Hamilton Depression Rating Scale factors from a double-blind, placebo-controlled trial of fluoxetine in geriatric major depression. *Int Clin Psychopharmacol* 8(4):253–259.

Unutzer, J., Katon, W., Callahan, C.M., Williams, J.W., Jr., Hunkeler, E., Harpole, L., Hoffing, M., Della Penna, R.D., Noel, P.H., Lin, E.H., Arean, P.A., Hegel, M.T., Tang, L., Belin, T.R., Oishi, S., and Langston, C. (2002) Collaborative care management of late-life depression in the primary care setting: A randomized controlled trial. *JAMA* 288(22):2836–2845.

Vaillant, G.E., Orav, J., Meyer, S.E., McCullough Vaillant, L., and Roston, D. (1996) 1995 IPA/Bayer Research Awards in Psychogeriatrics. Late-life consequences of affective spectrum disorder. *Int Psychogeriatr* 8(1):13–32.

Vallejo, J., Gasto, C., Catalan, R., and Salamero, M. (1987) Double-blind study of imipramine versus phenelzine in melancholias and dysthymic disorders. *Br J Psychiatry* 151:639–642.

Vanelle, J., Attar-Levy, D., Poirier, M., Bouhassira, M., Blin, P., and Olie, J. (1997) Controlled efficacy study of fluoxetine in dysthymia. *Br J Psychiatry* 170:345–350.

Versiani, M., Amrein, R., and Stabl, M. (1997) Moclobemide and imipramine in chronic depression (dysthymia): An international double-blind, placebo-controlled trial. International Collaborative Study Group. *Int Clin Psychopharmacol* 12:183–193.

Waern, M., Runeson, B.S., Allebeck, P., Beskow, J., Rubenowitz, E., Skoog, I., and Wilhelmsson, K. (2002) Mental disorder in elderly suicides: a case-control study. *Am J Psychiatry* 159(3):450–455.

Waring, E.M., Chamberlaine, C.H., McCrank, E.W., Stalker, C.A., Carver, C., Fry, R., and Barnes, S. (1988) Dysthymia: A randomized study of cognitive marital therapy and antidepressants. *Can J Psychiatry* 33(2):96–99.

Weissman, M.M., Leaf, P.J., Bruce, M.L., and Florio, L.P. (1988) The epidemiology of dysthymia in five communities: Rates risks, comorbidity, and treatment. *Am J Psychiatry* 145:815–819.

Wells, K.B., Sherbourne, C., Schoenbaum, M., Duan, N., Meredith, L., Unutzer, J., Miranda, J., Carney, M.F., and Rubenstein, L.V. (2000) Impact of disseminating quality improvement programs for depression in managed primary care: A randomized controlled trial. *JAMA* 12;283(2):212–220.

Wells, K.B., Stewart, A., Hays, R.D., Burnam, M.A., Rogers, W., Daniels, M., Berry, S., et al. (1989) The functioning and well-being of depressed patients. *JAMA* 262:914–919.

Williams, J.W., Jr., Barrett, J., Oxman, T., Frank, E., Katon, W., Sullivan, M., Cornell, J., and Sengupta, A. (2000) Treatment of dysthymia and minor depression in primary care: A randomized controlled trial in older adults. *JAMA* 284:1519–1526.

World Health Organization. (1996) *The Global Burden of Disease.* A comprehensive assessment of mortality and disability from diseases, injuries, and risk factors in 1990 and projected to 2020. Murray, C.J., and Lopez, A.D., eds. Geneva, International: World Health Organization.

# 6 | Nonmajor clinically significant depression in the elderly

ANAND KUMAR, HELEN LAVRETSKY, AND
VIRGINIA ELDERKIN-THOMPSON

Clinical depression in the elderly is associated with striking medical and psychosocial consequences. These include more frequent visits to physicians' offices, absenteeism, use of tranquilizers, and suicide attempts. Amplification of associated medical and cognitive difficulties together with a substantial decline in overall productivity are also hallmarks of mood disorders in late life (Lavretsky and Kumar, 2002; Lebowitz et al., 1997). While major depressive disorder (MDD) is the best recognized and characterized depressive syndrome in the elderly, other depressive syndromes and subsyndromal disorders are also associated with significant functional impairment and disability (Beck and Koenig, 1996; Beekman 1997; Geiselmann and Bauer, 2000; Judd et al., 1996; Koenig et al., 1997). These clinical categories have received minimal attention in the psychiatric literature.

This chapter focuses on clinically significant depression that does not meet established criteria for MDD. This category encompasses several clinical subtypes with subtle distinctions between them (Blazer et al., 1989; Tannock and Katona, 1995). We begin by discussing the clinical heterogeneity and nosological complexities of these disorders as currently described in the literature. We describe the phenomenological, neurobiological, and neuropsychological features associated with these groups of disorders. We also integrate information from the elderly with data from nongeriatric adult patients with comparable clinical impairment. Finally, we draw conclusions about the validity of this clinical category based on the published literature and recommend criteria for the diagnosis of these disorders.

## NOSOLOGICAL AND DIAGNOSTIC COMPLEXITIES

Only a few of the several depressive syndromes described in DSM-IV (American Psychiatric Association, 1994) are widely recognized and commonly used in clinical discourse. These include major depression, dysthymic disorder, mood disorder due to a general medical condition, substance-induced mood disorder, adjustment disorder(s), and depressive disorder not otherwise specified (NOS). The last category encompasses several very different and conceptually evolving subcategories including minor depressive disorder, premenstrual dysphoric disorder, and recurrent brief depressive disorder. According to DSM-IV, minor depression may be subsumed within dysthymia and adjustment disorder within depressed mood or depression NOS. Recognizing these ambiguities and overlap, DSM-IV has published tentative criteria sets for minor depressive disorder, recurrent brief depressive disorder (RBD), and mixed anxiety-depressive disorder. This exhaustive list of mood disorders does not, however, cover all categories of clinically significant depression.

The existing clinical and semantic overlap makes any assumptions about the true prevalence of nonmajor depression somewhat questionable. For example, the term *minor depression* is commonly used to denote all clinically significant forms of depression that fail to meet the criteria for major depression rather than the specific syndrome described in DSM-IV. The term *subthreshold major depression* emerged to classify patients with fewer than five clinically significant depressive symptoms, thereby not meeting the criteria for the diagnosis of major depression. This patient group was found to have significant impairment in social and occupational functioning in two epidemiological surveys (Broadhead et al., 1990; Wells et al., 1989). While these disorders are receiving increasing recognition, data are sparse on the clinical course, the outcome, and the risk of suicide in patients diagnosed with these conditions.

## HISTORICAL PERSPECTIVE

The classification of mental disorders has posed a fundamental challenge to clinicians and researchers in psychiatry and the behavioral sciences. The basic presumption in medicine that a classification based on etiology is the most valid is not yet applicable in psychiatry given the lack of clarity about the etiology of nearly all mental disorders (Kendell, 1989). Descriptive categorization of psychiatric syndromes remains the principal approach to classifying and understanding mental illnesses (Kendell, 1988, 1989). A syndrome may be operationally defined as a cluster of related symptoms and signs with a characteristic time course (Kendell, 1988, 1989). These may consist of abnormal behaviors, subjective experiences, or a combination of the two (Kendell, 1989). By definition, primary psychiatric disorders are idiopathic syndromes in which no defined disease processes are known to cause the manifest symptoms and signs (Caine et al., 1994; Wiggings and Schwartz, 1994). Syndromes are often treated as distinct from one another, and this approach forms the basis of both the *Diagnostic and Statistical Manual* (DSM) and the *International Classification of Diseases* (ICD) for psychiatric disorders. The DSM and ICD systems operationalize diagnostic concepts, standardize nomenclature (Guze, 1992), and provide the principal dialects for communication in psychiatry and the behavioral sciences around the world (Guze, 1992; Wiggings and Schwartz, 1994). However, a purely categorical approach has fundamental limitations, potentially impeding our understanding of the nature of these disorders. It is based on the assumption that the psychiatric syndromes are largely distinct from one another and mutually exclusive. Currently existing depressive constructs frequently overlap or coexist, and often fail to predict the disease course and/or the treatment outcome (van Praag, 1990, 1993, 1998).

In their classical paper, Robins and Guze (1970) proposed criteria for the validation of clinical syndromes. These comprise identification and description of the syndrome, either by *clinical intuition* or by cluster analysis; demonstration of the natural boundaries or *points of rarity* between related syndromes by discriminant function analysis, latent class analysis, and other statistical approaches; follow-up studies establishing a distinctive course and outcomes; therapeutic trials establishing a distinctive treatment response; family studies establishing that the syndrome *breeds true*; and association with some more fundamental abnormality—histological, psychological, biochemical, or molecular.

Few, if any, syndromes or disorders in the DSM classification have been validated using standardized criteria. The majority of clinical studies are based on narrowly defined samples that exclude much of the variability of the affective phenomena under consideration (Caine et al., 1994). They include psychiatric patients with categorically defined depressive disorders, and one must be especially cautious when concluding that different samples of depressed patients are phenomenologically distinct from one another.

The dimensional approach to classifying psychiatric disorders is an alternative described in research studies (Gallo, 1995; Gallo et al., 1994, 1999; Goldberg and Huxley, 1992; Grayson et al., 1987a, 1987b; Tien and Gallo, 1997). This approach conceptualizes behavioral syndromes as occurring along more than one dimension. For example, depression and anxiety may be conceptualized as two *parallel* dimensions, as opposed to distinct, mutually exclusive categories (Grayson et al., 1987a). Also, the vegetative and *psychic* or cognitive aspects of mood may be treated as two coexisting dimensions in patients with clinical depression. Psychometric techniques, such as latent trait analysis, have been used to model the relationship between variables and to identify clusters of symptoms forming a dimension (Grayson et al., 1987b; Parker et al., 1995a–1995c, 1996). This approach incorporates two measures of any particular symptom: the threshold of a symptom, which represents a measure of severity, and the slope of a symptom, which represents the discriminatory power of the symptom to distinguish individuals with the same symptom from one another and from normals (Goldberg and Huxley, 1992; Grayson et al., 1987b). The widely used categorical approach is useful when considering specific interventions for individual disease states. The dimensional approach more accurately captures symptoms and syndromes as overlapping clinical phenomena that reflect underlying traits and core psychopathological processes of mental illnesses (Vollebergh et al., 2001). It also helps us understand the contribution of specific variables and the interactions between biological and psychosocial factors in affective disorders.

## STABILITY OF SYNDROMES AND PSYCHIATRIC DIAGNOSES

The instability of psychiatric diagnoses over time has raised questions about the validity of contemporary diagnostic classification systems of depression. Angst and colleagues (Angst and Merikangas, 1997; Angst et al., 2000) reported that there is little stability among the specific subtypes of depression experienced by those who continue to manifest depression during the follow-up period. Changes in the clinical presentation and severity of depression are frequently encountered over time. This supports the notion of a *spectrum* depressive disorder rather than a set of discrete subtypes. Categories such as *subsyndromal, subclinical,* or *subthreshold* depression have been described to denote clinically significant symptoms of depression that linger over a period of time (Angst and Merikangas, 1997; Angst et al., 2000; Judd et al., 1997, 1998).

The results of the 1996 International College of Neuropsychopharmacology President's Workshop supported the conclusion that unipolar major depressive disorder is a pleiomorphic mood disorder consisting of a cluster of depressive subtypes existing in a relatively homogeneous, symptomatic clinical continuum. This extends from subsyndromal depressive symptomatology through minor depressive episode, dysthymic disorder, MDD, and double depression. The workshop argued (Judd, 1997) that subsyndromal and minor depression represent clinically significant depressive subtypes commonly observed during the course of illness in patients with unipolar major depressive illness. Also, some investigators (Judd et al., 1998) have observed in their prospective, naturalistic follow-up study of patients initially diagnosed with MDD that depressive symptoms at threshold for minor depression (27%), and subthreshold depressive symptoms (17%) were more common than MDD (15%).

It is clear from the emerging literature that clinically significant depression that does not meet criteria for MDD is responsible for considerable psychosocial and functional compromise (Angst and Merikangas, 1997; Blazer, 1994; Judd et al., 1997, 1998; Koenig et al., 1997; Rollman and Reynolds, 1999). Also, the relationship of these categories to MDD is dynamic and tends to change over time. Prospective longitudinal data from the studies of young adult patients reveal that subthreshold depression, and other forms, may be both antecedent to and sequelae of MDD, thereby providing evidence for the validity of the spectrum concept of the depression (Angst and Merikangas, 1997). Further, in the elderly, depression may also be the first symptom of a neurodegenerative disorder in addition to being part of the clinical profile of patients diagnosed with clinical dementia (Lavretsky and Kumar, 2002; Lebowitz et al., 1997). Despite their broad impact and clinical relevance, information on the natural course, neurobiological correlates, and treatment response of nonmajor depression is fragmentary at present. Several nosological entities may be subsumed under the rubric of nonmajor clinically significant depression, thereby complicating the overall picture both conceptually and clinically.

## DIFFERENTIAL DIAGNOSIS: MINOR DEPRESSION

Minor depressive disorder is now included in DSM-IV as a *potential category* with a set of diagnostic research criteria proposed for further studies (American Psychiatric Association, 1994). The essential feature of minor depression is one or more periods of depressive symptoms that are identical to major depressive episodes in duration (2 weeks or longer) but that involve fewer symptoms and less impairment. An episode involves either a sad/depressed mood or loss of interest/pleasure in nearly all activities. In total, at least two but fewer than five additional symptoms must be present. During the episode, these symptoms cause clinically significant distress or impairment in social, occupational, or other important areas of functioning. In some individuals, there may be near-normal functioning, but this is accomplished with significantly increased effort. The diagnosis of minor depression is excluded if there is a history of a major unipolar or bipolar mood disorder, a disorder belonging to the schizophrenia spectrum, or any other psychotic illness. Using this construct, minor depression may be conceptualized as part of a depressive spectrum defined by the number of symptoms and their severity, as well as the duration of the episode.

The recommended DSM-IV criteria notwithstanding, definitions of minor depression vary among different investigators, which contributes to the confusion when dealing with this group of disorders. Broadhead and associates (1990) defined minor depression with mood disturbance as the presence of depressed mood or anhedonia plus one or more other symptoms of depression for 2 weeks. Minor depression without mood disturbance is defined as one or more symptoms of depression for 2 weeks without depressed mood or anhedonia (Beck and Koenig, 1996; Blazer, 1994). Minor depression without mood disturbance was included because of a concern that individuals with depressive symptoms may have a depressive spectrum disorder without depressed mood or anhedonia. Bruce and colleagues (1990) defined *dysphoria* as 2 weeks or more of feeling "sad, blue, depressed, or when you lose all interest and pleasure in things you usually cared about or enjoyed." Skodol and colleagues (1994) defined minor depression as the presence of one or more symptoms of depression, one of which must be dysphoria or anhedonia. Diagnoses of major depression or dysthymia must be excluded (Beck and Koenig, 1996).

Little is known about the natural history of minor depression. About 20% of those diagnosed with minor depression had a lifetime diagnosis of major depression (Judd et al., 1996). As many as one-third to one-half of patients with major depressions did not have full recovery and had residual symptoms consistent with minor depressive syndrome (Beck and Koenig, 1996; Judd et al., 1996). Minor depression is associated with considerable discomfort, disability, and morbidity (Rosen et al., 2000), as well as the excessive use of non–mental health services (Beekman et al., 1997). Despite the obvious mental and public health significance of this group of disorders, only a few studies have focused on minor depression. These existing studies consistently report undertreatment of depressed elderly individuals in primary care and nursing home settings, underlining the importance of recognizing nonmajor clinically significant depression (Geiselmann and Bauer, 2000; Katz, 1998; Lyness et al., 1996; Mulsant and Ganguli, 1999; Rosen et al., 2000; Williams et al., 2000).

## DIFFERENTIAL DIAGNOSIS: SUBSYNDROMAL DEPRESSIVE SPECTRUM

*Subsyndromal depressive spectrum* (SSD) disorders have been proposed by different investigators in their longitudinal studies of large populations of adult and geriatric patients. *Subsyndromal depression* was operationally defined as any two or more concurrent symptoms of depression (DSM), present for most or all of the time, for at least 2 weeks, associated with evidence of social dysfunction occurring in individuals who do not meet criteria for the diagnosis of minor depression, major depression and/or dysthymia. It was initially subcategorized into SSD with and without depression. The former overlapped considerably with the DSM-IV category of minor depression. Therefore, the revised criteria only included patients who did not meet criteria for minor depression, that is, those without the 14-day depressed mood/anhedonia requirement. The investigators (Judd, 1997) suggested that the most common SSD symptoms include insomnia, feeling tired, recurrent thoughts of death, and trouble concentrating. They also proposed that the symptomatic course is dynamic and changeable, thus representing a symptomatic continuum of a single disease category. Further, SSD, which results in significant psychosocial impairment, may, together with subthreshold anxiety, represent a risk factor for rapid relapse of depression (Judd, 1997).

In an earlier paper based on the National Institute of Mental Health (NIMH) Epidemiological Catchment Area (ECA) study involving 10,526 community respondents (Judd et al., 1997), two different phenomena of SSD were observed. One occurred as an integral component of the course of unipolar MDD, and the other occurred spontaneously in nonunipolar depressed subjects. In both instances, subthreshold depression was associated with significant dysfunction, increased prevalence of a past history of major depressive episodes, and a high prevalence of suicide attempts.

## DIFFERENTIAL DIAGNOSIS: OTHER DIAGNOSTIC CATEGORIES

A number of mood disorders may be considered in the differential diagnosis of nonmajor clinically significant depression (DSM-IV) (American Psychiatric Association, 1994). Adjustment disorder with depressed mood is diagnosed if the depressive symptoms occur in response to a psychosocial stressor. Criteria for depressive disorder NOS differ from those for MDD in the number of presenting symptoms; that is, fewer than five symptoms can be present. Depressive symptoms occurring in response to the loss of a loved one are considered bereavement. Substance-induced mood disorder

is due to the direct physiological effects of a drug of abuse or to the side effects of a medication (e.g., steroids). Mood disorder due to a general medical condition is diagnosed when depression is considered to be the direct effect of a general medical condition. Recurrent brief depressive disorder is defined as an episode lasting less than 2 weeks but longer than 2 days that recurs at least once a month for 12 consecutive months. In summary, the same combination of signs and symptoms, occurring in the context of diverse antecedents (medical and psychosocial), has been classified and categorized as distinct clinical entities in standard psychiatric nosology.

## DOES GERIATRIC NONMAJOR CLINICALLY SIGNIFICANT DEPRESSION DIFFER FROM DEPRESSION IN YOUNGER ADULTS?

Clear similarities exist in phenomenology and disease course, especially in those patients who have had depression since their young adulthood. However, there are also important differences between adults and the elderly in the symptomatology of depressive disorders (Gottfries, 1998; Post, 1962; Roth, 1955). Elderly people, in general, tend to report depressed mood less frequently (Gallo and Rabins, 1999). A high rate of anxiety is seen in elderly patients with MDD compared with younger depressive patients. Depression in elderly people is often masked by somatic symptoms, either because of somatization or because of the accentuation of symptoms of the concomitant illness (Gallo and Rabins, 1999). Cognitive impairment, caused by depression and usually referred to as *pseudodementia* or *dementia syndrome of depression*, occurs more commonly in elderly than in younger patients (Gottfries, 1998). Moreover, the etiology of depression is more heterogeneous in elderly people than in younger ones. Genetic factors have been reported to be less influential in elderly patients, especially in cases of late-onset depression (Lavretsky and Kumar, in press; Lebowitz et al., 1997). However, biochemical and neurodegenerative changes in the aging brain may further reduce the threshold for depression in the elderly. Psychosocial factors are also important. Widowhood, retirement, loss of independence, or a caregiving role all increase the risk of depression (Lavretsky and Kumar, 2002; Lebowitz et al., 1997).

Unlike major depression, with its preponderance of biological and melancholic features, the clinical presentation of minor depression is variable. Blazer and colleagues (1989) identified a symptom cluster profile unique to people over 60 years of age characterized by depressed mood, psychomotor retardation, poor concentration, constipation, and poor self-perception of health. This cluster was associated with cognitive deficits and physical illness and did not correspond to any particular DSM category. The spectrum of geriatric depression also extends to patients with underlying medical or progressive dementing illnesses who may develop depression during the course of their illness as a psychological reaction to the illness or as a disorder that is related to the underlying pathophysiology of the primary condition. Although not unique to the elderly, depression associated with spousal bereavement, loss of independence, functional disability, medical illness, or cognitive impairment is more common among older adults.

In studies of spousal bereavement, the prior history of syndromal or subsyndromal depression predicted major depression following bereavement, as well as future depression throughout the unipolar depressive spectrum (Zisook et al., 1997). Subsyndromal and minor depression stood between major depression and no depression in terms of their effect on the overall adjustment to widowhood. The authors found this to be additional evidence in support of the spectrum concept. Prigerson and colleagues (1995) identified distinct patterns of symptoms in complicated grief and bereavement-related depression. Seven symptoms constituted complicated grief: searching, yearning, preoccupation with thoughts of the deceased, crying, disbelief regarding the death, feeling stunned by the death, and lack of acceptance of the death. These symptoms were associated with enduring functional impairment.

Several investigators have identified clinical features of dysthymia that are clearly different in the elderly compared with younger adults with the disorder (Devanand et al., 1994; Kocsis, 1998). These features include late onset, associated medical co-morbidity, cognitive deterioration, and frequent adverse life events. Geriatric dysthymia also appears to be less frequently associated with psychiatric co-morbidity, thereby suggesting that dysthymia in the elderly may be a different disorder (Devanand et al., 1994; Kirby et al., 1999). Older patients with dysthymia typically present to primary care settings rather than to specialized behavioral services, which requires a heightened awareness of this disorder by primary care providers. Although depressive syndromes are common in older patients, dysthymia occurs less frequently in the elderly than in younger adults. This finding may be the consequence of the DSM criteria that do not capture the unique features of depression in older adults.

## EPIDEMIOLOGY AND CLINICAL FEATURES

The nebulous nosological status of minor depression together with the variability in diagnostic criteria contributes to the differences in prevalence estimates of these disorders (Gallo, 1995; Henderson et al., 1993, 1997). Relevant factors include differences in diagnostic systems, severity threshold, and the duration of illness required for the diagnosis of various affective states/disorders (Beekman et al., 1999; Newman et al., 1998). Despite these methodological considerations, there is broad consensus on the prevalence and clinical impact of nonmajor forms of mood disorders in both the community and more specialized clinical settings.

### Community Samples

Minor and other nonmajor forms of clinical depression are more prevalent in adult and elderly populations than MDD. Reanalyzing the ECA data, Judd and colleagues (1997) reported a 1-year prevalence of SSD of 11.8% using the criterion of more than two symptoms for at least 2 weeks. This figure exceeds the 9.5% 1-year combined prevalence for all the DSM-defined mood disorders. Tannock and Katona (1995) suggested that depressive symptoms or subsyndromal cases of minor or mild depression are very common in the elderly population. Blazer and Williams (1980) found that 14.7% of their community sample over age 65 had "substantial depressive symptoms." Despite methodological differences, there is an emerging consensus that the prevalence of minor depression changes with age: there is an increase in symptoms in people in their 30s, a decrease in middle age, a steady increase in old age, and a very steep increase in people over 80 (Beck and Koenig, 1996; Ernst and Angst, 1995). This phenomenon appears unrelated to the increased mortality, somatization, or increased institutionalization of depressed elderly (Beck and Koenig, 1996; Koenig et al., 1997). There is also a suggestion of mitigation of severe depression with age (Ernst and Angst, 1995; Jorm, 2000). Caine et al. (1994) argue that much of the affective spectrum of symptomatology in elderly community populations is not captured by our current diagnostic entities. Most, though not all studies, also suggest that prevalence rates are higher in women and among older people living in adverse socioeconomic circumstances (Copeland et al., 1986; Steffens et al., 2000).

### Long-Term Care Settings

The prevalence rates of minor depression have been estimated in special populations and settings. For example, it affects up to 50% of residents in long-term care facilities and up to 25% of patients in primary care settings (Parmelee et al., 1989; Rosen et al., 2000). In all settings, the prevalence of depressive symptoms is two- to fourfold greater than that of major depression (Mulsant et al., 1999; Parmelee et al., 1989). Among institutionalized elderly, up to 70% feel "depressed, sad, or blue" at least enough to cause minor problems in their day-to-day activities (Mulsant and Ganguli, 1999). Elderly nursing home and congregate apartment residents were screened for symptoms of depression. Of 708 survey respondents, 12.4% met the DSM-III-R criteria for major depression. Another 30.5% of the total sample reported less severe but nonetheless marked depressive symptoms. Such minor depressive syndromes were much more common among congregate housing than nursing home residents. Possible MDD was more prevalent among newly admitted residents of both housing components.

## Medical Settings

Most patients with mental illness are seen exclusively in primary care settings (Beck and Koenig, 1996; Broadhead et al., 1990; Wells et al., 1989). Primary care settings have therefore been the recent focus of studies of minor depression. Studies of depression in the medically ill usually report on the negative impact of depression on the rate and speed of recovery, as well as its overall impact on disability and the increased cost of care (Beck and Koenig, 1996; Koenig, 1998; Lyness et al., 1996; Pennix et al., 1998; Rovner and Ganguli, 1998; Viinamaki et al., 1995; Whooley et al., 1999). It is estimated that 3% to 16% of medical outpatients suffer from minor depression. Up to 64% of medical outpatients complain of depressed mood (Beck and Koenig, 1996). These patients often present with medically unexplained somatic symptoms and have at least twice as many health visits as nondepressed patients.

## Geriatric Depression in the Medically Ill

A review of the literature from 1965 to 1995 found the reported prevalence of minor depression in medical outpatients to be between 3% and 16% (Beck and Koenig, 1996; Koenig, 1998; Pennix et al., 1998; Rovner and Ganguli, 1998; Viinamaki et al., 1995; Whooley et al., 1999). Up to 64% of medical inpatients complained of depressed mood, and mood disturbances are associated with a broad spectrum of medical disorders. In a study of 542 patients age 60 and older, Koenig (1998) reported higher rates of major and minor depression associated with congestive heart failure (CHF) compared with cardiac patients without CHF (ratio of 1.5–2:1). When the major and minor depression groups were compared directly, no significant differences were observed between them on salient clinical and psychosocial measures (Koenig, 1998). Depression is associated with excess disability in visually impaired patients (Rovner and Ganguli, 1998), with poor treatment in elderly patients with non-insulin-dependent diabetes (type 2) (Viinamaki et al., 1995), and with increased risk of falls and fractures (Whooley et al., 1999). Chronic depression, when present for at least 6 years, may also increase the risk of

cancer in elderly women according to a recent epidemiological study (Penninx et al., 1998).

## Depression in Patients with Degenerative and Neurological Disorders

Many diseases of the central nervous system (CNS) are associated with an increased prevalence of depression. Mood disturbances are commonly observed in neurodegenerative disorders, including probable Alzheimer's disease (AD) and Parkinson's disease (PD), and following ischemic injury to the brain—poststroke depression. However, depression is not invariably seen in all degenerative disorders, and the prevalence and profile of the mood and behavioral aberrations are relatively disease specific (Cummings and Masterman, 1999; Devanand, 1997; Devanand et al., 1997; Harwood et al., 1999; Kumar and Cummings, 2001; Lyketsos et al., 2000; Mendez et al., 1998; Menza et al., 1995; Parikh et al., 1987; Simpson et al., 1999). This suggests that specific neurobiological mechanisms and pathways may be responsible for mood disorders across conditions (Kumar and Cummings, 2001; Parikh et al., 1987; Simpson et al., 1999).

In AD, both MDD and other clinically significant forms of depression that do not meet the threshold for major depression have been described (Devanand, 1997; Devanand et al., 1997; Harwood et al., 1999; Kumar and Cummings, 2001; Lyketsos et al., 2000). In certain study samples, clinically significant minor depression and depressive symptoms are more prevalent than MDD and have been reported in 20%–40% of patients diagnosed with AD (Devanand, 1997; Devanand et al., 1997; Harwood et al., 1999; Lyketsos et al., 2000). Prevalence estimates of depression in AD vary widely from zero to as high as 86% in some samples. Estimates of depression in PD also vary widely. Studies using more stringent criteria for the diagnosis of depression suggest that its true prevalence in PD may be between 20% and 40% (Cummings and Masterman, 1999). Approximately half of these patients meet criteria for MDD, and the rest present with features consistent with minor depression and dysthymia. Differences in diagnostic instruments and in the clinical methods used to diagnose depression (patient interviews as opposed to caregiver reports) probably contribute to these discrepant findings (Kumar and Cummings, 2001). Also, the overlap in clinical features between AD, PD, and affective disorders complicates the diagnosis of depression in these disorders (Kumar and Cummings, 2001).

Depression following vascular injury to the cerebral hemispheres is now a well-recognized clinical entity. Poststroke depression may present as minor or major depression and may occur within 12–24 months of the cerebrovascular accident (Burvill et al., 1997). Clearly, major as well as less severe forms of depression occur in patients with neurodegenerative and vascular diseases. This observation, together with the absence of any biological rationale to treat these categories as distinct entities, lends credence to the notion that major and other forms of depression may represent a clinical continuum rather than distinct clinical entities. Impairments in neurotransmitter function and selective atrophy in the forebrain nuclei have been offered as explanations for the depression in neurodegenerative disorders (Mendez et al., 1998; Menza et al., 1995).

Representative studies of nonmajor clinically significant depression are summarized in Table 6.1.

## GENETICS

The results of the association studies in behavioral genetics have been inconsistent. The explanations of these inconsistencies include the lack of the diagnostic precision in defining phenotypes, as well as biases from population stratification (the mixture of individuals from heterogeneous genetic backgrounds) (Sher, 2000). These artifacts may occur because population stratification (or admixture) due to ethnic or other confounding factors can generate significant population differences in marker allele frequencies (Remick et al., 1996; Roses and Saunders, 1994). Sher (2000) suggested that a major problem of association studies in psychiatric diseases is that psychiatric diagnoses are not biologically real disease entities: syndromal psychiatric diagnosis such as depression includes etiologically, pathologically, and prognostically heterogeneous disorders. For this reason, genetic studies have not yet addressed subsyndromal depressive spectrum disorders.

On the syndromal level, traditional familial studies, designed to study heritability of depression, have found a relationship between MDD, bipolar depression, schizoaffective disorders, alcoholism, panic disorder, eating disorders, and personality disorders, thereby establishing a rather broad range of related spectrum disorders (Ramachandran et al., 1996; Small et al., 1996; Yaffe et al., 1997; Zubenko et al., 1996). Remick and colleagues (1996) examined first-degree relatives of probands with the diagnoses of minor depression, MDD, dysthymia, and double depression in adults. When morbidity risks were calculated for the first-degree relatives using the maximum likelihood approach, the results showed comparable risks of depression in first-degree relatives of probands with MDD, minor depression, and dysthymia. It was concluded that from a genetic perspective, MDD, recurrent depression, minor depression, and double depression were indistinguishable.

There are no published genetic studies examining the relationship of MDD to other forms of mood disturbances in the elderly. The few genetic studies of depression in the elderly have focused primarily on the apolipoprotein E genotype, a known risk factor for AD (Lavretsky et al., 2000; Levy et al., 1999; Mauricio et al., 2000; Papassotiropoulos et al., 1999; Ramachandran et al., 1996; Roses and Saunders, 1994; Small et al., 1996; Yaffe et al., 1997; Zubenko et al., 1996) and its relationship to late-onset depression (Kumar et al., 1993) and cerebrovascular disease in late-life depression (Lavretsky et al., 2000). However, the results of these studies are inconsistent, and many investigators do not find any relationship between the apolipoprotein E genotype and behavioral symptoms such as depression in either cognitively intact or impaired patients (Levy et al., 1999; Mauricio et al., 2000; Papassotiropoulos et al., 1999). Therefore, genetic studies of affective disorders (Levy et al., 1999; Mauricio et al., 2000; Papassotiropoulos et al., 1999), although limited, appear to support the concept of a continuum of depressive disorders and suggest that further studies should also include milder forms of clinically significant depression.

## NEUROIMAGING, AND NEUROPSYCHOLOGICAL AND POLYSOMNOGRAPHIC STUDIES

Most neuroimaging studies in mood disorders are largely restricted to patients with MDD (Kumar et al., 1993, 1998; Nobler et al., 1999). Magnetic resonance imaging studies demonstrate that patients with late-life MDD have smaller focal brain volumes and larger high-intensity lesion volumes in the neocortical and subcortical regions compared with controls (Kumar et al., 1993, 1998). The focal reductions in brain volume have been identified in the prefrontal region, hippocampus, and caudate nucleus. The physiological correlates of MDD in late life include widespread reductions in glucose metabolism and cerebral blood flow on positron emission tomography (PET), Xenon-133 inhalation, and single photon emission computed tomography (SPECT) (Nobler et al., 1999). Glucose hypometabolism in MDD occurred in neocortical and subcortical regions (Kumar et al., 1993). Cerebral blood flow and metabolism were reduced in prefrontal cortical regions, superior temporal areas, and anterior parietal areas (Kumar et al., 1993; Nobler et al., 1999) (Fig. 6.1).

Our recent study (Kumar et al., 1998) demonstrated that patients with late-onset minor depression had smaller prefrontal lobe volumes compared with age-matched nondepressed controls. Our findings indicate that patients with minor depression present with specific neuroanatomical abnormalities comparable to those of the MDD group but significantly different from those of controls (Kumar et al., 1998). Normalized prefrontal lobe volumes showed a significant linear trend with the severity of depression, with volumes

TABLE 6.1. *Summary of Representative Studies of Nonmajor Clinically Significant Depression*

| Area of Research | Authors | Study Design | Sample | Depressive Subtype | Results |
|---|---|---|---|---|---|
| *Epidemiology* | | | | | |
| 1. Community samples | Beekman et al., (1999) | Literature review by the level of casesness | Review of 16 community studies of geriatric depression in 22,794 patients | Major depression; minor depression; depressive symptoms | Weighted average prevalence of major depression, 1.8%; minor depression, 9.8%; depressive symptoms, 13.5%. |
| | Steffens et al. (2000) | 90% of Cache County (Utah) elderly community sample | 4559 individuals age 65–100 years | Major, minor, subclinical depression | Prevalence of major depression was 4.4% in women and 2.7% in men. Lifetime prevalence was 20.4% in women and 9.6% in men, decreasing with age. Only 35.7% of those with MDD were treated with antidepressants. |
| | Newman et al., 1998 | Community survey in Edmonton, Canada | 1119 community residents age 65 and older were administered the Geriatric Mental State (GMS) questionnaire and compared to the DSM-III-R diagnoses | Major and minor depression | Prevalence of GMS-AGECAT depression (11.4%) was higher than the DSM-III-R diagnosis of major (0.86%) or minor depression (3.6%), which was determined mainly by the proportion of dysphoric symptoms in the instrument. |
| | Henderson et al. (1993) | Cross-sectional prevalence and clinical correlates | ICD-10 and DSM-III-R depressive diagnoses | Depressive disorder versus symptoms | Elderly had many depressive symptoms that did not increase with age. The number of depressive symptoms correlated with neuroticism, poor physical health, disability, and prior depression. |
| 2. Medical illness | Koenig (1998) | Prevalence of depression in patients with congestive heart failure | 542 consecutive medical patients | Major and minor depression | Major depression rate was 36.5% in patients with CHF compared to 25.5% in patients without CHF. The rate of minor depression was 21.5% in patients with CHF compared to 17% in patients without CHF. |
| 3. Neurological illness | Burvill et al. (1997) | Risk factors for poststroke depression over 4 months of follow-up | 191 first-ever stroke patients were followed for 4 months | Major and minor depression | 17% had major and 11% minor depression at 4 months poststroke. Predictors of depression included functional impairment, living in a nursing home, and being divorced. |

*(continued)*

TABLE 6.1. *Summary of Representative Studies of Nonmajor Clinically Significant Depression (Continued)*

| Area of Research | Authors | Study Design | Sample | Depressive Subtype | Results |
|---|---|---|---|---|---|
| | Menza et al., (1995) | Cross-sectional comparison of patients with PD and PSP | 19 patients with PSP and 42 with PD | Depressive symptoms | 42% of the PSP group had mild to moderate depression; 52% of patients had some degree of dementia. |
| | Grayson et al. (1987a) | Four diagnostic systems for dementia and depression were compared by using Latent Trait Analysis | 274 community-dwelling elderly persons | Depression and dementia | DSM-III, Gurland's system and AGECAT, and clinicians' ratings were used. Two distinct clusters of symptoms were identified, and the level of severity (threshold) was identified. |
| Phenomenology | Geiselmann and Bauer (2000) | Epidemiological Berlin Aging Study (BASE) | Community sample | Subthreshold depression, dysthymia, major depression | Subthreshold depression produced fewer symptoms with less continuity; with fewer suicidal ideations, thoughts of guilt or worthlessness. |
| Outcomes | Beekman et al. (1997) | Cross-sectional association study of depression and disability | 646 community-dwelling older adults age 55–85 years | Major and minor depression | Associations of major and minor depression with disability and reduced well-being remained significant after controlling for chronic disease and functional limitations. Adequate treatment was often not administered, even to subjects with major depression. Major and minor depression were associated with excessive use of non–mental health services. |
| | Penninx et al. (1998) | Epidemiological follow-up of community samples (the established populations for epidemiologic studies of the elderly) | 4825 persons age 71 years and older followed up at 3 and 6 years | Chronic depression (CES-D) based on cutoff criteria | When present for at least 6 years, depression was associated with a generally increased risk of cancer after controlling for age, sex, race, disability, hospital admissions, alcohol intake, and smoking. |
| Neuroimaging | Kumar et al. (1998) | Cross-sectional quantitative MRI study—whole brain volumes and normalized measures of prefrontal and temporal volumes | 18 subjects with minor depression, 35 patients with late-onset major depression, and 30 normal controls | Major and minor depression | Normalized prefrontal lobe volumes showed a significant linear trend with severity of depression, with volumes decreasing with volume severity. |

*(continued)*

TABLE 6.1. *Summary of Representative Studies of Nonmajor Clinically Significant Depression (Continued)*

| Area of Research | Authors | Study Design | Sample | Depressive Subtype | Results |
|---|---|---|---|---|---|
| Genetics | Remick et al. (1996) | Family study | Examined first-degree relatives of probands with depressive-spectrum diagnosis | Probands with minor depression, major depression, dysthymia, and double depression | When morbidity risks were calculated for first-degree relatives using the maximum likelihood approach, the results showed no significant differences in morbidity risk calculations to first-degree relatives. |
| Interventions | Rosen et al. (2000) | 6-week open-label study of sertraline treatment of minor depression | 12 nursing home residents | Minor depression | 75% achieved remission, and all tolerated medication well. |
| | Williams et al. (2000) | Randomized 11-week effectiveness trial | Comparing paroxetine to placebo and problem-solving therapy in primary care (PST-PC) | Minor depression, dysthymia | The paroxetine group showed greater resolution of symptoms than the placebo group in patients with dysthymia and minor depression. Patients treated with PST-PC did not show more improvement than placebo-treated patients, but their symptoms improved more rapidly. |

*Note.* Representative studies of late-life major and nonmajor depression, as well as genetic studies addressing the depressive spectrum, have been included. CES-D, Center for Epidemiologic Studies-Depression scale; GMS-AGECAT, Geriatric Mental State-Automated Geriatric Examination for Computer-Assisted Taxonomy; MDD, major depressive disorders; MRI, magnetic resonance imaging; PD, Parkinson's disease; PSP, progressive supranuclear palsy.

decreasing as the illness became more severe. Whole brain volumes did not differ significantly among the groups. These findings suggest common neurobiological substrates for all clinically significant forms of depression with a late onset and support the spectrum hypothesis of depression. Neuroanatomical abnormalities may represent one aspect of a broader neurobiological diathesis to mood disorders in late life. However, while these findings are intriguing, they clearly need to be replicated before more definitive conclusions can be drawn. Additional studies combining neuroimaging with focused postmortem and other neurochemical studies are also required to further elucidate the biological basis of late-life mood disorders. Studies are underway to examine the extent to which structural abnormalities of the brain, such as hyperintensities on MRI, covary with functional deficits.

The early anatomical findings introduce the secondary question of whether or not minor depressives also share cognitive features. Impairment in a number of cognitive domains, particularly executive functioning and information processing, is well documented among geriatric patients with MDD. Approximately 15% of minor depressives go on to develop a major depressive episode within 2 years (Beck and Koenig, 1996), so a decrease in executive functioning and psychomotor slowing, which increases the risk of relapse for major depressives (Akiskal et al., 1997), and a poor response to pharmacological therapy (Alexopoulos et al., 2000), might also predict a poor prognosis for minor depressives. Use of the Mini-Mental State Examination as a measure of cognitive functioning in patients with minor and major depression has not shown a difference between either group of depressives and healthy controls (Kalayam and Alexopoulos, 1999), but the lack of significance is undoubtedly due to the lack of sensitivity of the test because of the well-documented cognitive deficits among major depressives.

A longitudinal study of aging identified persons with depressive symptoms, as described in the ninth revision of the ICD-9 (Van et al., 2000), and reported depressive symptoms to be more common among those with low cognitive scores than among patients with high scores. Overall, elderly individuals who initially had low scores were also more likely to experience depressive episodes than those with high scores. Another large epidemiological study on the social and role dysfunction of SSD did not examine cognition per se (Judd et

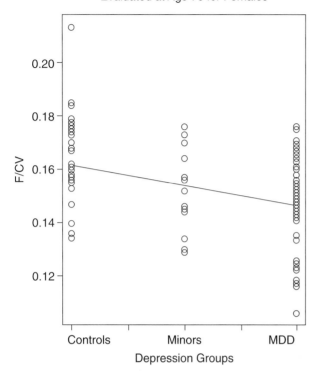

$R^2 = 0.23$, p value for group = 0.0003

Adjusted for Age, Gender, Age*Gender
Evaluated at Age 70 for Females

FIGURE 6.1 A regression plot for normalized prefrontal volume in all three groups after age and gender corrections. F/CV, prefrontal volume/cranial volume; MDD, major depressive disorder.
*The interaction between age and gender.

al., 1997), but it did report an elevated risk of suicide attempts, which have been associated with neuropsychological impairment, particularly executive dysfunction (World Health Organization, 1979).

Our research team recently completed a preliminary study on the pattern of cognitive functioning among minor and major depressives. Five domains emerged from a factor analysis in which minor depressives scored intermediate between major depressives and healthy controls in four of the five domains: verbal learning and recall, maintenance of set, working memory, and nonverbal recognition—the same pattern observed in the neuroimaging studies (Figure 6.2). In the one exception of executive functioning, minor depressives had slightly lower scores than major depressives. As Figure 6.2 shows, the difference in scores between the performance of minor depressives and controls was significant. The similarity in performance between major and minor depressives occurred despite a high percentage of hospitalized major depressives in the sample. As would be expected, major depressives showed a strong trend toward a significant difference from controls in the other factors. In what might appear to be a contradiction, severity of symptoms, as measured by the Hamilton Depression Rating Scale (HDRS), did not prove to be a good indicator of cognitive functioning because of subgroup fluctuations. For example, women with minor depression demonstrated a strong correlation with severity of symptoms in executive functioning, but men with minor depression showed a strong correlation between symptomatology and nonverbal

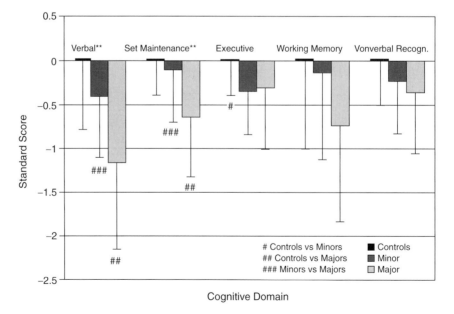

FIGURE 6.2 Cognitive factor scores in minor and major depression and controls. All scores were normalized to the mean and standard deviation of the control subjects, so the controls have zero values. Significant comparisons are noted and represent a $p$ value of $\leq 0.05$.
**Overall MANCOVA $p < .01$.

functioning. Even though overall performance levels of the three groups showed a pattern of deteriorating ability, there were differences within the domains that were not captured by the HDRS. Preliminary information, then, indicates that cognition appears to be compromised with minor levels of depression and that executive functioning and verbal and nonverbal recall are the domains most strongly affected. The possibility of a relationship between impaired cognition and anatomical and physiological changes in the prefrontal cortex warrants continued research because executive, verbal, and nonverbal abilities are closely associated with the functioning of the prefrontal cortex.

Polysomnographic findings in adult patients with subthreshold depression demonstrated shortened rapid eye movement (REM) latency, increased REM sleep, redistribution of REM to the first part of the night, classic diurnality, a frequent family history of mood disorders, and a positive response to antidepressant medication and sleep deprivation. Among primary care patients referred to a sleep disorders center, short REM latency was found in a large number of those without subjective mood change but with somatic manifestation of depression. Rather than being incidental, the REM disturbances in the foregoing studies appear consistently in the subthreshold affective group, which suggests a common neurophysiological substrate for subthreshold and melancholic depression (Akiskal et al., 1997). Functional imaging studies of subsyndromal mood disorders in late life are lacking, but could provide additional information about the pathophysiology of these conditions compared to syndromal depression.

## TREATMENT

Studies of the treatment of nonmajor depressive disorders are limited. Very little is known about treatment strategies in clinically significant nonmajor depression. Most studies focus on dysthymia and minor depression and are primary care based (Bruce and Pearson, 1999; Katz, 1998; Katz and Coyne, 2000; Rollman and Reynolds, 1999).

Descriptive studies have established that in treating depression, primary care providers use one or more of three modalities: watchful waiting, medication, and referral to the specialty sector (Barret et al., 1999). Used most commonly, watchful waiting return visits provided sympathetic listening and a show of interest, and in some cases brief commonsense counseling and tension-reducing suggestions (Barrett et al., 1999). Return visits also permitted the provider to monitor the patient's level of symptomatology. Approximately 50% of the time when a referral to a specialist was considered, the patient refused to accept it because of cost, possible stigma, or

problems with access (Barrett et al., 1999). The use of medication is virtually the only active treatment provided by primary care providers, but evidence of the efficacy of psychopharmacological interventions in nonmajor clinically significant depression is lacking.

### Treatment of Depression in Patients with Neurological and Degenerative Disorders

Although a high prevalence of clinically significant depression has been reported in many neurological and neurodegenerative disorders, there have been only 13 placebo-controlled trials of antidepressants, of which only 3 enrolled more than 10 subjects (Rummans et al., 1999). Positive results were reported in trials of citalopram in depressed patients with Alzheimer's disease and poststroke depression, and in the use of desipramine in patients with multiple sclerosis and brain injury (Rummans et al., 1999). Nearly half of the trials did not report drug–placebo differences. These studies examined the use of imipramine, maprotiline, or clomipramine in depressed patients with Alzheimer's disease, trazodone in patients with poststroke depression, and amitriptyline in patients with depression and epilepsy. Beneficial effects of nortriptyline were complicated by significant orthostatic hypotension (Rummans et al., 1999). Delirium and cardiovascular morbidity occurred in patients taking nortriptyline for poststroke depression (Rummans et al., 1999). Although it is clear that depression co-morbid with neurological illness compounds disability and worsens outcomes, clear evidence in support of effective pharmacological approaches is lacking.

### Psychotherapy and Combined Treatments

In the United Kingdom, with its general practice–based health-care delivery system, attention has been paid to developing brief, practical psychological treatments that could be provided in the primary care setting itself. Problem-solving therapy (PST) is based on behavioral medicine principles and teaches a patient that there can be a relationship between problems experienced and emotional symptoms, particularly depression and anxiety (Gath and Catalan, 1986; Mynors-Wallis, 1996). It is a collaborative treatment, with the therapist and patient focusing on regaining a sense of control over life's problems, which are likely to be important factors in resolving emotional symptoms. Gath (Gath, 1986; Gath and Catalan, 1986) and Mynors-Wallis (1996) at Oxford reported a high level of patient acceptance and satisfaction with the treatment, as patients readily understood and accepted the practical value of acquiring problem-solving skills. The British investigators concluded that PST was an effective alternative to medication treatment in their primary care patients based on the fact that it performed better than placebo and was as effective as amitriptyline (Mynors-Wallis et al., 1995). In a recent U.S. randomized 11-week effectiveness trial comparing paroxetine to placebo and PST in primary care (PST-PC), the paroxetine group showed greater symptom resolution than the placebo group. Paroxetine showed a moderate benefit for depressive symptoms and mental health functioning in elderly patients with dysthymia and more severely impaired elderly patients with minor depression. The benefits of PST-PC were smaller, had slower onset, and were more subject to site differences than those of paroxetine. Patients treated with PST-PC did not show more improvement than those given a placebo, but their symptoms improved more rapidly than those of placebo patients during the latter treatment weeks. Placebo–PST-PC differences were more pronounced in the minor depression group than in patients with dysthymia (Williams et al., 2000).

## Current Trials of Pharmacological and Combined Treatment of Depression in Primary Care Settings

Several ongoing collaborative trials are addressing the effectiveness of pharmacological and nonpharmacological treatments of depression in the primary care setting. Two current collaborative trials include the NIMH-supported Prevention of Suicide in the Primary Care Elderly Collaborative Trial (PROSPECT) study (Bruce and Pearson, 1999) and the Hartford Foundation–supported Improving Mood: Promoting Access to Collaborative Treatment for Late Life Depression (IMPACT) study; both are evaluating the effectiveness of models in practices by nurse health specialists (Katz and Coyne, 2000). The PROSPECT study was designed to evaluate the extent to which interventions targeting depression in older primary care patients could reduce risk factors for suicide, including suicidal ideation, hopelessness, and depression. Both trials included patients with nonmajor depression.

At present, treatment approaches to nonmajor clinically significant depression remain unclear. However, the results of a large multisite trial for minor depression and dysthymia in primary care (Williams et al., 2000) offer some hope for improving the outcomes of depression. In the absence of evidence to the contrary, antidepressant medications and psychotherapeutic interventions, alone or combined, are currently the recommended course of action.

## CONCLUSIONS

There are similarities and differences in the clinical manifestations of clinically significant depressive disorders. There is an emerging consensus from epidemiological, longitudinal, and genetic studies supporting the idea of a continuum of depressive disorders, ranging from the very mild subthreshold disorders to major unipolar and bipolar disorders. Evidence from neuroimaging and neuropsychological studies lends additional support to this thesis. All forms of clinically significant depression are associated with considerable economic and psychosocial consequences. Current approaches to studying affective illness, which adhere to traditional nosological categories, may no longer be adequate for the next generation of studies on the biological and psychosocial correlates of this group of disorders. Rigid definitions of the phenotype, without full integration of clinical realities, greatly limit the scope of studies aimed at elucidating the true biological basis of mood disorders.

Applying the classical criteria outlined by Robins and Guze (1970) for the validity of a diagnostic category, one would be hard pressed to draw meaningful distinctions between major and nonmajor forms of depression in elderly and nongeriatric adults with depression. Dividing patients with these forms of affective illness into rigid categories would ignore clinical and scientific realities for the sake of nosological simplicity. Mood disorders need to be conceptualized and studied along multiple dimensions including severity, duration of illness, and treatment response. In addition, while there are similarities between geriatric and nongeriatric depression with regard to phenomenology and other clinical features, there are also important differences that make the independent study of elderly patients crucial to our understanding of depression in late life.

Our desire to draw sharp boundaries between serious mental disorders and transient states of distress has contributed to our neglect of the biological and psychosocial basis of nonmajor forms of depression. Clearly, the sustained and more extreme forms of mood disturbances are easier to conceptualize as clinical disorders. The precise distinction between mood changes as a normal emotional response to the vicissitudes of life and depression as a clinical disorder is more nebulous in mild depressive states. Defining a condition operationally is often a necessary first step in trying to establish its clinical and biological correlates and demarcating its boundaries from other conditions and normality. However, any operational definition needs to be clinically meaningful and should reflect all relevant dimensions of the condition. Defining a minimum *floor effect* for the severity of depression, duration of symptoms, and overall psychosocial functioning and integrating these domains cohesively would be an important first step in defining a plausible phenotype. In the elderly, cognitive and medical aspects are additional dimensions that need to be considered. A phenotype encompassing all of the relevant dimensions could then serve as the basis for genetic, neurobiological, and psychoneuropharmacological studies.

Recently, we proposed clinical criteria for the diagnosis of clinically significant nonmajor depression in the elderly (Table 6.2) (Lavretsky and Kumar, 2002). These criteria are consistent with operational definitions of minor depression used in other clinical studies but broader in clinical and methodological scope (World Health Organization, 1979). We believe this is

an important first step in understanding and elucidating the phenomenological and neurobiological basis of clinically significant mood disorders, especially in the elderly.

Traditional approaches to classifying psychiatric disorders may no longer be adequate for the next generation of studies on the biological correlates and treatment approaches to patients with these groups of disorders. As more evidence accumulates from well-designed multicenter studies, we will be in a position to make more definitive statements and recommend more precise guidelines for both the diagnosis and management of these complex groups of disorders.

### TABLE 6.2. *Proposed Diagnostic Criteria*

1. Presence of low mood and/or loss of interest in all activities most of the day, nearly every day, and

2. At least two additional symptoms from the DSM checklist:
    a. Significant weight loss when not dieting or weight gain (e.g., a change of more than 5% of body weight in a month), or a decrease or increase in appetite nearly every day
    b. Insomnia or hypersomnia nearly every day
    c. Psychomotor retardation or agitation nearly every day (observable by others, not merely subjective feelings of restlessness or being slowed down)
    d. Fatigue or loss of energy nearly every day
    e. Feelings of worthlessness or excessive or inappropriate guilt (which may be delusional) nearly every day (not merely self-reproach or guilt about being sick)
    f. Diminished ability to think or concentrate, or indecisiveness, nearly every day (either by subjective account or as observed by others)
    g. Recurrent thoughts of death (not just fear of dying), recurrent suicidal ideation without a specific plan, or a suicide attempt or a specific plan for committing suicide

3. The symptoms cause clinically significant distress or impairment in social and occupational functioning

4. A 17-item Hamilton Depression Scale Score of 10 or greater, or Geriatric Depression Scale Score of 12 or greater (Yesavage, 1988)

5. Duration of at least 1 month; duration subtypes: 1–6 months; 6–24 months; greater than 24 months

6. The symptoms may be associated with precipitating events (e.g., loss of significant other)

7. Organic criteria:
    a. Objective evidence from physical and neurological examinations and laboratory tests, and/or a history of cerebral disease, damage, or dysfunction, or of systemic physical disorder known to cause cerebral dysfunction, including hormonal disturbances and drug effects
    b. A presumed relationship between the development or exacerbation of the underlying disease and clinically significant depression;
    c. Limitation of the disturbance to the direct psychological effect of alcohol or substance use
    d. Disappearance or significant improvement of the depressive symptoms following removal or improvement of the underlying presumed cause

8. Exclusion criteria: there has never been:
    a. An episode of mania or hypomania
    b. A chronic psychotic disorder, such as schizophrenia or delusional disorder
    c. A prior history of major depressive episode is not an exclusion criterion

ACKNOWLEDGMENTS
This work was supported in part by Grants MH55115, MH 61567 and KO2-MH02043 (AK), a NARSAD Young Investigator Award and Grant K23-MH01948 to Dr. Lavretsky, and Training Grant T32-MH17140 to Dr. Elderkin-Thompson.

REFERENCES

Akiskal, H.S., Judd, L.L., Gillin, J.C., et al. (1997) Subthreshold depressions: Clinical and polysomnographic validation of dysthymic, residual and masked forms. *J Affect Disord* 45:53–63.

Alexopoulos, G.S., Meyers, B.S., Young, R.C., et al. (2000) Executive dysfunction and long-term outcomes of geriatric depression. *Arch Gen Psychiatry* 57:285–290.

American Psychiatric Association. (1994) *Diagnostic and Statistical Manual of Mental Disorders: DSM-IV.* 4th ed. Washington, DC: American Psychiatric Press.

Angst, J. and Merikangas, K. (1997) The depressive spectrum: Diagnostic classification and course. *J Affect Disord* 45:31–39.

Angst, J., Sellaro, R., and Merikangas, K.R. (2000) Depressive spectrum diagnoses. *Compr Psychiatry* 41:39–47.

Barrett, J.E., Williams, J.W., Jr., Oxman, T.E., et al. (1999) The treatment effectiveness project. A comparison of the effectiveness of paroxetine, problem-solving therapy, and placebo in the treatment of minor depression and dysthymia in primary care patients: Background and research plan. *Gen Hosp Psychiatry* 21:260–273.

Beck, D.A. and Koenig, H.G. (1996) Minor depression: A review of the literature. *Int J Psychiatry Med* 26:177–209.

Beekman, A.T., Copeland, J.R., and Prince, M.J. (1999) Review of community prevalence of depression in later life. *Br J Psychiatry* 174:307–311.

Beekman, A.T., Deeg, D.J., Braam, A.W., et al. (1997) Consequences of major and minor depression in later life: A study of disability, well-being and service utilization. *Psychol Med* 27:1397–1409.

Blazer, D.G. (1994) Epidemiology of late-life depression. In: Schneider, L.S., ed. *Diagnosis and Treatment of Depression in Late Life: Results of the NIH Consensus Development Conference.* Washington, DC: American Psychiatric Press, pp. 9–20.

Blazer, D. and Williams, C.D. (1980) Epidemiology of dysphoria and depression in an elderly population. *Am J Psychiatry* 137:439–444.

Blazer, D., Woodbury, M., Hughes, D.C., et al. (1989) A statistical analysis of the classification of depression in a mixed community and clinical sample. *J Affect Disord* 16:11–20.

Broadhead, W.E., Blazer, D.G., George, L.K., et al. (1990) Depression, disability days, and days lost from work in a prospective epidemiologic survey. *JAMA* 264:2524–2528.

Bruce, M.L., Kim, K., Leaf, P.J., et al. (1990) Depressive episodes and dysphoria resulting from conjugal bereavement in a prospective community sample. *Am J Psychiatry* 147:608–611.

Bruce, M.L., and Pearson, J.L. (1999) Designing an intervention to prevent suicide: PROSPECT (Prevention of Suicide in Primary Care Elderly: Collaborative Trial) *Dialog Clin Neurosci* 1:100–112.

Burvill, P., Johnson, G., Jamrozik, K., et al. (1997) Risk factors for post-stroke depression. *Int J Geriatr Psychiatry* 12:219–226.

Caine, E.D., Lyness, J.M., King, D.A., et al. (1994) Clinical and etiological heterogeneity of mood disorders in elderly patients. In: Schneider, L.S., Reynolds, C.F., Lebowitz, B.D., and Friedhoff, A.J., eds. *Diagnosis and Treatment of Depression in Late Life: Results of the NIH Consensus Development Conference.* Washington, DC: American Psychiatric Press, pp. 21–54.

Copeland, J.R., Dewey, M.E., and Griffiths-Jones, H.M. (1986) A computerized psychiatric diagnostic system and case nomenclature for elderly subjects: GMS and AGECAT. *Psychol Med* 16:89–99.

Cummings, J.L. and Masterman, D.L. (1999) Depression in patients with Parkinson's disease. *Int J Geriatr Psychiatry* 14:711–718.

Devanand, D.P. (1997) Behavioral complications and their treatment in Alzheimer's disease. *Geriatrics* 52(suppl 2):S37–S39.

Devanand, D.P., Jacobs, D.M., Tang, M.X., et al. (1997) The course of psychopathologic features in mild to moderate Alzheimer disease. *Arch Gen Psychiatry* 54:257–263.

Devanand, D.P., Nobler, M.S., Singer, T., et al. (1994) Is dysthymia a different disorder in the elderly? *Am J Psychiatry* 151:1592–1599.

Ernst, C. and Angst, J. (1995) Depression in old age. Is there a real decrease in prevalence? A review. *Eur Arch Psychiatry Clin Neurosci* 245:272–287.

Gallo, J.J. (1995) Epidemiology of mental disorders in middle age and late life: Conceptual issues. *Epidemiol Rev* 17:83–94.

Gallo, J.J., Anthony, J.C., and Muthen, B.O. (1994) Age differences in the symptoms of depression: A latent trait analysis. *J Gerontol* 49:251–264.

Gallo, J.J. and Rabins, P.V. (1999) Depression without sadness: Alternative presentations of depression in late life. *Am Fam Physician* 60:820–826.

Gallo, J.J., Rabins, P.V., and Anthony, J.C. (1999) Sadness in older persons: 13-year follow-up of a community sample in Baltimore, Maryland. *Psychol Med* 29:341–350.

Gath, D. and Catalan, J. (1986) The treatment of emotional disorders in general practice: Psychological methods versus medication. *J Psychosom Res* 30:381–386.

Geiselmann, B. and Bauer, M. (2000) Subthreshold depression in the elderly: Qualitative or quantitative distinction? *Compr Psychiatry* 41:32–38.

Goldberg, D.P., and Huxley, P. (1992) *Common Mental Disorders: A Bio-social Model.* London and New York: Tavistock/Routledge.

Gottfries, C.G. (1998) Is there a difference between elderly and younger patients with regard to the symptomatology and aetiology of depression? *Int Clin Psychopharmacol* 13(suppl 5):S13–S18.

Grayson, D.A., Bridges, K., Duncan-Jones, P., et al. (1987a) The relationship between symptoms and diagnoses of minor psychiatric disorder in general practice. *Psychol Med* 17:933–942.

Grayson, D.A., Henderson, A.S., and Kay, D.W. (1987b) Diagnoses of dementia and depression: A latent trait analysis of their performance. *Psychol Med* 17:667–675.

Guze, S.B. (1992) *Why Psychiatry Is a Branch of Medicine.* New York: Oxford University Press.

Harwood, D.G., Barker, W.W., Ownby, R.L., et al. (1999) Association between premorbid history of depression and current depression in Alzheimer's disease. *J Geriatr Psychiatry Neurol* 12:72–75.

Henderson, A.S., Jorm, A.F., MacKinnon, A., et al. (1993) The prevalence of depressive disorders and the distribution of depressive symptoms in later life: A survey using Draft ICD-10 and DSM-III-R. *Psychol Med* 23:719–729.

Henderson, A.S., Korten, A.E., Jacomb, P.A., et al. (1997) The course of depression in the elderly: A longitudinal community-based study in Australia. *Psychol Med* 27:119–129.

Jorm, A.F. (2000) Does old age reduce the risk of anxiety and depression? A review of epidemiological studies across the adult life span. *Psychol Med* 30:11–22.

Judd, L.L. (1997) Pleomorphic expressions of unipolar depressive disease: Summary of the 1996 CINP President's Workshop. *J Affect Disord* 45:109–116.

Judd, L.L., Akiskal, H.S., Maser, J.D., et al. (1998) A prospective 12-year study of subsyndromal and syndromal depressive symptoms in unipolar major depressive disorders. *Arch Gen Psychiatry* 55:694–700.

Judd, L.L., Akiskal, H.S., and Paulus, M.P. (1997) The role and clinical significance of subsyndromal depressive symptoms (SSD) in unipolar major depressive disorder. *J Affect Disord* 45:5–17.

Judd, L.L., Paulus, M.P., Wells, K.B., et al. (1996) Socioeconomic burden of subsyndromal depressive symptoms and major depression in a sample of the general population. *Am J Psychiatry* 153:1411–1417.

Kalayam, B. and Alexopoulos, G.S. (1999) Prefrontal dysfunction and treatment response in geriatric depression. *Arch Gen Psychiatry* 56:713–718.

Katz, I.R. (1998) What should we do about undertreatment of late life psychiatric disorders in primary care? *J Am Geriatr Soc* 46:1573–1575.

Katz, I.R. and Coyne, J.C. (2000) The public health model for mental health care for the elderly. *JAMA* 283:2844–2845.

Keilp, J.G., Sackeim, H.A., Brodsky, B.S., et al. (2001) Neuropsychological dysfunction in depressed suicide attempters. *Am J Psychiatry* 158:735–741.

Kendell, R.E. (1988) What is a case? Food for thought for epidemiologists. *Arch Gen Psychiatry* 45:374–376.

Kendell, R.E. (1989) Clinical validity. *Psychol Med* 19:45–55.

Kirby, M., Bruce, I., Coakley, D., et al. (1999) Dysthymia among the community-dwelling elderly. *Int J Geriatr Psychiatry* 14:440–445.

Kocsis, J.H. (1998) Geriatric dysthymia. *J Clin Psychiatry* 59(suppl 10):13–15.

Koenig, H.G. (1997) Differences in psychosocial and health correlates of major and minor depression in medically ill older adults. *J Am Geriatr Soc* 45:1487–1495.

Koenig, H.G. (1998) Depression in hospitalized older patients with congestive heart failure. *Gen Hosp Psychiatry* 20:29–43.

Koenig, H.G., George, L.K., Peterson, B.L., et al. (1997) Depression in medically ill hospitalized older adults: Prevalence, characteristics, and course of symptoms according to six diagnostic schemes. *Am J Psychiatry* 154:1376–1383.

Kumar, A., and Cummings, J.L. (2001) Depression in neurodegenerative disorders and related conditions. In: Gauthier, S., and Cummings, J.L., eds. *Alzheimer's Disease and Related Disorders Annual 2001.* London: Martin Dunitz Ltd., pp. 123–142.

Kumar, A., Jin, Z., Bilker, W., et al. (1998) Late-onset minor and major depression: Early evidence for common neuroanatomical substrates detected by using MRI. *Proc Natl Acad Sci USA* 95:7654–7658.

Kumar, A., Newberg, A., Alavi, A., et al. (1993) Regional cerebral glucose metabolism in late-life depression and Alzheimer disease: A preliminary positron emission tomography study. *Proc Natl Acad Sci USA* 90:7019–7023.

Lavretsky, H., and Kumar, A. (2002) Non-major clinically significant depression: Old concepts, new insights. *Am J Geriatr Psychiatry* 10:239–255.

Lavretsky, H., Lesser, I.M., Wohl, M., et al. (2000) Apolipoprotein-E and white-matter hyperintensities in late-life depression. *Am J Geriatr Psychiatry* 8:257–261.

Lebowitz, B.D., Pearson, J.L., Schneider, L.S., et al. (1997) Diagnosis and treatment of depression in late life. Consensus statement update. *JAMA* 278:1186–1190.

Levy, M.L., Cummings, J.L., Fairbanks, L.A., et al. (1999) Apolipoprotein E genotype and noncognitive symptoms in Alzheimer's disease. *Biol Psychiatry* 45:422–425.

Lyketsos, C.G., Steinberg, M., Tschanz, J.T., et al. (2000) Mental and behavioral disturbances in dementia: Findings from the Cache County Study on Memory in Aging. *Am J Psychiatry* 157:708–714.

Lyness, J.M., Bruce, M.L., Koenig, H.G., et al. (1996) Depression and medical illness in late life: report of a symposium. *J Am Geriatr Soc* 44:198–203.

Mauricio, M., O'Hara, R., Yesavage, J.A., et al. (2000) A longitudinal study of apolipoprotein-E genotype and depressive symptoms in community-dwelling older adults. *Am J Geriatr Psychiatry* 8:196–200.

Mendez, M.F., Perryman, K.M., Miller, B.L., et al. (1998) Behavioral differences between frontotemporal dementia and Alzheimer's disease: A comparison on the BEHAVE-AD rating scale. *Int Psychogeriatr* 10:155–162.

Menza, M.A., Cocchiola, J., and Golbe, L.I. (1995) Psychiatric symptoms in progressive supranuclear palsy. *Psychosomatics* 36:550–554.

Mulsant, B.H. and Ganguli, M. (1999) Epidemiology and diagnosis of depression in late life. *J Clin Psychiatry* 60(Suppl 20):9–15.

Mynors-Wallis, L. (1996) Problem-solving treatment: Evidence for effectiveness and feasibility in primary care. *Int J Psychiatry Med* 26:249–262.

Mynors-Wallis, L.M., Gath, D.H., Lloyd-Thomas, A.R., et al. (1995) Randomised controlled trial comparing problem solving treatment with amitriptyline and placebo for major depression in primary care. *Br Med J* 310:441–445.

Newman, S.C., Sheldon, C.T., and Bland, R.C. (1998) Prevalence of depression in an elderly community sample: A comparison of GMS-AGECAT and DSM-IV diagnostic criteria. *Psychol Med* 28:1339–1345.

Nobler, M.S., Pelton, G.H., and Sackeim, H.A. (1999) Cerebral blood flow and metabolism in late-life depression and dementia. *J Geriatr Psychiatry Neurol* 12:118–127.

Papassotiropoulos, A., Bagli, M., Jessen, F., et al. (1999) Early-onset and late-onset depression are independent of the genetic polymorphism of apolipoprotein E. *Dementia Geriatr Cogn Disord* 10:258–261.

Parikh, R.M., Lipsey, J.R., Robinson, R.G., et al. (1987) Two-year longitudinal study of post-stroke mood disorders: Dynamic changes in correlates of depression at one and two years. *Stroke* 18:579–584.

Parker, G., and Hadzi-Pavlovic, D. (1996) *Melancholia: A Disorder of Movement and Mood: A Phenomenological and Neurobiological Review.* Cambridge and New York: Cambridge University Press.

Parker, G., Hadzi-Pavlovic, D., Austin, M.P., et al. (1995a) Sub-typing depression, I. Is psychomotor disturbance necessary and sufficient to the definition of melancholia? *Psychol Med* 25:815–823.

Parker, G., Hadzi-Pavlovic, D., Brodaty, H., et al. (1995b) Sub-typing depression, II. Clinical distinction of psychotic depression and non-psychotic melancholia. *Psychol Med* 25:825–832.

Parker, G., Hadzi-Pavlovic, D., Hickie, I., et al. (1995c) Sub-typing depression, III. Development of a clinical algorithm for melancholia and comparison with other diagnostic measures. *Psychol Med* 25:833–840.

Parmelee, P.A., Katz, I.R., and Lawton, M.P. (1989) Depression among institutionalized aged: Assessment and prevalence estimation. *J Gerontol* 44:M22–M29.

Penninx, B.W., Guralnik, J.M., Pahor, M., et al. (1998) Chronically depressed mood and cancer risk in older persons. *J Natl Cancer Inst* 90:1888–1893.

Post, F. (1962) *The Significance of Affective Symptoms in Old Age, a Follow-up Study of One Hundred Patients.* London and New York: Oxford University Press.

Prigerson, H.G., Frank, E., Kasl, S.V., et al. (1995) Complicated grief and bereavement-related depression as distinct disorders: Preliminary empirical validation in elderly bereaved spouses. *Am J Psychiatry* 152:22–30.

Ramachandran, G., Marder, K., Tang, M., et al. (1996) A preliminary study of apolipoprotein E genotype and psychiatric manifestations of Alzheimer's disease. *Neurology* 47:256–259.

Remick, R.A., Sadovnick, A.D., Lam, R.W., et al. (1996) Major depression, minor depression, and double depression: Are they distinct clinical entities? *Am J Med Genet* 67:347–353.

Robins, E. and Guze, S.B. (1970) Establishment of diagnostic validity in psychiatric illness: Its application to schizophrenia. *Am J Psychiatry* 126:983–987.

Rollman, B.L. and Reynolds, C.F., III. (1999) Minor and subsyndromal depression: Functional disability worth treating. *J Am Geriatr Soc* 47:757–758.

Rosen, J., Mulsant, B.H., and Pollock, B.G. (2000) Sertraline in the treatment of minor depression in nursing home residents: A pilot study. *Int J Geriatr Psychiatry* 15:177–180.

Roses, A.D. and Saunders, A.M. (1994) APOE is a major susceptibility gene for Alzheimer's disease. *Curr Opin Biotech* 5:663–667.

Roth M. (1955) The natural history of mental disorder in old age. *J Ment Sci* 101:281–301.

Rovner, B.W. and Ganguli, M. (1998) Depression and disability associated with impaired vision: The MoVies Project. *J Am Geriatr Soc* 46:617–619.

Rummans, T.A., Lauterbach, E.C., Coffey, C.E., et al. (1999) Pharmacologic efficacy in neuropsychiatry: A review of placebo- controlled treatment trials. A report of the ANPA Committee on Research. *J Neuropsychiatry Clin Neurosci* 11:176–189.

Sher, L. (2000) Psychiatric diagnoses and inconsistent results of association studies in behavioral genetics. *Med Hypotheses* 54:207–209.

Simpson, S., Allen, H., Tomenson, B., et al. (1999) Neurological correlates of depressive symptoms in Alzheimer's disease and vascular dementia. *J Affect Disord* 53:129–136.

Skodol, A.E., Schwartz, S., Dohrenwend, B.P., et al. (1994) Minor depression in a cohort of young adults in Israel. *Arch Gen Psychiatry* 51:542–551.

Small, G.W., Komo, S., La Rue, A., et al. (1996) Early detection of Alzheimer's disease by combining apolipoprotein E and neuroimaging. *Ann NY Acad Sci* 802:70–78.

Steffens, D.C., Skoog, I., Norton, M.C., et al. (2000) Prevalence of depression and its treatment in an elderly population: The Cache County study. *Arch Gen Psychiatry* 57:601–607.

Tannock, C. and Katona, C. (1995) Minor depression in the aged. Concepts, prevalence and optimal management. *Drugs Aging* 6:278–292.

Tien, A.Y. and Gallo, J.J. (1997) Clinical diagnosis: A marker for disease? *J Nerv Ment Dis* 185:739–747.

Van, D.B., Oldehinkel, A.J., Brilman, E.I., et al. (2000) Correlates of symptomatic, minor and major depression in the elderly. *J Affect Disord* 60:87–95.

van Praag, H.M. (1990) The DSM-IV (depression) classification: To be or not to be? *J Nerv Ment Dis* 178:147–149.

van Praag, H.M. (1993) Diagnosis, the rate-limiting factor of biological depression research. *Neuropsychobiology* 28:197–206.

van Praag, H.M. (1998) Inflationary tendencies in judging the yield of depression research. *Neuropsychobiology* 37:130–141.

Viinamaki, H., Niskanen, L., and Uusitupa, M. (1995) Mental well-being in people with non-insulin-dependent diabetes. *Acta Psychiatr Scand* 92:392–397.

Vollebergh, W.A., Iedema, J., Bijl, R.V., et al. (2001) The structure and stability of common mental disorders: the NEMESIS study. *Arch Gen Psychiatry* 58:597–603.

Wells, K.B., Stewart, A., Hays, R.D., et al. (1989) The functioning and well-being of depressed patients. Results from the Medical Outcomes Study. *JAMA* 262:914–919.

Whooley, M.A., Kip, K.E., Cauley, J.A., et al. (1999) Depression, falls, and risk of fracture in older women. Study of Osteoporotic Fractures Research Group. *Arch Intern Med* 159:484–490.

Wiggings, O.P., and Schwartz, M.A. (1994) The limits of psychiatric knowledge and the problem of classification. In: Sadler, J.Z., Wiggins, O.P., and Schwartz, M.A., eds. *Philosophical Perspectives on Psychiatric Diagnostic Classification.* Baltimore: Johns Hopkins University Press, pp. 89–103.

Williams, J.W., Jr., Barrett, J., Oxman, T., et al. (2000) Treatment of dysthymia and minor depression in primary care: A randomized controlled trial in older adults. *JAMA* 284:1519–1526.

World Health Organization. (1979) *International Classification of Diseases*, 9th ed. Geneva: World Health Organization.

Yaffe, K., Cauley, J., Sands, L., et al. (1997) Apolipoprotein E phenotype and cognitive decline in a prospective study of elderly community women. *Arch Neurol* 54:1110–1114.

Yesavage, J.A. (1988) Geriatric Depression Scale. *Psychopharmacol Bull* 24:709–711.

Zisook, S., Paulus, M., Shuchter, S.R., et al. (1997) The many faces of depression following spousal bereavement. *J Affect Disord* 45:85–94.

Zubenko, G.S., Henderson, R., Stiffler, J.S., et al. (1996) Association of the APOE epsilon 4 allele with clinical subtypes of late-life depression. *Biol Psychiatry* 40:1008–1016.

# 7 | Mixed cognitive and depressive syndromes

HELEN LAVRETSKY AND GARY W. SMALL

Depression and dementia are the most frequently occurring psychiatric syndromes in elderly populations (Blazer and Williams 1980; Caine et al., 1994). The two disorders often coexist. There are multiple streams of evidence for a relationship between affective and cognitive symptoms and syndromes in elderly persons. However, our understanding of the pathophysiology and possible common pathways of both disorders is limited.

Because of the growing evidence of a clinical overlap between depression and dementia, several nosological classifications have been proposed based on the sequence of the onset of the affective and cognitive symptoms (Emery and Oxman, 1992). Reifler (1998) supports a classification involving a continuum of mixed cognitive and depressive symptoms based on the severity of cognitive impairment and the duration of illness. Type 1, a purely depressive disorder, is characterized by the relatively recent onset of illness and mild cognitive impairment, which is mostly subjective in nature. Type 2 is characterized by depression superimposed on a progressive dementing illness of several years' duration, where depression has occurred more recently. An intermediate type of depressive disorder is typified by the unclear onset of cognitive and affective symptoms, where cognitive impairment may be mild but confirmed by objective testing. In the face of the increasing number of tools and approaches aiding in the early detection and prevention of Alzheimer's disease (AD) and related dementias, it becomes increasingly important to differentiate between nonprogressive cognitive impairment associated with late-life depression and depressive manifestations of progressive neurodegenerative dementias.

Despite intense research efforts, the existing data remain tentative and poorly integrated. Although the most straightforward evidence of the relationship between depression and cognitive impairment comes from research on depression in AD, we do not yet understand the nature of the link between affective and cognitive dementias in the older person. We do not know the incidence of dementia (e.g., AD or vascular) in depressed elderly patients. There is no consensus on the pattern of cognitive impairment in patients with late-life major depression. We do not yet have a complete grasp of the relationship between vascular and neurodegenerative processes in the aging brain and their effect on cognitive disturbances observed in patients with late-life depression. The available treatment options are still palliative. Large epidemiological studies must be conducted to clarify the widely debated dilemma of late-onset depression with onset in late middle and old age that is frequently accompanied by cognitive impairment: Does it represent a precursor of dementia or is it a separate disorder? If it is a prodrome of a dementing illness, what dementia subtype will likely develop later in the course of the illness? If it is not a prodrome of dementia, what will happen to the cognitive impairment over time? Will it improve with antidepressant treatment or will it remain unchanged even in the face of improvement in depressed mood? Researchers have only recently started to address these complicated questions.

In this chapter, we will review the main concepts and the existing data in the field of mixed cognitive and depressive disorders. We will limit our review to late-life unipolar depression and will not discuss cognitive syndromes associated with geriatric mania or anxiety disorders that deserve a separate review. We will describe parallel lines of evidence linking geriatric depression and cognitive disturbance derived from the epidemiological studies in different populations. We will also examine naturalistic follow-up and case-control studies indicative of causality, as well as cross-sectional studies documenting an association between the two disorders. First, we will review the rates and phenomenology of depression in dementia. Then we will describe the pattern of cognitive impairment in the context of geriatric depression, along with the historically important and relevant concept of *pseudodementia*. We will also provide an overview of recent advances in the neuropsychology of late-life depression and discuss a newer understanding of cognitive disturbances associated with geriatric depression, such as changes in cognition over time and in the response to various treatment modalities. We will then describe recent advances in the search for biomarkers of depression and dementia and outline future directions for research in this challenging area.

## DEPRESSION IN DEMENTIA

Many diseases of the central nervous system (CNS) are associated with an increased prevalence of depression (Lavretsky and Kumar, 2002b). Mood disturbances are commonly observed in patients with neurodegenerative disorders including probable AD and Parkinson's disease (PD), as well as ischemic injury to the brain, referred to as *poststroke depression* (Lavretsky and Kumar, 2002b). However, depression is not invariably seen in all degenerative disorders, and the prevalence and profile of the mood and behavioral aberrations are relatively disease specific. This suggests that particular neurobiological mechanisms and pathways may be responsible for mood disorders across conditions (Kumar and Cummings, 2001; Robinson et al., 1987; Simpson et al., 1999).

Depressive symptoms have been found in as many as 50% of patients with dementia (Reifler et al., 1982). Close to 17% of patients with dementia meet criteria for major depression (Reifler et al., 1982). Epidemiological evidence demonstrates that depression is a common feature of AD (Olin et al., 2002a,b). Reports vary concerning the prevalence of major depression in AD, with investigators reporting rates as low as 2% and as high as 85% (Cummings, 2000). Reported rates of dysthymia range from 25% to 50% (Cummings, 2000; Lyketsos et al., 1997; Vida et al., 1994). However, the observed rates of depression in dementia vary in the different studies due to variability in the methodology of epidemiological studies, including patient selection, diagnostic criteria, and duration of follow-up. Some studies suggest that depression may be a risk factor for dementia, while others indicate an association of geriatric depression and dementia (Schweitzer et al., 2002).

Affective symptoms are frequently reported by patients with dementia and by their caregivers. These symptoms range from anxiety to low energy, apathy, depression, and weight loss. However, guilt and suicidal ideations are uncommon (Weiner et al., 1997). Patients with a family history of an affective disorder are more likely to experience a depressive episode in the course of AD (Pearlson et al., 1990). The role of the age of onset of depression in the development of AD is still debated (Lawlor et al., 1994; Steffens et al., 1997). Both early and late onset have been implicated as risk factors for AD, but the data are still inconclusive (Heun et al., 2002).

Depression is regarded as a cause of excess disability in persons with dementia and contributes to their overall functional decline, as well as their diminished rehabilitation potential (Espiritu et al., 2001; Gillen et al., 2001). However, depression does not appear to worsen cognitive impairment in patients with AD to a significant degree (Berger et al., 2002). Depressed patients with AD do not exhibit greater impairment of attention, language, memory, or visual-spatial functioning than patients without mood changes (Cummings, 2000).

Awareness of dementia does not appear to be associated with the risk of depression, nor is there a consistent association between severity of cognitive impairment and the risk of depression (Olin et al., 2002a,b). Depression in the context of dementia is similar to a major depressive episode, but the signs and symptoms may be less severe. Symptoms can also include social isolation, withdrawal, and irritability (Olin et al., 2002b; Vida et al., 1994). Apathy, as defined by loss of drive, motivation, or lack of emotional response, is a common feature of the behavioral disturbances in patients with dementia. It is easily confused with depression and frequently is treated as such (Assal and Cummings, 2002; Lavretsky and Kumar, 2002a; Levy et al., 1998). Apathy is associated with executive dysfunction but not with other neuropsychological deficits (McPherson et al., 2002). The commonly coexisting symptoms of apathy and dysphoria in geriatric patients make it more difficult to differentiate related cognitive impairments.

## PUTATIVE COMMON NEUROBIOLOGICAL MECHANISMS OF DEMENTIA AND DEPRESSION

Although the psychosocial stress of receiving the diagnosis of dementia and associated functional decline is sufficient to cause depression in patients with dementia, there is also strong evidence of neurobiological commonalities between the two phenomena. The overlapping clinical features make the differential diagnosis difficult in some cases. The underlying disturbance usually resides within one or several of five principal frontal-subcortical circuits linking the specific areas of the frontal cortex to the striatum, basal ganglia, and thalamus (Tekin and Cummings, 2002). Specific chemoarchitecture and multiple interactions modulate the functional activity of each circuit (Tekin and Cummings, 2002). Dorsolateral-prefrontal circuit lesions cause executive dysfunction; orbitofrontal circuit lesions lead to personality changes characterized by disinhibition; and anterior cingulate lesions present with apathy (Tekin and Cummings, 2002).

The disruption of the frontal-subcortical circuit may occur at cortical and subcortical levels. In AD and frontal-temporal dementia (FTD), the pathological process occurs in the cortex. In PD or Huntington's disease (HD), the damage occurs at the subcortical level. In depression or stroke, pathological processes involve both cortical and subcortical areas (Lavretsky and Kumar, 2002a; Tekin and Cummings, 2002). However, at the behavioral level, these illnesses may have similar presentations. The overlap occurs with the disruption of the dorsolateral prefrontal circuit, resulting in executive dysfunction and such clinical features as mood and personality changes, retrieval-type deficits, and motor abnormalities such as dysarthria and gait abnormalities, as well as poor recall with preserved recognition (Tekin and Cummings, 2002). Apathy results from the disruption of anterior cingulate subcortical connections, lesions in the basal ganglia, and ventrolateral and dorsomedial thalamic nuclei. In addition to the neurodegenerative processes, cerebrovascular disease, clinical (i.e., stroke) or subclinical, is another common pathophysiological mechanism of disruption in brain neurocircuitry and neurochemistry implicated in broad cognitive and neuropsychiatric symptoms of late life (Lavretsky and Kumar, 2002a).

## CEREBROVASCULAR DISEASE AND DEPRESSION IN DEMENTIA

A subset of patients with neurodegenerative dementing illnesses also has coexisting cerebrovascular disease. Although mostly nonspecific, the presence of cerebrovascular disease is likely to contribute to the cognitive and behavioral symptoms of dementia. The growing evidence linking changes in white matter to depressive illness in late life (Kumar et al., 2000, 2002; Lavretsky and Kumar, 2002; Steffens and Krishnan, 1998) has stimulated similar explorations among dementia patients (Barber et al., 1999; Starkstein et al., 1997; Sultzer et al., 1993). In a cross-sectional study of patients diagnosed with dementia of Lewy bodies, AD, vascular dementia, and normal controls, periventricular hyperintensities were positively correlated with age and were more severe in all dementia groups compared with the control group (Barber et al., 1999). Total hyperintensity scores, including hyperintensities in deep white matter and basal ganglia (WMHs and BGHs) were significantly higher in all dementia groups than in the control subjects, and were higher in patients with vascular dementia than in those with dementia of Lewy bodies or AD. In all dementia patients, frontal WMHs were associated with higher depression scores. In another study of consecutive patients with probable AD (Starkstein et al., 1997), the presence of leukoareosis on magnetic resonance imaging (MRI) was associated with increased apathy and extrapyramidal signs, as well as bilateral hypoperfusion in the basal ganglia, thalamus, and frontal lobes compared to AD patients without leukoareosis. However, no differences were found

between groups in age, duration of illness, depression scores, severity of delusions, or deficits on neuropsychological tasks. Lopez and colleagues (1997) reported a significant correlation between global scores on deep white matter lesions and cognitive components of depression (low self-esteem and suicidal ideations) in patients with AD. The highest regional correlations were found between symptoms and lesions in the frontal lobe white matter. Functional neuroimaging has been somewhat inconsistent in identifying regional correlates of depression (Cummings, 2000). In an MRI and a positron emission tomography (PET) study of 11 subjects without cortical lesions who were diagnosed with vascular depression, subcortical MRI lesions were associated with cortical metabolic dysfunction, increased anxiety, depression, and greater overall severity of neuropsychiatric symptoms (Sultzer et al., 1993). Sultzer and colleagues (1995) found an association between depression and reduced metabolism in the parietal lobes. However, Hirono et al. (1998) showed a relationship between depression and hypometabolism in the superior frontal cortex bilaterally and the left anterior cingulate cortex. Unfortunately, only a few studies have attempted to integrate the impact of cerebrovascular disease on depression and other neuropsychiatric symptoms across dementia subtypes.

### Other Biological Markers of Depression in Dementia: Postmortem Studies and Behavioral Genetics

Postmortem studies of patients with AD and major depression have consistently shown reductions in locus ceruleus cell populations (Forstl et al., 1992). Zubenko and colleagues (1990) documented neurochemical changes in postmortem samples of patients with AD and depression. Dopamine levels were increased in the enthorhinal cortex of depressed compared to nondepressed AD patients. Serotonin levels were reportedly normal in AD patients with depression (Chen et al., 1996).

Exploration of the behavioral genetics of dementia is still rudimentary. It is mainly limited to AD, with the main focus on apolipoprotein E-4 allele (APOE-4). Although the APOE-4 allele is a known risk factor for AD and results in more severe language and memory impairment, most investigators have failed to show an association between the presence of APOE-4 and neuropsychiatric symptoms (Cummings, 2000). Lesch and Mossner (1998) proposed that a polymorphism in the 5′-flanking regulatory region of the serotonin (5-HTT) gene that results in allelic variation of 5-HTT expression may influence the risk of developing affective disorders. Disturbances in functional 5-HTT expression are also likely to play a role in the pathophysiology of neurodegenerative disorders, particularly late-onset AD and related cognitive and affective syndromes. Although the existing database is still limited, this is a promising and rapidly growing research area (Merikangas et al., 2002).

## COGNITION IN LATE-LIFE DEPRESSION

Despite numerous studies describing cognitive functioning in late-life depression, neuropsychology of late-life depression is poorly understood. Heterogeneity of the research data stems from the differences in methodological approaches, diagnostic criteria, assessment instruments, and patient populations (Butters et al., 2000; Lockwood et al., 2000). The patient populations differ in their medication status (treated or untreated), history of electroconvulsive therapy (ECT), inclusion of unipolar and bipolar depressed patients, age, and level of education. Only a few studies employed a comprehensive assessment of cognitive domains (Butters et al., 2000). The reported cognitive deficits in depressed outpatients are generally mild to moderate. Depressed elderly patients may exhibit some cognitive impairment, with deficits in attention and concentration, executive functioning, and memory that often resembles dementia.

From 18%–57% of depressed patients present with a syndrome resembling dementia or the dementia syndrome of depression that subsides after remission of depressive symptomatology (Emery, 1988; Kral and Emery, 1989). In most cases, the cognitive changes are less debilitating than the depressive symptoms. However, longitudinal follow-up studies of patients with combined affective and cognitive impairment demonstrate that 50%–91% of these patients develop dementia over time (Kral, 1983).

## IS "PSEUDODEMENTIA" REAL?

The term *pseudodementia* has been used historically to describe impairment in memory and other cognitive domains resembling dementia but caused by *functional* psychiatric disorders such as depression (Lavretsky and Kumar, 1999). In these disorders the cognitive impairments were considered reversible with appropriate treatment; therefore, the underlying dementia was characterized as not real. This nosological distinction was also useful in conceptually separating psychiatric diseases from the classical neurodegenerative disorders that typically involve progression and irreversibility of the cognitive aberrations (Caine, 1981; Cummings and Benson, 1992; Kiloh, 1961; Reynolds and Hoch, 1989; Wells, 1979). The concept of pseudodementia has evolved since Kiloh (1961) coined the term (Lavretsky and Kumar, 1999). Several other terms have been used since to describe this widely observed phenomenon, including *dementia syndrome of depression, coexisting dementia and depression, cognitive affective disorder, depression-induced cognitive dysfunction,* and most, recently, *depression-executive dysfunction syndrome of late life* (DED). These terms are often used interchangeably in the literature, although they represent efforts to find a unifying term to describe a relatively complex clinical phenomenon (Emery, 1988; McGuire and Rabins, 1994; Raskind, 1998; Reichman, 1994).

Four essential criteria have been proposed to define pseudodementia (Caine, 1981; Reynolds and Hoch, 1989). (*1*) There must be evidence of a primary psychiatric disorder accompanied by intellectual impairment. (*2*) The cognitive features of the disorder must resemble those typically found in degenerative brain disorders with neuropathological confirmation. (*3*) The intellectual deficit should reverse with psychiatric treatment. (*4*) There must be no evidence supporting the diagnosis of a primary neurodegenerative disorder (Caine, 1981; Lavretsky and Kumar, 1999; Reichman, 1994).

The pseudodementia phenomenon, although extensively studied, remains controversial. The controversy stems from the following three unresolved issues pertaining to the definition of pseudodementia: (*1*) whether the cognitive deficits are detectable or undetectable; (*2*) the functional versus organic origins of these deficits; (*3*) the reversibility or irreversibility of the deficits (Alexopoulos et al., 1993; Nussbaum, 1994; Reifler, 1982; Shraberg, 1978). One central criticism of the concept is based on the lack of a validated test or battery of tests to differentiate depression-related cognitive dysfunction from irreversible and progressive conditions such as AD and vascular dementia. In addition, recent developments in the understanding of the pathophysiology of depression have added to the criticisms of the implied *nonorganic* nature of the cognitive deficits associated with depression. Cummings and Benson (1992) classified depression-related cognitive impairment as a mild form of subcortical dementia with impairment in frontal executive function and psychomotor speed. Recent evidence from more sophisticated longitudinal studies and modern neuroimaging approaches has led to a reappraisal of the original term *pseudodementia* (Lavretsky and Kumar, 1999).

The classical description of depressive pseudodementia involves an elderly patient who presents with the typical features of depression including psychomotor retardation, neurovegetative signs, and feelings of worthlessness and guilt together with poor attention and concentration. These are frequently accompanied by decreased immediate recall of newly learned information, often helped by *cuing* (Alexopoulos et al., 1993; Lamberty and Bieliauskas, 1993). While this presentation is still observed in a subgroup of patients, patients with mixed cognitive and affective symptoms are more frequently encountered clinically.

The question still remains of whether cognitive impairment of late-life depression is the result of brain aging, ultimately leading to the development of dementia, or is a product of depression or a combination of both. The most recent evidence stemming from studies comparing elderly depressed persons to normal controls points to the likelihood of the combined effect of depression and aging on cognition (Boone et al., 1995; Butters et al., 2000; Nebes et al., 2001a). A definitive study attempting to answer this question would require a longitudinal follow-up from young adulthood to old age of a large population of subjects, both depressed and nondepressed, matched by age, gender, and education, with periodic comprehensive cognitive, neuroimaging, and neuropsychiatric assessment. This rigorous and expensive study has not been done yet, but there are many smaller comparative studies that may shed light on the underlying processes. These are reviewed below. In addition, we are likely to learn more in the near future from the large collaborative studies of various health initiatives, which include longitudinal cognitive and behavioral assessments such as the Cardiovascular Health Study and the Women's Health Initiative.

## NEUROPSYCHOLOGICAL STUDIES OF COGNITION IN LATE-LIFE DEPRESSION

In a number of neuropsychological studies, attempts have been made to characterize the cognitive changes in depression and to help differentiate depression from dementia based on clinical evidence. To some degree, variability in the tests and in the samples studied limits the conclusions that can be drawn from these studies. Collectively, they suggest that the cognitive disturbance in depression, especially in mild to moderate forms of the disorder, is not severe, and is typically characterized by impaired attention and recall (LaRue, 1992; Lezak, 1995). Although research findings on cognitive functioning in elderly patients with depression have been inconsistent, there is evidence of deficits in right hemisphere abilities and frontal executive functions (Boone et al., 1995; Lesser et al., 1996). Further, some studies of the depressed elderly have reported declines in memory, attention, language, and executive skills (Alexopoulos et al., 1993; LaRue, 1992; Lezak, 1995). Severity of depression has been related primarily to declines in information processing speed but has not been related specifically to memory impairment (Boone et al., 1995). Studies have shown that older depressed men exhibit a different pattern of cognitive deficits than older depressed women. While men demonstrate a more lateralized pattern, women display a pattern suggestive of bilateral hemispheric dysfunction (Boone et al., 1992, 1995; LaRue, 1992).

Among the severely depressed elderly, other factors such as functional impairment, poor physical health, and polypharmacy may influence cognitive impairment and decline. LaRue (1992) reported differences between severely depressed patients and control subjects on tests of learning and recall, as well as on tests of visual-spatial processing. On memory tests, impairments in nonverbal recall and retrieval were found in the mild to moderate range. Compared to demented patients, depressed patients performed much better on tests of verbal information (comprehension and vocabulary), verbal learning, and recall. Dudley et al. (2002) reported differences in the Emotional Stroop task response pattern in patients with AD compared to nondemented patients with major depression and normal controls. Generally depressed patients and those with AD were both slower than the controls on the task. However, the depressed group alone showed a statistically significant and specific increase in response time when naming the colors of negative-emotion words. The other two groups did not demonstrate such an increase in pattern and color, and named neutral, positive, and negative words equally quickly.

Nebes and colleagues (2000) reported impairment in working memory and processing speed in patients with geriatric major depression compared to normal controls. The processing resources in depressed elderly patients appeared to be decreased, which mediated impairments in several cognitive domains including episodic memory and visual-spatial performance. The resource decrement persisted after remission of the depression. In another report, Nebes et al. (2001a) demonstrated that working memory in performing dual tasks, as expressed in the ability to coordinate the simultaneous performance of multiple tasks, was impaired in patients before antidepressant treatment commenced and persisted after the remission of depression. This suggested that executive dysfunction may be a trait phenomenon.

Alexopoulos and colleagues (2002) underscored the importance of executive dysfunction in geriatric depression by coining the term *depression-executive dysfunction syndrome of late life*. They observed that at least a proportion of patients with geriatric depression experienced executive dysfunction, including disturbances in planning, sequencing, organizing, abstracting, and retrieving information, but with relative preservation of recognition memory. In addition, patients with the DED syndrome evidenced reduced verbal fluency, impaired visual naming, paranoia, loss of interest in activities, and psychomotor retardation but showed a rather mild vegetative syndrome (Alexopoulos et al., 2002b; Kalayam and Alexopoulos, 1999). Alexopoulos (2001) summarized studies that employed diverse neuroimaging, neurocognitive, and neuropathological techniques by identifying frontostriatal and limbic dysfunction as putative underlying mechanisms predisposing to, precipitating and perpetuating geriatric depression.

## COGNITIVE IMPAIRMENT ASSOCIATED WITH SUBCLINICAL CEREBROVASCULAR DISEASE IN LATE-LIFE DEPRESSION

Subclinical cerebrovascular disease in late-life depression and normal aging documented on structural neuroimaging, computed tomography (CT), or MRI has been confirmed in multiple studies (Lavretsky and Kumar, 2002a). Cognitive impairment associated with subclinical cerebrovascular disease may be observed in healthy control subjects with a large volume of hyperintensities reaching a *threshold effect*. Deficits in attention, motor speed, and executive function have been reported in these patients (Boone et al., 1992). Lesser et al. (1996) compared patients diagnosed with late-onset depression (beginning at age 50 and older) with those with early-onset depression (beginning before age 35) and normal controls. The late-onset group had greater deep white matter hyperintensities (DWMHs) than either of the other groups. Cognitive deficits were most marked in the late-onset group and pertained to nonverbal intelligence, nonverbal memory, constructional ability, executive function, and speed of processing. Patients with more severe DWMHs had significantly poorer executive function. A *vascular* depression hypothesis described a syndrome associated with striato-frontal impairment expressed in executive dysfunction, psychomotor retardation, apathy, reduced agitation, guilt, and insight (Alexopoulos, 2002; Alexopoulos et al., 1997; Krishnan, 2002; Krishnan et al., 1997).

Simpson and associates (1997) conducted neuropsychological assessment following treatment of an elderly major depressive disorder (MDD) sample. Hyperintensities in the pons were associated with reduced psychomotor speed. Additionally, basal ganglia hyperintensities were linked to impaired category production, an executive function test, and periventricular hyperintensities (PVHs) were associated with impaired delayed recall. In a retrospective casenote analysis of 38 patients with MRI scans performed 3 years earlier, a poor outcome was associated with lesions in the pons. Pontine raphe lesions and confluent periventricular lesions were associated with later dementia and with reduced survival of cardiovascular disease. Men had a higher incidence of recurrences than women and a lower survival rate.

Nebes et al. (2001) reported that hyperintensities in the deep white matter, but not in the periventricular white matter, were associated with depressive symptoms, especially impaired motivation, concentration, and decision making. The relationship was particularly strong in the APOE-4 allele carriers compared to non-

carriers. Cahn-Weiner et al. (1996) reported that age, depression severity, and subcortical hyperintensities on MRI scans accounted for 53% of the variance in activities of daily living (ADL) functioning. Severity of hyperintensities accounted for an additional 18% of the variance.

In a recent study of cognition in patients with remitted unipolar major depression, those with silent cerebral infarctions had a greater impairment in psychomotor speed, as well as in total, verbal, and performance IQ, compared to those without silent infarctions (Yamashita et al., 2002). These findings indicate that silent infarctions contribute to cognitive impairment even during remission of depression.

## OTHER MARKERS OF COGNITIVE IMPAIRMENT AND DECLINE IN GERIATRIC DEPRESSION: NEUROPSYCHOLOGICAL MEASURES

Visser and colleagues (2000) indicated that age and memory performance on the test of delayed recall, as well as verbal fluency, were predictive of future AD in patients with depression and preclinical AD in 111 elderly patients followed up to 5 years. The specificity of these predictors was 94% and sensitivity was 90%. The positive predictive value was 90% and the negative predictive value was 94%. In contrast, although the tests of executive function predict a poor outcome of geriatric depression, their results are not consistently associated with cognitive decline (Alexopoulos, 2002).

A number of reports indicate that subjective memory complaints could predict the development of dementia (Gron et al., 2002; St. John and Montgomery, 2002). This prediction appears to be independent of depressive symptoms, although depression increases the rates of subjective memory complaints in non-APOE-4 carriers (Small et al., 2001).

## OTHER MARKERS: STRUCTURAL NEUROIMAGING

Neuroimaging technology has provided unprecedented opportunities for elucidating the anatomical correlates of major depression (Drevets, 2001; Krishnan, 2002). The knowledge gained from imaging research has shifted our conceptualization of mood disorders as illnesses that involve abnormalities of brain structure and function. They particularly support a role for dysfunction within the prefrontal cortical and striatal system that normally modulates limbic and brain stem structures in mediating emotional behavior in the pathogenesis of depressive symptoms (Drevets, 2001). The overlap of structural brain changes in cognitive and mood disorders serves as a neurobiological substrate of the cognitive-emotional manifestations of mood disorders. This process is likely to become more pronounced with aging.

One brain structure that may mediate the relationship between depression and dementia is the hippocampus (Steffens et al., 2002). It has been established that the hippocampus is involved in memory and is significantly affected in AD (Petersen et al., 2000). Small hippocampal size has been observed in depression of longer duration (Sheline et al., 1999) and may serve as a marker for incipient dementia and cognitive decline (Steffens et al., 2002). Other structural changes potentially involved in the pathogenesis of both cognitive and mood symptoms include generalized atrophy and white and gray matter MRI signal hyperintensities. Their role is described in the sections discussing the role of cerebrovascular disease in depression and dementia in this chapter.

## OTHER MARKERS: FUNCTIONAL NEUROIMAGING

The existing evidence from functional imaging studies in younger and mixed-age, nondemented subjects implicates the dorsolateral prefrontal cortex and the anterior cingulate, particularly in the right hemisphere, as key brain structures in emotion–cognition interaction in depression (Liotti and Mayberg, 2001).

In an attempt to address the question of whether depressive pseudodementia represents an early stage of AD, Cho and colleagues (2002) compared subjects with depressive pseudodementia to depressed subjects free of cognitive impairment, healthy comparison subjects, and patients with AD by using 99m-hexamethypropyleneminexoxime single photon emission computed tomography (99m-HMPAO SPECT) scanning. The depressive pseudodementia group showed significant decreases of cerebral blood flow (CBF) in the right temporal and biparietal regions compared with the depression group. The depression group showed significantly decreased CBF in the left frontal region compared with the control group. The AD group showed significantly decreased CBF in the right temporal, bifrontal, and biparietal regions compared with the depressive pseudodementia group. The authors concluded that the depressive pseudodementia group had a decreased CBF pattern similar to that in AD but not to that in depression, which increased the likelihood of pseudodementia being a prodrome of AD. However, they could not conclude from a cross-sectional comparison of depressed subjects whether the observed pattern was a state or a trait marker (Cho et al., 2002). Reed and colleagues (2001) reported that bilateral and right hemisphere dorsolateral frontal metabolism significantly predicted cognitive decline, with right dorsolateral frontal metabolism explaining 19% of the variance. They concluded that cognitive decline in pa-

tients with lacunas may result in part from progressive vascular compromise in subcortical frontal circuits.

Small and colleagues (1995), along with other investigators, have reported improved accuracy of the dementia diagnosis with PET (Small, 1998). They combined the use of the apolipoprotein E genotype and PET to further improve early detection of AD (Small et al., 1996). Recently, Small and colleagues (Shoghi-Jadid et al., 2002) used a hydrophobic radiofluorinated derivative of 2-(1-[6-(dimethylamino)-2-naphthyl]ethylidene) malononitrile (DDNP), in conjunction with PET, to determine the localization and load of neurofibrillary tangles (NFTs) and beta-amyloid senile plaques (APs) in the brains of living AD patients. Greater accumulation and slower clearance were observed in AP- and NFT-dense brain areas and correlated with lower memory performance scores. This noninvasive technique for monitoring AP and NFT development is expected to facilitate early diagnostic assessment of patients with AD and assist in response monitoring during experimental treatments. Functional MRI (fMRI) is another promising tool using cognitive probes that can help in the early detection of AD (Bookheimer et al., 2000). These neuroimaging techniques can be particularly helpful in difficult diagnostic dilemmas such as mixed cognitive-affective syndromes.

## OTHER MARKERS: GENETIC MARKERS

Genetic markers of AD and other degenerative dementias could be used to identify individuals with an increased risk of developing dementia. In only a few neurodegenerative illnesses, such as HD, is the presence of a single gene necessary and sufficient for the development of the illness. However, in the majority of multifactorial disorders, such as AD, the presence of genetic markers merely increases the risk of developing the disease. The apolipoprotein E-4 allele is the best-known risk factor for AD that has been tested in geriatric depression and in mild cognitive decline. No clear relationship with late-life depression, its age of onset (Papassotiropoulos et al., 1999), or cognitive decline has been identified. Zubenko and colleagues (1996) did not find a relationship between the APOE-4 allele and cognitive impairment in patients with geriatric depression, but they identified a higher frequency of the allele among those with psychotic depression.

Small and colleagues (2001) reported an association between depressive symptoms and memory self-appraisal in APOE-4 noncarriers in a cross-sectional study. However, in our recent report of a longitudinal follow-up of nondemented older adults, APOE-4 was associated with cognitive decline but not mild depressive symptoms (Lavretsky et al., 2003). In a follow-up study of 16 subjects, we found an association of APOE-4 with an increase in the volume of WMH (Lavretsky et al., 2000). Other genetic markers of the serotonin neurotransmitter system have been tested in geriatric depression as markers of depression or treatment response (Pollock et al., 2000).

A recent study of aging twins reported interesting evidence for genetic mediation of executive control. The shared executive control factor had a heritability of 79% and accounted for 10%–56% of the genetic variance in performance on four tests of executive function (Swan and Carmelli, 2002). Digit symbol substitution appeared to be the marker of executive control with the largest genetic component, whereas verbal fluency stood out as displaying a pattern of genetic and environmental influences (Swan and Carmelli, 2002).

At present, there are no strong genetic markers for either late-life depression or the cognitive impairment associated with it. However, it will remain an area of great research interest in the next decade.

## OTHER MARKERS: STRESS HORMONES AND OTHER PERIPHERAL BIOCHEMICAL MARKERS

Hypothalamic-pituitary-adrenal (HPA) axis dysregulation has been the most consistent and reproducible biological finding in affective disorders (Nemeroff, 2002; Rubinow et al., 1984). The brain's limbic system, particularly the hippocampus and amygdala, is also intimately involved in the stress response. Chronically elevated corticosteroid levels induced by persistent stress may adversely affect hippocampal structure and function, producing deficits of both memory and cognition (Vanitallie, 2002). State-related cortisol abnormalities have been described in depressed patients but also have been implicated in the pathophysiology of hippocampal atrophy, potentially leading to the development of dementia of Alzheimer's type. In a series of reports, hypercortisolemia has been linked to cognitive impairment associated with depression (Rubinow et al., 1984); it also increased the risk of cognitive impairment following ECT (Neylan et al., 2001). Higher cerebrospinal fluid (CSF) cortisol concentrations were associated with an increased frequency of APOE-4 and a decreased frequency of APOE-2 in AD subjects relative to control subjects (Peskind et al., 2001). This effect of the APOE genotype on HPA axis activity may be related to the increased risk of AD in persons carrying APOE-4 and the decreased risk of AD in persons carrying APOE-2 (Peskind et al., 2001).

Cerebrospinal fluid markers for AD such as CSF total tau protein, A-beta 42 protein, and phosphorylated tau protein have been identified as markers for AD. They can be particularly helpful in differentiating AD from age-appropriate memory impairment, other primary and secondary dementias, and depression.

Despite the growing database, no laboratory tests have emerged that are considered appropriate for routine use in the clinical evaluation of patients with suspected AD and/or depression. Several promising avenues are being pursued, including neuroimaging, neuropsychological predictors of decline, genotyping and biomarkers, or any combination of these methods.

## COURSE AND OUTCOME OF DEPRESSION WITH COGNITIVE IMPAIRMENT

Studies of the course and outcome of geriatric depression with cognitive impairment suggest that this syndrome is heterogeneous. While the early studies emphasized a total, or near-total, reversal of cognitive disturbances with successful treatment of depression, more recent studies indicate a more complex picture. Cognitive dysfunction may develop during an episode of geriatric depression and then diminish in varying degrees once the depressive symptoms remit (Alexopoulos and Chester, 1992). Recent follow-up data demonstrates that patients with pseudodementia develop dementia at a rate 9% to 25% per year (Alexopoulos and Chester, 1992). In an epidemiological community study of dementia, Devanand and colleagues (1996) demonstrated that a depressed mood was common in subjects with cognitive impairment who did not meet the criteria for dementia. In addition, the baseline depressed mood in these subjects was associated with a moderately increased risk of incident dementia at follow-up. Chen et al. (1999) followed a large group of subjects for development of depressive symptoms and cognitive decline, and found that depression did not increase the risk of dementia but was an early manifestation of dementia. In a large meta-analysis, Jorm et al. (1991) found that a history of depression was associated with onset of AD after age 70 only if depressive symptoms had appeared within 10 years before the onset of dementia. In this report, depression was considered a risk factor for AD and not a prodromal symptom if the onset was more than 10 years prior to the onset of AD.

Geriatric depression, accompanied by the reversible dementia syndrome of depression or depressive pseudodementia, leads to irreversible dementia at a rate 2.5 to 6 times higher than that in the general geriatric population. Thus, recent evidence clearly demonstrates that geriatric depression, especially when associated with objective evidence of cognitive dysfunction, is a significant risk factor for dementia.

In addition, the presence of cognitive impairment, particularly executive dysfunction in patients with geriatric major depression, leads to worse outcomes expressed in greater disability (Alexopoulos et al., 1996a), chronicity and slow time to recovery (Alexopoulos et al., 1996b), and higher rates of relapse and recurrence

(Alexopoulos et al., 2002b). In depressed elderly patients, executive dysfunction was the cognitive impairment most likely to result in impairment of instrumental activities of daily living (IADLs) (Alexopoulos et al., 1996a, 2000; Kiosses et al., 2000, 2001). Moreover, depression was found to contribute to IADL impairment mainly in patients with executive dysfunction, whereas it had a nonsignificant effect in patients without impaired executive functioning (Kiosses et al., 2000, 2001). In addition, executive impairment predicted a poor or delayed antidepressant response in geriatric major depression. Executive dysfunction and cerebrovascular disease have been reported in association with a poor or delayed antidepressant response, relapse and with recurrence of depression. Unlike executive dysfunction, neither memory impairment nor disability, medical burden, lack of social support, or the number of previous episodes have been shown to influence the course of geriatric depression (Alexopoulos et al., 2000).

## EFFECTS OF ANTIDEPRESSANT TREATMENT ON COGNITIVE FUNCTIONS

Few studies have addressed the effect of antidepressants on cognitive function. Despite the existing notion that cognitive symptoms associated with depression improve with reduction of depression severity, very few studies have demonstrated this relationship. Butters and colleagues (2000) reported that elderly depressed patients showed a small improvement in overall cognitive functioning after treatment. However, in patients with cognitive impairment at baseline, performance on the Mattis Dementia Rating scale domains of conceptualization and initiation/perseveration improved significantly relative to the performance of depressed patients with normal cognition at baseline. Despite the improvement following treatment, the overall level of cognitive functioning in patients with cognitive impairment at baseline remained mildly impaired, particularly in memory and executive functions. Nebes and colleagues (2000) reported some improvement in processing speed and working memory with successful treatment of depression, but the improvement was not greater than that seen in the control subjects with repeat testing.

In the majority of studies, improvement in cognitive performance was associated with improvement in mood (Butters et al., 2000; Stoudemire et al., 1991). While the cognitive functions in patients treated for depression often show improvement with treatment of depression, in a recent report treatment with paroxetine resulted in a slight increase in anticholinergicity but did not result in impaired cognitive function even in patients with a preexisting cognitive impairment (Nebes et al., 1999). Similar reports of the lack of negative effects of psychotropic medications on cognition have been reported for other tricyclic medications and ECT (Butters et al., 2000; Stoudemire et al., 1991). Although ECT is clearly associated with an increase in cognitive impairment during acute treatment—more so with bilateral compared to unilateral electrode placement (Sackeim et al., 1987)—in longitudinal studies cognitive impairment was substantially and significantly less than that observed before ECT (Abrams and Taylor, 1985). A high dosage of right unilateral ECT is as effective as a robust form of bilateral ECT, but it produces less severe and less persistent cognitive effects (Sackeim et al., 2000). Bifrontal electrode placement in ECT has been reported to have less treatment-induced intellectual dysfunction than unilateral and bilateral electrode placement (Delva et al., 2000). In a recent report on the effect of vagus nerve stimulation on cognitive performance in patients with treatment-resistant depression, Sackeim and colleagues (2001) observed improvement in motor speed, psychomotor function, language, and executive functions.

In conclusion, cognitive function should improve with successful treatment and reduction of depressive symptoms. However, some residual impairment may persist, especially impaired performance on tests of executive function. If only minimal improvement in cognition occurs, a cognitive disorder must be ruled out.

## DIAGNOSIS AND DIFFERENTIAL DIAGNOSIS

Diagnosis in a case of mixed depressive and cognitive disorder needs to be approached in a systematic manner. It should always begin with a careful history from both the patient and family or another reliable observer, accompanied by a thorough and detailed mental status examination (Emery and Oxman, 1992). On the basis of available clinical information, a new scale has recently been developed allowing the differentiation of the two conditions (Yousef et al., 1998). The Pseudodementia Scale represents the first systematic attempt to standardize the clinical assessment of pseudodementia. It consists of 44 characteristic features covering the areas of history, clinical data, insight, and performance in the form of questions with "yes" or "no" answers. Additionally, comprehensive neuropsychological testing may be necessary at baseline and at follow-up, approximately 1 year later, to document or rule out a progression in cognitive decline. Tests of delayed recall and recognition are most sensitive in differentiating between AD and depression (Albert, 1996). A complete medical and neurological exam is required, together with appropriate laboratory testing, to further investigate the possible secondary causes of symptoms (Alexopoulos, 1998; Alexopoulos et al., 2002a). Laboratory testing typically includes complete and differential blood counts, hepatic, renal, and thyroid screens, and serum electrolytes (Knopman et al., 2001). Commonly occurring in the elderly, vitamin $B_{12}$ deficiency, hypothyroidism, depression, and (in case of the present risk factors) syphilis and human immunodeficiency virus infection may cause reversible dementia. Routine screening is recommended for these causes (Knopman et al., 2002). Neuroimaging, both structural and functional, may also be required to rule out underlying dementing illnesses or other neuropsychiatric disorders that may be contributing to cognitive impairment. According to the practice guidelines on the diagnosis of dementia (Knopman et al., 2002), no neuroimaging or laboratory test was recommended for routine use, with the exception of the CSF 14-3-3 protein for confirmation of the diagnosis of Creutzfeldt-Jakob disease. Clinical diagnosis remains the gold standard of clinical practice (Knopman et al., 2002). However, with the appearance of more reliable neuroimaging techniques such as PET and in vivo amyloid imaging, the accuracy of the early diagnosis of dementia in confusing cases will improve and allow early detection and intervention to prevent dementia. In cases where no identifiable medical causes are evident for the cognitive impairment, and where clinical depression or other psychiatric features predominate, the diagnosis of pseu-

dodementia may be seriously entertained and the treatment of depression needs to be attempted.

In summary, we have reviewed the existing data supporting a continuum of clinical features and outcomes between depression and cognitive disorders of late life. There is clear evidence for late-life cognitive-affective spectrum disorders ranging from the commonly observed mild to moderate cognitive deficits in geriatric depression to depressive symptoms in the context of a neurodegenerative or vascular dementia. It is also clear that this group of patients is heterogeneous in the pattern of cognitive impairment and corresponding etiologies. Some will go on to develop AD, and their pattern of neuropsychological deficits may be different from that of those who will develop vascular dementia or will not meet the diagnosis of dementia. In the longitudinal Canadian Study of Health and Aging, however, patients with an initial vascular cognitive impairment but no dementia developed incident dementia after 5 years. Low baseline scores on tests of memory and category fluency were associated with incident dementia, which is not different from that seen in AD (Ingles et al., 2002).

More rigorous and systematic integration of the data from different areas of neuropsychiatric research is needed to establish a consensus on the patterns of cog-

TABLE 7.1. *Differential Diagnosis of Cognitive and Clinical Features of Late-life Depression and of Neurodegenerative and Vascular Dementias*

| | Depression | Neurodegenerative Dementia | Vascular |
|---|---|---|---|
| Onset and course | Relatively acute and nonprogressive | Insidiously progressive | Stepwise progressive |
| Affect | Symptoms and signs of depression predominate | Depressive symptoms are generally mild | Depressive symptoms range from mild to severe |
| Sequence | Typically, affective symptoms precede cognitive complaints | Cognitive symptoms precede affective symptoms | Cognitive symptoms precede affective symptoms |
| Executive Function | Attention and concentration impairment common | May be preserved early on | Impairment is common |
| Psychomotor retardation | Common | Uncommon | Common |
| Language | Typically preserved | May be impaired | May be impaired |
| Praxis | Preserved | May be impaired | May be impaired |
| Visual-Spatial | Generally mild | May be seriously compromised | May be impaired |
| Memory | Retrieval may be impaired | Immediate and delayed recall compromised early on | Retrieval may be impaired early on |
| Orientation | Generally intact | Compromised, especially in more advanced cases | May be impaired |
| EEG | Typically normal | Regional/diffuse slow-wave activity | Regional/patchy areas of slow-wave activity |
| MRI | Mild atrophy | Progressive diffuse atrophy | Cortical and subcortical strokes |
| PET Glucose Metabolism | Widespread hypometabolism | Temporal-parietal hypometabolism | Patchy cortical and subcortical hypometabolism |
| Response of Cognitive Impairment to Treatment of Depression | Cognitive features typically improve with treatment | Minimal improvement with treatment | Minimal improvement with treatment |

EEG, electroencephalogram; MRI, magnetic resonance imaging; PET, positron emission tomography.

nitive impairment in geriatric depression, associated biological markers, and response to treatment. Such tools as functional and structural imaging, along with genetic testing, may aid in establishing guidelines for the diagnosis and treatment of cognitive impairment. Identification of early predictors of the incipient dementia can help in the differential diagnosis and early detection and prevention of dementing illnesses.

Table 7.1 compares the patterns of cognitive impairment, as well as the clinical features of depression, to those of neurodegenerative and vascular dementia syndromes.

ACKNOWLEDGMENTS

This work was supported in part by the Fran and Ray Stark Foundation Fund for Alzheimer's Disease Research; NIH grants MH52453, AG10123, and AG13308 (Dr. Small); and the NARSAD Young Investigator Award and Grant K23-MH01948 (Dr. Lavretsky).

REFERENCES

Abrams, R., and Taylor, M.A. (1985) A prospective follow-up study of cognitive functions after electroconvulsive therapy. *Convulsive Ther* 1(1):4–9.

Albert, M.S. (1996) Cognitive and neurobiologic markers of early Alzheimer disease. *Proc Natl Acad Sci USA* 93:13547–13551.

Alexopoulos, G.S. (1998) The assessment and treatment of depressed-demented patients. In Nelson, J.C., ed. *Geriatric Psychopharmacology*. New York, Basel, and Hong Kong: Marcel Dekker, pp. 223–245.

Alexopoulos, G.S. (2001) New concepts for prevention and treatment of late-life depression. *Am J Psychiatry* 158:835–858.

Alexopoulos, G.S., Borson, S., Cuthbert, B.N., Devanand, D.P., Mulsant, B.H., Olin, J.T., and Oslin, D.W. (2002a) *Assessment of late-life depression*. Biol Psychiatry 52:164–174.

Alexopoulos, G.S. and Chester, J.G. (1992) Outcomes of geriatric depression. *Clin Geriatr Med* 2:363–376.

Alexopoulos, G.S., Kiosses, D.N., Klimstra, S., Kalayam, B., and Bruce, M.L. (2002b) Clinical presentation of the depression-executive dysfunction syndrome of late life. *Am J Geriatr Psychiatry* 10:98–106.

Alexopoulos, G.S., Meyers, B.S., Young, R.C., et al. (1993) The course of geriatric depression with "reversible dementia": A controlled study. *Am J Psychiatry* 150:1693–1699.

Alexopoulos, G.S., Meyers, B.S., Young, R.C., et al. (1996b) Recovery in geriatric depression. *Arch Gen Psychiatry* 53:305–312.

Alexopoulos, G.S., Meyers, B.S., Young, R.C., et al. (1997) "Vascular depression" hypothesis [see comments]. *Arch Gen Psychiatry* 54:915–922.

Alexopoulos, G.S., Meyers, B.S., Young, R.C., et al. (2000) Executive dysfunction and long-term outcomes of geriatric depression. *Arch Gen Psychiatry* 57:285–290.

Alexopoulos, G.S., Vrontou, C., Kakuma, T., et al. (1996a) Disability in geriatric depression. *Am J Psychiatry* 153:877–885.

Assal, F., and Cummings, J.L. (2002) Neuropsychiatric symptoms in the dementias. *Curr Opin Neurol* 15:445–450.

Barber, R., Gholkar, A., Scheltens, P., et al. (1999) Apolipoprotein E epsilon4 allele, temporal lobe atrophy, and white matter lesions in late-life dementias. *Arch Neurol* 56:961–965.

Berger, A.K., Fahllander, K., Wahlin, A., and Backman, L. (2002) Negligible effects of depression on verbal and spatial performance in Alzheimer's disease. *Dementia Geriatr Cogn Disord* 13:1–7.

Blazer, D.M. and Williams, C.D. (1980) Epidemiology of dysphoria and depression in an elderly population. *Am J Psychiatry* 137:439–444.

Bookheimer, S.Y., Strojwas, M.H., Cohen, M.S., Saunders, A.M., Pericak-Vance, M.A., Mazziotta, J.C., and Small, G.W. (2000) Patterns of brain activation in people at risk for Alzheimer's disease. *N Engl J Med* 17;343(7):450–456.

Boone, K.B., Lesser, I.M., Miller, B., et al. (1995) Cognitive functioning in older depressed outpatients: Relationship of presence and severity of depression to neuropsychological test scores. *Neuropsychology* 9:390–398.

Boone, K.B., Miller, B.L., Lesser, I.M., et al. (1992) Neuropsychological correlates of white matter lesions in healthy elderly subjects. *Arch Neurol* 49:549–554.

Butters, M.A., Becker, J.T., Nebes, R.D., et al. (2000) Changes in cognitive functioning following treatment of late-life depression. *Am J Psychiatry* 157:1949–1954.

Cahn-Weiner, D.A., Malloy, P.F., Boyle, P.A., et al. (2000) Prediction of functional status from neuropsychological tests in community-dwelling elderly individuals. *Clin Neuropsychol* 14:187–195.

Caine, E. (1981) Pseudodementia. *Arch Gen Psychiatry* 38:1359–1364.

Caine, E.D., Lyness, J.M., King, D.A., et al. (1994) Clinical and etiological heterogeneity of mood disorders in elderly patients. In Shneider, L.S., Reynolds, C.F., Lebowitz, B.D., and Friedhoff, A.J., eds. *Diagnosis and Treatment of Depression in Late Life: Results of the NIH Consensus Development Conference*. Washington, DC: American Psychiatric Association, pp. 21–54.

Chen, C.P.L.-H., Adler, J.T., Bowen, D.M., Esiri, M.M., McDonald, B., Hope, T., Jobst, K.A., and Francis, P.T. (1996) Presynaptic serotonergic markers in community-acquired cases of Alzheimer's disease: Correlations with depression and neuroleptic medication. *J Neurochem* 66:1592–1598.

Cho, M.J., Lyoo, I.K., Lee, D.W., Kwon, J.S., Lee, J.S., Lee, D.S., Jung, J.K., and Lee, M.C. (2002) Brain single photon emission computed tomography findings in depressive pseudodementia patients. *J Affect Disord* 69(1–3):159–166.

Cummings, J.L. (2000) Cognitive and behavioral heterogeneity in Alzheimer's disease: Seeking the neurobiological basis. *Neurobiol Aging* 21:845–861.

Cummings, J.L. and Benson, D.F. (1992) *Dementia. A Clinical Approach*, 2nd ed. Boston: Butterworth-Heinemann.

Delva, N.J., Brunet, D., Hawken, E.R., Kesteven, R.M., Lawson, J.S., Lywood, D.W., Rodenburg, M., and Waldron, J.J. (2000) Electrical dose and seizure threshold: Relations to clinical outcome and cognitive effects in bifrontal, bitemporal, and right unilateral ECT. *J ECT* 16(4):361–369.

Devanand, D.P., Sano, M., Tang, M.X., et al. (1996) Depressed mood and the incidence of Alzheimer's disease in the elderly living in the community. *Arch Gen Psychiatry* 53:175–182.

Drevets, W.C. (2001) Neuroimaging and neuropathological studies of depression: Implications for the cognitive-emotional features of mood disorders. *Curr Opin Neurobiol* 11(2):240–249.

Dudley, R., O'Brien, J., Barnett, N., et al. (2002) Distinguishing depression from dementia in later life: A pilot study employing the emotional Stroop task. *Int J Geriatr Psychiatry* 17:48–53.

Elderkin-Thompson, V., Kumar, A., Gur, R.E., et al. (2002, February) Neuropsychological deficits among patients with late-onset minor and major depression. *Abstract ML4*. Presented at the annual meeting of the American Association for Geriatric Psychiatry, Orlando, FL.

Emery, V.O.B. (1998) Pseudodementia: A theoretical and empirical discussion. *Western Reserve Geriatric Education Center Interdisciplinary Monograph Series*. Cleveland: Case Western Reserve University School of Medicine.

Emery, V.O.B., and Oxman, T.E. (1992) Update on the dementia spectrum of depression. *Am J Psychiatry* 149:305–317.

Espiritu, D.A., Rashid, H., Mast, B.T., et al. (2001) Depression, cognitive impairment and function in Alzheimer's disease. *Int J Geriatr Psychiatry* 16:1098–1103.

Forstl, H., Burns, A., Luthert, P., Cairns, N., Lantos, P., and Levy, R. (1992) Clinical and neuropathological correlates of depression in Alzheimer's disease. *Psychol Med* 22:877–884.

Gillen, R., Tennen, H., McKee, T.E., et al. (2001) Depressive symptoms and history of depression predict rehabilitation efficiency in stroke patients. *Arch Phys Med Rehabil* 82:1645–1649.

Heun, R., Kockler, M., and Ptok, U. (2002) Depression in Alzheimer's disease: Is there a temporal relationship between the onset of depression and the onset of dementia? *Eur Psychiatry* 17:254–258.

Hirono, N., Mori, E., Ishii, K., Ikejiri, Y., Imamura, T., Shimomura, T., Hashimoto, M., Yamashita, H., and Sasaki, M. (1998) Frontal lobe hypometabolism and depression in Alzheimer's disease. *Neurology* 50:380–383.

Ingles, J.L., Wentzel, C., Fisk, J.D., and Rockwood, K. (2002) Neuropsychological predictors of incipient dementia in patients with vascular cognitive impairment without dementia. *Stroke* 33(8):1999–2002.

Kalayam, B. and Alexopoulos, G.S. (1999) Prefrontal dysfunction and treatment response in geriatric depression. *Arch Gen Psychiatry* 56:713–718.

Kiloh, L.G. (1961) Pseudodementia. *Acta Psychiatr Scand* 37:336–351.

Kiosses, D.N., Alexopoulos, G.S., and Murphy, C. (2000) Symptoms of striatofrontal dysfunction contribute to disability in geriatric depression. *Int J Geriatr Psychiatry* 15:992–999.

Kiosses, D.N., Klimstra, S., Murphy, C., and Alexopoulos, G.S. (2001) Executive dysfunction and disability in elderly patients with major depression. *Am J Geriatr Psychiatry* 9:269–274.

Knopman, D.S., DeKosky, S.T., Cummings, J.L., Chui, H., Corey-Bloom, J., Relkin, N., Small, G.W., Miller, B., and Stevens, J.C. (2001) Practice parameter: Diagnosis of dementia (an evidence-based review). Report of the Quality Standards Subcommittee of the American Academy of Neurology. *Neurology* 56(9):1143–1153.

Kral, V.A. (1993) The relationship between senile dementia (Alzheimer's type) and depression. *Can J Psychiatry* 34:445–446.

Kral, V.A. and Emery, O.B. (1989) Long-term follow-up of depressive pseudodementia of the aged. *Can J Psychiatry* 34:445–446.

Krishnan, K.R., Hays, J.C., and Blazer, D.G. (1997) MRI-defined vascular depression. *Am J Psychiatry* 154:497–501.

Kumar, A., Bilker, W., Jin, Z., and Udupa, J. (2000) Atrophy and high intensity lesions: Complementary neurobiological mechanisms in late-life major depression. *Neuropsychopharmacology* 22:264–274.

Kumar, A. and Cummings, J.L. (2001) Depression in neurodegenerative disorders and related conditions in Alzheimer's disease and related conditions. In: Gothier, S., and Cummings, J.L., eds. *Alzheimer's Disease and Related Disorders, Annual 2001*. London: Martin Dunitz, Ltd., pp. 123–141.

Kumar, A., Mintz, J., Bilker, W., and Gottlieb, G. (2002) Autonomous neurobiological pathways to late-life major depressive disorder: Clinical and pathophysiological implications. *Neuropsychopharmacology* 26:229–236.

Lamberty, G.J. and Bieliauskas, L.A. (1993) Distinguishing between depression and dementia in the elderly: A review of neuropsychological findings. *Arch Clin Neuropsychol* 8:149–170.

LaRue, A. (1992) *Aging and Neuropsychological Assessment*. New York and London: Plenum Press.

Lavretsky, H. and Kumar, A. (1999) Depression and pseudodementia. Differential diagnosis and treatment issues. *Alzheimer's Dis Mgmt Today* 2:3–8.

Lavretsky, H. and Kumar, A. (2002a) Depressive disorders and cerebrovascular disease. In: Chiu, E., Ames, D., and Katona, C., eds. *Vascular Disease and Affective Disorders*. London: Martin Dunitz Ltd., pp. 127–148.

Lavretsky, H. and Kumar, A. (2002b) Clinically significant non-major depression: Old concepts, new insights. *Am J Geriatr Psychiatry* 10(3):239–255.

Lavretsky, H., Lesser, I.M., Miller, B.L., and Wohl, M. (1998) The relationship of age, age of onset and sex to depression in older adults. *Am J Geriatr Psychiatry* 6:248–256.

Lavretsky, H., Small, G.W., Ercoli, L.M., et al. (2001) APO E-4 tatus, depressive symptoms, and cognitive decline in elderly non-demented persons. *Am J Geriatr Psychiatry* 9:76–77 (No. SaG12).

Lawlor, B.A., Ryan, T.M., Schmeidler, J., Mohs, R.C., and Davis, K.L. (1994) Clinical symptoms associated with age at onset in Alzheimer's disease. *Am J Psychiatry* 151:1646–1649.

Lesch, K.P., and Mossner, R. (1998) Genetically driven variation in serotonin uptake: Is there a link to affective spectrum, neurodevelopmental, and neurodegenerative disorders? *Biol Psychiatry* 44(3):179–192.

Lesser, I.M., Boone, K.B., Mehringer, C.M., et al. (1996) Cognition and white matter hyperintensities in older depressed patients. *Am J Psychiatry* 153:1280–1287.

Levy, M.L., Cummings J.L., Fairbanks, L.A., Masterman, D., Miller, B.L., Craig, A.H., Paulsen, J.S., and Litvan, I. (1998) Apathy is not depression. *J Neuropsychiatry Clin Neurosci* 10:314–319.

Lezak, M.D. (1995) *Neuropsychological Assessment*, 3rd ed. New York and Oxford: Oxford University Press.

Liotti, M. and Mayberg, H.S. (2001) The role of functional neuroimaging in the neuropsychology of depression. *J Clin Exp Neuropsychol* 23(1):121–136.

Lockwood, K.A., Alexopoulos, G.S., Kakuma, T., and Van Gorp, W.G. (2000) Subtypes of cognitive impairment in depressed older adults. *Am J Geriatr Psychiatry* 8(3):201–208.

Lopez, O.L., Becker, J.T., Reynolds, I., Jungreis, C.A., Weinman, S., and DeKosky, S.T. (1997) Psychiatric correlates of MR deep white matter lesions in probable Alzheimer's disease. *J Neuropsychiatry Clin Neurosci* 9:246–250.

Lyketsos, C.G, Steele, C., Baker, L., Galik, E., Kopunek, S., Steinberg, M., and Warren, A. (1997) Major and minor depression in Alzheimer's disease: Prevalence and impact. *J Neuropsychiatry Clin Neurosci* 9:556–561.

McGuire, M.H. and Rabins, P.V. (1994) Mood disorders. Neuropsychiatric aspects of psychiatric disorders in the elderly. In: Coffey, C.E. and Cummings, J.L., eds. *Textbook of Geriatric Neuropsychiatry*. Washington, DC, and London: American Psychiatric Press; pp. 243–261.

McPherson, S., Fairbanks, L., Tiken, S., Cummings, J.L., and Back-Madruga, C. (2002) Apathy and executive function in Alzheimer's disease. *J Int Neuropsychol Soc* 8:373–381.

Merikangas, K.R., Chakravarti, A., Moldin, S.O., Araj, H., Blangero, J.C., Burmeister, M., Crabbe, J., Jr., Depaulo, J.R., Jr., Foulks, E., Freimer, N.B., Koretz, D.S., Lichtenstein, W., Mignot, E., Reiss, A.L., Risch, N.J., and Takahashi, J.S. (2002) Future of genetics of mood disorders research. *Biol Psychiatry* 52(6):457–477.

Nebes, R.D., Butters, M.A., Houck, P.R., et al. (2001a) Dual-task performance in depressed geriatric patients. *Psychiatry Res* 102:139–151.

Nebes, R.D., Butters, M.A., Mulsant, B.H., et al. (2000) Decreased working memory and processing speed mediate cognitive impairment in geriatric depression. *Psychol Med* 30:679–691.

Nebes, R.D., Pollock, B.G., Mulsant, B.H., Butters, M.A., Zmuda, M.D., and Reynolds, C.F., 3rd (1999) Cognitive effects of paroxetine in older depressed patients. *J Clin Psychiatry* 60(suppl 20):26–29.

Nebes, R.D., Pollock, B.G., Mulsant, B.H., et al. (1997) Low-level serum anticholinergicity as a source of baseline cognitive heterogeneity in geriatric depressed patients. *Psychopharmacol Bull* 33:715–720.

Nebes, R.D., Vora, I.J., Meltzer, C.C., et al. (2001b) Relationship of deep white matter hyperintensities and apolipoprotein E genotype to depressive symptoms in older adults without clinical depression. *Am J Psychiatry* 158:878–884.

Nemeroff, C.B. (2002) New directions in the development of antidepressants: The interface of neurobiology and psychiatry. *Human Psychopharmacol* 17(suppl 1):S13–S16.

Neylan, T.C., Canick, J.D., Hall, S.E., Reus, V.I., Sapolsky, R.M., and Wolkowitz, O.M. (2001) Cortisol levels predict cognitive impairment induced by electroconvulsive therapy. *Biol Psychiatry* 50(5):331–336.

Nussbaum, P.D. (1994) Pseudodementia: A slow death. *Neuropsychol Rev* 4:71–90.

Olin, J.T., Katz, I.R., Meyers, B.S., Schneider, L.S., and Lebowitz, B.D. (2002a) Provisional diagnostic criteria for depression of Alzheimer disease: Rationale and background. *Am J Geriatr Psychiatry* 10(2):129–141.

Olin, J.T., Schneider, L.S., Katz, I.R., Meyers, B.S., Alexopoulos, G.S., Breitner, J.C., Bruce, M.L., Caine, E.D., Cummings, J.L., Devanand, D.P., Krishnan, K.R., Lyketsos, C.G., Lyness, J.M., Rabins, P.V., Reynolds, C.F., 3rd, Rovner, B.W., Steffens, D.C., Tariot, P.N., and Lebowitz, B.D. (2002b) Provisional diagnostic criteria for depression of Alzheimer disease. *Am J Geriatr Psychiatry* 10:125–128.

Papassotiropoulos, A., Bagli, M., Jessen, F., Rao, M.L., Schwab, S.G., and Heun, R. (1999) Early-onset and late-onset depression are independent of the genetic polymorphism of apolipoprotein E. *Dementia Geriatr Cogn Disord* 10(4):258–261.

Pearlson, G.D., Ross, C.A., Lohr, W.D, Rovner, B.W., Chase, G.A., and Folstein, M.F. (1990) Association between family history of affective disorder and the depressive syndrome of Alzheimer's disease. *Am J Psychiatry* 147:452–456.

Peskind, E.R., Wilkinson, C.W., Petrie, E.C., Schellenberg, G.D., and Raskind, M.A. (2001) Increased CSF cortisol in AD is a function of APOE genotype. *Neurology* 56(8):1094–1098.

Petersen, R.C., Jack, C.R., Jr., Xu, Y.C., Waring, S.C., O'Brien, P.C., Smith, G.E., Ivnik, R.J., Tangalos, E.G., Boeve, B.F., and Kokmen, E. (2000) Memory and MRI-based hippocampal volumes in aging and AD. *Neurology* 54(3):581–587.

Pollock, B.G., Ferrell, R.E., Mulsant, B.H., Mazumdar, S., Miller, M., Sweet, R.A., Davis, S., Kirshner, M.A., Houck, P.R., Stack, J.A., Reynolds, C.F., and Kupfer, D.J. (2000) Allelic variation in the serotonin transporter promoter affects onset of paroxetine treatment response in late-life depression. *Neuropsychopharmacology* 23(5):587–590.

Raskind, M.A. (1998) The clinical interface of depression and dementia. *J Clin Psychiatry* 59(suppl. 10):9–12.

Reed, B.R., Eberling, J.L., Mungas, D., Weiner, M., and Jagust, W.J. (2001) Frontal lobe hypometabolism predicts cognitive decline in patients with lacunar infarcts. *Arch Neurol* 58(3):493–497.

Reichman, W.E. (1994) Nondegenerative dementing disorders. In: Coffey, C.E. and Cummings, J.L., eds. *Textbook of Geriatric Neuropsychiatry*. Washington, DC, and London: American Psychiatric Press, pp. 284–310.

Reifler, B.V. (1982) Arguments for abandoning the term pseudodementia. *J Am Geriatr Soc* 30:665–668.

Reifler, B.V. (1998) Detection and treatment of mixed cognitive and affective symptoms in the elderly: Is it dementia, depression, or both? *Clin Geriatr* 6:17–33.

Reynolds, C.F. and Hoch, C.C. (1998) Differential diagnosis of depressive pseudodementia and primary degenerative dementia. *Psychiatr Ann* 17:743–749.

Robinson, R.G., Bolduc, P.L., and Price, T.R. (1987) Two-year longitudinal study of post-stroke mood disorders: Diagnosis and outcome at one and two years. *Stroke* 18:579–584.

Rubinow, D.R., Post, R.M., Savard, R., and Gold, P.W. (1984) Cortisol hypersecretion and cognitive impairment in depression. *Arch Gen Psychiatry* 41(3):279–283.

Sackeim, H.A., Decina, P., Kanzler, M., Kerr, B., and Malitz, S. (1987) Effects of electrode placement on the efficacy of titrated, low-dose ECT. *Am J Psychiatry* 144(11):1449–1455.

Sackeim, H.A., Keilp, J.G., Rush, A.J., George, M.S., Marangell, L.B., Dormer, J.S., Burt, T., Lisanby, S.H., Husain, M., Cullum, C.M., Oliver, N., and Zboyan, H. (2001) The effects of vagus nerve stimulation on cognitive performance in patients with treatment-resistant depression. *Neuropsychiatry Neuropsychol Behav Neurol* 14(1):53–62.

Sackeim, H.A., Prudic, J., Devanand, D.P., Nobler, M.S., Lisanby, S.H., Peyser, S., Fitzsimons, L., Moody, B.J., and Clark, J. (2000) A prospective, randomized, double-blind comparison of bilateral and right unilateral electroconvulsive therapy at different stimulus intensities. *Arch Gen Psychiatry* 57(5):425–434.

Schweitzer, I., Tuckwell, V., O'Brien, J., and Ames, D. (2002) Is late onset depression a prodrome to dementia? *Int J Geriatr Psychiatry* 17:997–1005.

Sheline, Y.I., Sanghavi, M., Mintun, M.A., and Gado, M.H. (1999) Depression duration but not age predicts hippocampal volume loss in medically healthy women with recurrent major depression. *J Neurosci* 19(12):5034–5043.

Shoghi-Jadid, K., Small, G.W., Agdeppa, E.D., Kepe, V., Ercoli, L.M., Siddarth, P., Read, S., Satyamurthy, N., Petric, A., Huang, S.C., and Barrio, J.R. (2002) Localization of neurofibrillary tangles and beta-amyloid plaques in the brains of living patients with Alzheimer disease. *Am J Geriatr Psychiatry* 10(1):24–35.

Shraberg, D. (1978) The myth of pseudodementia: Depression and the aging brain. *Am J Psychiatry* 135:601–603.

Simpson, S.N., Allen, H., Tomenson, B., et al. (1999) Neurological correlates of depressive symptoms in Alzheimer's disease and vascular dementia. *J Affect Disord* 53:129–136.

Simpson, S.W., Jackson, A., Baldwin, R.C., and Burns, A. (1997) IPA/Bayer Research Awards in Psychogeriatrics. Subcortical hyperintensities in late-life depression: Acute response to treatment and neuropsychological impairment. *Int Psychogeriatr* 9:257–275.

Small, G.W., Chen, S.T., Komo, S., et al. (2001) Memory self-appraisal and depressive symptoms in people at genetic risk for Alzheimer's disease. *Int J Geriatr Psychiatry* 16:1071–1077.

Small, G.W., Komo, S., La Rue, A., Saxena, S., Phelps, M.E., Mazziotta, J.C., Saunders, A.M., Haines, J.L., Pericak-Vance, M.A., and Roses, A.D. (1996) Early detection of Alzheimer's disease by combining apolipoprotein E and neuroimaging. *Ann NY Acad Sci* 802:70–78.

Small, G.W., Mazziotta, J.C., Collins, M.T., Baxter, L.R., Phelps, M.E., Mandelkern, M.A., Kaplan, A., La Rue, A., Adamson, C.F., Chang, L., et al. (1995) Apolipoprotein E type 4 allele and cerebral glucose metabolism in relatives at risk for familial Alzheimer disease. *JAMA* 273(12):942–947.

Starkstein, S.E., Sabe, L., Vazquez, S., et al. (1997) Neuropsychological, psychiatric, and cerebral perfusion correlates of leukoaraiosis in Alzheimer's disease. *J Neurol Neurosurg Psychiatry* 63:66–73.

Steffens, D.C. and Krishnan, K.R. (1998) Structural neuroimaging and mood disorders: Recent findings, implications for classification, and future directions. *Biol Psychiatry* 43:705–712.

Steffens, D.C., Payne, M.E., Greenberg, D.L., Byrum, C.E., Welsh-Bohmer, K.A., Wagner, H.R., and MacFall, J.R. (2002) Hippocampal volume and incident dementia in geriatric depression. *Am J Geriatr Psychiatry* 10(1):62–71.

Steffens, D.C., Plassman, B.L., Helms, M.J., Welsh-Bohmer, K.A., Saunders, A.M., and Breitner, J.C.S. (1997) A twin study of late-onset depression and apolipoprotein E e4 as risk factors for Alzheimer's disease. *Biol Psychiatry* 41:851–856.

Stoudemire, A., Hill, C.D., Morris, R., Martino-Saltzman, D., Markwalter, H., and Lewison, B. (1991) Cognitive outcome following tricyclic and electroconvulsive treatment of major depression in the elderly. *Am J Psychiatry* 148(10):1336–1340.

Sultzer, D.L., Levin, H.S., Mahler, M.E., et al. (1993) A comparison of psychiatric symptoms in vascular dementia and Alzheimer's disease. *Am J Psychiatry* 150:1806–1812.

Swan, G.E. and Carmelli, D. (2002) Evidence for genetic mediation of executive control: A study of aging male twins. *J Gerontol Ser B Psychol Sci Soc Sci* 57:133–143.

Tekin, S. and Cummings, J.L. (2002) Frontal-subcortical neuronal circuits and clinical neuropsychiatry: An update. *J Psychosom Res* 53:647–654.

Vanitallie, T.B. (2002) Stress: A risk factor for serious illness. *Metabolism* 51(6 suppl 1):40–45.

Vida, S., Des Rosiers, P., Carrier, L., and Gauthier, S. (1994) Prevalence of depression in Alzheimer's disease and validity of research diagnostic criteria. *J Geriatr Psychiatry Neurol* 7:238–244.

Visser, P.J., Verhey, F.R., Ponds, R.W., Kester, A., and Jolles, J. (2000) Distinction between preclinical Alzheimer's disease and depression. *J Am Geriatr Soc* 48(5):479–484.

Weiner, M.F., Svetlik, D., and Risser, R.C. (1997) What depressive symptoms are reported in Alzheimer's patients? *Int J Geriatr Psychiatry* 12:648–652.

Wells, C. (1979) Pseudodementia. *Am J Psychiatry* 136:895–900.

Yamashita, H., Fujikawa, T., Yanai, I., et al. (2002) Cognitive dysfunction in recovered depressive patients with silent cerebral infarction. *Neuropsychobiology* 45:12–18.

Yousef, G., Ryan, W.J., Lambert, T., and Kellett, J. (1998) A preliminary report: A new scale to identify the pseudodementia syndrome. *Int J Geriatr Psychiatry* 13:389–399.

Zubenko, G.S., Henderson, R., Stiffler, J.S., Stabler, S., Rosen, J., and Kaplan, B.B. (1996) Association of the APOE epsilon 4 allele with clinical subtypes of late-life depression. *Biol Psychiatry* 40(10): 1008–1016.

Zubenko, G.S., Moossy, J., and Kopp, U. (1990) Neurochemical correlates of major depression in primary dementia. *Arch Neurol* 47:209–214.

# 8 | Suicide

YEATES CONWELL

Rates of suicide in later life are higher than at any other point in the life course. In May 2001 the National Strategy for Suicide Prevention was released by the Office of the Surgeon General of the United States, acknowledging suicide as a major public health concern and articulating specific goals and objectives for action (U.S. Public Health Service, 2001). Reduction of suicide in elders is an important component of that agenda. Older adults not only have higher rates of suicide than younger cohorts (National Center for Health Statistics, 2001) but are also the fastest-growing segment of the population. These patterns, in general, pertain worldwide. As increasing numbers of people age into the stage of life that carries the greatest risk, demographers anticipate that the absolute number of seniors who take their own lives will increase dramatically (Haas and Hendin, 1983).

The goal of this chapter is to provide an overview of factors in the biological, psychological, and social domains that place older adults at risk for suicide, and to consider their implications for the design and implementation of prevention and treatment strategies.

## METHODOLOGICAL ISSUES

The study of suicide in older adults, as in younger cohorts, faces a number of unique methodological challenges. The terms used to describe suicidal behaviors are often ill defined and loosely applied, complicating the interpretation of findings. Further, the boundaries between suicidal ideation (SI), attempted suicide (AS), and completed suicide (CS) are overlapping and uncertain (Linehan, 1986). Therefore, studies of SI or AS cannot be assumed to apply directly to CS.

Both CS and AS have a low base rate in the elderly population, making difficult the acquisition of sample sizes necessary to yield meaningful results in research. Although prospective cohort studies may be the optimal means to study risk factors and the efficacy and effectiveness of preventive interventions, suicide's low base rate makes them prohibitively expensive. The case-control method is better suited to the examination of rare outcomes (Gordis, 2000).

When applied to the study of suicide, the retrospective case control method is known as the *psychological autopsy* (PA) (Hawton et al., 1998). The PA method is limited by its retrospective nature, with potential for acquisition and informant bias. Recent articulation of standardized methods and demonstration of their validity, however, have made the PA approach an increasingly powerful tool for determining risk factors where prospective data collection would be impractical (Clark and Horton-Deutsch, 1992; Conner et al., 2001a, 2001b; Kelly and Mann, 1996). Large, methodologically sound PA studies of older adults have recently been completed in four countries (Beautrais, 2002; Conwell et al., 2001; Harwood et al., 2001; Waern et al., 2002). All used standardized methods, suicides and controls sampled from carefully defined populations, and analytic approaches enabling quantification of the risk associated with factors in a variety of domains (principally odds ratios).

Finally, suicide is a complex, multidetermined behavior described well by Havens (1965) as "the final common pathway of diverse circumstances, of an interdependent network rather than an isolated cause, a knot of circumstances tightening around a single time and place." Ultimately, our understanding of suicide in older adults must reflect that complexity as well.

## PREVALENCE OF SUICIDAL BEHAVIORS IN LATE LIFE

Surveys of SI consistently report lower rates in elders than in younger adults (Blazer et al., 1986; Duberstein et al., 1999; Gallo et al., 1994). Representative figures for elders are presented in Table 8.1. Estimates vary from 1% to 36%, reflecting differences in methodology and in the populations sampled. Also, some investigators distinguish between active or passive SI or between SI and death ideation (DI; thoughts of death without suicidal intent), while others do not.

Because there is no systematic surveillance mechanism in the United States for AS, data on its incidence and prevalence are far fewer and less reliable than those for CS. Like SI, AS is less common among elders than in younger age groups (Moscicki, 1997). The ratio of AS to CS in the general population is estimated to range from 8:1 to 36:1 (Crosby et al., 1999; Paykel et al.,

TABLE 8.1. *Studies of Suicidal and Death Ideation in Older Adults*

| Study[*] | Location | Age | Sample Size | Time Frame | Suicidal (SI) and Death (DI) Ideation | |
|---|---|---|---|---|---|---|
| | | | | | Prevalence | Correlates |
| Forsell et al. (1997) | Kungsholmen, Sweden | ≥75 | 969 | 2 weeks | SI: 10.1 fleeting, 2.5% frequent | Major depression (50% of those with frequent SI), institutionalization, functional disability, visual problems |
| Callahan et al. (1996) | Indiana, USA | ≥60 | 301 primary care depressives | 1 week | SI: 4.6% | Depressive illness, functional impairment. |
| Crosby et al. (1999) | U.S.A. (nationwide telephone survey) | ≥65 | 760 | 1 year | SI: 1.0% | Older age |
| Rao et al. (1997) | Cambridge, U.K. | ≥81 | 125 | 2 years | SI: 7% DI: 20% | Female gender, depression symptoms and diagnosis dementia |
| Linden and Barnow (1997) | Berlin, Germany | ≥70 | 516 | 1 week | SI: 1% DI: 21.1% | Major depressive disorder (50%–75%). |
| Jorm et al. (1995) | Canberra, Australia | ≥70 | 923 | 2 weeks | SI/DI: 2.3% | Depressive disorder, poor health, disability, vision and hearing impairments, unmarried, in residential care |
| Skoog et al. (1996) | Gothenberg, Sweden | ≥85 | 345 | 1 month | SI/DI: 15.9% | Major depression, psychotic disorders, heart and peptic ulcer disease, use of anxiolytics, neuroleptics |
| Shah et al. (2000) | West Middlesex, U.K. | ≥65 | 55 medical inpatients | 1 month | SI: 36% DI: 33% | Depressive symptoms and diagnosis, antidepressants |
| Paykel et al. (1974) | Connecticut, U.S.A. | ≥60 | 156 | 1 year | SI/DI: 9.0% | (Analyzed for all subjects ≥18) Psychiatric symptoms, social isolation, other adverse life events |
| Scocco et al. (2001) | Padua, Italy | ≥65 | 611 | 1 month 1 year Lifetime | SI/DI: 6.5% 9.2% 17.0% | Depression, anxiety, hostility, hypnotic use |

[*]All studies used in-person interviews except that of Crosby et al. (2001), which used a telephone survey.

1974); the ratio among adolescents may be 200:1 or more (Fremouw et al., 1990). In contrast, studies estimate that there are three or four ASs for each CS in later life (Parkin and Stengel, 1965). Self-destructive behaviors in older people more often result in death because of their greater physical frailty (reduced resistance to the insult), greater likelihood that they live alone (decreased likelihood of discovery and rescue), and greater lethality of intent (Conwell et al., 1998). Elders give fewer warnings to others of their suicidal plans, more often use firearms, and use greater planning and resolve. These findings indicate the critical importance of early recognition of elders at risk in order to prevent development of a suicidal crisis.

Unlike SI and AS, rates of CS increase with age in the United States, a pattern accounted for by the elevated risk among white males. Figure 8.1 illustrates rates of suicide in the United States as a function of age, race, and sex. Whereas the suicide rate for the general population was 10.7/100,000 in 1999, the rate among those 65 years of age and over was 15.9/100,000. The group at highest risk was white males aged 85 and over, whose rate of 54.9/100,000 was almost six times the nation's age-adjusted rate. In contrast, midlife is the time of highest suicide risk for women in the United States. Rates peak for white women at ages 50–54 (7.5/100,000) and for black women at slightly younger ages (40–44 years; 3.3/100,000). Rates among women of both races show a slight decline in older age.

The United States has a somewhat unusual pattern with regard to gender differences in suicide risk. In most other countries that report suicide statistics to the World Health Organization, later life is the time of highest risk for both men and women (Pearson and Conwell, 1995). In China, for example, rates of suicide among women peak at over 62/100,000 in old old age.

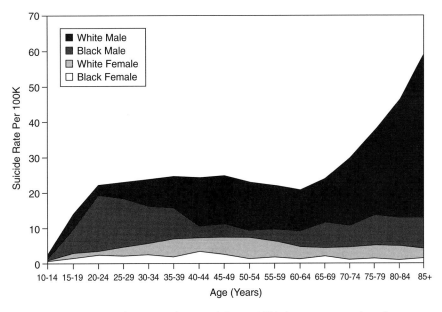

FIGURE 8.1 Suicide rates in the United States, 1999, by age, race, and gender.

The fact that suicide rates rise with age in both men and women in most cultures raises the possibility that aging-related biological and/or psychological processes may contribute to an increased risk of suicide in older adults. The observation that the late-life suicide risk is similar for men and women in some countries and races, while differing dramatically in others, underscores the importance of sociocultural factors in determining risk. The following sections review evidence in the biological, psychological, and social domains, first noting correlative and descriptive data, followed by reference to studies in which sufficiently rigorous methodologies were used and control samples were included to enable quantification of risk.

## NEUROBIOLOGY OF LATE-LIFE SUICIDE

The association between low cerebrospinal fluid (CSF) levels of the primary serotonin metabolite, 5-hydroxyindolacetic acid (5-HIAA), and aggressive, impulsive behavior is one of the most consistent and replicated findings in biological psychiatry (see Stoff and Mann, 1997, for a representative review). This association has been noted in suicide attempters with depression and other diagnoses, arsonists, and other violent offenders.

Postmortem studies of brain tissue from suicides and controls reinforce the potential importance of serotonergic dysfunction and self-destructive behaviors. Representative findings include low CSF concentrations of serotonin and 5-HIAA, increased postsynaptic 5-hydroxytryptamine (5-HT) receptor binding and decreased presynaptic binding at $5\text{-HT}_1$ receptor sites and at the serotonin transporter. Taken together, these findings suggest a presynaptic deficit and a postsynaptic compensatory response in impulsive, aggressive individuals. Mann and colleagues (1999) have presented a stress-diathesis model in which individuals with low serotonergic activity, either on a genetic or an environmental basis, are more prone to act impulsively and aggressively in the face of dysphoria, hopelessness, and emergent suicidal ideation in the depressed state. Noradrenergic, dopaminergic, and other neuroendocrine and neurochemical systems have been implicated as well (see Mann and Stoff, 1997 for a representative review).

The dramatic rise in suicide rates with age among men in the United States suggests that aging and possibly gender-related changes in these or other neurobiological systems may contribute to the suicide risk in older adults as well. Preliminary evidence indicates that age-related effects on serotonergic and other monoamine systems may be more pronounced in men (Mann and Stoff, 1997), and the finding of lower CSF levels of 5-HIAA in elderly depressed patients who had attempted suicide compared to elderly depressed controls suggests that the model may apply in later life as well (Jones et al., 1990). However, high rates of medication use and medical co-morbidity in elderly suicides greatly complicate the interpretation of neurochemical and receptor assays. As a consequence, very few studies have included elderly subjects.

Other investigators, however, have correlated structural and functional abnormalities in the aging brain with suicidal behaviors. Neuropsychological testing indicates abnormalities in the executive function of SAs compared with controls (Keilp et al., 2001), including in older adults (King et al., 2000). Our group reported significantly greater hippocampal neurofibrillary pathology in postmortem analysis of elderly suicides than controls (Rubio et al., 2001), while Ahearn and colleagues (2001) found that elderly depressives with lifetime histories of suicide attempts had significantly more subcortical gray matter hyperintensities on magnetic resonance imaging (MRI) than did carefully matched depressives with no previous suicide attempt. The particular mechanisms that may result in suicidal behavior remain unclear. However, these findings raise the possibility that suicide in later life may be associated with destruction of neural pathways critical to the regulation of mood, cognition, and behavior. Additional research is necessary to confirm and extend these functional and neuroanatomical findings, define their neurochemical correlates, and establish whether they represent early, subtle presentations of vascular or other degenerative neuropathology. Unfortunately, there is no neurobiological marker of suicide risk in older or younger adults.

## MENTAL HEALTH

Psychological autopsy studies including suicides in later life found that 71% to 95% had a diagnosable major psychiatric disorder at the time of death (Table 8.2). Affective disorders were the most frequent psychopathology among suicides in all studies. They are typically of moderate severity and are infrequently associated with co-morbid substance use disorders, suggesting the likelihood of a response to standard therapies (Conwell et al., 1996). Primary psychotic illnesses, including schizophrenia, schizoaffective illness, and delusional disorder, play a relatively smaller role in suicide among the elderly than at younger ages. Similarly,

personality disorders and anxiety disorders are uncommon in samples of older suicides. Alcoholism and other drug use disorders are present in 3%–43%, a smaller proportion than at younger ages. The risk that delirium and dementia pose for suicidal behaviors in older adults is unclear. Depressive symptoms are common in individuals with mild to moderate dementia, suggesting that they may also be at elevated risk for suicide. At more advanced stages of the disease, however, patients require greater supervision and may be less able to effectively conceptualize and carry through a suicidal act.

More recent studies have included control samples that enable quantification of the risk of suicide associated with specific late-life disorders. They include one prospective nonclinical cohort study and five case-control PA studies.

In the only prospective cohort study to date that has examined the outcome of suicide in older adults, Ross and colleagues (1990) followed almost 12,000 retirement community residents for 5 years. Nineteen died by suicide. In a nested case-control design, they found that self-rated depressive symptom severity was the strongest predictor of case status. Subjects with the greatest depressive symptomatology were 23 times more likely to take their own lives than asymptomatic subjects. In addition, drinking three or more alcoholic beverages and sleeping 9 or more hours per night were associated with a significantly increased risk of suicide (OR = 3.5 and OR = 4.6, respectively) in multivariate analysis.

Five methodologically sound case-control PA studies have shown that the presence of any Axis I disorder is clearly and powerfully associated with an elevated risk of suicide in older adults (Beautrais, 2002; Conwell et

TABLE 8.2. *Axis I Diagnoses Made by Psychological Autopsy in Studies of Late-Life Suicide*

| Study | Location | Age | Sample Size | Diagnosis: % with | | | | | |
| | | | | Major Dep | Other Mood D/O | Alcohol Use D/O | Other Drug Use D/O | Nonaffective Psychosis | No Dx[*] |
| --- | --- | --- | --- | --- | --- | --- | --- | --- | --- |
| Barraclough (1971) | West Sussex, UK | ≥65 | 30 | 87 | | 3 | | 0 | 13 |
| Clark (1991) | Chicago, USA | ≥65 | 54 | 54 | 11 | 19 | | 0 | 24 |
| Conwell et al. (1991) | Monroe County, USA | ≥50 | 18 | 67 | 17 | 42 | | 0 | 11 |
| Carney et al. (1994) | San Diego, USA | ≥60 | 49 | 54 | | 22 | | | 14 |
| Henriksson et al. (1995) | Finland | ≥60 | 43 | 44 | 21 | 25 | 5 | 12 | 9 |
| Conwell et al. (1996) | Monroe County, USA | 55–74 | 36 | 47 | 17 | 43 | 3 | 6 | 8 |
| | | 75–92 | 14 | 57 | 21 | 27 | 7 | 0 | 29 |
| Beautrais (2002) | New Zealand | ≥55 | 31 | 86 | | 14 | | | 9 |
| Conwell et al. (2001) | Western New York, USA | ≥50 | 73 | 71 | | 18 | | 7 | 12 |
| Harwood et al. (2001) | Central England | ≥60 | 100 | 63 | | 5 | 5 | 4 | 23 |
| Waern et al. (2002) | Goteborg, Sweden | ≥65 | 85 | 46 | 36 | 27 | | 8 | 5 |

[*]Includes cases with insufficient data to allow diagnosis (dx).

al., 2000, 2001; Harwood et al., 2001; Waern et al., 2002). Odds ratios ranged from 27.4 to 113.1, reflecting differences in the samples selected and the diagnostic criteria employed. Mood disorders were particularly prominent risk factors. Waern and colleagues (2002) found that recurrent major depression was associated with the greatest relative risk in multivariate analyses, although single-episode major depression, dysthymia, and minor depression were also significant predictors of suicide.

Three studies found no significant differences in the proportions of suicides and controls with dementia (Conwell et al., 2000, 2001; Waern et al., 2002), and none found that anxiety disorders were associated with elevated risk after controlling for depression in multivariate analyses. The results for substance use disorders were mixed, with three of the five studies showing a statistically significant elevation of risk, with ORs ranging from 4.4 to 43.1 (Beautrais, 2002; Conwell et al., 2000; Waern et al., 2002).

### Other Psychological Factors

Hopelessness has been shown to be a significant predictor of SI (Beck et al., 1993), suicidal intent (Beck et al., 1974), and eventual suicide (Beck et al., 1985, 1990) in mixed-age samples. However, the construct has been less thoroughly studied in older adults. Shneidman and Farberow (1957) found that elders were more likely to express hopelessness than anger or guilt in suicide notes. Hopelessness was found to be predictive of SI in older outpatient depressives in one study (Hill et al., 1988), and in Ross and colleagues' (1990) prospective cohort study, a single-item hopelessness measure was a significant predictor of eventual suicide.

Among elderly depressives, hopelessness may represent both a trait and a state marker of increased risk. Szanto and colleagues (1998) found that hopelessness remained significantly higher, even after treatment to resolution of a depressive syndrome, in elderly patients with major depression and a lifetime history of SA than among either persons with SI only or nonsuicidal elderly patients.

As well, hopelessness is theoretically linked to other constructs, such as self-efficacy (Bandura, 1977) and locus of control (Rodin and Salovey, 1989; Rowe and Kahn, 1987), each of which may, in turn, have specific implications for the design of preventive intervention strategies. Cognitive behavioral therapies may be particularly applicable. These relationships and potential therapeutic interventions have yet to be tested specifically with regard to suicide behavior and risk in later life, however.

Although personality disorder diagnoses have not been systematically examined in studies of late-life suicide, descriptive studies have linked elder suicide with the personality traits of timidity and shy seclusiveness (Batchelor and Napier, 1953), hypochondriasis, hostility, and a rigid, independent style (Batchelor et al., 1953; Clark, 1993; Farberow and Shneidman, 1970). Duberstein and colleagues (Duberstein, 1995) have stressed the importance of high Neuroticism (N) and lower scores on the Openness to Experience (OTE) factor of the NEO Personality Inventory (Costa and McCrae, 1992). Both factors statistically distinguished suicides aged 50 years and over from matched controls. Low OTE describes a constellation of characteristics that include muted affective and hedonic responsiveness, a limited range of interests, and comfort with the familiar. We have hypothesized that low OTE places elders at risk both because it leaves them less well equipped socially and psychologically to manage the challenges of aging and because elders low in OTE are less likely to experience or express SI, thus escaping detection and lifesaving interventions (Duberstein, 2001). This theory helps resolve the seemingly contradictory finding that low OTE has also been associated with *decreased* reporting of SI (Duberstein et al., 1999). Relationships of these traits to the depressive conditions so common in older suicide victims, and their potential role as moderators of other putative risk and protective factors present (e.g., stressful events and social supports), remain to be studied.

## PHYSICAL HEALTH AND FUNCTION

Although it is commonly assumed that physical illness and functional impairment place older adults at increased risk for suicide, relatively few data are available with which to quantify that risk. Harris and Barraclough (1994) demonstrated, in a comprehensive review of over 60 medical disorders and their treatments, that the illnesses for which there was evidence of increased risk were, in general, more characteristic of middle-aged or young-old than old-old adults. These included human immunodeficiency virus/acquired immune deficiency syndrome (HIV/AIDS), Huntington's disease, multiple sclerosis, renal disease, peptic ulcer disease, spinal cord injury, and systemic lupus erythematosus. Record linkage studies have convincingly demonstrated that malignant neoplasms (with the exception of skin cancer) are associated with increased risk. Seizure disorders, other central nervous system (CNS) conditions, cardiopulmonary complications, and urogenital diseases in men have been implicated by other authors as well (Mackenzie and Popkin, 1987; Whitlock, 1986).

Given the strong association between mood disorders and suicide in older adults, and the association between physical illness and depression, any demonstrated risk of suicide associated with medical conditions may be mediated by affective disorders. Perhaps only those who become clinically depressed in the face of medical illness become suicidal. Two groups have reported that SI among seriously ill people was rare in the absence of clinically significant mood disturbance (Brown et al., 1986; Chochinov et al., 1995). Our group compared CSs aged 60 years and over who died within 30 days of contact with their primary care provider with a demographically matched sample of living primary care patients (Conwell et al., 2000). Physical illness burden and the presence of one or more serious physical conditions significantly distinguished the two groups. However, after controlling for mood disorders, physical health and functional measures were no longer predictive. Waern and colleagues (2002) did find that serious physical illness in any organ category was an independent risk factor for suicide even after controlling for psychiatric diagnosis. When the sexes were analyzed separately, however, illness represented a risk factor only in men. Beautrais (2002) found that neither serious physical illness nor the likelihood of a visit to a primary care provider in the previous month was associated with an increased risk of suicide in her case-control study of New Zealand elders. While physical illness is clearly an important factor in determining the risk of suicide in later life, the mediating influence of depressive disorders is also critical to consider.

## SOCIAL FACTORS

The stressful life events associated with suicide in older adults differ from those at younger ages. Whereas suicides in young and middle adulthood typically occur in the context of interpersonal discord, and legal, financial, and occupational problems, old-age suicides are more often associated with physical illness and other losses (Carney et al., 1994; Conwell et al., 1990; Heikkinen et al., 1995), including bereavement (Duberstein et al., 1998). These observations may only reflect the relative prevalence of stressful events at various points in the life course. Two case-control PA studies examined the associations of specific stressors with suicide in later life. Financial and relationship problems and family discord (Beautrais, 2002; Rubenowitz et al., 2001) distinguished elder suicides from matched community controls in univariate analyses. When other factors, including depression, were controlled for in multivariate analyses, however, only family discord remained predictive. Findings are mixed with regard to the role that social isolation and support may play as risk and protective factors in late-life suicide. Barraclough (1971) used census data for comparison with elder suicides, concluding that cases were more likely to live alone than their peers in the community. Of three case-con-

trol PA studies that examined this question, however, only one found that elder suicides were more likely to live alone (unadjusted OR = 5.1) (Conwell et al., 2001). Social support is a complex construct that incorporates the type, frequency, and quality of the interactions and help provided. Although research in late-life suicide has not reached this level of methodological sophistication, a number of controlled studies allow preliminary conclusions. In their analyses of the Established Populations for Epidemiologic Studies of the Elderly (EPESE) database, Turvey and colleagues (2002) reported that having a greater number of friends and relatives in whom to confide was associated with a significantly reduced suicide risk. In his PA study of men in Arizona, Miller (1978) also reported that matched community controls were significantly more likely than elder male suicides to have had a confidant. In unadjusted analyses, our group found that controls received significantly greater help with the practical tasks of day-to-day life, and had more frequent social interactions, than suicides (Conwell et al., 2001). Lack of social interaction was also a significant risk factor for elder suicide in the New Zealand sample (OR = 4.5), even after adjustment for physical and mental health variables (Beautrais, 2002).

Because the rate of suicide for women is so much lower than that for men, no PA study to date has included sufficient samples of older U.S. women to examine what factors may be either protective or place them at risk. We are left to speculate, therefore, that women's greater ability than men to establish and maintain supportive interpersonal relationships may play a protective role. Another possibility is that older women may die by suicide less often than men, despite having higher rates of SA, because they tend to choose less immediately lethal means—for example, ingestion of drugs rather than use of firearms.

## ACCESS TO LETHAL MEANS

A higher proportion of late-life suicides used a firearm than suicides at younger ages. This observation holds true for both men and women (McIntosh, 2002), although older men remain far more likely to take their lives with a gun than are women. Miller (1978) found no difference between male suicides and controls in the proportion who owned a firearm. However, a significantly greater proportion of suicides than controls had acquired the weapon within the past year. Our group has recently reported that the presence of a handgun in the home significantly increased the risk of suicide in elderly men but not women (Conwell et al., 2002). Among those subjects who kept a gun in the home, storing the weapon loaded and unlocked were independent predictors of suicide as well.

## SUMMARY OF RISK

Epidemiological evidence is strong that older age, male gender, white race, and unmarried status are associated with an increased risk of suicide. Further evidence for risk factors in suicide must be drawn either from prospective cohort or retrospective case-control (PA) studies that adequately account for base rates of the hypothesized factors in the population. Stressful life events, in particular bereavement and family discord, appear to increase the suicide risk in later life; their influence may be modified in part by social support and depressive disorders. Social support variables may act as both risk enhancers and protective factors. Physical illness augments the risk of suicide, although its effect may largely be mediated by depressive disorders. Personality traits may also influence the risk. Interactions of these variables within an older individual determine his or her vulnerability at a particular point in time. For example, the tendency to become depressed and suicidal in the face of physical illness may be higher among individuals low in OTE, but only in the absence of social supports that act to buffer the functional or financial impact of the illness. Examination of more complete multivariate models is important for increasing our understanding of these myriad potential interactions.

At the same time, it is abundantly clear that affective illness is a powerful independent determinant of suicide risk in older adults. Every study to date has reinforced the association of either depressive symptomatology or an affective disorder diagnosis with CS in elders, all at considerably greater odds than for any other risk factor. Population attributable risk (PAR) is a statistic indicating the proportional reduction in suicide that would result from elimination of a confirmed risk factor from the population. Based on her study of suicide and life-threatening SA in elders, Beautrais (2002) calculated that elder suicides would be reduced by 74% if mood disorders were eliminated from the population. While this goal may be difficult to attain, it provides clear and compelling direction for the design and implementation of prevention efforts.

## APPROACHES TO PREVENTION

A general tenet of prevention science is that complex, multilevel intervention strategies that target a variety of risk factors are more successful at reducing an adverse outcome than is any isolated prevention strategy. The recommended approach to suicide prevention in late life, therefore, should be one that combines universal, selective, and indicated preventive interventions (NAMHC Workgroup on Mental Disorders Prevention Research, 1998). Table 8.3 lists the target populations for each approach, with objectives and examples of their

application to the reduction of late-life suicidal behaviors. The evidence base for defining risk factors, as reviewed previously, is in its early stages. Very few prevention programs in fact target suicide in elders (Mercer, 1989), and virtually none of them has rigorously demonstrated efficacy or effectiveness. The following recommendations, therefore, remain largely theoretical.

## UNIVERSAL PREVENTION

Universal suicide prevention strategies address the entire population, irrespective of any individual's age or risk status. They constitute broad initiatives that typically target more distal risk factors with the anticipation of large downstream effects. Their importance is underscored by Rose's (1985) theorem "that a large number of people at small risk may give rise to more cases of disease and a small number who are at high risk." Even a small impact in a large population, therefore, may have a large impact on those at greatest risk.

No universal preventive interventions have been tested that specifically target suicidal behaviors in later life. One approach that should be considered is the restriction of access to handguns, given indications that their presence in the homes of elders increases the risk. Similar findings and recommendations have been made concerning firearm access by adolescents and younger adults as well (Brent, 2001), suggesting that suicide rates across the life span might be expected to decrease as a result.

Universal prevention should also include education of the general population and health care providers about the myths and realities of depression and suicide in older adults. General awareness is low, for example, that depressive syndromes and SI are not normal for the aged, but rather that they may indicate disorders highly responsive to treatment. Culturally ingrained biases against aging and the aged represent another important target for universal education interventions.

## SELECTIVE PREVENTION

Selective preventive interventions target subgroups or individual elders who may be placed at increased risk for suicide by vulnerability to, rather than the presence of, more proximal risk factors. Isolated elders lacking social supports are an example, for whom a selective preventive intervention might include outreach services to provide supportive interactions. The Center for Elder Suicide Prevention offers such a program. Called the Friendship Line, this 24-hour telephone service provides emotional support and referral information to older adults. In addition, it supports an outreach program to provide counseling and more intensive mental

TABLE 8.3. *The Language of Prevention Science Applied to Suicide in Later Life*

| Intervention Terminology | Approach | Target | Objectives | Examples of Possible Prevention Efforts |
|---|---|---|---|---|
| Universal Prevention | Population | Entire population, not identified based on individual risk | Implement broadly directed initiatives to prevent suicide-related morbidity and mortality through reducing risk and enhancing protective factors | Education of the general public, clergy, the media, and health-care providers concerning normal aging, ageism, and stigmas regarding mental illness, pain, and disability, management of depression, and suicidal behaviors; restriction of access to lethal means, such as handguns |
| Selective Prevention | Population; high-risk | Asymptomatic or presymptomatic individuals or subgroups who have distal risk factors for suicide or a higher than average risk of developing mental disorders or other, more proximal risk factors | Prevent suicide-related morbidity and mortality through addressing specific characteristics that place elders at risk | Promote church-based and community programs to contact and support isolated elders; focus medical and social services on reducing disability and enhancing independent functioning; increase access to home care and rehabilitation services; improve access to pain management and palliative care services |
| Indicated Prevention | High risk | Individuals with detectable symptoms and/or other proximal risk factors for suicide | Treat individuals with precursor signs and symptoms to prevent development of disorder or the expression of suicidal behavior | Train gatekeepers to recognize symptomatic and at-risk elders; link outreach and gatekeeper services to comprehensive evaluation and health management services in a continuum of care; implement strategies to provide more accessible, acceptable, and affordable mental health care to elders; treat elders with chronic pain syndromes more effectively; increase screening/treatment in primary care settings for elders with depression, anxiety, and substance misuse; improve providers' assessment and restrict access to lethal means |

health services for those at greater risk (an *indicated* intervention) (Fiske and Arbore, 2000).

The documented associations between physical health and functional impairment, depressive disorders, and suicide in later life indicate a wide range of other possible selective prevention strategies. They should include programs that enhance the independent functioning of older adults; improve access to home care and rehabilitative services that decrease the need for hospitalization and institutional care; and improve access to pain management and palliative care services.

## INDICATED PREVENTION

Indicated preventive interventions address high-risk individuals with diagnosable mental illness and/or other proximal risk factors for suicide. Pharmacological and psychotherapeutic approaches to the treatment of de-

pression are prominent examples that are well reviewed elsewhere in this volume. There is no study, however, in which either approach has been specifically applied to the treatment or prevention of suicidality in older adults. More attention has been paid to the contexts in which elders at risk can be recognized, diagnosed, and treated.

A large majority of elder suicides had an active relationship with a primary care provider at the time of death. Up to three-quarters of older suicide victims saw a primary care provider within 30 days of death and up to half within 1 week of their suicides (Luoma et al., 2002), the majority of whom had actively symptomatic affective illnesses (Conwell et al., 2000). For a variety of reasons related to the patient, the physician, and the primary care setting, depressive disorders often go unrecognized and inadequately treated by primary care providers. Physicians spend less time with older patients (Keeler et al., 1982), who are in turn less likely to volunteer SI (Duberstein et al., 1999) or the ideational and affective symptoms of depression (Gallo et al., 1994; Lyness et al., 1995). The presentation of affective distress in somatic terms is common (Heithoff, 1995; Knauper and Wittchen, 1994). Physicians often lack the knowledge and experience, as well as the necessary time in a given appointment, to distinguish psychiatric disorders from their frequent and often complex medical co-morbidities (Callahan et al., 1992; Rost et al., 1994). These observations suggest the need for more uniform application of screening tools for depression and other psychiatric syndromes in primary care offices (Lyness et al., 1997), as well as programs to improve the effectiveness of primary care physicians in their diagnosis and aggressive treatment.

A study carried out on the island of Gotland in Sweden tested the hypothesis that education of primary care physicians in the recognition and treatment of mood disorders would result in lower suicide rates (Rutz et al., 1989). All primary care physicians on the island were given intensive training in two sessions during 1983 and 1984. In the following year, the suicide rate on Gotland was significantly lower than in other areas of Sweden and significantly lower than the island's rates preceding the intervention. These findings were best accounted for by reductions in the proportions of suicides with affective illness. As well, the educational program was associated with reduced sick leave for depressive disorders, decreased inpatient care days for depression, and increased numbers of antidepressant prescriptions (Rihmer et al., 1995). However, the program's benefit waned after several years, suggesting the need for periodic reinforcement of the educational lessons (Rutz et al., 1992). Furthermore, the effect was more pronounced for women than men (Rutz et al., 1995), the group at greatest risk in later life. Because the study did not use a randomized, controlled design, its findings have been questioned and require replication.

Although not designed specifically for older adults, other models of collaborative care have been tested in randomized, controlled designs and show promise to provide better outcomes of depression in primary care practices. As indicated interventions, therefore, they should be expected to reduce suicide as well. Schulberg and colleagues (1996) found that the provision of mental health services in the primary care office to young adults and middle-aged depressives yielded significantly better outcomes than treatment as usual. Katon and colleagues (1996, 1997) tested a combined intervention that involved patient and physician education, cognitive behavioral therapy delivered by study psychologists, antidepressant therapy prescribed by physicians, and regular ongoing consultation between the two disciplines. Patients with major depressive disorder showed significant improvement at lower cost compared to care as usual. More recently, a number of care-

fully designed clinical trials have been initiated to test the effectiveness of collaborative care models in reducing SI, depression, and anxiety symptoms in primary care elders (Alexopoulos and The PROSPECT Group, 2001; Bartels et al., 2002; Unutzer et al., 2002). The results of these studies will provide guidance for the design of future intervention strategies for these highest-risk elders.

In addition to indicated prevention in primary care, community outreach is necessary to identify at-risk elders who lack access to, or avoid, health-care visits. The Elder Services Division of the Spokane Mental Health Center offers one instructive model that combines identification of vulnerable elders with evaluation and care through a comprehensive clinical case management system (Florio et al., 1996). For identification of elders at risk for suicide, the Center recruited *gatekeepers* whom they educated regarding depression and suicide in later life. Gatekeepers are individuals who observe older adults at home and in the community as a routine part of their jobs, such as postal workers, pharmacists, bank personnel, and custodians. When concerned about an older adult, the gatekeeper may refer him or her to the clinical case management program, which is equipped to respond with clinical referrals; in-home medical, psychiatric, family, and nutritional assessments; medication management and respite services; and crisis intervention. Although components of the program have been described (Florio et al., 1998), no controlled trials have been published of gatekeeper and case management models with which to evaluate their impact on suicide and other related outcomes in older adults.

## CONCLUSION

Suicide in later life is a significant public health problem that in coming decades is likely to account for an even larger number of deaths. Although substantial progress has been made in the definition of factors that place elders at risk, far more work remains to be done. The next generation of research should include larger representative samples of elder suicides and comparison groups to enable testing of more complex models. An understanding not only of causal risk factors, but also of the mediating and moderating effects of correlates, will provide far better guidance for the design of preventive interventions, particularly for high-risk groups. At the same time, population-based preventive strategies are critical to implement and evaluate. Even as research goes on, elders continue to die by their own hands. The National Strategy for the Prevention of Suicide has set an ambitious agenda for clinicians, researchers, policy makers, and the general population (U.S. Public Health Service, 2001). Its goals, nonetheless, are attainable.

REFERENCES

Ahearn, E.P., Jamison, K.R., Steffens, D.C., Cassidy, F., Provenzale, J.M., Lehman, A., et al. (2001) MRI correlates of suicide attempt history in unipolar depression. *Biol Psychiatry* 50:266–270.

Alexopoulos, G.S. and The PROSPECT Group. (2001) Interventions for depressed elderly primary care patients. *Int J Geriatr Psychiatry* 16:553–559.

Bandura, A. (1977) Self-efficacy: Toward a unifying theory of behavioral change. *Psychol Rev* 84:191–215.

Barraclough, B.M. (1971) Suicide in the elderly: Recent developments in psychogeriatrics. *Br J Psychiatry Spec Suppl.* #6 87–97.

Bartels, S.J., Coakley, E., Oxman, T.E., Constantino, G., Oslin, D., Chen, H., et al. (2002) Suicidal and death ideation in older primary care patients with depression, anxiety, and at-risk alcohol use. *Am J Geriatr Psychiatry* 10:417–427.

Batchelor, I.R.C. and Napier, M.B. (1953) Attempted suicide in old age. *Br Med J* 2:1186–1190.

Beautrais, A.L. (2002) A case control study of suicide and attempted suicide in older adults. *Suicide Life Threat Behav* 32:1–9.

Beck, A.T., Brown, G., Berchick, R.J., Stewart, B.L., and Steer, R.A. (1990) Relationship between hopelessness and ultimate suicide: A replication with psychiatric outpatients. *Am J Psychiatry* 147:190–195.

Beck, A.T., Steer, R.A., Beck, J.S., and Newman, C.F. (1993) Hopelessness, depression, suicidal ideation, and clinical diagnosis of depression. *Suicide Life-Threat Behav* 23:139–145.

Beck, A.T., Steer, R.A., Kovacs, M., and Garrison, B. (1985) Hopelessness and eventual suicide: A 10-year prospective study of patients hospitalized with suicidal ideation. *Am J Psychiatry* 142:559–563.

Beck, A.T., Weissman, A., Lester, D., and Trexler, L. (1974) The measurement of pessimism: The hopelessness scale. *J Consult Clin Psychol* 42:861–865.

Blazer, D.G., Bahn, A.K., and Manton, K.G. (1986) Suicide in late life: Review and commentary. *J Am Geriatr Soc* 34:519–525.

Brent, D.A. (2001) Firearms and suicide. *Ann NY Acad Sci* 932:225–239.

Brown, J.H., Henteleff, P., Barakat, S., and Rowe, C.J. (1986) Is it normal for terminally ill patients to desire death? *Am J Psychiatry* 143:208–211.

Callahan, C.M., Hendrie, H.C., Nienaber, N.A., and Tierney, W.M. (1996) Suicidal ideation among older primary care patients. *J Am Geriatr Soc* 44:1205–1209.

Callahan, C.M., Nienaber, N.A., Hendrie, H.C., and Tierney, W.M. (1992) Depression of elderly outpatients: Primary care physicians' attitudes and practice patterns. *J Gen Intern Med* 7:26–31.

Carney, S.S., Rich, C.L., Burke, P.A., and Fowler, R.C. (1994) Suicide over 60: The San Diego study. *J Am Geriatr Soc* 42:174–180.

Chochinov, H.M., Wilson, K.G., Enns, M., Mowchun, N., Lander, S., Levitt, M., et al. (1995) Desire for death in the terminally ill. *Am J Psychiatry* 152:1185–1191.

Clark, D.C. (1991) *Suicide among the Elderly. Final Report to the AARP Andrus Foundation.* Washington, DC: AARP.

Clark, D.C. (1993) Narcissistic crises of aging and suicidal despair. *Suicide Life-Threatening Behav* 23:21–26.

Clark, D.C. and Horton-Deutsch, S.L. (1992) Assessment in absentia: The value of the psychological autopsy method for studying antecedents of suicide and predicting future suicides. In: Maris, R.W. and Berman, A.L., eds. *Assessment and Prediction of Suicide.* New York: Guilford Press, pp. 144–182.

Conner, K., Conwell, Y., and Duberstein, P. (2001a) The validity of proxy-based data in suicide research: A study of patients 50 years of age and older who attempted suicide. II. Life events, social support and suicidal behavior. *Acta Pscyhiatr Scand* 104:452–457.

Conner, K.R., Duberstein, P.R., and Conwell, Y. (2001b) The validity of proxy-based data in suicide research: A study of patients 50 years of age and older who attempted suicide. I. Psychiatric diagnoses. *Acta Psychiatr Scand* 104:204–209.

Conwell, Y., Duberstein, P.R., Conner, K.R., Eberly, S., Cox, C., and Caine, E.D. (2002) Access to firearms and risk for suicide in middle aged and older adults. *Am J Geriatr Psychiatry* 10:407–416.

Conwell, Y., Duberstein, P.R., Cox, C., Herrmann, J.H., Forbes, N.T., and Caine, E.D. (1996) Relationships of age and axis I diagnoses in victims of completed suicide: A psychological autopsy study. *Am J Psychiatry* 153:1001–1008.

Conwell, Y., Duberstein, P.R., Cox, C., Herrmann, J., Forbes, N., and Caine, E.D. (1998) Age differences in behaviors leading to completed suicide. *Am J Geriatr Psychiatry* 6:122–126.

Conwell, Y., Duberstein, P., DiGiorgio, A., Cox, C., Forbes, N.T., and Caine, E.D. (2001) *Risk Factors for Suicide in Later Life.* Lorne, Australia: International Psychogeriatric Association.

Conwell, Y., Lyness, J.M., Duberstein, P., Cox, C., Seidlitz, L., DiGiorgio, A., et al. (2000) Completed suicide among older patients in primary care practices: A controlled study. *J Am Geriatr Soc* 48:23–29.

Conwell, Y., Olsen, K., Caine, E.D., and Flannery, C. (1991) Suicide in later life: Psychological autopsy findings. *Int Psychogeriatr* 3:59–66.

Conwell, Y., Rotenberg, M., and Caine, E.D. (1990) Completed suicide at age 50 and over. *J Am Geriatr Soc* 38:640–644.

Costa, P.T. and McCrae, R.R. (1992) *Revised NEO Personality Inventory and NEO Five Factor Inventory: Professional Manual.* Odessa, FL: PAR.

Crosby, A.E., Cheltenham, M.P., and Sacks, J.J. (1999) Incidence of suicidal ideation and behavior in the United States, 1994. *Suicide Life Threat Behav* 29:131–140.

Duberstein, P.R. (1995) Openness to experience and completed suicide across the second half of life. *Int Psychogeriatr* 7:183–198.

Duberstein, P.R. (2001) Are closed-minded people more open to the idea of killing themselves? *Suicide Life Threat Behav* 31:9–14.

Duberstein, P.R., Conwell, Y., and Cox, C. (1998) Suicide in widowed persons. A psychological autopsy comparison of recently and remotely bereaved older subjects. *Am J Geriatr Psychiatry* 6:328–334.

Duberstein, P.R., Conwell, Y., Seidlitz, L., Lyness, J.M., Cox, C., and Caine, E.D. (1999) Age and suicidal ideation in older depressed inpatients. *Am J Geriatr Psychiatry* 7:289–296.

Farberow, N.L. and Shneidman, E.S. (1970) Suicide among patients with malignant neoplasms. In: Shneidman, E.S., Farberow, N.L., and Litman, R.E., eds. *The Psychology of Suicide.* New York: Science House, pp. 324–344.

Fiske, A. and Arbore, P. (2000) Future directions in late life suicide prevention. *Omega—J Death Dying* 42:37–53.

Florio, E.R., Jensen, J.E., Hendryx, M.S., Raschko, R., and Mathieson, K. (1998) One year outcomes of older adults referred for aging and mental health services by community gatekeepers. *J Case Manage* 7:1–10.

Florio, E.R., Rockwood, T.H., Hendryx, M.S., Jensen, J.E., Raschko, R., and Dyck, D.G. (1996) A model gatekeeper program to find the at-risk elderly. *J Case Manage* 5:106–114.

Forsell, Y., Jorm, A.F., and Winblad, B. (1997) Suicidal thoughts and associated factors in an elderly population. *Acta Psychiatr Scand* 95:108–111.

Fremouw, W.J., dePerczel, M., and Ellis, T.E. (1990) *Suicide Risk: Assessment and Response Guidelines.* New York: Pergamon Press.

Gallo, J.J., Anthony, J.C., and Muthen, B.O. (1994) Age differences in the symptoms of depression: A latent trait analysis. *J Gerontol* 49:251–264.

Gordis, L. (2000) *Epidemiology*, 2nd ed. Philadelphia: W.B. Saunders Co.

Haas, A.P. and Hendin, H. (1983) Suicide among older people: Projections for the future. *Suicide Life-Threatening Behav* 13:147–154.

Harris, E.C. and Barraclough, B.M. (1994) Suicide as an outcome for medical disorders. *Medicine* 73:281–296.

Harwood, D., Hawton, K., Hope, T., and Jacoby, R. (2001) Psychiatric disorder and personality factors associated with suicide in older people: A descriptive and case-control study. *Int J Geriatr Psychiatry* 16:155–165.

Havens, L. (1965) The anatomy of a suicide. *N Engl J Med* 272:401–406.

Hawton, K., Appleby, L., Platt, S., Foster, T., Cooper, J., Malmberg, A., et al. (1998) The psychological autopsy approach to studying suicide: A review of methodological issues. *J Affect Disord* 50:269–276.

Heikkinen, M.E., Isometsä, E.T., Aro, H.M., Sarna, S.J., and Lönnqvist, J.K. (1995) Age-related variation in recent life events preceding suicide. *J Nerv Ment Dis* 183:325–331.

Heithoff, K. (1995) Does the ECA underestimate the prevalence of late-life depression? *J Am Geriatr Soc* 43:2–6.

Henriksson, M.M., Marttunen, M.J., Isometsa, E.T., Heikkinen, M.E., Aro, H.M., Kuoppasalmi, K.I., et al. (1995) Mental disorders in elderly suicide. *Int Psychogeriatr* 7:275–286.

Hill, R.D., Gallagher, D., Thompson, L.W., and Ishida, T. (1988) Hopelessness as a measure of suicide intent in the depressed elderly. *Psychol Aging* 3:230–232.

John A. Hartford Foundation, C.H.F. (2002) IMPACT: Improving Care for Depression in Late Life. Available online at http://www.impact.ucla.edu/

Jones, J.S., Stanley, B., Mann, J.J., Frances, A.J., Guido, J.R., Traskman-Bendz, L., et al. (1990) CSF 5-HIAA and HVA concentrations in elderly depressed patients who attempted suicide. *Am J Psychiatry* 147:1225–1227.

Jorm, A.F., Henderson, A.S., Scott, R., Korten, A.E., Christensen, H., and Mackinnon, A.J. (1995) Factors associated with the wish to die in elderly people. *Age Ageing* 24:389–392.

Katon, W., Robinson, P., Von Korff, M., Lin, E., Bush, T., Ludman, E., et al. (1996) A multifaceted intervention to improve treatment of depression in primary care. *Arch Gen Psychiatry* 53:924–932.

Katon, W., Von Korff, M., Lin, E., Simon, G., Walker, E., Bush, T., et al. (1997) Collaborative management to achieve depression treatment guidelines. *J Clin Psychiatry* 58(suppl 1):20–23.

Keeler, E.M., Solomon, D.H., Beck, J.C., Mendenhall, R.C., and Kane, R.L. (1982) Effect of patient age on duration of medical encounters with physicians. *Med Care* 20:1101–1108.

Keilp, J.G., Sackeim, H.A., Brodsky, B.S., Oquendo, M.A., Malone, K.M., and Mann, J.J. (2001) Neuropsychological dysfunction in depressed suicide attempters. *Am J Psychiatry* 158:735–741.

Kelly, T.M. and Mann, J.J. (1996) Validity of DSM-III-R diagnosis by psychological autopsy: A comparison with clinician antemortem diagnosis. *Acta Psychiatr Scand* 94:337–343.

King, D.A., Conwell, Y., Cox, C., Henderson, R.E., Denning, D.G., and Caine, E.D. (2000) A neuropsychological comparison of depressed suicide attempters and nonattempters. *J Neuropsychiatry Clin Neurosci* 12:64–70.

Knauper, B. and Wittchen, H.U. (1994) Diagnosing major depression in the elderly: Evidence for response bias in standardized diagnostic interviews? *J Psychiatr Res* 28:147–164.

Linden, M. and Barnow, S. (1997) 1997 IPA/Bayer Research Awards in Psychogeriatrics. The wish to die in very old persons near the end of life: A psychiatric problem? Results from the Berlin Aging Study. *Int Psychogeriatr* 9:291–307.

Linehan, M.M. (1986) Suicidal people: One population or two? In Mann, J.J., and Stanley, M., eds. *The Psychobiology of Suicidal Behavior.* New York: New York Academy of Sciences, pp. 16–33.

Luoma, J.B., Pearson, J.L., and Martin, C.E. (2002) Contact with mental health and primary care prior to suicide: A review of the evidence. *Am J Psychiatry* 159:909–916.

Lyness, J.M., Cox, C., Curry, J., Conwell, Y., King, D.A., Caine, et al. (1995) Older age and the underreporting of depressive symptoms. *J Am Geriatr Soc* 43:216–221.

Lyness, J.M., Noel, T.K., Cox, C., King, D.A., Conwell, Y., Caine,

E.D., et al. (1997) Screening for depression in elderly primary care patients. A comparison of the Center for Epidemiologic Studies—Depression Scale and the Geriatric Depression Scale. *Arch Intern Med* 157:449–454.

Mackenzie, T.B. and Popkin, M.K. (1987) Suicide in the medical patient. *Int J Psychiatry Med* 17:3–22.

Mann, J.J. and Stoff, D.M. (1997) A synthesis of current findings regarding neurobiological correlates and treatment of suicidal behavior. *Ann NY Acad Sci* 836:352–363.

Mann, J.J., Waternaux, C., Haas, G.L., and Malone, K.M. (1999) Toward a clinical model of suicidal behavior in psychiatric patients. *Am J Psychiatry* 156:181–189.

McIntosh, J.L. (2002) U.S.A Suicide: 1999 Official Final Statistics. NCHS/CDC. Available online at http://www.iusb.edu/~jmcintos/SuicideStats.html

Mercer, S.O. (1989) *Elder Suicide: A National Survey of Prevention and Intervention Programs* (Rep. No. 8904). Washington, DC: American Association of Retired Persons Public Policy Institute.

Miller, M. (1978) Geriatric suicide: The Arizona study. *Gerontologist* 18:488–495.

Moscicki, E.K. (1997) Identification of suicide risk factors using epidemiologic studies. *Psychiatr Clin North Am* 3:499–517.

NAMHC Workgroup on Mental Disorders Prevention Research. (1998) *Priorities for Prevention Research at NIMH: A Report by the National Advisory Council Workgroup on Mental Disorders Prevention Research.* Washington, DC: National Institutes of Health.

National Center for Health Statistics (2001) Death rates for 72 selected causes by 5-year age groups, race, and sex: United States, 1979–1998. http://www.cdc.gov/datawh/statab/unpubd/mortabs/gmwk291.htm [Online]. Available at http://www.cdc.gov/datawh/statab/unpubd/mortabs/gmwk291.htm

Parkin, D. and Stengel, E. (1965) Incidence of suicidal attempts in an urban community. *Br Med J* 2:133–138.

Paykel, E.S., Myers, J.K., Lindenthal, J.J., and Tanner, J. (1974) Suicidal feelings in the general population: A prevalence study. *Br J Psychiatry* 124:460–469.

Pearson, J.L. and Conwell, Y. (1995) Suicide in late life: Challenges and opportunities for research. Introduction. *Int Psychogeriatr* 7:131–136.

Rao, R., Dening, T., Brayne, C., and Huppert, F.A. (1997) Suicidal thinking in community residents over eighty. *Int J Geriatr Psychiatry* 12:337–343.

Rihmer, Z., Rutz, W., and Pihlgren, H. (1995) Depression and suicide on Gotland. An intensive study of all suicides before and after a depression-training programme for general practitioners. *J Affect Disord* 35:147–152.

Rodin, J. and Salovey, P. (1989) Health psychology. *Annu Rev Psychol* 40:533–579.

Rose, G. (1985) Sick individuals and sick populations. *Int J Epidemiol* 14:32–38.

Ross, R.K., Bernstein, L., Trent, L., Henderson, B.E., and Paganini-Hill, A. (1990) A prospective study of risk factors for traumatic death in the retirement community. *Prev Med* 19:323–334.

Rost, K., Smith, R., Matthews, D.B., and Guise, B. (1994) The deliberate misdiagnosis of major depression in primary care. *Arch Fam Med* 3:333–337.

Rowe, J.W. and Kahn, R.L. (1987) Human aging: Usual and successful. *Science* 237:143–149.

Rubenowitz, E., Waern, M., Wilhelmsson, K., and Allebeck, P. (2001) Life events and psychosocial factors in elderly suicides—a case control study. *Psychol Med* 31:1193–1202.

Rubio, A., Vestner, A.L., Stewart, J.M., Forbes, N.T., Conwell, Y., and Cox, C. (2001) Suicide and Alzheimer's pathology in the elderly: A case-control study. *Biol Psychiatry* 49:137–145.

Rutz, W., von Knorring, L., Pihlgren, H., Rihmer, Z., and Walinder (1995) Prevention of male suicides: Lessons from Gotland study [letter]. *Lancet* 345:524.

Rutz, W., von Knorring, L., and Walinder, J. (1989) Frequency of suicide on Gotland after systematic postgraduate education of general practitioners. *Acta Psychiatr Scand* 80:151–154.

Rutz, W., von Knorrring, L., and Walinder, J. (1992) Long-term effects of an educational program for general practitioners given by the Swedish Committee for the Prevention and Treatment of Depression. *Acta Pscyhiatr Scand* 85:414–418.

Schulberg, H.C., Block, M.R., Madonia, M.J., Scott, C.P., Rodriguez, E., Imber, S.D., et al. (1996) Treating major depression in primary care practice. Eight-month clinical outcomes. *Arch Gen Psychiatry* 53:913–919.

Scocco, P., Meneghel, G., Caon, F., Dello, B.M., and De Leo, D. (2001) Death ideation and its correlates: Survey of an over-65-year-old population. *J Nerv Ment Dis* 189:210–218.

Shah, A., Hoxey, K., and Mayadunne, V. (2000) Suicidal ideation in acutely medically ill elderly inpatients: Prevalence, correlates and longitudinal stability. *Int J Geriatr Psychiatry* 15:162–169.

Shneidman, E.S. and Farberow, N.L. (1957) *Clues to Suicide*. New York: McGraw-Hill.

Skoog, I., Aevarsson, O., Beskow, J., Larsson, L., Palsson, S., Waern, M., et al. (1996) Suicidal feelings in a population sample of nondemented 85-year-olds. *Am J Psychiatry* 153:1015–1020.

Stoff, D.M. and Mann, J.J. (1997) The neurobiology of suicide: From the bench to the clinic. *Ann NY Acad Sci* 836:1–365.

Szanto, K., Reynolds, C.F. III, Conwell, Y., Begley, A.E., and Houck, P. (1998) High levels of hopelessness persist in geriatric patients with remitted depression and a history of attempted suicide. *J Am Geriatr Soc* 46:1401–1406.

Turvey, C.L., Conwell, Y., Jones, M.P., Phillips, C., Simonsick, E.M., Pearson, J.L., et al. (2002) Risk factors for late life suicide: A prospective community-based study. *Am J Geriatr Psychiatry* 10:398–406.

Unutzer, J., Katon, W., Callahan, C.M., Williams, J.W., Jr., Hunkeler, E., Harpole, L., et al. (2002) IMPACT investigators. Improving mood-promoting access to collaborative treatment: collaborative care management of late-life depression in the primary care setting—a randomized controlled trial. *JAMA* 288:2836–2845.

U.S. Public Health Service (2001) *National Strategy for Suicide Prevention: Goals and Objectives for Action*. Rockville, MD: U.S. Public Health Service.

Waern, M., Runeson, B., Allebeck, P., Beskow, J., Rubenowitz, E., Skoog, I., et al. (2002) Mental disorder in elderly suicides. *Am J Psychiatry* 159:450–455.

Whitlock, F.A. (1986) Suicide and physical illness. In Roy, A., ed. *Suicide*. Baltimore: Williams and Wilkins, pp. 151–170.

# 9 | Bereavement and depression

PAULA J. CLAYTON

The loss of a loved one is an unavoidable human experience. By the time American women reach the age of 65 (Carr et al., 2001), almost half will be widowed, whereas at the same age, only 14% of men are widowed. Besides this notable loss, there may have been losses of children, brothers, sisters, and parents, so older women and men have much experience with dying and death. Not surprisingly, the majority of elderly persons handle losses with minimal morbidity (Murrell et al., 1984, 1988, 1989). Still, significant loss may lead to increased doctors' visits for new or worsening medical illnesses, increased use of substances such as alcohol, benzodiazepines, hypnotics, and cigarettes, the development of chronic depression, complicated grief, and increased mortality.

Therefore, to understand the more pathological outcomes, it is necessary to be aware of the normal or expected reaction in the immediate postbereavement period and the year or so following it. Once these distinctions are made, consideration of interventions or treatments is appropriate.

## STAGES

Almost everyone who has studied the recently bereaved prospectively has delineated the stages of bereavement as three: numbness, depression, and recovery.

The first stage is *numbness*. Men and women are dazed; they do what they have to do, but without much awareness. Their functions are automatic. Much of what is said and done is poorly remembered. Funeral directors are aware of this and compensate by writing important things down. Anxiety and depressive symptoms may begin here. A recent study of survivors of the September 11 terrorist attack reported that the early occurrence of a panic attack predicted later psychopathology, mainly the development of depression or posttraumatic stress disorders (PTSD) (Galea et al., 2002). This stage lasts for hours to days, seldom weeks.

The second stage is *depression*, which quickly follows the first stage. This stage lasts for a few weeks to a year, sometimes longer. It is during this stage that all the common depressive symptoms are prominent. For most, recovery begins in the first 4 months, with only one or two lingering symptoms remaining after 1 year. However, mood is almost always noticeably disturbed on holidays, anniversaries, the birthday of the deceased, the anniversary of the death, and other personal meaningful events. It may partially be the cause of the much discussed *Christmas depression*.

The last stage is *recovery*. Here the bereaved accepts the death and returns to the predeath level of functioning. For some, this means simply strengthening the role they held before the death, while for others it means seeking out new roles and new relationships. This varies by age and by gender, as well as for other reasons, such as the survivor's health. The process is well described in older adults by Lund et al. (1986, 1990, 1993). They emphasize that the outcome depends on the survivor's personal competence and positive self-esteem.

## PSYCHOLOGICAL AND SOMATIC DEPRESSIVE SYMPTOMS AND COURSE OF BEREAVEMENT

At this point, there have been numerous longitudinal follow-up studies of recently bereaved individuals. The majority deal with the widowed, although there are excellent studies of children who have lost a parent and of parents who have lost a child. Despite the fact that the mode of selection, response rate, gender, age group, time since the death to the first interview, comparison groups, and the selection of instruments and outcome measures differ greatly from study to study, the similarities of outcome outweigh the differences. Our own data highlight the major outcomes, although important additional findings have been identified and there are still areas of controversy.

In studying relatives' reactions to the loss of a significant person, we collected data on three different samples. The first sample (Clayton et al., 1968) was a group of 40 bereaved relatives of people who had died at a general hospital in St. Louis. The second sample (Clayton et al., 1971) was a random sample of 109 widows and widowers (96 and 33, respectively) chosen from the death certificates and seen at 1, 4, and 13 months after the deaths of their spouses. Their average age was 61.5 (range, 20–89). The third sample (Clayton and Darvish

TABLE 9.1 *Frequency of Depressive Symptoms at 1 and 13 Months*

| | $n = 149^a$ | |
|---|---|---|
| Symptom | 1 month % + | 13 months % + |
| Crying | 89 | 33[d] |
| Sleep disturbance | 76 | 48[d] |
| Low mood | 75 | 42[d] |
| Loss of appetite | 51 | 16[d] |
| Fatigue | 44 | 30[c] |
| Poor memory | 41 | 23[d] |
| Loss of interest | 40 | 23[d] |
| Difficulty concentrating | 36 | 16[d] |
| Weight loss of 2.25 kg or more | 36 | 20[c] |
| Feeling guilty | 31 | 12[d] |
| Restlessness ($n = 89$) | 48 | 45 |
| Reverse diurnal variation | 26 | 22 |
| Irritability | 24 | 20 |
| Feels someone is to blame | 22 | 22 |
| Diurnal variation | 17 | 10 |
| Death wishes | 16 | 12 |
| Feeling hopeless | 14 | 13 |
| Hallucinations | 12 | 9 |
| Suicidal thoughts | 5 | 3 |
| Fear of losing mind | 3 | 4 |
| Suicide attempts | 0 | 0 |
| Feeling worthless | 6 | 11 |
| Feels angry about death | 13 | 22[b] |
| Depressive syndrome | 42 | 16[d] |

[a]$n$ varies from symptom to symptom.
[b]Significant by McNemar's chi-square. $df = 1$, $p \le .02$.
[c]Significant by McNemar's chi-square. $df = 1$, $p \le .01$.
[d]Significant by McNemar's chi-square. $df = 1$, $p \le .001$.
*Source:* Clayton, P.J. Breavement. In: Raykel, E.S., ed. *Handbook of Affective Disorders.* London: Churchill Livingstone, p. 404.

1979) was a consecutive series of 62 young (under 45 years old) widowed individuals also seen within a month after the death and again at 1 year. There were 34 women and 28 men. The last two samples were matched through the voter registry with married people of the same age and sex who had not had a first-degree relative die and who were also followed prospectively to ascertain their morbidity and mortality. The findings are presented in Table 9.1, which displays the depressive symptoms that were endorsed at 1 and 13 months. In the first month, a large majority of the sample experienced depressed mood, anorexia, and the beginning of weight loss, insomnia that was initial, middle, and terminal, marked crying, some fatigue, and loss of interest in their surroundings but not necessarily in the people around them, restlessness, and guilt. The guilt that these people expressed was different from the guilt seen in the depressed patient. For the most part, it was guilt of omission surrounding either the terminal illness or the death. The ru-

minative guilt of the depressed patient is rare, as is morbid cultivation or mummification of the deceased, as practiced by Queen Victoria (Longford, 1964). Irritability was common, but overt anger was uncommon. Suicidal thoughts and ideas were rare. Hallucinations were not uncommon. Many widows and widowers, when asked, admitted that they had felt touched by their dead spouse or had heard his or her voice, had seen a vision of him or her, or had smelled his or her presence. The misidentification of their dead spouses in a crowd was extremely common.

We matched some of our older subjects with well-studied hospitalized depressives (Clayton et al., 1974) and found, as Freud (1959) suggested, that symptoms such as feeling hopeless, worthless, a burden, psychomotor retardation, wishing to be dead, and thinking of suicide differentiated the depressed from the bereaved. The average number of depressive symptoms in the patients was 15, compared to 7 in the bereaved. Patients with depression experienced their condition as a change, not as their usual selves, which led them to seek help and to define themselves as patients, whereas

TABLE 9.2. *Frequency of Depressive Symptoms at Any Time in the First Year of Bereavement and in Controls*

| Symptom | Probands (%) ($n = 149^a$) | Controls (%) ($n = 131^a$) |
|---|---|---|
| Crying | 90 | 14[e] |
| Sleep disturbance | 79 | 35[e] |
| Low mood | 80 | 18[e] |
| Loss of appetite | 53 | 4[e] |
| Fatigue | 55 | 23[e] |
| Poor memory | 50 | 22[e] |
| Loss of interest | 48 | 11[e] |
| Difficulty concentrating | 40 | 13[e] |
| Weight loss of 2.25 kg or more | 47 | 24[e] |
| Feeling guilty | 38 | 11[e] |
| Restlessness | 63 | 27[e] |
| Irritability | 35 | 21[b] |
| Diurnal variation | 22 | 14 |
| Death wishes | 22 | 5[e] |
| Feeling hopeless | 19 | 4[d] |
| Hallucinations | 17 | 2[e] |
| Suicidal thoughts | 8 | 1[c] |
| Fear of losing mind | 7 | 5 |
| Suicide attempts | 0 | 0 |
| Worthlessness | 14 | 15 |
| Depressive syndrome | 47 | 8[d] |

[a]$n$ varies from symptom to symptom.
[b]Significant by chi-square. $df = 1$, $p < .05$.
[c]Significant by chi-square. $df = 1$, $p < .01$.
[d]Significant by chi-square. $df = 1$, $p < .0005$.
[e]Significant by chi-square, $df = 1$, $p < .0001$.
*Source:* Clayton, P.J. Breavement. In: Raykel, E.S., ed. *Handbook of Affective Disorders.* London: Churchill Livingstone, p. 405.

the bereaved considered their responses normal and understandable. These findings were confirmed by Breckenridge et al. (1986), who reported that in 196 elderly, recently (2 months) bereaved and 145 comparison individuals, self-deprecatory cognitions occurred with similar frequency. We never observed a retarded depression in a bereaved person, a finding similar to those of Lindemann (1944) and Parkes (1970).

By the end of the first year, the somatic symptoms of depression had greatly improved. Low mood (usually associated with specific events or holidays), restlessness, and poor sleep continued. In fact, some subjects worried that the insomnia would become entrenched. The few psychological symptoms of depression, although rare, resolved less easily. In our studies, the symptoms were as frequent in men as in women, in people who had lost a spouse suddenly or after a lingering death, in people who had good or bad marriages, and in people who were religious or nonreligious. There was no relationship between income and outcome. By 1 year, most bereaved individuals could discuss the dead person with equanimity. A severe reaction to the first anniversary of the death (Bornstein and Clayton 1972; Jacobs et al., 1987b) was rare and indicated a poor outcome. Asking about it is a good way for a clinician to assess the survivor's clinical state 1 year after the death.

As Table 9.2 shows, when the frequency of depressive symptoms was compared to the community controls, all symptoms were found to be more common among the bereaved. These findings were nicely replicated in Grimby's (1993) longitudinal study of an older group. He found that low mood, loneliness, and crying were the cardinal symptoms of bereavement, with loneliness persisting the longest. He did not include sleep disturbance as a possible symptom. Anxiety, identified as feelings of restlessness and nervousness but not as anxiety attacks, was also common. Grimby felt that restlessness represented a search for the lost object. He and Rees (1971) also found that hallucinations were reported by the bereaved. Delusions were rarely reported, although they were inquired about.

When depressive symptoms reported at 13 months were examined by those with symptoms for the entire year and by those who had just developed them, the percentage who had new symptoms was found to be similar to the percentage reported by the controls who had had no deaths. This is shown in Table 9.3. Those who were disturbed early were more likely to be disturbed later. Delayed grief, like delayed PTSD, may be an interesting ideological concept but remains unproven. It is also counterintuitive since the usual recognized reaction to a physical or psychological insult is an immediate injury with a gradual resolution. This is also confirmed by Byrne and Raphael (1994) and is nicely duplicated in the studies of North et al. (1997, 1999) dealing with the reactions of survivors of trauma, especially terrorism.

TABLE 9.3. *Frequency of Depressive Symptoms at 13 Months*

| Symptom | Those with Symptoms at 13 Months | | Those without Symptoms at 1 Month (New Symptoms) | |
|---|---|---|---|---|
| | % + | n | % + | n |
| Crying | 36 | 132 | 6 | 16 |
| Sleep disturbance | 59 | 113 | 11 | 35 |
| Low mood | 49 | 111 | 22 | 37 |
| Loss of appetite | 28 | 76 | 4 | 72 |
| Fatigue | 45 | 65 | 19 | 83 |
| Poor memory | 34 | 61 | 15 | 88 |
| Loss of interest | 40 | 57 | 12 | 84 |
| Difficulty concentrating | 33 | 52 | 6 | 94 |
| Weight loss of 2.25 kg or more | 22 | 51 | 17 | 92 |
| Feeling guilty | 25 | 49 | 6 | 97 |
| Restlessness | 63 | 43 | 28 | 46 |
| Reverse diurnal variation | 39 | 38 | 17 | 109 |
| Irritability | 37 | 35 | 15 | 113 |
| Feels someone is to blame | 63 | 32 | 11 | 111 |
| Diurnal variation | 24 | 25 | 7 | 122 |
| Death wishes | 33 | 24 | 7 | 124 |
| Feeling hopeless | 55 | 20 | 6 | 128 |
| Hallucinations | 29 | 17 | 6 | 131 |
| Suicidal thoughts | 0 | 8 | 3 | 139 |
| Fear of losing mind | 0 | 5 | 4 | 143 |
| Suicide attempts | 0 | 0 | 0 | 147 |
| Feeling worthless | 56 | 9 | 8 | 139 |
| Feels angry about death | 63 | 19 | 16 | 128 |
| Depressive syndrome | 27 | 63 | 8 | 86 |

*Source:* Clayton, P.J. Bereavement. In: Paykel, E.S., ed. *Handbook of Affective Disorders.* London: Churchill Livingstone, p. 405.

## PHYSICAL SYMPTOMS, SUBSTANCE USE, AND MEDICAL TREATMENT

We systematically ask about physical symptoms, usually associated with major depression, in both the recently widowed and controls. They are depicted in Table 9.4. In general, physical symptoms were not more frequent in the recently bereaved and the controls. Nor did they change much over the year. The largest difference was recorded in "other pains" in the elderly bereaved and consisted of arthritis-type pains. In our studies, there were no more physician visits or hospitalizations in the year following the bereavement. This finding is controversial.

The most striking finding of this research is illustrated in this table. After a significant stress like bereavement, the use of alcohol, tranquilizers, and hypnotics significantly increased. For the most part, these were not new users but people who had used them be-

TABLE 9.4. *Frequency of Physical Symptoms in 1 Year in Breaved and Controls*

| Symptom | Probands (%) (n = 149[a]) | Controls (%) (n = 131[a]) |
|---|---|---|
| Headaches | 36 | 27 |
| Dysmenorrhea | 38 | 20 |
| Other pains | 44 | 18[e] |
| Urinary frequency | 30 | 23 |
| Constipation | 27 | 24 |
| Dyspnea | 27 | 16[a] |
| Abdominal pain | 26 | 11[c] |
| Blurred vision | 22 | 13 |
| Anxiety attacks | 15 | 8 |
| Alcohol use | 19 | 9[d] |
| Tranquilizers | 46 | 8[d] |
| Hypnotics | 32 | 2[d] |
| Physician visits | 79 | 80 |
| 3 or more | 45 | 48 |
| 6 or more | 27 | 29 |
| Hospitalizations | 22 | 14 |
| General poor health | 10 | 7 |

Note: *n* varies slightly from symptom to symptom.
[a]Significant by chi-square. *df* = 1, *p* < .05.
[b]Significant by chi-square. *df* = 1, *p* < .005.
[c]Significant by chi-square. *df* = 1, *p* < .001.
[d]Significant by chi-square. *df* = 1, *p* < .0001.
*Source:* Clayton, P.J. (1986) Breavement and its relation to clinical depression. In: Hippius et al., eds. *New Results in Depression*. Berlin and Heidelberg: Springer-Verlag, p. 64.

fore. Cigarette smoking also increased. The morbidity and mortality of bereavement may be related to these changes in behavior. It also highlights how people behave after significant stress.

A separate study (Frost and Clayton, 1977) examined 249 psychiatric in-patients and similarly matched hospital controls and found that there were no significant differences between the groups for the loss of a first-degree relative or spouse in the 6 months or 1 year prior to admission to the hospital. In each case only 2% reported such a loss in the 6 months prior and 3% or 4% in the 7–12 months prior to the hospitalization. In the psychiatric patients, the major diagnosis was a mood disorder. There were diagnoses of alcoholism in both the bereaved psychiatric patients and bereaved hospitalized controls related to their increased drinking after the death.

## MORTALITY

In more recent years, the method of study (collecting health data on a large cohort of men and women, following them prospectively to ascertain the point of widowhood, and using the portional Cox hazards regression module to estimate the effect of bereavement on

mortality while controlling for the effects of other covariates) has greatly improved the validity of the mortality data. Nevertheless, controversies remain (Clayton, 1998). Three recent studies have used this method. De Leon et al. (1993) reported that elderly, young-old (65–74 years), and old-old men (more than 74 years) showed increased mortality in the first 6 months of widowhood. But because there was an age difference between the future widowed and nonwidowed, when they were age adjusted the death rate fell to a nonsignificant level. Among young-old women there was also an increased risk of death in the first 6 months, which decreased only slightly after the age adjustment but enough to make it of borderline significance. The authors suggested that the "true risk period" may be even shorter than 6 months. Schaefier et al. (1995) also reported that mortality following bereavement was significantly elevated in both men and women after adjusting for age, education, and other predictors of mortality. Here, the highest mortality rates occurred 7–12 months following the bereavement. Lusyne et al. (2001) confirmed the excess mortality in early (6-month) widowhood, which was higher for men than women. They found, as many others had, that in men it is highest for the youngest bereaved (<60 years of age), and drops with each age group, and disappears almost completely for the oldest old. This is probably because older men who survive their spouses are usually in better health than married men of the same age. To their surprise, the more highly educated had an excess mortality. There is also a recent twin study of mortality after spousal bereavement (Lichtenstein et al., 1998). Without stating whether the twins were monozygotic or dizygotic, the authors found an increased mortality for young-old (under 70 years) men and women during the first year of bereavement. The death hazard diminished the longer the bereaved were followed. The authors analyzed their data for smoking status, excessive alcohol consumption, education, body mass, cardiovascular disease, respiratory disease, and other chronic illnesses and found that these did not affect the relative hazard estimates. Other studies show that remarriage, which is much more likely to occur in men, protects men from death, either because the healthier remarry or because the remarriage itself is protective. The death rate of those who remarry is similar to that of married men of the same age. Taken as a whole, these studies support the conclusion that there is probably an increased mortality in men and women under age 74 in the first year after bereavement.

These studies reveal no clear tendency toward increased mortality from any one cause, such as cancer or cardiovascular disease. The most frequent causes are accidents and suicides, although in smaller samples, most of those who committed suicide were psychiatrically ill prior to their spouses' deaths. A recent well-done case-control study (Rubenowitz et al., 2001) of 100 elderly suicides confirmed the latter but not the former. That is, for elderly suicides, the major independent risk factors were family discord and mental disorders (mainly depression and substance abuse). Recent bereavement was not an important risk factor.

## PSYCHIATRIC DISORDERS—DEPRESSION, ANXIETY, AND MANIA

In our first study of widowhood, 35% of the subjects had a depressive syndrome at 1 month, 25% at 4 months, and 17% at 1 year. Forty-five percent were depressed at some point during the year, and 11% were depressed for the entire year. Adding the second younger sample, 42% were depressed at 1 month and 16% met the criteria at 1 year. Forty-seven percent were depressed at some time during the year compared to 8% of controls and, again, 11% for the entire year. These findings are remarkably similar to those of a study extensively reported by Zisook and Shuchter (1991, 1993a, 1993b). They identified a large sample of widows and widowers from death certificates and solicited volunteers to be interviewed. The demographics of the final sample were very similar to those of the first widowed sample reported here. The authors reported that 24% of their sample were depressed at 2 months, 23% at 7 months, 16% at 13 months, and 14% at 25 months. Seven percent were chronically depressed, which is very similar to the 8.8% reported by Byrne and Raphael (1994). In all of these studies, the best predictor of depression at 13 months was depression at 1 month. In the Zisook and Shuchter studies, a past history of depression also predicted depression at 1 year. In our own studies, because we did not have enough depressives, it was any psychiatric morbidity prior to the death that predicted depression at 1 year. The other common correlate of depression at 1 year was poor physical health prior to the death of the spouse. Thus, prior poor physical or mental health predicted a poor outcome at 13 months.

Although there are methodological issues in defining both anticipation of a death (e.g., expected versus unexpected) and outcomes (depression, death, remarriage, etc.) (Clayton et al., 1980a, 1980b), in our data unexpected deaths produced more severe immediate responses but the differences disappeared by 13 months. The same was true for Byrne and Raphael (1994). A recent prospective longitudinal study by Carr et al. (2001) on older adults from a larger study, entitled "Changing Lives of Older Couples" confirmed that forewarning did not affect depression, anger, shock, or overall grief at 6 or 18 months after the loss. Unlike the above findings, using the best definitions of unexpected death—a death in a healthy individual that occurred in less than 2 hours—Lundin (1984a) compared such bereaved to those bereaved after longer terminal illnesses and found that morbidity, especially psychiatric morbidity as measured in physician visits, significantly increased in the sudden death survivors. However, he did not give the average age of the groups. The survivors ($n = 32$) were spouses and parents, of whom at least 5 had experienced sudden infant death; and, as a group, their health was poor prior to the death. Even years later, they had higher ratings on a number of grief symptoms (Lundin 1984b). It may be that instantaneous death in a younger population produces a more immediate and prolonged reaction, but for the majority, especially the older bereaved, forewarning has little effect.

In more than one study, about 24% of the recently bereaved met criteria for some anxiety disorder immediately following bereavement. More than half, however, had generalized anxiety disorder, which correlated with the severity of the depressive disorder (Jacobs et al., 1990). Surtees (1995) also showed that anxiety disorders were rare after bereavement. In another study, since anxiety scores did not vary by circumstance or timing of bereavement, Hays et al. (1994) also concluded that it is possible that anxiety is encompassed in the concept of *grief*.

There are occasional reports of persons developing a manic episode after a bereavement, hence the *merry widow*. Given this possibility, it is conceivable that this could occur in a bipolar-prone person or one with only previous episodes of depression. In our own study, in retrospect, a policeman's widow who had a previous history of depression was probably hypomanic at our first interview. Two recent articles (Morgan et al., 2001; Onishi et al., 2000) reported such an occurrence. Although the authors discussed precipitating factors, the most obvious one, the poor sleep associated with bereavement, was not noted. Yet, if there is any known reliable precipitant for mania, it is sleep deprivation (Winokur and Clayton, 1994).

## COMPLICATED OR TRAUMATIC BEREAVEMENT

Lindemann (1944) probably wrote the first papers on bereavement that dealt with prospective observations of 13 bereaved subjects who were hospitalized at Massachusetts General Hospital after the Coconut Grove fire. He combined those observations with those of his own patients who had lost a relative during treatment, with relatives whom he saw of patients who died at the hospital, and with surviving relatives of members of the armed forces. Although he considered his observations to be of normal grief, many of them were probably pathological responses. More recently, investigators have begun to quantify pathological responses.

Prigerson and colleagues (1995) have developed an inventory of complicated grief and shown it to be related to the severity of depressive symptoms, but with distinct symptoms. Building on earlier inventories such as the Texas Grief Inventory (Fashingbauer et al., 1987) and the Grief Measurement Scale (Jacobs et al., 1986), they took symptoms such as preoccupation with death, crying, searching and yearning for the deceased, disbelief about the death, being stunned, and not accepting the death and added questions about preoccupation with thoughts of the deceased, anger, distrust, detachment, avoidance, replication of symptoms that the deceased experienced, auditory and visual hallucinations, guilt, loneliness, bitterness, and envy of others who had not lost someone close. Their instrument was shown to be reliable and to have criterion validity. Many of the symptoms are seen in normal early bereavement. Whether this is just a definition of the most severe form of depression or a PTSD outcome remains to be seen. Modifying the Grief Measurement Scale in accordance with the above symptoms, Prigerson et al. (1997) looked at a previously ascertained sample of bereaved individuals (average age, 62) who were followed from before the death until 25 months afterward. They found that if they identified bereaved persons at 6 months who scored high on their inventory, at 13 months there was a correlation between high scores and changes in smoking and eating, depression, and elevated systolic blood pressure. At 25 months, these widowed persons had an increased risk of developing heart trouble and cancer and more often expressed suicidal ideation, as ascertained on a single item. When the authors tried to separate the sample based on traumatic grief at 2 months, they could not predict unfavorable outcomes. Using a similar approach, Burnett et al. (1997) have also measured bereavement phenomena and developed a scale for core bereavement items. This scale also measures images and thoughts surrounding the death, yearning and pining about the death, and some grief symptoms such as sadness, loneliness, longing, tearfulness, and loss of enjoyment. Their inventory was developed using parents of deceased children, bereaved spouses, and bereaved adult children who scored high, in descending order, on the inventory. However, they have not yet correlated the questionnaire findings with the outcome. Horowitz et al. (1997) also defined a set of symptoms for a complicated grief disorder in a younger sample of volunteers bereaved for about 6 months.

Some of the symptoms in all of these inventories seem similar to symptoms that occur in PTSD, and it is difficult to justify a new category except that in the bereaved the death was not usually traumatic. Clearly, these investigators are defining an important bereavement response that defines survivors with a poorer outcome.

## PREDICTORS OF PATHOLOGICAL OUTCOMES

Before reviewing the predictors of pathological outcomes, it should be noted that all studies of widowhood, including those on mortality, emphasize that psychological stability predicts a good outcome, although unfortunately, no one has measured personality traits prior to entry into widowhood. Good health predicts a better outcome, as does having no sleep difficulty or having low scores on depression ratings in the first month of bereavement (Clayton, 2000).

There are many ways to assess outcome. Loneliness is the most characteristic outcome following bereavement. In many, it persists for years. In terms of psychological morbidity, chronic depression, as measured a year after the death, and complicated bereavement both lead to significant morbidity. Physical morbidity is another outcome. The mortality noted after bereavement still needs further study.

There are very few definitive predictors of chronic depression. A past history of psychiatric illness, particularly depression, poor physical health, and depression at 1 month after the bereavement, definitely predicts it. The bereavement that follows an instantaneous and totally unexpected death may predict it in younger bereaved individuals, but in the elderly it is usually not predictive. A recent prospective study of older adults (Carr et al., 2000) and controls found that regardless of the quality of the marital relationship, the loss of the partner led to depression, whereas anxiety occurred mainly when the loss was accompanied by changes in daily responsibilities and burdens. All the other variables—gender, education, perceived lack of social supports, and socioeconomic status or income—did not predict it. Gender is important to note, because major depression is overwhelmingly more common in women then in men but chronic depression after bereavement is not. Stress-related depression affects both genders equally and occurs equally in those with or without a family history of depression.

## TREATMENT

The vast majority of people who experience a loss will recover gradually without any interventions. In those who become chronically depressed or have traumatic grief, an intervention at 6 months after the bereavement is indicated. Interpersonal therapy (ITP) was designed as a therapy that concentrates on loss, so it seems a likely psychotherapeutic tool. Antidepressants have also been used and shown to be efficacious.

There have been three open drug trials treating the depression of widowhood (Jacobs et al., 1987a; Pasternak et al., 1991; Zisook et al., 2001) and one placebo-controlled study, which included an arm of IPT (Reynolds et al., 1999). All showed the efficacy of antidepressants in treating this depression. In the first trial (Jacobs et al., 1987a), 10 widows/widowers aged 26–65 with a major depressive disorder were treated for 1–2 years after their spouses' deaths with 75–150 mg desipramine for 4 weeks. Those who improved and wanted to continue the medication were referred to their family physicians for further treatment. Their mean Hamilton Depression Rating Scale-21 (HDRS-21) scores fell 2 to 6 points, although no statistics were done because of the small numbers. Seven of the 10 were rated as much or very much improved.

In the second open trial (Pasternak et al., 1991), 13 widows/widowers aged 61–78 were treated for 2–25 months after their spouses' deaths with 25–75 mg of nortriptyline (NT). The criterion for response was a Hamilton Rating Scale for Depression (HAM-D) rating of $\leq 10$ for $\geq 3$ weeks after a therapeutic level (50–150 ng/ml) of NT had been achieved. After acute treatment, subjects were allowed to continue the treatment for 16 weeks. The median response time was 6.4 weeks. Their mean 17-item HAM-D scores fell from 22 to 7, a decrease of 67.9% ($p < .001$).

In the third study (Zisook et al., 2001), 22 widows/widowers aged 21–69 who developed a major depressive disorder within 6 months preceding the death or 6 months after the death were treated in an open trial with bupropion SR at a dose of 150–300 mg for 8 weeks. The 14 completers had HAM-D scores that fell from a mean of 16.5 to 4.5 ($p < .001$). Even the intent-to-treat sample of 22 had HAM-D median scores that fell from 16.77 to 7.73, again significant at the $p < .001$ level.

In the last study (Reynolds et al., 1999), which was the only double-blind trial, 80 men and women 50 years of age or older whose major depressive disorder began 6 months before or in the 12 months following the death of a spouse or significant other were treated with NT alone or with IPT, or with placebo alone or with IPT. Remission was defined as having a 17-item HAM-D score of less than 7 for 3 consecutive weeks. The remission rate with NT alone was 56%, and for NT with IPT it was 68%, compared to remission rates for placebo of 45% and placebo plus IPT of 29%. The remission occurred 49.5–76.5 days after the beginning of treatment. The overall dichotomous outcome (remission/no remission) detected a significant drug effect ($p < 0.03$) but not a main effect for IPT. Subjects who achieved remission were allowed an additional 16 weeks of treatment to ensure stability and then the medication was gradually tapered. They were followed for 2 years. The rate of relapse into major depression during the continuation therapy was low for all groups (5%).

Finally, a post hoc comparison of paroxetine or NT for bereaved persons with traumatic grief showed that both medications decreased depressive and traumatic grief symptoms by more than 50% (Zymont et al., 1998).

Thus, bereavement-related depression appears to respond well to treatment with antidepressant medication (Rosenweig et al., 1996). It is also important to remember that should the patient be psychotic or suicidal, electroconvulsive therapy is probably indicated.

## SUMMARY

The death of someone close is a significant event, even to the elderly. Almost every bereaved individual experiences some depressive symptoms. In the majority of survivors, these symptoms resolve over the first year. About 10% develop a chronic major depression, and an unknown percentage develops a more severe PTSD-like syndrome labeled *complicated grief*. These latter outcomes are more likely to occur if the person has had a previous mood disorder or a history of substance abuse or is in poor physical health. There is an increased mortality in widowed men, especially young-old (<75 years) men, in the first 6 months of bereavement. On the other hand, dating and remarriage do occur. Whether treatment with an antidepressant would improve the outcome is unproved but seems likely.

## REFERENCES

Bornstein, P.E. and Clayton, P.J. (1972) The anniversary reaction. *Dis Nerv Syst* 33:470–472.

Breckenridge, J.N., Gallagher, D., Thompson, L.W., et al. (1986) Characteristic depressive symptoms of bereaved elders. *J Gerontol* 41:163–168.

Burnett, P., Middleton, W., Raphael, B., and Martiner, N. (1997) Measuring core bereavement phenomena. *Psychol Med* 27:49–57.

Byrne, G.J.A. and Raphael, B. (1994) A longitudinal study of bereavement phenomena in recently widowed elderly men. *Psychol Med* 24:411–421.

Carr, D, House, J.S., Kessler, R.C., Nesse, R.M., Sonnega, J., and Wortman, C. (2000) Marital quality and psychological adjustment to widowhood among older adults: A longitudinal analysis. *J Gerontol Soc Sci* 55B(4):S197–S207.

Clayton, P.J. (1998) *Adversity, Stress and Psychopathology* (Dohrenwend, B., ed.). Oxford University Press.

Clayton, P.J. (2000) Bereavement. In: Fink, G., ed. *Encyclopedia of Stress*. San Diego: Academic Press, pp. 304–311.

Clayton, P.J. and Darvish, H.S. (1979) Course of depressive symptoms following the stress of bereavement. In: Barrett, J.E., ed. *Stress and Mental Disorder*. New York; Raven Press, pp. 121–136.

Clayton, P., Demarais, L., and Winokur, G. (1968) A study of normal bereavement. *Am J Psychiatry* 125(2):168–178.

Clayton, P.J., Halikas, J.A., and Maurice, W.L. (1971) The bereavement of the widowed. *Dis Nerv Syst* 32(9):597–604.

Clayton, P.J., Herjanic, M., Murphy, G.E., and Woodruff, R.A., Jr. (1974) Mourning and depression, their similarities and differences. *Can Psychiatr Assoc J* 19:309–312.

Clayton, P.J., Parilla, R.H., Jr., and Bieri, M.D. (1980a) Methodological problems in assessing the relationship between acuteness of death and the bereavement outcome. In: Reiffe, S., et al., eds. *The Psychosocial Aspects of Cardiovascular Disease: The Patient, the Family and the Staff*. New York: Columbia University Press, pp. 267–275.

Clayton, P.J., Parilla, R.H., Jr., and Bieri, M.D. (1980b) Survivors of cardiovascular and cancer deaths. In Reiffe, J., et al., eds. *Psychosocial Aspects of Cardiovascular Disease: The Patient, the Family, and the Staff*. New York: Columbia University Press, pp. 277–293.

Fashingbauer, T.R., Zisook, S., and DeVaul, R. (1987) The Texas Revised Inventory of Grief. In: Zisook, S., ed. *Biopsychosocial Aspects of Bereavement*. Washington, DC: American Psychiatric Press, pp. 109–124.

Freud, S. (1959) *The Complete Psychological Works of Sigmund Freud*, XIV. London: Hogarth Press, pp. 243–258.

Frost, N.R. and Clayton, P.J. (1977) Bereavement and psychiatric hospitalization. *Arch Gen Psychiatry* 34:1172–1175.

Galea, S., Resnick, H., Kilpatrick, D., Bucuvalas, M, Gold, J., and Vlahov, D. (2002) Psychological sequelae of the September 11 terrorist attacks in New York City. *N Engl J Med* 346(13):982–987.

Grimby, A. (1993) Bereavement among elderly people: Grief reactions, post-bereavement hallucinations and quality of life. *Acta Psychiatr Scand* 87:72–80.

Hays, J.C., Kasl, S.V., and Jacobs, S.C. (1994) The course of psychological distress following threatened and actual conjugal bereavement *Psychol Med* 24:917–927.

Horowitz, M.J., Seige, B., Holen, A., Bonanno, G.A., Milbrath, C., and Stinson, C.H. (1997) Diagnostic criteria for complicated grief disorder. *Am J Psychiatry* 154(7):904–910.

Jacobs, S.C., Hansen, F., Kasl, S., et al. (1990) Anxiety disorders during acute bereavement: Risk and risk factors. *J Clin Psychiatry* 51:269–274.

Jacobs, S.C., Kasl, S.V., Ostfeld, A.M., Berkman, L., Kosten, T.R., and Charpentier, P. (1986) The measurement of grief: bereaved versus non-bereaved. *Hosp J* 2(4):21–36.

Jacobs, S.C., Nelson, J.C., and Zisook, S. (1987a) Treating depressions of bereavement with antidepressants, a pilot study. *Psychiatr Clin North Am* 10:501–510.

Jacobs, S.C., Schaefer, C.A., Ostfeld, A.M., et al. (1987b) The first anniversary of bereavement. *Isr J Psychiatry Relat Sci* 24:77–85.

Lichtenstein, P., Gatz, M., and Berg, S. (1998) A twin study of mortality after spousal bereavement. *Psychol Med* 28:635–643.

Lindeman, E. (1944) Symptomatology and management of acute grief. *Am J Psychiatry* 101:141–148.

Longford, E. (1964) Queen Victoria: Harper & Row Publishers, 1964.

Lund, D.A., Caserta, M.S., and Dimond, M.F. (1986) Gender differences through two years of bereavement among the elderly. *Gerontologist* 26(3):314–320.

Lund, D.A., Caserta, M.S., and Dimond, M.F. (1993) The course of spousal bereavement in later life. In: Stroebe, M.S., Stroebe, W., and Hansson, R.O., eds. *Handbook of Bereavement*. Cambridge: Cambridge University Press, pp. 241–254.

Lund, D.A., Caserta, M.S., Van Pelt, J. and Gass, K.A. (1990) Stability of social support networks after later-life spousal bereavement. *Death Sci* 14:53–73.

Lundin, T. (1984a) Morbidity following sudden and unexpected bereavement. *Br J Psychiatry* 144:84–88.

Lundin, T. (1984b) Long-term outcome of bereavement. *Br J Psychiatry* 145:423–428.

Lusyne, P., Page, H., and Lievens, J. (2001) Mortality following conjugal bereavement, Belgium 1991–96: The unexpected effect of education. *Pop Studies* 55:281–289.

Mendes de Leon, C.F.M., Kasl, S.F., and Jacobs, S. (1993) Widowhood and mortality risk in a community sample of the elderly: A prospective study. *J Clin Epidemiol* 46(6):519–527.

Morgan, J.F., Beckett, J., and Zolese, G. (2001) Psychogenic mania and bereavement. *Psychopathology* 34:265–267.

Murrell, S.A. and Himmelfarb, S. (1989) Effects of attachment bereavement and pre-event conditions on subsequent depressive symptoms in older adults. *Psychol Aging* 4(2):166–172.

Murrell, S.A., Himmelfarb, S., and Phifer, J.F. (1988) Effects of bereavement/loss and pre-event status on subsequent physical health in older adults *Int J Aging Hum Dev* 27(2):89–107.

Murrell, S.A., Norris, F.H., and Hutchins, G.L. (1984) Distribution and desirability of life events in older adults; population and policy implications. *J Commun Psychol* 12:301–311.

North, C.S., Nixon, S.J., Shariat, S., Mallonee, S., McMillen, J., Spitznagel, L., and Smith, M. (1999) Psychiatric disorders among survivors of the Oklahoma City bombing. *JAMA* 282(8):755–762.

North, C.S., Smith, E.M., and Spitznagel, E.L. (1997) One-year follow-up of survivors of a mass shooting. *Am J Psychiatry* 154:1696–1702.

Onishi, H., Miyashita, A., and Kosaka, K. (2000) A manic episode associated with bereavement in a patient with lung cancer. *Support Care Cancer* 8:339–340.

Pasternak, R.E., Reynolds, C.F., Schlernitzauer, M., et al. (1991) Acute open-trial nortriptyline therapy of bereavement-related depression in late life. *J Clin Psychiatry* 52:307–310.

Parkes, C.M. (1970) The first year of bereavement: A longitudinal study of the reaction of London widows to the deaths of their husbands. *Psychiatry* 33:444–467.

Prigerson, H.G., Bierhals, A.J., Kasl, S.V., Reynolds, C.F., III, Shear, K., Day, N., Beery, L.C., Newsom, J.T., and Jacobs, S. (1997) Traumatic grief as a risk factor for mental and physical morbidity. *Am J Psychiatry* 154(5):616–623.

Prigerson, H.G., Maciejewski, P.K., Reynolds, C.F., III, Bierhals, A.J., Newsom, J.T., Fasiczka, A., Frank, E., Doman, J., and Miller, M. (1995) Inventory of Complicated Grief. A scale to measure maladaptive symptoms of loss. *Psychiatry Res* 59:65–79.

Rees, W.D. (1971) The hallucinations of widowhood. *Br Med J* 4:39–41.

Reynolds, C.F., III, Miller, M.D., Pasternak, R.E., Frank, E., Perel, J.M., Cornes, C., Houck, P.R., Mazumdar Des, M.A., and Kupfer, D.J. (1999) Treatment of bereavement-related major depressive episodes in later life: A controlled study of acute and continuation treatment with nortriptyline and interpersonal psychotherapy. *Am J Psychiatry* 156:202–208.

Rosenweig, A.S., Pasternak, R.E., Prigerson, H.G., Miller, M.D., and Reynolds, C.F. (1996) Bereavement-related depression in the elderly. *Drugs Aging* 8(5):323–328.

Rubenowitz, E., Waern, M, Wilhelmson, K., and Allebeck, P. (2001) Life events and psychosocial factors in elderly suicides—a case-control study. *Psychol Med* 31(7):1193–1202.

Schaefier, C., Quesenberry, J.C.P., Jr., and Wi, S. (1995) Mortality following conjugal bereavement and the effects of a shared environment. *Am J Epidemiol* 141(12):1142–1152.

Surtees, P.G. (1995) In the shadow of adversity: The evolution and resolution of anxiety and depressive disorder. *Br J Psychiatry* 166:583–594.

Winokur, G. and Clayton, P. (1994) *The Medical Basis of Psychiatry*. Philadelphia: W.B. Saunders Co.

Zisook, S. and Shuchter, S.R. (1991) Depression through the first year after the death of a spouse. *Am J Psychiatry* 148:1346–1352.

Zisook, S. and Shuchter, S.R. (1993a) Major depression associated with widowed. *Am J Geriatr Psychiatry* 1:316–326.

Zisook, S. and Shuchter, S.R. (1993b) Uncomplicated bereavement. *J Clin Psychiatry* 54:365–372.

Zisook, S., Shuchter, S.R., Pedrelli, P., Sable, J., and Deacluc, S.C. (2001) Bupripion sustained release for bereavement: Results of an open trail. *J Clin Psychiatry* 62:227–230.

Zygmont, M., Prigerson, H.G., Houck, P.R., Miller, M.D., Shear, M.K., Jacobs, S., and Reynolds C.F., III (1998) A post hoc comparison of paroxetine and nortriptyline for symptoms of traumatic grief. *J Clin Psych* 59(5):241–245.

# III | THE PSYCHOBIOLOGY OF LATE-LIFE DEPRESSION

IN the Department of Psychiatry at Columbia University, as probably in many other university departments, a prominent saying is that "the brain is the organ of the mind." Traditionally, one dimension of psychobiology has been the translation of mental processes, as represented by thought, mood, and emotion, into aspects of brain function, characterized by localization, physiology, and connectivity. Linkages between brain and behavior have been derived from the characterization of the behavioral deficits accompanying brain lesions and the behavioral phenomena interfered with or released during brain stimulation or spontaneous seizures. Recent techniques have relied on the fact that under normal circumstances the energy supply to and consumption of the brain are determined on a regional basis by level of activity. Thus, the basic assumption is that the physical work of the brain, as expressed in blood supply or glucose and oxygen consumption, reflects levels of the mental activity. In vivo research studies, based on positron emission tomography or functional magnetic resonance imaging methods, use this assumption to study the physiological bases of cognitive and affective processes, whether experimentally manipulated or as manifested in health and disease states. This work has generated considerable new information about the localization of mental functions and the distributed networks that subserve elemental and complex psychological processes. Beyond providing circuit maps, the next task for brain imaging research is to describe the biochemistry that fuels these pathways. For example, only in recent years have we had confirmation that accentuating or depleting the dopamine concentration in the human has a direct effect on the expression of psychosis. This part reviews the changes in brain structure and function, neurotransmitter, and endocrine systems associated with aging and depression.

The interpretations offered for psychobiological research often reflect an uncertainty about whether causal inferences are justified or whether findings simply reflect correlations that may be epiphenomena. In the clinical situation, behavioral phenomena are complex and multifaceted. Late-life depression can impact a host of processes, including diverse aspects of thinking (e.g., learning and memory), mood regulation, neurovegetative processes (e.g., sleep and appetite), and motor behavior (e.g., retardation, agitation). Thus even at the level of establishing correlations, it is often difficult to know what features of a complex illness are responsible for the relationship with an abnormality in brain function. The problem of complexity in interpreting correlations also applies to understanding treatment mechanisms. For example, a medication may be documented to be effective. However, given that most psychotropics have multiple effects on diverse transmitter and receptor systems, identifying the mechanism of therapeutic action is problematic. This difficulty applies to identifying the *active ingredient* in virtually any clinical trial, whether of somatic treatments or psychotherapy.

Psychobiological research can establish that an illness, symptom pattern, or behavior is correlated with a biological variable; however, correlation is not proof of causation, and such data are often misrepresented as the biology *causing* the thought, feeling or behavior. To establish causation requires that the putative causal agent be added and/or subtracted and result consistently and specifically in the hypothesized change in behavior. Unfortunately, many of our most critical hypotheses about factors that cause late-life depression, such as the aging process, genetic factors, personality dimensions, and so on, involve variables that cannot be experimentally manipulated. This limitation, to a large extent true of many medical disorders, underscores the need for skepticism in definitive acceptance of theories of etiology.

# 10 | Neuropsychological assessment of late-life depression

WILFRED G. VAN GORP, JAMES C. ROOT, AND HAROLD A. SACKEIM

The incidence and prevalence of mental disorders, specifically depression, in the general population has received considerable attention given their social, financial, and vocational impact. With respect to depressive disorders, U.S. statistics combined from the Epidemiological Catchment Area (ECA) study of the early 1980s and the National Co-morbidity Survey (NCS) of the early 1990s have produced a best estimate of a 6.5% 1-year prevalence for major depressive episodes, 5.3% for unipolar major depression, and 1.6% for dysthymia (Mental Health: A Report of the Surgeon General, 1999). Depressive spectrum disorders continue to evidence high prevalence rates in our elderly population. For older adults, aged 65 and over, prevalence rates have been estimated as 3.8% for a major depressive episode, 3.7% for unipolar major depression, and 1.6% for dysthymia. Given that the makeup of our population is projected to become increasingly older in coming decades, the understanding and treatment of depressive spectrum disorders in the elderly is especially significant.

Initially based on anecdotal and clinical observation (Caine, 1981), depression has long been associated with decreased cognitive abilities. As neuropsychology gained prominence in psychiatry and clinical psychology, efforts to delineate the effects of depression on cognitive functioning became increasingly refined. Several studies sought to characterize the hallmarks of cognitive decline associated with depression compared to other psychiatric and neurological conditions (see Keilp et al., 2001; King and Caine, 1996; King et al., 1995, for reviews). The neuropsychological investigation and analysis of cognitive functioning in depression has been aided by a more complex understanding of brain–behavior relationships and the use of standardized instruments. In addition, recent advances in normative research have allowed for more accurate comparisons of individuals' performance with their appropriate age- and education-matched cohort.

We review three issues in the assessment of cognitive functioning in the elderly—age-appropriate cognitive decline, the profile of cognitive decline related to depression in the nonelderly, and the interaction of age and depression on cognitive functioning. A sample battery of neuropsychological instruments will be discussed, both for situations in which a comprehensive assessment is required and for situations in which conditions do not allow for a comprehensive examination, either as a result of time constraints or because of physical/sensory limitations often present in the elderly.

Cognitive impairments secondary to depression will be referred to as *depression-associated cognitive decline* (DACD), which we believe is preferable to the terms *pseudodementia* or *dementia syndrome secondary to depression*—the former because of the idiopathic, syndromal nature of dementia and the latter because the cognitive decline associated with depression rarely meets criteria for a diagnosis of dementia but nonetheless may significantly impact on functioning.

## THE EFFECT OF AGE ON NEUROPSYCHOLOGICAL FUNCTIONING: AGE-APPROPRIATE COGNITIVE DECLINE

Elderly individuals present for neuropsychological assessment with a variety of cognitive difficulties, with increased forgetfulness and distractibility being primary complaints. The clinician must often tease apart the relative contributions of depression and a possible dementing condition in relation to such functional complaints. This differential diagnosis is complicated by variations in the profile and progression of age-appropriate cognitive decline (Crook et al., 1986), which may also be confused with the early stages of a primary dementia or the sequelae of a depressive disorder.

Several rules of thumb have been offered in determining age-appropriate cognitive decline. Ratcliff and Saxton (1998) suggested preliminary criteria consisting of objective findings of performance one standard deviation below the mean in comparison to healthy young adults, together with self-reported memory complaints,

117

preserved vocabulary, and no indication of a primary neurological disorder that could account for the abnormalities.

Analysis of Wechsler Adult Intelligence Scale III/Wechsler Memory Scale-III (WAIS-III/WMS-III) performance, presented below, partially supports a one standard deviation threshold for detecting a decline in elderly cognitive performance. The following analysis uses normative data from the recent WAIS-III/WMS-III standardization in comparing cognitive performance in the elderly to that of the age group between 20 and 54. Table 10.1 presents the average performance of individuals 70 to 74 years of age compared to those of individuals in younger age groupings on WAIS-III subtests. Scaled scores for younger age groups were derived by identifying the raw score performance of 70- to 74-year-olds that corresponded to a scaled score of 10 (average performance, 50th percentile) and calibrating for this level of performance in five other age groups. For example, a scaled score of 10 (average performance) for an individual 70–74 years of age on the Picture Completion subtest corresponds to a scaled score of 7 (one standard deviation below the mean) for an individual 20–24 years of age.

Table 10.1 demonstrates that in group data, cognitive decline can be readily demonstrated in neurologically intact 70- to 74-year-olds compared to younger cohorts. A similar pattern and level of deficit characterize the 65- to 69-year-old age group. Significantly, subtests sampling verbal abilities and semantic memory (Vocabulary, Similarities, Information) showed a relatively constant level of performance across age groups. In contrast, tests of attention and working memory (Digit Span, Letter-Number Sequencing), vi-

suospatial functioning (Block Design, Matrix Reasoning, Picture Completion), and processing speed (Digit Symbol, Symbol Search) declined by one standard deviation or more. Processing speed was particularly affected (Digit Symbol, Symbol Search), with a decrease of more than one standard deviation in the elderly compared to younger age groups.

Table 10.2 presents the average performance of these age groups on selected subtests of the WMS-III. Scaled scores for the age groups were derived in the same manner as for the WAIS-III. For example, a scaled score of 10 (average performance) for an individual 70–74 years of age on the Family Pictures Immediate Recall subtest corresponds to a scaled score of 6 (more than one standard deviation below the mean) for an individual 20–24 years of age.

Individuals, aged 70 to 74, and to a lesser extent, those aged 65 to 69, exhibited performance roughly one standard deviation below that of younger groups on select subtests. Structured verbal recall is mostly consistent across groups, while performance in most other memory subdomains exhibited an advantage for younger individuals. Interestingly, the difference between immediate and delayed recall was slight, arguing against a differential impact of age on encoding and retrieval abilities.

Thus, it is evident that test performance is closely linked to age. Individuals 70–74 years of age performed up to one standard deviation below levels reached in young adulthood (20–24) on select tests. This effect may be noted even in relatively younger, elderly cohorts (65–69). As noted above, it is not clear whether this disparity is owing to cohort effects such as education and environmental demands, or to actual changes in

TABLE 10.1. *Scaled Scores on WAIS-III Subtests Corresponding to 50th Percentile Performance for Various 70–74 Age Groups*

| WAIS Subtest | 20–24 | 25–29 | 30–34 | 45–54 | 65–69 | 70–74* |
|---|---|---|---|---|---|---|
| Vocabulary | 11 | 11 | 10 | 9 | 10 | 10 |
| Similarities | 9 | 9 | 9 | 9 | 10 | 10 |
| Arithmetic | 10 | 10 | 10 | 9 | 10 | 10 |
| Digit Span | 8 | 8 | 9 | 9 | 9 | 10 |
| Information | 11 | 11 | 11 | 10 | 10 | 10 |
| Comprehension | 11 | 11 | 10 | 9 | 10 | 10 |
| Letter-Number Seq. | 7 | 7 | 7 | 8 | 9 | 10 |
| Picture Completion | 7 | 7 | 7 | 7 | 10 | 10 |
| Digit Symbol | 6 | 6 | 6 | 7 | 10 | 10 |
| Block Design | 8 | 8 | 8 | 9 | 10 | 10 |
| Matrix Reasoning | 6 | 6 | 6 | 7 | 9 | 10 |
| Picture Arrangement | 6 | 6 | 6 | 8 | 10 | 10 |
| Symbol Search | 6 | 6 | 6 | 8 | 10 | 10 |
| Object Assembly | 7 | 7 | 7 | 8 | 10 | 10 |

*Seventy- to 74-year-old performance is the reference for all other derived scores.
WAIS-III, Wechsler Adult Intelligence Scale-III.

TABLE 10.2. *Scaled Scores on WMS-III Subtests Corresponding to 50th Percentile Performance for Various 70–74 Age Groups*

| WMS-III Subtest | 20–24 | 25–29 | 30–34 | 45–54 | 65–69 | 70–74* |
|---|---|---|---|---|---|---|
| Logical Memory I | 9 | 9 | 9 | 9 | 10 | 10 |
| Faces I | 7 | 8 | 8 | 8 | 9 | 10 |
| Verbal Paired I | 7 | 8 | 8 | 9 | 10 | 10 |
| Family Pictures I | 6 | 6 | 7 | 8 | 10 | 10 |
| Logical Memory II | 8 | 8 | 8 | 9 | 10 | 10 |
| Faces II | 7 | 7 | 8 | 8 | 9 | 10 |
| Verbal Paired II | 8 | 8 | 8 | 8 | 10 | 10 |
| Family Pictures II | 6 | 6 | 7 | 7 | 10 | 10 |

*Seventy- to 74-year-old performance is the reference for all other derived scores.
WMS-III, Wechsler Memory Scale III.

cognitive ability over the lifespan. Nonetheless such an analysis does suggest unique cognitive profiles in relation to sample age. Such findings are also in agreement with the distinction between fluid and crystallized intelligence (Horn, 1970), in which knowledge gained throughout the lifespan (e.g., verbal abilities) is retained, while processes dependent on current physiological integrity (e.g., psychomotor speed, visuospatial processing, attention) may be expected to decline with advancing age. Thus, one must question whether age appropriate cognitive decline is significantly affected by the presence of a depressive disorder.

## PROFILE OF DEPRESSION-ASSOCIATED COGNITIVE DECLINE

Two main theories have offered differing accounts about the source of the cognitive dysfunction secondary to depression. The first account focused primarily on the motivational deficits often observed in depressed individuals. Given the ostensible primacy of motivational deficits in the phenomenology of depression, performance on neuropsychological instruments with strong effort and motivation demands—such as free recall versus cued recall or recognition—was predicted to be especially impaired in depressed individuals. In other words, when individuals lack interest and make little effort, they are not expected to perform well on effortful tasks. While such findings were observed in a variety of studies (Hartlage et al., 1993; Miller, 1975) and appear to be a consistent source of decreased performance in depressed individuals, the depth and breadth of cognitive impairment observed in major depression remained to be explained.

A number of studies have challenged the purely motivational hypothesis, as depressed individuals exhibit wide-ranging deficits on effortful and noneffortful tasks alike. Flor-Henry (1979, 1983) served as an exponent of a theory emphasizing more immediate, parallel dysfunction in depression, consisting of both the commonly observed symptoms of dysphoria, anhedonia, amotivation, and fatigue, as well as wide-ranging cognitive deficits across several domains, and postulated right hemisphere dysfunction as the source. Numerous research investigations followed, examining the parallel nature of the cognitive decline in major depression, the right hemisphere hypothesis, and the profile of such impairment (Caine et al., 1993; Christensen et al., 1997; Fromm-Auch, 1983; King et al., 1991b, 1993; Niederhe and Camp; 985; Richards and Ruff, 1989). While a differential effect of hemispheric dysfunction has been questioned, the main outcome of such observations has been to focus more specifically on the profile of cognitive impairment in depression and the differentially affected cognitive domains. This research also has as its aim a better understanding of the specific neural substrates of clinical depression.

Broadly, neurocognitive functioning traditionally has been divided into five partially qualitatively distinct domains: attention, verbal processing, visuospatial processing, psychomotor speed, and executive functioning; memory is dealt with separately. These domains represent functional distinctions but appear to have partially overlapping neuroanatomical correlates.

## ATTENTION

Attention represents a somewhat heterogeneous set of functions as it is described in the literature, with the subdomains of simple, complex, divided, and sustained attention falling within the same domain. We focus on those tasks that measure simple attention—that is, those that require the individual to briefly retain small amounts of information, as well as working memory and selective, divided, and sustained attention measures, although the latter functions may more accurately be included in the domain of executive functioning.

Simple attentional performance (reporting back five ± two items) does not appear to be significantly affected in depressive individuals. In a carefully controlled, conservative meta-analysis of depressive cognitive function, Veiel (1997) found that simple attention performance of depressives (Digit Span-Forward, Spatial Span-Forward) differed from that of controls by an average standardized difference of .18, or approximately one-sixth of a standard deviation. Impaired performance (2nd percentile and below) on simple attentional tasks occurred in only 2.8% of depressed individuals, representing the least sensitive indicator of depressive cognitive decline.

A meta-analysis conducted by Zakzanis et al. (1999) reached similar conclusions, with 72% of depressive simple attention scores overlapping with those obtained by nondepressed, control subjects. Similarly, working memory performance yielded 78% overlap with control performance. Likewise, and somewhat surprisingly, divided attention performance yielded roughly 78% overlap with that of controls. Together, performance in simple attention, working memory, and divided attention distinguished no more than one-third of depressed performance from that of controls (meaning that about 66% of depressed and control individuals performed approximately equally in most attentional tasks). The most sensitive indicator of attentional decline in depressed individuals was the Letter Cancellation Task, a speeded measure of selective, sustained attention, yielding a relatively low overlap between depressed and control performance of 46%, suggesting that over half of depressed individuals performed more poorly than controls in selective sustained attention.

## VERBAL PROCESSING

Verbal abilities have been traditionally measured by means of verbal fluency and confrontation naming tasks. Verbal fluency is tested by having individuals generate words in response to a specific cue (i.e., words beginning with a certain letter or words belonging to a particular semantic category). Verbal fluency is most commonly assessed with the FAS Controlled Oral Word Association Task (words beginning with *F*, *A*, or *S*) and the Animal Naming Task. Naming on the basis of letter and category may reflect only partially overlapping capacities, as there is some evidence that the former (phonemic fluency) is disrupted most by frontal lesions, whereas temporal lesions may disrupt category naming. Confrontation naming consists of the ability to name visually presented stimuli of increasing difficulty and has often been assessed with the Boston Naming Test.

Veiel's (1997) meta-analysis surveyed verbal abilities as measured solely by verbal fluency tasks, and found an average standardized difference of .55 between depressed and nondepressed groups, with 11% of depressed individuals obtaining scores at the 2nd percentile or below. While the subdomains of phonemic and semantic fluency were not analyzed separately, a recent study of verbal fluency in depression (Fossati et al., 2003) found that fluency performance varied in relation to task demands. Performance on a semantic fluency measure, in which subjects were required to generate animal names, was found to be significantly lower in depressed individuals, while phonemic fluency was not impaired. The authors also measured the total number of *switches* in semantic and phonemic fluency performance, that is, the number of times the generated words reflected a switch from one semantic or phonemic clustering (pets–insects, foot–frank), and found that the depressed sample had decreased switching but only in the semantic fluency task. They related this finding to a theory that depressed individuals tend to become *stuck* in a particular mental set, with a corresponding decrease in set shifting. Similar deficits in semantic fluency were found in other studies (Calev et al., 1989; Fossati et al., 2003; Tarbuck and Pakel, 1995), suggesting that verbal fluency, and specifically semantic fluency, is particularly subject to a performance deficit in depressed individuals. Zakzanis et al.'s (1999) meta-analysis supports the semantic–phonemic distinction suggested by Fossati et al., with depressive semantic fluency performance being considerably lower than phonemic fluency performance.

Confrontation naming has rarely been assessed in samples of depressed patients. One study of anomia in major depression (Georgieff et al., 1998) found that depressed individuals exhibited a significantly greater number of word-finding errors than nondepressed controls. Depressed individuals were able to arrive at semantically related incorrect words but had difficulty finding the correct word in relation to pictured test items. This suggested that the deficit pertained particularly to the phonological representation stage of confrontation naming. Zakzanis et al.'s survey of the literature, however, found confrontation naming to be a relatively insensitive indicator of depression, with approximately one-quarter of depressed individuals being accurately identified. Thus, while studies of confrontation naming suggest a statistically significant difference in performance, relative effect sizes reported in larger meta-analyses suggest that this may not be a common or especially marked deficit.

## VISUOSPATIAL PROCESSING

The assessment of visuospatial function concerns the ability to observe, manipulate, reason about, and construct nonverbal, spatially represented information. Typical assessment includes the Rey-Osterreith Complex Figure Test, Block Design, Matrix Reasoning, Picture Completion, and Mental Rotation. With the revision of the WAIS-III, a Perceptual Organization Index was constructed, consisting of Block Design, Picture Completion, and Matrix Reasoning, all found to be highly intercorrelated and partially distinct from other tested abilities.

Veiel's (1997) analysis of visuospatial ability (Rey-O Complex Figure, Block Design, and Object Assembly subtests) in depression found an average standardized difference of .81 between depressed and nondepressed samples, with 15% of depressed individuals at the 2nd percentile or below. Interpretation of performance on these instruments is qualified regarding their ability to measure a *process pure* visuospatial ability, as the majority of visuospatial tasks are timed tasks, and psychomotor slowing may contribute to deficits. Significantly, when analyzed separately, timed and untimed visuospatial tasks were found to accurately identify 40% and 25% of depressed individuals, respectively, supporting the notion that the speeded nature of a subset of visuospatial tasks contributes to the performance deficit.

## MEMORY

Learning and memory tasks in neuropsychological assessment cover a wide range of abilities. Typical tasks include the short-term retrieval of verbal or visuospatial information, as well as the ability to retain and retrieve this information over longer intervals (20–30 minutes to 24 hours). Stimuli in such tasks may be structured (e.g., semantically or structurally related) or unstructured (e.g., unrelated supraspan lists of verbal stimuli or visual information such as abstract figures). Individuals may be required to retrieve such information in free recall paradigms or in response to cueing (e.g., semantic groupings) or forced-choice recognition paradigms.

Decreased memory performance in depression has been well documented and is frequently subject to subjective complaint in depressed individuals (see Burt et al., 1995; Jorm et al., 2001; Kindermann and Brown, 1997; King and Caine, 1996, for reviews). Memory functioning in depression has typically been divided between *effortful* and *noneffortful* remembering relying on Hasher and Zacks' (1979) distinction between automatic and effortful memory processes (Kaszniak and Christenson, 1995; Nussbaum, 1998). The distinction between these two forms of learning and memory is suggested by studies of implicit and explicit memory, as well as by experimental dissociations between free recall and recognition, in which depressives have been noted to perform worse on the former but similar to controls on the latter (Bazin et al., 1994; Danion et al., 1991; Hartlage et al., 1993). Early studies of memory functioning in depression provide several examples of the effects of relative effort in particular learning and memory tasks, both in comparing recall and recognition performance and in structured versus unstructured

learning situations (Cummings and Benson, 1983; Niederhe and Camp, 1985; Weingartner et al., 1981). However, other studies have observed equally impaired recall *and* recognition in depressives' performance (Elliot and Greene, 1992; Hart et al., 1987a; La Rue, 1989; Richards and Ruff, 1989; Watkins et al., 1992), and represent contradictory findings.

Zakzanis et al. (1999) reported that measures of delayed recall performance were most successful in distinguishing depressed individuals from healthy controls. One measure of serial verbal list learning, delayed recall on the Rey Auditory Verbal Learning Test, was particularly sensitive in distinguishing depressed samples (correctly identifying 77% of depressed individuals). This contrasted with poorer sensitivity when using a similar task, the California Verbal Learning Test (CVLT) (which correctly identified only 37% of depressed individuals). This difference between these tasks may be related to their relative difficulty, as the Rey Auditory-Verbal Learning Test (RAVLT) uses stimuli that are semantically unrelated, while the CVLT word items are composed of semantically related subgroups and thus may require less effortful remembering.

A deficit in delayed recall is a rather coarse characterization of a memory deficit, as it may result from more specific deficits in the encoding, retention, or retrieval of information and may pertain to specific types of information. However, in the case of major depression, such specificity, suggesting a particular profile of memory disturbance, has not been identified. Several studies found that global memory performance is significantly impacted in depressed individuals. Burt et al. (1995) conducted a meta-analysis using relatively less stringent controls in study selection than those used in other meta-analyses, generating a larger study sample. Memory performance of depressed samples was generally decreased relative to that of controls, and recognition and recall performance were not found to vary consistently between the groups, suggesting a more generalized deficit.

Veiel (1997) found that depressed individuals performed, on average, nearly one standard deviation below that of controls in both verbal and nonverbal learning and memory tasks. Of note, however, significant variability was exhibited between studies that were analyzed, such that the range of depressive memory performance compared to that of controls was found to vary considerably.

Summarizing the above findings, depression does appear to exert a significant effect on memory functioning across wide-ranging tasks and the subdomains of learning and memory. However, a specific neurocognitive profile of memory impairment in depression does not appear consistently. While several studies found significant effects of motivation and effort in depressive memory performance (Zakzanis et al., 1999), other studies did not replicate this effect (Burt et al., 1995;

Veil, 1997). Meta-analytic reviews documented a significant (on average, up to one standard deviation) decline in depressive memory performance but did not find a consistent or distinct profile of memory impairment, either for effortful versus noneffortful remembering or for verbal versus nonverbal recall. Perhaps the most parsimonious interpretation of this literature is that deficits in remembering new information stem largely from deficient learning or acquisition. In particular, impairments in attention and concentration may lead to reduced immediate memory (learning as the principle source of impairment) (Steif et al., 1986). The attentional disturbance may also contribute to milder difficulties with effortful retrieval, making delayed recall measures the most sensitive due to the additivity of sources of diminished performance.

## PROCESSING SPEED

Speed of processing measures usually focuses on the speed of motor responses, functionally defined as thought tied to action. In the recent revision of the WAIS-III, a Processing Speed Index was defined, consisting of two measures of information processing and motor response (Digit Symbol Coding and Symbol Search). Other common measures of processing speed include visual tracking and sequencing (Trail Making Test A), fine-motor dexterity (Grooved Pegboard), and simple motor speed (Finger Tapping).

Deficits in processing speed (i.e., psychomotor slowing) have been linked historically to the depressed state (Sobin and Sackeim, 1997) and are one criterion for the formal diagnosis of a major depressive episode (American Psychiatric Association, 1994). In Veil's (1997) review, the domain of scanning/visuomotor tracking (Trail Making Test Part A and the WAIS-R Digit Symbol subtest) best encompassed the concept of processing speed. The performance of depressed samples on these two measures averaged a standardized difference of 0.93 compared to controls, and 18.2% of depressed individuals score at or below the 2nd percentile, representing a quite sensitive indicator of cognitive dysfunction in depressed individuals. Zakzanis et al. (1999) found speed of processing measures to be moderately discriminating, although not as consistently as suggested by Veil. These findings indicated that there was heterogeneity among processing speed measures (Digit Symbol = 40% overlap; Trail Making Test Part A = 85% overlap), suggesting that different aspects of processing speed are not equally affected.

Similar results have been found in studies investigating *processing resources* (Nebes et al., 2000) in which general factors such as processing speed have been found to be associated with, and contributory to, dysfunction in higher-order processing (e.g., memory,

executive functioning). The source of the sometimes marked slowing in information processing and motor response in depressed individuals remains unclear.

The distinction of cognitive and motor speed as composite sources of variability in processing speed tasks was highlighted by Sobin and Sackeim (1997), and has been investigated using specialized paradigms that attempt to segregate these components. Results of such studies reveal both longer cognitive *decision* time and slower motor movements following cognitive processing (Ghozlan and Widlocher, 1989) and have shown some promise in subtyping depressive conditions more accurately (LaPierre and Butter, 1980). In studies analyzing motor speed with minimal cognitive loads, Sabbe et al. (1999) used a simple speeded drawing task in which subjects' motor speed was monitored by computer. They found significant motor slowing in depressed individuals relative to controls throughout motor movement, which involved longer duration, significant pauses, and slower speed of movement, consistent with the results of several other studies (Caligiuri and Ellwanger, 2000; Cornell and Suarez, 1984; Rogers et al., 1987; Sabbe et al., 1996a).

In comparing depressed individuals' performance with that of individuals diagnosed with probable dementia of the Alzheimer's type (DAT) (Nebes et al., 1998), a differentiating pattern of cognitive and motor slowing was found between the two groups, consisting of uniform slowing across both cognitive and motor components in the DAT group and greater motor slowing in the depressed group. While such results are promising in their suggestion of a unique pattern of processing speed deficits, further research is necessary to establish the reliability of this finding.

Thus, processing speed decrements have been associated both clinically and experimentally with depressive episodes. Objective findings of slowed processing speed are often corroborated by findings of psychomotor retardation and slowed thinking in gross examination. However, while meta-analytic findings suggest that the processing speed impairment is a sensitive marker of cognitive dysfunction in depression, such retardation lacks specificity as to pathoetiology. In addition, standard tasks assessing psychomotor speed require that individuals perform quickly. There is evidence that depressed patients show considerably greater deficits when asked to perform at their preferred speed as opposed to performing quickly (Sackeim and Steiff, 1988).

## EXECUTIVE FUNCTIONING

Executive functioning represents a somewhat heterogeneous group of functional abilities and is typically associated with processes subserved by prefrontal cortex. Broadly defined, three partially overlapping neural substrates have been associated with executive functioning (Lezak, 1995). Dorsolateral (convexity) aspects of the prefrontal cortex have generally been linked with the control and regulation of cognitive function. Orbital areas (anterior-inferior) are associated with inhibition of response, impulse control, and maintenance of set. Medial aspects, particularly involving the anterior cingulate gyrus, have been associated with maintenance of drive, and with emotional regulation and tone. The term *executive functions* subsumes the cognitive operations subserved by these areas; thus, measurement of function associated with frontal areas is necessarily diverse and heterogeneous.

The analysis of frontal/executive function in depressive disorders is receiving increasing attention. Renewed interest in the association of frontal lobe functioning and depression results from the exquisite interconnected and reciprocal nature of neural projections from frontal areas to diverse areas of the cerebrum, as well as recent investigations of frontal areas and their association with regulation of emotion and motivation (Davidson, 1995). Veiel's meta-analysis of executive functioning in depression examined the findings with measures of mental control and flexibility (Trail Making Test–Part B, Stroop Color-Word Naming Test). Performance on these measures was found to be the most sensitive indicator of cognitive dysfunction in depression, with an average standardized difference of 2.0 and with 50.2% of depressed samples falling at the 2nd percentile or below. While this finding suggests a differential deficit, its interpretation is confounded by the timed and effortful nature of both tasks. It is not clear whether impaired performance on measures of mental control and flexibility reflects poor inhibition of the dominant response and cognitive rigidity (both associated with impaired executive functioning) or incorporates a generalized slowing in speed of processing. Furthermore, as with the finding of impairment in processing speed, it is noted that both measures have been shown to be sensitive, but not necessarily specific, indicators of cognitive dysfunction. As such, Veiel's finding of impaired mental control and flexibility awaits further investigation of the potentially distinct processes that contribute to performance on each task. The review by Zakzanis et al. (1999) lends further support to the contribution of processing speed to deficits in presumably executive tasks. In contrast to impaired performance on the above timed tasks, the authors reported that higher-order abstraction (Similarities) and untimed cognitive flexibility performance (Wisconsin Card Sorting Task) showed no consistent impairment relative to controls, with depressed and control performance overlapping by 88% on the former and by 77% on the latter. Thus, the concept of executive function is rather nebulous, encompassing a set of diverse capabilities with differing anatomical referents. The findings are inconsistent regarding the extent to which depression is associated with a general or specific deficit in executive functions.

## THE INTERACTION OF AGE AND DEPRESSION ON NEUROPSYCHOLOGICAL FUNCTIONING

The neurocognitive effects of depression and age necessarily intersect in the depressed elderly. The following discussion surveys the available literature examining the potential ways in which age and depression may interact and result in either qualitatively or quantitatively distinct profiles of cognitive performance. In addition, the question of whether the age-of-onset of depression in the elderly is associated with a different neurocognitive profile is also addressed.

In research examining the interaction of depression and age on cognitive functioning (Raskin, 1986), depressed elderly (up to age 70) were found to be significantly slower in information processing, and exhibited a loss of cognitive flexibility and abstraction compared to that of controls. Decreased functioning has also been found in select measures of visuospatial processing (Hart et al., 1987), WAIS Performance IQ (Sackeim et al., 1992), and executive functioning (Geffen et al., 1993).

Building on these findings and other research (King et al., 1991a), King and colleagues (1995) conducted a cross-sectional analysis of elderly depressive patients' functioning using a wide variety of neuropsychological instruments. They suggested that relative to matched controls, the depressed elderly had a distinct neuropsychological profile. Specifically, in addition to the neuropsychological impairment commonly associated with depression and described above, the depressed elderly exhibited significant difficulty in a task of visual tracking and set shifting (Trails B), as well as on tasks of visuospatial praxis and reasoning (Rey-O Complex Figure, Hooper Visual Organization Test). Medicated, depressed elderly had more difficulty in confrontation naming than unmedicated, depressed elderly, which could be due to the neurocognitive effects of certain psychotropics or to more severe disease in the patients who received medication. Thus, in addition to the more commonly associated effects of depression and cognitive functioning, King et al. found decreased ability in visuospatial processing and set shifting. While the particular measure of set shifting in this study relied on a speeded task, thus potentially confounding the effects of depression on processing speed and higher-order executive functioning, the finding of decreased visuospatial ability is particularly significant, as such functioning is typically preserved in younger depressed groups.

Another study of the combined effects of age and depression on cognitive functioning reported a bimodal distribution of neurocognitive performance, suggesting an interaction of severity of depression and cognitive functioning in the depressed elderly (Boone et al., 1995). Specifically, Boone et al. found that, regardless of disease severity, the depressed elderly exhibited deficits in study-defined nonverbal intelligence (Picture

Completion, Block Design, Picture Arrangement, Object Assembly) and visual memory at both the encoding and retrieval stages. Notably, disease severity exerted a significant influence on test performance, with more depressed individuals exhibiting decreased performance on tasks of information processing speed (Stroop, Digit Symbol) and executive skills (Wisconsin Card Sort, Stroop Interference, Auditory Consonant Trigrams, Controlled Oral Word Fluency). These findings suggested that severity of depressive symptoms may modulate neuropsychological performance in the depressed elderly in a manner distinct from that observed in younger depressed samples.

However, several studies have not found a distinct impairment in cognitive functioning, either globally or in regard to memory performance, when comparing midlife and elderly depressed groups. In regard to memory impairment, Kindermann and Brown (1997) conducted a meta-analysis of memory functioning in the elderly depressed, surveying 40 studies. Interestingly, and in line with Burt et al.'s (1995) findings, elderly depressed memory performance, while significantly different from that of controls, exhibited smaller effect sizes in regard to learning and memory than did the performance of younger samples. There was a distinctly bimodal distribution of scores, with more negative effect sizes (poorer performance among the elderly depressed) being associated with heterogeneous depressive groups (mixed unipolar and bipolar patients), underscoring the importance of inclusion criteria and the possibility of disease heterogeneity. The findings of less severe age-adjusted impairment in the depressed elderly compared to younger depressed groups may suggest a partial floor effect. It is conceivable that with increasing age, the gap between age-appropriate memory decline and the deficits associated with depressive illness is lessened. Palsson et al. (2000) examined the effects of depression on the cognitive functioning of individuals 85 years of age. They found a profile of impairment typical of that reported in younger adult depressed samples (deficits in delayed recall, processing speed, and performance on tasks requiring increased effort and concentration) but found no evidence of a distinct profile of cognitive dysfunction in the depressed elderly.

## THE INTERACTION OF AGE-AT-ONSET AND DEPRESSIVE COGNITIVE DECLINE

Among the potential subtypes of major depression in the elderly, age-at-onset may be especially important in accounting for heterogeneity in neurocognitive performance. Individuals with late-onset major depression are thought to have a less frequent family history of affective disorder, a higher rate of magnetic resonance

imaging (MRI) abnormalities compatible with a cerebrovascular disease (CVD) process, and a higher rate of treatment resistance and a deteriorating course with respect to both affective and cognitive symptoms. On the other hand, the elderly with onset of mood disorder early in life typically have had considerably greater exposure to psychiatric treatments and a longer duration of mood disturbance. There is some evidence that cumulative lifetime days in a depressed state is associated with extent of hippocampal volume reduction (Shelline et al., 1996) and verbal memory deficits (Shelline et al., 1999). Burt et al. (2000) compared elderly and younger adult patients with either bipolar or unipolar depression on a variety of memory tests. Among the younger sample, the bipolar patients tended to have superior performance, while the elderly bipolar patients had considerably larger deficits than the elderly unipolar patients. This finding was compatible with an iatrogenic neurocognitive effect of the illness, since the elderly patients with bipolar disorder were also distinct in having a greater number and longer duration of lifetime episodes of depression and more frequent psychiatric hospitalizations. Therefore, given these distinct literatures, late age-at-onset, usually taken as more than 50–60 years of age, can be hypothesized as linked to either preserved or deficient neuropsychological performance.

Age-at-onset has been associated with a distinct cognitive profile in a few studies (Cole and Hicking, 1976; Steingart and Herrmann, 1991). However, the bulk of the studies described in the preceding sections either did not report such an effect (Boone et al., 1995; Kindermann and Brown, 1997) or had negative findings (King et al., 1991a; Palsson et al., 2000). The inconsistency and lack of clear differentiation are compatible with reports arguing that while etiological factors may be distinct in early- and late-onset depression, these groups show considerable overlap in functional, symptomatic, and neurocognitive measures (Brodaty et al., 2001).

Of note, the failure to find age-at-onset differences in the neurocognitive literature may be partly related to the selection criteria used to generate the patient samples or, in the case of meta-analysis, study groups. These studies have typically excluded individuals with suspected neurological disease, including subcortical changes, probable DAT, Parkinson's disease, and traumatic brain injury. These exclusions lead to the selection of samples in which depression is a primary diagnosis with minimal neurological co-morbidity. Thus, this approach may inadvertently identify individuals who are indistinguishable phenotypically from those with early-onset depression.

In contrast, significant age-at-onset findings in other work may be partly driven by the inclusion of individuals in whom neurological illness is incipient or subsyndromal, but in whom the stigmata of primary neurological illness have not yet manifested. As individuals grow older, the incidence of neurological illness rises exponentially, with the prevalence of Alzheimer's disease, vascular dementias, and idiopathic dementias roughly doubling every 5 years and rising to a prevalence of 53% between the ages of 90 and 95 (Jorm and Jolley, 1998). Significantly, such disorders very often present with changes in mood, including heightened anxiety and depression, both of which may be manifestations of a neurological insult as well as reactions to perceived functional decline. In addition, depressive symptoms are often observed in advance of a formal diagnosis of dementia, leading many to question whether depression represents a prodromal symptom of dementia, lowers the threshold at which dementia symptoms are manifested, and/or is neuropathologically associated with dementing illnesses (Jorm, 2001). While several primary neurological conditions may present with depressive symptoms in the elderly, cerebrovascular pathology has been a subject of renewed interest of late, due both to its prevalence in the elderly depressed and to advances in neuroimaging technologies allowing detection of lacunar hyperintensities that previously may have remained undetected.

## NEUROPSYCHOLOGICAL ASSESSMENT OF LATE-LIFE DEPRESSION

Neurocognitive investigation of patients with late-onset depression may be helpful in detecting an underlying neuropathological process, commonly some form of CVD or a dementing illness. In addition, while far from established, it is likely that elderly depressed patients with clear-cut cognitive impairment are among the most likely to have a deteriorating cognitive course. Therefore, neuropsychological assessment can be useful to detect and clarify underlying central nervous system dysfunction, as well as to predict the disease course. A preliminary neuropsychological test battery is presented in Table 10.3 to aid the clinician in delineating cognitive dysfunction related to depression.

This battery uses a mixed flexible and fixed approach to neuropsychological assessment. While a fixed battery approach (i.e., the same tests for all individuals) offers complete and uniform evaluation of neurocognitive function, several difficulties are present in using a fixed battery across several disparate clinical situations. Elderly individuals present for assessment in a variety of clinical contexts—both inpatient and outpatient—and often may not be capable of meaningfully engaging in a full assessment. In the assessment of the elderly, time and physical limitations are salient. As such, while certain measures are used in nearly all clinical contexts, additional measures may or may not be used given the needs of both the patient and the referring clinician.

When time and physical circumstances allow, a candidate test battery should sample all areas of cognitive functioning, including overall intellectual ability (current and premorbid), attention, verbal abilities, visuospatial function, learning and memory, psychomotor and motor functioning, and executive functions. Table 10.3 organizes the tests in relation to these cognitive domains.

TABLE 10.3. *Neuropsychological Test Battery to Identify Cognitive Deficits in Depression*

| Cognitive Domain | Neuropsychological Measure |
| --- | --- |
| Intellectual functioning (current, premorbid) | Wechsler Adult Intelligence Scale-III (WAIS-III), Wechsler Test of Adult Reading (WTAR) |
| Attentional functioning (simple, complex, divided, sustained) | Trail Making Test A, Digit Span, Letter Number Sequencing, Arithmetic, Auditory Consonant Trigrams (ACT), Paced Auditory Serial Addition Test (PASAT), Continuous Performance Test (CPT) |
| Verbal functioning (phonemic and semantic fluency, confrontation naming) | FAS Controlled Oral Word Association Test (FAS-COWAT), Animal Naming Test (ANT), Boston Naming Test (BNT) |
| Visuospatial functioning (visual construction, nonverbal reasoning) | Picture Completion, Matrix Reasoning, Block Design, Rey-Osterreith Complex Figure Test |
| Learning and memory (structured and unstructured, verbal and nonverbal, immediate, delayed, and recognition) | California Verbal Learning Test-II (CVLT-II), Wechsler Memory Scale-III, Rey-Osterreith Complex Figure Test |
| Psychomotor and motor functioning (psychomotor speed, fine motor dexterity, motor strength) | Digit Symbol, Symbol Search, Grooved Pegboard, Finger Tapping, Hand Dynamometer |
| Executive functioning (concept acquisition, maintenance and flexibility, set-shifting, inhibition of dominant response) | Wisconsin Card Sorting Test (WCST), Trail Making Test Part B, FAS, Stroop, Auditory Consonant Trigrams (ACT), Paced Auditory Serial Addition Test (PASAT), Continuous Performance Test (CPT) |
| Personality and psychological functioning | Minnesota Multiphasic Personality Inventory-2, Personality Assessment Inventory, Beck Depression Inventory |

TABLE 10.4. *Abbreviated Neuropsychological Test Battery to Identify Cognitive Deficits in Depression*

| Cognitive Domain | Neuropsychological Measure |
|---|---|
| Intellectual functioning (current, premorbid) | Wechsler Abbreviated Scale of Intellelligence (WASI), Wechsler Test of Adult Reading (WTAR) |
| Attentional functioning (simple, complex, divided, sustained) | Trail Making Test A, Digit Span, Letter Number Sequencing |
| Verbal functioning (phonemic and semantic fluency, confrontation naming) | FAS Controlled Oral Word Association Test (FAS-COWAT), Animal Naming Test (ANT), Boston Naming Test (BNT) |
| Visuospatial functioning (visual construction, nonverbal reasoning) | Matrix Reasoning, Block Design, Rey-Osterreith Complex Figure Test |
| Learning and Memory (structured and unstructured, verbal and nonverbal, immediate, delayed, and recognition) | California Verbal Learning Test-II (CVLT-II), Rey-Osterreith Complex Figure Test |
| Psychomotor and Motor Functioning (psychomotor speed, fine motor dexterity, motor strength) | Digit Symbol, Symbol Search |
| Executive functioning (concept acquisition, maintenance and flexibility, set-shifting, inhibition of dominant response) | Wisconsin Card Sorting Test-Short Form (WCST-64), Trail Making Test Part B, FAS, Stroop |
| Personality and psychological functioning | Personality Assessment Inventory; Beck Depression Inventory |

In situations in which significant fatigue, sensory limitations, or physical circumstances do not allow for comprehensive assessment, the battery may be modified to achieve a minimally adequate sampling of each cognitive domain. Table 10.4 outlines a modified test battery that should be helpful for brief assessment.

In both the comprehensive and brief formats, the suggested measures have been restricted to those for which age- and, in a subset of measures, education-appropriate normative data exist. The Wechsler measures—WAIS-III, and WMS-III—include normative data up to the age of 89 years. Measures included in the original Halstead-Reitan battery—Wisconsin Card Sorting Test, Trails A, Trails B, Grooved Pegboard, Finger Tapping, and so on—offer both age- and education-matched normative data up to 80 years of age and 18 years of education (Heaton et al., 1991).

## CONCLUSION

This chapter has outlined issues pertaining to the neurocognitive assessment and sequelae of geriatric depression. Beginning with the neurocognitive presentation of depression in the nonelderly, it is clear that depression can exert significant and characteristic effects on cognitive functioning. It is further suggested that such deficits, while compounded by poor motivation and effort, likely represent an immediate symptom of depression, existing in parallel with mood and motivational deficits. In other words, neurocognitive impairment can be considered part of the phenomenology of depression. As such, depressed individuals exhibit decreased functioning on a wide range of cognitive measures—both effortful and noneffortful—with particular impact on the domains of processing speed, learning, and memory. While a specific neuropsychological profile has been investigated in presentations of depression, there is no single cognitive-pathological hallmark of the depressive condition. While certain distinctions in depressive cognitive functioning hold out promise for future research directions—such as preserved phonemic fluency versus impaired semantic fluency, preserved recognition versus impaired recall, and preserved cognitive speed versus impaired motor speed—such distinctions, while in some cases statistically significant, do not yet offer significant clinical utility for diagnosis or determination of prognosis. Likewise, analysis of cognitive functioning in the depressed elderly is typified by generally poor performance over a wide range of measures, with no one cognitive hallmark being evident. Expression of a specific profile is likely hampered by age-appropriate cognitive decline, which may exert a partial floor effect on cognitive functioning and in comparison to which depressive cognitive decline may appear to be less significant. Promising areas for further exploration in late-life depression include the findings of significantly poorer performance in measures of cognitive flexibility and visuospatial functioning. However, as with younger cohorts, these deficits do not suggest a pathologically distinct profile by which the cognitive effects of depression may be distinguished.

Of special promise is the research suggesting that subclinical CVD may impact on or produce depressive symptoms and cognitive dysfunction in the elderly. Several studies suggest that, to the extent that neurocognitive functioning differs in early- and late-onset depression, these differences may result from a CVD process, a condition to which the elderly are particularly prone. While the effects of stroke on cognitive and affective functions are well documented, more recent research has shown significant neurocognitive and depressive deterioration in the presence of subsyndromal *microvascular* disease. Determining whether subcortical white matter MRI abnormalities are associated with a specific cognitive profile in the elderly with depression, the reversibility of these deficits, their neuroanatomical and functional brain activity correlates, and their prognostic value will be issues addressed in the years to come.

## REFERENCES

American Psychiatric Association. (1994) *Diagnostic and Statistical Manual of Mental Disorders*. Fourth Edition. Washington, D. C.: American Psychiatric Association.

Bazin, N., Perruchet, P., De Bonis, M., and Feline, A. (1994) The dissociation of explicit and implicit memory in depressed patients. *Psychol Med* 24:239–245.

Boone, K.B., Lesser, I.M., Miller, B.L., Wohl, M., Berman, N., Lee, A., Palmer, B., and Back, C. (1995) Cognitive functioning in older depressed outpatients: relationship of presence and severity of depression to neuropsychological test scores. *Neuropsychology* 9:390–398.

Brodaty, H., Luscombe, G., Parker, G., Wilhelm, K., Hickie, I., Austin, M.P., and Mitchell, P. (2001) Early and late onset depression in old age: different aetiologies, same phenomenology. *J Affect Disord* 66:225–236.

Burt, D.B., Zembar, M.J. and Niederehe, G. (1995) Depression and memory impairment: a meta-analysis of the association, its pattern, and specificity. *Psychol Bull* 117:285–305.

Burt, D.B., Zembar, M.J., and Niederehe, G. (1995) Depression and memory impairment: a meta-analysis of the association, its pattern, and specificity. *Psychol Bull* 117:285–305.

Burt, T., Prudic, J., Peyser, S., Clark, J., and Sackeim, H.A. (2000) Learning and memory in bipolar and unipolar major depression: effects of aging. *Neuropsychiatry Neuropsychol Behav Neurol* 13:246–253.

Caine, E.D. (1981) Pseudodementia. Current concepts and future directions. *Arch Gen Psychiatry* 38:1359–1364.

Caine, E.D., Lyness, J.M., and King, D.A. (1993) Reconsidering depression in the elderly. *Am J Geriatric Psychiatry* 1:4–20.

Calev, A., Nigal, D., and Chazan, S. (1989) Retrieval from semantic memory using meaningful and meaningless constructs by depressed, stable bipolar and manic patients. *Br J Clin Psychol* 28:67–73.

Caligiuri, M. and Ellwanger, J. (2000) Motor and cognitive aspects of motor retardation in depression. *J Affect Disord* 57:83–93.

Christensen, H., Griffiths, K., Mackinnon, A., and Jacomb, P. (1997) A quantitative review of cognitive deficits in depression and Alzheimer-type dementia. *J Int Neuropsychol Soc* 3:631–651.

Cole, M. and Hicking, T. (1976) Frequency of minor organic signs in elderly depressives. *Can Psychiatric Assoc* 21:7–12.

Cornell, D., Suarez, R., and Berent, S. (1984) Psychomotor retardation in melancholic and nonmelancholic depression: Cognitive and motor components. *J Abnorm Psychol* 93:150–157.

Crook, T.H. Bartus, R.T. Ferris, S.H. Whitehouse, P. Cohen, and G.D. Gershon, S. (1986) Age-associated memory impairment: proposed diagnostic criteria and measures of clinical change. Report of a National Institute of Mental Health work group. *Devel Neuropsychol* 2:261–276.

Cummings, J.L. and Benson, D.F. (1983) *Dementia: A Clinical Approach*. Boston: Butterworth.

Danion, J.M., Willard-Schroeder, D., Zimmermann, M.A., Grange, D., Schlienger, J.L., and Singer, L. (1991) Explicit memory and repetition priming in depression. Preliminary findings. *Arch Gen Psychiatry* 48:707–711.

Davidson, R.J. (1995) Cerebral asymmetry, emotion, and affective style. In: Davidson, R.J., and Hugdahl, K., eds. *Brain Asymmetry* Cambridge, MA: MIT Press, pp. 361–387.

Elliott, C.L., and Greene, R.L. (1992) Clinical depression and implicit memory. *J Abnorm Psychol* 101:572–574.

Flor-Henry, P. (1979) On certain aspects of the localization of the cerebral systems regulating and determining emotion. *Biol Psychiatry* 14:677–698.

Flor-Henry, P. (1983) Neuropsychological studies in patients with psychiatric disorders. In: Heilman, K. and Satz, P., eds. *Neuropsychology of Human Emotion*. New York: Guilford Press, pp. 193–220.

Fossati, P., Guillaume, Le.B., Ergis, A.M., and Allilaire, J.F. (2003) Qualitative analysis of verbal fluency in depression. *Psychiatry Res* 117:17–24.

Franke P., Maier W., Hardt J, Frieboes R., Lichtermann D., Hain C. (1993) Assessment of frontal lobe functioning in schizophrenia and unipolar major depression. *Psychopathology* 26:76–84

Fromm-Auch, D. (1983) Neuropsychological assessment of depressed patients before and after drug therapy: Clinical profile interpretation. In: Flor-Henry, P. and Gruzelier, J., eds. *Laterality and Psychopathology*. Amsterdam: Elsevier, pp. 83–102.

Geffen, G.M., Bate, A., Wright, M.J., and Geffen, L.B. (1993) A comparison of cognitive impairments in dementia of the Alzheimer's type and depression in the elderly. *Dementia* 4:294–300.

Georgieff, N., Dominey, P.F., Michel, F., Marie-Cardine, M., and Dalery, J. (1998) Anomia in major depressive state. *Psychiatry Res* 77:197–208

Ghozlan, A. and Widlocher, D. (1989) Decision time and movement time in depression: differential effects of practice before and after clinical improvement. *Percept Mot Skills* 68:187–192.

Hart, R.P., Kwentus, J.A., Hamer, R.M., and Taylor, J.R. (1987) Selective reminding procedure in depression and dementia. *Psych Aging* 2:111–115.

Hart, R.P., Kwentus, J.A., Taylor, J.R., and Harkins S.W. (1987) Rate of forgetting in dementia and depression. *J Consult Clin Psychol* 55:101–105.

Hartlage, S., Alloy, L.B., Vazquez, C.V., and Dykman, B.M. (1993) Automatic and effortful processing in depression. *Psychol Bull* 113:247–278.

Hartlage, S., Alloy, L.B., Vazquez, C.V., and Dykman, B.M. (1993) Automatic and effortful processing in depression. *Psychol Bull* 113:247–278.

Heaton, R.K., Grant, I., and Matthews, C.G. (1991) *Comprehensive norms for an expanded Halstead-Reitan Battery* Odessa: Psychological Resources Inc.

Jorm, A.F. (2001) History of depression as a risk factor for dementia: an updated review. *Aust NZ J Psychiatry* 35:776–781.

Jorm, A.F. and Jolley, D. (1998) The incidence of dementia: a meta-analysis. *Neurology* 51:728–733.

Jorm, A.F., Christensen, H., Korten, A.E., Jacomb, P.A., and Henderson, A.S. (2001) Memory complaints as a precursor of memory impairment in older people: a longitudinal analysis over 7–8 years. *Psychol Med* 31:441–449.

Kaszniak, A.W. and Christenson, G.D. (1994) Differential diagnosis of dementia and depression. In: Storandt, M., and and Vanden-Bos, G.R., eds. *Neuropsychological Assessment of Dementia and Depression in Older Adults: A Clinician's Guide*. Washington, DC: American Psychological Association, pp. 81–117.

Keilp, J.G., Sackeim, H.A., Brodsky, B., Oquendo, M.A., Malone, K.M., and Mann, J.J. (2001) Neuropsychological dysfunction in depressed suicide attempters. *Am J Psychiatry* 158:735–741.

Kinderman, S.S. and Brown G.G. (1997) Depression and memory in the elderly: A meta-analysis. *J Clin Exp Neuropsychol* 19:625–642.

Kindermann, S.S., Kalayam, B., and Brown, G.G. (2000) Executive functions and P300 latency in elderly depressed patients and control subjects. *Am J Geriatr Psychiatry* 8:57–65.

King, D.A. and Caine, E.D. (1996) Cognitive impairment in major depression. In: Grant, I., and Adams, K.M., eds. *Neuropsychological Assessment of Neuropsychiatric Disorders*, Second Edition ed. New York: Oxford University Press, pp. 200–217.

King, D.A., Caine, E.D., Conwell, Y., and Cox, C. (1991a) The neuropsychology of depression in the elderly: a comparative study of normal aging and Alzheimer's disease. *J Neuropsychiatry Clin Neurosci* 3:163–168.

King, D.A., Caine, E.D., Conwell, Y., and Cox, C. (1991b) Predicting severity of depression in the elderly at six month follow-up: A neuropsychological study. *J Neuropsychiatry Clin Neurosci* 3:64–66.

King, D.A., Caine, E.D., and Cox, C. (1993) Influence of depression and age on selected cognitive functions. *Clin Neuropsychol* 7:443–453.

King, D.A., Cox, C., Lyness, J.M., and Caine, E.D. (1995) Neuropsychological effects of depression and age in an elderly sample: A confirmatory study. *Neuropsychology* 9:399–408.

La Rue, A. (1989) Patterns of performance on the Fuld Object Memory Evaluation in elderly inpatients with depression or dementia. *J Clin Exp Neuropsychol* 11:409–422.

Lezak, M.D. (1995) *Neuropsychological Assessment*. New York: Oxford University Press.

Miller, W.R. (1975) Psychological deficit in depression. *Psychol Bull* 82:238–260.

Nebes, R.D., Butters, M.A., Mulsant, B.H., Pollack, B.G., Zmuda, M.D., Houck, P.R., and Reynolds, C.F., III (2000) Decreased working memory and processing speed mediate cognitive impairment in geriatric depression. *Psychol Med* 30:679–691.

Niederhe, G. and Camp, C.J. (1985) Signal detection analysis of recognition memory in depressed elderly. *Exp Aging Res* 11:207–213.

Nussbaum, P.D. (1998) General assessment issues for a geriatric population. In: Nussbaum, P.D., and Snyder, P.J., eds. *Clinical Neuropsychology: Pocket handbook of Assessment*. American Psychological Association: Washington D.C, pp. 122–130.

Palsson, S., Johansson, B., Berg, S., and Skoog, I. (2000) A population study on the influence of depression on neuropsychological functioning in 85-year-olds. *Acta Psychiatr Scand* 101:185–193.

Raskin, A. (1986) Partialing out the effects of depression and age on cognitive functions: Experimental data and methodologic issues. In: Poon, L.W., ed. *Handbook for Clinical Memory Assessment of Older Adults*. Washington, DC: American Psychological Association, pp. 244–256.

Richards, P.M. and Ruff, R.M (1989) Motivational effects on neuropsychological functioning: Comparison of depressed versus nondepressed individuals. *J Consult Clin Psychol* 57:396–402.

Rogers, J., Lees, A.J., Smith, E., Trimble, M., and Stern, G.M. (1987) Bradyphrenia in Parkinson's disease and psychomotor retardation in depressive illness. An experimental study. *Brain* 110:761–776.

Sabbe, B.G.C., Hulstijn, W., Van Hoof, J.J.M., Tuynman-Qua, H.G., and Zitman, F.G. (1999) Retardation in depression: assessment by means of simple motor tasks. *J Affect Disord* 55:39–44.

Sackeim, H.A., Freeman, J., McElhiney, M., Coleman, E., Prudic, J., and Devanand, D.P. (1992) Effects of major depression on estimates of intelligence. *J Clin Exp Neuropsychol* 14:268–288.

Sackeim, H.A., and Steif, B.L. (1988) The neuropsychology of depression and mania. In: Georgotas, A. and and Cancro, R., eds. *Depression and Mania*. New York: Elsevier, pp. 265–289.

Shelline, Y.I., Sanghavi, M., Mintun, M.A., and Gado, M.H. (1999) Depression duration but not age predicts hippocampal volume loss in medically healthy women with recurrent major depression. *J Neurosci* 19:5034–5043.

Shelline, Y.I., Wang, P.W., Gado, M.H., Csernansky, J.G., and Vannier, M. (1996) Hippocampal atrophy in recurrent major depression. *Proc Natl Acad Sci USA* 93:3908–3913.

Sobin, C. and Sackeim, H.A. (1997) Psychomotor symptoms of depression. *Am J Psychiatry* 154:4–17.

Steif, B.L., Sackeim, H.A., Portnoy, S., Decina, P., and Malitz, S. (1986) Effects of depression and ECT on anterograde memory. *Biol Psychiatry* 21:921–930.

Steingart, A. and Herrmann, N. (1991) Major depressive disorder in the elderly: The relationship between age of onset and cognitive impairment. *Int J Geriatr Psychiatry* 6:593–598.

Tarbuck, A.F. and Paykel, E.S. (1995) Effects of major depression on the cognitive function of younger and older subjects. *Psychol Med* 25:285–295.

U.S. Department of Health and Human Services. (1999) *Mental Health: A Report of the Surgeon General*. Rockville, MD: U.S. Department of Health and Human Services, Substance Abuse and Mental Health Services Administration, Center for Mental Health Services, National Institutes of Health, National Institute of Mental Health.

Veiel, H.O.F. (1997) A preliminary profile of neuropsychological deficits associated with major depression. *J Clin Exp Neuropsychol* 19:587–603.

Weingartner, H., Cohen, R.M., Murphy, D.L., Martello, J., and Gerdt, C. (1981) Cognitive processes in depression. *Arch Gen Psychiatry* 38:42–47.

Zakzanis, K. K., Leach, L., and Kaplan, E. (1999) *Neuropsychological Differential Diagnosis*. Swets and Zeitlinger: Lisse, The Netherlands.

# 11 | Structural and functional brain imaging in late-life depression

HAROLD A. SACKEIM

Depressive syndromes carry a lifetime risk, as they can be experienced for the first time at any age. Furthermore, the identification, diagnosis, and treatment of depressive disorders in the elderly can be problematic given the age-related changes in the profile of depressive symptoms, the frequency of co-morbid medical conditions, medication intolerance, and other factors (Lebowitz et al., 1997). Depression in late life has been viewed by some as a natural consequence of aging, and as often reflecting psychological reactions to incapacities and interpersonal loss. However, it is now well established that abnormalities in the structure and function of the brain are especially common in patients with late-life depression and that these deficits cannot be attributed to the normal aging process. Indeed, there are suggestions that some neuroanatomical and functional abnormalities are most frequent or severe in patients with late-onset major depression, that is, those who have their first episode after 50–60 years of age. This is of both conceptual and clinical importance.

At the conceptual level, the brain abnormalities observed in late-life depression might easily be attributed to the sequelae of a lifetime of repeated episodes of mood disorder and prolonged exposure to psychiatric interventions. Indeed, there is evidence, albeit controversial, suggesting that a greater cumulative lifetime experience of a depressed state is associated with a greater reduction in hippocampal volume (atrophy) and more marked verbal memory deficit (MacQueen et al., 2003; Sheline et al., 1996, 1999). These alterations are usually thought to arise from atrophic (neurotoxic) effects of excessive stimulation of glucocorticoid receptors during the depressed state as a result of hyperactivity of the hypothalamic-pituitary-adrenal (HPA) axis (Lupien et al., 1999; McEwen, 2001; McEwen and Lasley, 2003). In turn, since the HPA axis is a closed-loop endocrine system, with the hippocampus having an important role in its regulation, it is conceivable that a progressive downward spiral (negative feedback loop) is triggered, with states of depression producing the atrophic structural brain changes that lead to increased stress vulnerability, greater dyscontrol of glucocorticoid release,

and more frequent, severe, or treatment-resistant episodes of depression (Sheline, 2003).

In contrast, there are strong indications that some structural brain abnormalities, especially white matter hyperintensities on magnetic resonance imaging (MRI) examination, are more evident in elderly patients with late- than early-onset illness (see Sackeim, 2001a, for a review). Since patients with late-onset depression are often naive to psychiatric treatments and, by definition, have a limited history of being in the depressed state, it is likely that their pattern of brain abnormalities is more a reflection of the pathoetiological factors that produce the major depression than an adverse consequence of being depressed.

Thus, from the outset, it is important to entertain the possibility that biological *disturbances*, distinct in degree or kind, may characterize normal aging, the conditions that result in first episodes of depression late in life, and the sequelae of states of depression. In turn, our understanding of the nature of the biological abnormalities seen in late-life depression is leading to new perspectives on their prevention, diagnosis, and treatment.

## BRAIN STRUCTURAL ABNORMALITIES: MAGNETIC RESONANCE IMAGING HYPERINTENSITIES

Compared to healthy volunteers and other neuropsychiatric groups, high rates of abnormality have been consistently reported in MRI studies of individuals with late-life major depressive disorder (MDD) (see Sackeim et al., 2001a, for a review). The abnormal findings reflect areas of increased signal intensity in balanced, $T_2$-weighted, and fluid-attenuated inversion recovery (FLAIR) images. $T_1$-weighted sequences are used to maximize the contrast between gray and white matter, and they provide fine anatomical detail. In contrast, $T_2$-weighted and FLAIR sequences are particularly sensitive to water and readily identify fluid-filled areas. These fluid-filled areas appear as bright spots, accounting for the term *hyperintensity* (HI, an area of increased signal) and the original characterization of these abnormalities as *unidentified bright objects* (UBOs).

The abnormalities are classified into three major groups, although finer divisions are possible. Periventricular hyperintensities (PVH) are haloes or rims adjacent to ventricles that in severe forms invade the surrounding deep white matter. Caps at the top or bottom of the ventricles are normal variants and likely reflect cerebrospinal fluid (CSF) flow into the ventricles. A thin, hyperintense lining of the walls of the ventricles is also a normal variant.

Alternatively, single patchy or confluent foci may be observed in subcortical white matter (deep white matter hyperintensity: DWMH), with or without PVH. The deep white matter, composed of myelinated axons connecting cortical and subcortical regions, comprises a largely unmapped expanse. Hyperintensities in this region may be scattered and small in diameter or volume. They may also extend in mass from the lining of the ventricles into the deep white matter and may occupy signficant volume.

Hyperintensities may also be found in deep gray structures, particularly the basal ganglia, thalamus, and pons. There is no clear division between MRI findings of HIs in subcortical gray matter structures and silent lacunar infarction.

As a group, these abnormalities have been referred to as *leukoencephalopathy, leukoaraiosis, subcortical arteriosclerotic encephalopathy, encephalomalacia,* and UBOs. The preface *leuko* stems from the Greek for "white." But the abnormalities in late-life depression are not restricted to the white matter. The etiology of the HIs in MDD is not established, and they may have more than one set of determinants. Thus, their characterization as reflecting an arteriosclerotic encephalopathy is either premature or erroneous. Instead, the term *encephalomalacia* is used here.

Figure 11.1 illustrates a moderate to severe case of encephalomalacia. It consists of FLAIR images from a patient with late-onset, first-episode major depression treated at the Late-Life Depression Research Clinic of the New York State Psychiatric Institute and Columbia University. The image on the left illustrates PVH, with thick bands of high signal intensity (white) adjacent to the lateral ventricles. On the left side of this image, the HIs are extending into the deep white matter. The image on the right is at a higher MRI slice from the same patient and shows multiple confluent HIs through the deep white matter (DWMH). As discussed below, in patients presenting with these MRI findings, clinicians often receive radiological reports that emphasize small vessel ischemic disease.

This patient illustrates the difficulties in classifying the HIs. The DWMH seen in this patient is simply an extension of the HIs surrounding the ventricles. In three-dimensional space, the PVH and DWMH form

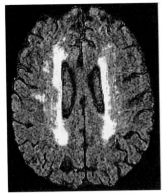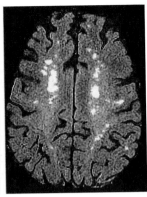

FIGURE 11.1 Magnetic resonance imaging (MRI) fluid-attenuated inversion recovery (FLAIR) images of a patient with late-onset major depression. White or bright areas show MRI hyperintensities. The image on the left demonstrates periventricular hyperintensities (PVH), with a broad band of increased signal adjacent to the lateral ventricles and invading the deep white matter. The image on the right, from the same patient at a higher level, shows multiple confluent foci of hyperintensities in the deep white matter (centrum semiovale).

single units, and classifying them as distinct phenomena seems questionable. In addition, there is keen interest in determining the anatomical specificity of the HIs in MDD (Greenwald et al., 1998). It would be of great interest if a specific set of fiber tracts were invaded in individuals who presented with MDD, while HIs in other deep white matter areas did not manifest with mood disorder. Unfortunately, most attempts to examine the anatomical specificity of HIs in MDD have had to resort to crude characterization in terms of brain quadrants, that is, anterior versus posterior and left versus right. This limitation results from an absence of clear-cut landmarks in the deep white matter or other means of establishing more refined localization.

In one of the largest and earliest prospective MRI series in MDD, all 51 elderly patients (age >60 years) referred for electroconvulsive therapy (ECT) presented with HIs, with over half of the patients rated as having moderate to severe encephalomalacia. Furthermore, 51% had lesions of subcortical gray nuclei (Coffey et al., 1990). These rates of abnormality greatly exceeded those found in a healthy control group, and basal ganglia HIs were the most discriminative (Figure 11.2). The depressed samples studied to date have often included patients with co-morbid medical illness and without adequate control for cerebrovascular disease (CVD) risk factors, medications, or drug abuse. Nonetheless, in the report by Coffey et al. (1990), when MDD patients with preexisting neurological conditions were excluded, the rate of encephalomalacia greatly exceeded that of normal controls. In a replication study, MDD patients had marked increases in the frequency of PVH, DWMH, and basal ganglia and thalamic HI relative to controls matched for CVD risk factors (Coffey et al.,

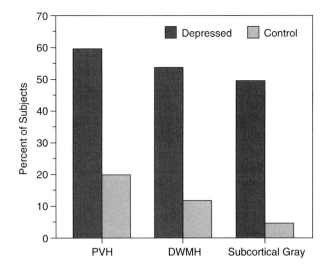

FIGURE 11.2 A representation of the findings of Coffey et al. (1990). The percentage of patients with major depression and control subjects are contrasted in rates of periventricular hyperintensities (PVH), deep white matter hyperintensities (DWMH), and hyperintensities in subcortical gray matter structures.

1993). The age-adjusted odds ratio for PVH was 5.32. In other, often large population studies of elderly healthy controls, when the halo or caps commonly at the top and bottom of the lateral ventricles are excluded, approximately 10%–30% present with MRI white matter abnormalities, with typically mild severity and low rates of subcortical gray matter abnormalities (e.g., Breteler et al., 1994a).

The rate or severity of encephalomalacia in late-life depression may equal or exceed that observed in Alzheimer's disease (AD) (e.g., Erkinjuntti et al., 1994) and may be comparable to that in multi-infarct dementia (e.g., Zubenko et al., 1990; see Sackeim et al., 2000, for a review). In considerably younger samples, several groups have reported that MRI HIs are more common among young bipolar patients than controls (e.g., Dupont et al., 1990, 1995; Swayze et al., 1990). Aylward et al. (1994) found that older (>38 years) and not younger bipolar patients had an excess of HIs. Brown et al. (1992) did not detect an excess in young bipolar patients, although they did observe that severe HIs were overrepresented in elderly patients with MDD.

In general, it important to note that excessive HIs may have different causes and associations in bipolar and unipolar mood disorders. Abnormal HIs are an age-related phenomenon in unipolar depression, and abnormalities are most manifest in late life. In contrast, abnormal HIs have been observed with some regularity in adolescent and young adult bipolar patients. In addition, as discussed below, in unipolar depression a central thread of findings suggests that abnormal HIs are linked to late-onset depression, a low rate of posi-

tive family history of mood disorder, and CVD risk factors. The initial studies in bipolar illness have not observed these associations. Thus, the possibility should be kept in mind that the etiological and pathophysiological meaning of HIs may differ in the two forms of affective illness.

## CLINICAL CORRELATES

Specific clinical and historical features of depressive illness appear to be associated with encephalomalacia. Coffey et al. (1990, 1993) were the first to suggest that medication-resistant patients and those with late-onset MDD (onset ≥60 years) were at increased risk. However, the patients in these studies were consecutive referrals to an ECT service and were atypical in that the rate of late-onset depression was found to be 80%. Further, 86% were said to be medication resistant. Many patients are incorrectly classified as having late-onset disease when formal interviews are not conducted with the patients and family members to detect episodes earlier in life. Similarly, the most common reason for referral to ECT, including patients with late-life depression, is resistance to antidepressant medication. However, when patient records are exhaustively examined and previous providers are contacted to document the treatment history, it is common to find that the majority of ECT recipients had not received a single adequate medication trial during the current episode. Indeed, the criteria for medication resistance used in the work by Coffey and colleagues were not consistent with current standards for medication dosage and duration (Sackeim, 2001b) and included medication-intolerant patients.

### Age-at-Onset

Several studies have found an association between encephalomalacia and age-at-onset of depressive illness. Lesser et al. (1991) reported an excess of large DWMH in patients with late-onset psychotic depression compared to normal controls. Figiel et al. (1991) found that a higher rate of caudate HI and large DWMH distinguished late- from early-onset MDD in a small sample of unipolar patients. In a larger sample, Hickie et al. (1995) found that late age-at-onset and a negative family history of mood disorder were associated with more severe DWMH. In relatively small samples of elderly MDD patients and controls with an equivalent frequency of CVD risk factors, Krishnan et al. (1993) found that late-onset illness was associated with smaller volumes of the caudate and lenticular nuclei and a greater frequency and severity of DWMH.

In a subsequent study, Krishnan et al. (1997) compared 32 elderly MDD patients with encephalomalacia to 57 MDD patients without encephalomalacia. After controlling for age, the group characterized by MRI abnormalities had later age-at-onset and tended to have a lower rate of positive family history for mood disorder. Lesser et al. (1996) also found that, independent of current age, patients with late-onset MDD had larger areas of white matter HI than patients with early-onset (<35 years) recurrent MDD. Fujikawa et al. (1994) found a higher rate of *silent cerebral infarctions* in late- compared to early-onset MDD. Patients with these large HIs also had a lower rate of family history of mood disorder. Dahabra et al. (1998) compared small groups of early- and late-onset elderly patients who had recovered from an episode of MDD. White matter HIs were more common in the late-onset group, as was ventricular enlargement. Salloway et al. (1996) compared 15 MDD patients with late onset (>60 years) to 15 MDD patients with early onset (<60 years) using semi-automated measures of DWMH and PVH area. A marked difference was observed, with the late-onset group having twice the subcortical HI of the early-onset group. O'Brien et al. (1996) also reported that DWMH were most common in severely affected inpatients with late-onset MDD.

Thus, a large number of independent investigations reported either a higher prevalence or a greater severity of encephalomalacia in late- relative to early-onset depression, with comparatively few negative findings (e.g., Dupont et al., 1995; Ebmeier et al., 1997; Greenwald et al., 1996). There is also a suggestion, less consistently observed, that MDD patients with these MRI abnormalities are less likely to have a positive family history of mood disorder.

## Severity and Nature of Depressive Symptoms

With notable exceptions, the MRI research on encephalomalacia in MDD has concentrated on inpatients with severe symptoms often referred for ECT. Generalizability to the far more common MDD in outpatients needs to be established, particularly since symptom severity has not been found to correlate with encephalomalacia. There is also no indication of a difference in rates or severity of encephalomalacia in psychotic and nonpsychotic depression. Indeed, Krishnan et al. (1997) reported that patients with encephalomalacia were less likely to have psychotic symptoms but more likely to present with anhedonia. Phenomenological differences as a function of encephalomalacia has rarely been examined.

## Treatment Response and Long-Term Outcome

Coffey et al. (1990) suggested that patients with encephalomalacia had a positive response to ECT, but improvement was evaluated retrospectively and only glob-

ally. In contrast, Hickie et al. (1995) reported that severe DWMH predicted a poorer outcome in patients with MDD treated with either heterogeneous pharmacological regimens or ECT. In a retrospective study, Fujikawa et al. (1996) found that patients with severe silent cerebral infarction (both perforating and cortical areas) had a longer hospital stay and a poorer response to antidepressant medications than MDD patients without infarction. In a study of 44 MDD patients between 65 and 85 years of age, Simpson et al. (1997) found that the globally assessed short-term clinical outcome was poorer in patients with DWMH and HIs in the basal ganglia or pons. Recently, the Duke University group that earlier had claimed to achieve a strong response to ECT in patients with encephalomalacia (Coffey et al., 1990) found that more severe HIs were associated with a poorer ECT outcome (Steffens et al., 2001). In particular, subcortical gray matter HIs, but not PVH or DWMH, were linked to the short-term outcome with ECT.

There has been no report of a prospective study testing the prognostic significance of these structural abnormalities and using a standardized pharmacological protocol, let alone a single medication. The available evidence is largely consistent, however, in suggesting that encephalomalacia is associated with a poorer short-term response to antidepressant treatments. Thus, particularly aggressive treatment regimens may be needed in patients with moderate or severe encephalomalacia.

In a sample of 37 patients followed for an average of 14 months, Hickie et al. (1997) provided the first evidence that encephalomalacia in MDD predicts a poor long-term outcome. Late age-at-onset, DWMH, and cerebrovascular risk factors were each associated with unremitting depressive symptoms (chronic depression) and cognitive decline, with a subgroup developing vascular dementia.

The linkage between encephalomalacia and a poor long-term outcome was supported in other work. O'Brien et al. (1998) followed 60 MDD patients over 55 years of age for an average of 32 months. Time to relapse of depressive symptoms and cognitive decline were the principal outcome measures. Patients with severe white matter HI at baseline (DWMH) had a median survival time of only 136 days compared to 315 days in those without severe HI. A 5-year follow-up of patients with MDD reported that the volume of gray matter HIs at baseline was three times greater in patients who later developed dementia than in patients without this finding (Steffens et al., 2000).

In light of the recurrent and often chronic nature of MDD, and given the evidence that depressive symptoms in the elderly may be prodromal or a risk factor for dementing conditions, further investigation of the prognostic significance of encephalomalacia is clearly needed.

## Adverse Side Effects

Elderly MDD patients with basal ganglia HIs may be prone to develop delirium when treated with antidepressant medications or ECT (Figiel et al., 1989, 1990). However, these reports by Figiel and colleagues were based on very small samples and did not examine the specificity of the relation with basal ganglia HIs by testing for associations with HIs in other subcortical or white matter areas.

Fujikawa et al. (1996) retrospectively assessed the relationships of silent cerebral infarction to adverse effects and the response to pharmacotherapy in MDD patients over the age of 50. Patients with silent infarctions had a higher incidence of central nervous system (CNS) adverse events, and the frequency of adverse events increased with the severity of infarction.

## Cognition and Neurological Signs

Some degree of encephalomalacia is common among normal, nonsymptomatic subjects, with the prevalence and severity of HIs strongly related to age. Initially, it had been unclear whether the limited degree of encephalomalacia in normal samples is associated with cognitive impairment, and there was a suggestion that there should be a threshold effect for HI volume (Boone et al., 1992). Nonetheless, there has been a concentration of replicated findings in normal and neurological samples associating encephalomalacia with deficits in attention, motor speed, and executive function (e.g., Breteler et al., 1994b; see Sackeim et al., 2000, for a review). These are hallmark areas of deficit in MDD in the elderly (Sackeim and Steif, 1988; Chapter 10 of this volume). In nonpsychiatric patient samples, the most common neurological abnormalities associated with encephalomalacia are gait disturbances, a tendency to fall, the extensor plantar reflex, and primitive reflexes.

Surprisingly, there has been limited investigation of the neuropsychological correlates of encephalomalacia in MDD. Ebmeier et al. (1997) found that severity of DWMH was inversely related to global cognitive function (Mini-Mental State scores) in elderly patients with MDD. In the most comprehensive study to date, Lesser et al. (1996) contrasted 60 late-onset (>50 years of age) MDD patients, 35 early-onset (<35 years of age) MDD patients, and 165 normal controls. All subjects were at least 50 years of age. The late-onset group had greater DWMH than either of the other groups. Cognitive deficits were most marked in the late-onset group and pertained to nonverbal intelligence, nonverbal memory, constructional ability, executive function, and speed of processing. Patients with greater severity of DWMH had significantly poorer executive function.

Jenkins et al. (1998) found that elderly MDD patients with HIs showed poorer performance on a number of learning and memory indices, with the pattern of deficits resembling that in subcortical degenerative disorders (i.e., Huntington's and Parkinson's diseases). Simpson et al. (1997) conducted neuropsychological assessment following treatment of an elderly MDD sample. Pontine HIs were associated with reduced psychomotor speed, basal ganglia HIs were linked to impaired category productivity (executive function), and PVH was associated with recall deficits. Since the severity of encephalomalacia in this study was also associated with the clinical outcome, the findings regarding neuropsychological correlates may have been confounded with the clinical state. There is clearly a need for comprehensive neuropsychological and neurological evaluations of elderly MDD patients in relation to structural and functional imaging deficits.

## ETIOLOGY OF ENCEPHALOMALACIA

### Neuropathology: Linkage to Cerebrovascular Disease

The pathogenesis of the MRI abnormalities in MDD is unknown. In other samples, these abnormalities usually have been attributed to ischemic CVD, with the HIs reflecting increased water content in the perivascular space, axon and myelin loss, astrocyte proliferation (gliosis), and/or frank infarction (e.g., Awad et al., 1986c; Chimowitz et al., 1992; Van Swieten et al., 1991). Typically, the HIs are in watershed areas supplied by small arterioles that branch off long, penetrating medullary and lenticulostriate arteries. These areas receive a limited collateral supply and are particularly vulnerable to vascular insult. In all the populations studied, including MDD patients and normal controls, age has been the most critical correlate. To a lesser extent, these abnormalities are also associated in these populations with hypertension, diabetes, coronary heart disease, or other vascular risk factors (e.g., Awad et al., 1986b; Breteler et al., 1994a; Coffey et al., 1990).

In a study of patients with AD, frank CVD at 1 year of follow-up was observed only in those patients with baseline CT white matter lucencies on computed tomography (CT) (Lopez et al., 1992). In 215 patients with lacunar infarction, prospective 3-year follow-up indicated that baseline encephalomalacia predicted subsequent stroke, new-onset dementia, and death (Miyao et al., 1992). Several other recent studies indicate that encephalomalacia predicts subsequent stroke, myocardial infarction, and vascular death (e.g., Tarvonen-Schroder et al., 1995). Boiten et al. (1993) found a considerably higher rate of encephalomalacia in patients with asymptomatic lacunar infarcts than in patients with symptomatic lacunar infarcts (odds ratio: 10:7). These groups differed in the location and implicated vascular territories of the infarcts, with the suggestion offered that ischemia due to arteriosclerosis leads to encephalomalacia and silent lacunar infarcts, while microatheromatosis more commonly produces symptomatic lacunar infarcts. There is also evidence of greater 24-hour variability in blood pressure among patients with HIs, suggesting periodic ischemic compromise.

The induction of similar-appearing $T_2$-weighted abnormalities in animals is now done via middle cerebral artery (MCA) occlusion. Awad et al. (1993) reported the first prospective de novo appearance of DWMH in humans. Despite full anticoagulation, four of eight patients undergoing therapeutic internal carotid artery (ICA) occlusion (detachable balloon technique) developed ipsilateral subcortical HIs. Overall, this large array of findings supports a vascular etiology for the HIs, and especially an ischemic process. Awad et al.'s (1986c) suggestion of état criblé is also compatible. Pulsation in ectatic or tortuous blood vessels, rigidified by arteriosclerosis, may mechanically increase water-filled perivascular spaces or produce the same effect, with parenchymal atrophy, due to ischemic substrate supply.

In contrast, some types of PVH may be due to CSF leakage into surrounding tissue. As indicated, caps at the horns of the lateral ventricles are common in normal persons, may not be age related, and may be due to interstitial flow into ventricles combined with low myelin content and ependymitis granularis. Therefore, including caps in encephalomalacia ratings can lead to high false-positive rates.

There has been considerable histopathological investigation of the HIs but only one study in MDD (Thomas et al., 2002). The findings generally support a vascular etiology, as areas of MRI HI in neurological and normal samples commonly show arteriolar hyalinization, ectasia, enlarged perivascular (Virchow-Robin) space, gliosis, spongiosis, and/or lacunar infarcts (e.g., Awad et al., 1986c; Chimowitz et al., 1992). Van Swieten et al. (1991) found that DWMH was invariably accompanied by demyelination and gliosis, and less consistently with increased perivascular space. The demyelination was strongly associated with increased wall thickness of small arterioles. The authors concluded that arteriosclerosis in small arterioles ($<150$ $\mu$m) is the primary cause, leading to demyelination followed by cell loss with progression. Munoz et al. (1993) suggested that some pathological changes could also be due to microaneurysm at the points of arteriole bifurcation resulting in leakage of serum proteins (edema). Fazekas et al. (1993) observed that the size and appearance of MRI-defined PVH and DWMH were strongly associated with the extent of ischemic tissue damage. Moody et al. (1995) offered the novel findings that venous collagenosis is strongly associated with encephalomalacia. They found marked thickening of periventricular postcapillary venules and collecting veins that provide drainage of the centrum semiovale,

and suggested that disordered venous drainage results in distal chronic ischemia and brain edema.

Thomas et al. (2002) conducted the first neuropathological investigation of encephalomalacia in individuals with a history of MDD. In vitro MRI scans were obtained from three sections of brain tissue, two sections in frontal regions and one occipital section. The tissues were derived from 20 elderly individuals with a history of major depression and 20 matched controls. The scans were rated blind to group membership, and the sections were subject to MRI under neuropathological examination and staining for microglia, macrophages, and astroglia. Specifically, HIs on the scans were identified in the tissue and classified into lesions reflecting ischemic and nonischemic processes.

Upon unblinding, Thomas et al. (2002) found that all the DWMH in the depressed sample were ischemic, compared to less than a third of these lesions among the controls ($p < .001$). The difference between the groups was largely attributable to small punctate, and not larger confluent, lesions ($<3$ mm). The small lesions, corresponding to small HIs often dismissed in radiological examination, were mostly ischemic in the depressed but not in the control sample. In contrast, larger lesions were commonly ischemic in both groups. Compared with the control sample, ischemic lesions in the depressed sample were more likely to be in the dorsolateral prefrontal cortex relative to either the anterior cingulate cortex or the occipital cortex. These investigators concluded appropriately that the study strongly supported the concept that an ischemic CVD process is common in late-life depression, with the implication that this process is of pathoetiological importance.

The notion that late-life depression is associated with ischemic vascular disease was recently supported in an earlier postmortem study focusing on the expression of intercellular adhesion molecule-1 (ICAM-1). This is a vascular marker of inflammation, whose expression is increased by ischemia. Thomas et al. (2000) assayed ICAM-1 in the dorsolateral prefrontal cortex (DLPFC) and occipital cortex in 20 deceased individuals over the age of 60 with a history of MDD and 20 comparison subjects. Expression of ICAM-1 was significantly greater in DLPFC gray and white matter of the depressed group, with no difference in occipital cortex. This finding, in addition to reinforcing the *vascular hypothesis* for late-life depression, is compatible with the well-replicated findings that the DLPFC is a common site for reduced regional cerebral blood flow (rCBF) and regional cerebral metabolic rate for glucose ($rCMR_{glu}$) in MDD (see below).

## Pathophysiology of Encephalomalacia

One way of testing the view that encephalomalacia reflects local ischemic damage is to quantify rCBF and other metabolic processes in the areas corresponding to MRI HIs. Until recently, no study had coregistered high-resolution functional and structural images and quantified perfusion and/or metabolism in the areas of asymptomatic MRI-defined HI. Such research is in progress by our group. However, in recent years, at least 20 studies have examined more general perfusion or metabolic abnormalities in samples characterized by varying degrees of encephalomalacia.

Meguro et al. (1990) conducted one of the key studies, using positron emission tomography (PET) with the $^{15}$O-PET steady-state method to quantify rCBF, cerebral metabolic rate for oxygen (rCMRO$_2$), oxygen extraction fraction (rOEF), and cerebral blood volume (rCBV) in 28 asymptomatic individuals with CVD risk factors. More severe PVH was associated with global reductions in gray matter CBF and in the CBF/CBV ratio, with the latter parameter free of partial volume effects (e.g., contamination of gray matter values by effects of nearby white matter and vice versa). In contrast, OEF tended to increase with severe PVH, and there was a trend for reduced global CMRO$_2$ only with increasing PVH. These effects were consistent across gray matter regions and, critically, suggested a compensatory mismatch between metabolism and CBF (*misery perfusion*). As CBF (tissue perfusion) declined, OEF (oxygen extraction) increased to maintain metabolic rate.

De Reuck et al. (1992), also using the $^{15}$O-PET steady-state method, reported similar findings. White matter CT lucencies were associated with reduced CBF in frontal and parietal gray and white matter in both demented and normal subjects. Particularly in frontal white matter, the encephalomalacia was associated with increased OEF, with greater reductions in rCBF than in rCMRO$_2$. Similarly, Hatazawa et al. (1997) compared 8 normal subjects without encephalomalacia and 15 asymptomatic individuals with white matter HIs using H$_2$$^{15}$O, C$^{15}$O, and $^{15}$O$_2$ PET. White matter HIs were associated with reduced CBF and increased OEF in the cerebral white matter and basal ganglia, without effects in the thalamus.

In the only similar study in MDD, Lesser et al. (1994) reported a tendency for patients with large areas of white matter HIs to have the greatest deficits in whole brain CBF. Of note, in this elderly sample (>60 years), whole brain CBF was markedly diminished across the MDD group and the subgroup with HIs had the largest deficit.

Promoting vasodilation through the use of a hypercapnic challenge (e.g., carbon dioxide inhalation) should be a particularly useful method to investigate the pathophysiology of encephalomalacia. Brown et al. (1990), using stable xenon CT, found that, compared to controls, CVD patients with encephalomalacia had a diminished white matter CBF response to acetazolamide, an inducer of hypercapnia. In 28 asymptomatic

subjects, Isaka et al. (1993) found that the extent of PVH was marginally related to global gray matter resting CBF ($r = -0.36$) but strongly related to global CBF after hypercapnic challenge with acetazolamide ($r = -0.78$), as well as to the CBF change between rest and hypercapnia ($r = -0.57$). This study linked PVH in asymptomatic individuals to a diffuse reduction in cerebrovascular dilatory capacity (i.e., hemodynamic reserve), suggesting that small vessel disease may not only characterize the territories of the subcortical HI, but may be widespread in the cortical gray matter. Similarly, in a study using technetium-99 hexamethyl propyleneamine oxime ($^{99m}$Tc-HMPAO or HMPAO) single photon computed tomography (SPECT) in patients with unilateral carotid occlusive disease, the severity of DWMH and PVH was linked to resting perfusion deficits, with the associations magnified following acetazolamide (hypercapnic) challenge (Isaka et al., 1997).

Virtually all of the 20 studies of diverse populations (with only 1 in MDD) found relations between MRI white matter HI and measures of perfusion. While CBF deficits in white matter were common, diffuse cortical gray matter deficits were also observed. The findings have consistently linked encephalomalacia to low CBF and increased OEF, suggesting that the relations between the structural and functional deficits are more marked for perfusion than metabolism measures. This has been observed in work assessing both CBF and CMRO$_2$ or CMR$_{glu}$.

It is not known if such uncoupling occurs in geriatric depression. Indeed, it is almost invariably assumed that rCBF deficits in mood disorders reflect disturbed patterns of neuronal activity and not a constrained vascular substrate. In contrast, there is sufficient evidence from other populations to hypothesize that this assumption is false in the case of late-life, or specifically late-onset, depression. Were this the case, one should observe in late-life depressed samples greater deficits in global CBF than global CMR, or at least more widely distributed regional deficits in CBF than in CMR. Further, the findings linking encephalomalacia to a reduced CBF response to hypercapnia suggest both that limited vasodilatory capacity may be an important correlate and that structure–function relations become magnified with hypercapnic (vasodilatory) challenge.

In research near completion at Columbia University, a sample of patients with late-onset major depression and a healthy control sample underwent repeated examinations with MRI and PET (fully quantified rCBF at rest and with hypercapnia and fully quantified rCMR$_{glu}$). The samples were carefully matched for CVD risk factors as well as the usual demographic variables, and both samples were free of psychotropics for at least 3 weeks prior to PET. The initial findings indicate that at pretreatment baseline, the differences between the two samples reflected reduced functional activity in the patients. Furthermore, these differences were more extensive and profound for resting rCBF than rCMR$_{glu}$. In particular, the metabolic deficits in the patient group pertained primarily to posterior cortical regions, while CBF deficits encompassed these areas but also involved extensive areas of prefrontal cortex. These preliminary findings support the notion that an ischemic vascular disease process is common in late-onset major depression and that such patients may manifest a mismatch between blood flow and metabolism. Of note, the patient and control groups did not differ in the volume of HIs. This lack of difference in HI volume may have been due to the careful matching of the patients to controls in CVD risk factors. A key question, not adequately addressed in the literature, is whether, at the epidemiological level, individuals with late-life depression have an excess of CVD risk factors, thus accounting for the presumed excess of HIs, or whether late-life depression presents with excessive HIs over and above any contribution from or associations with CVD risk factors. The preliminary findings from our study support the first possibility. Furthermore, they suggest that in vivo measurements of rCBF may be a better marker of the hypothesized ischemic disease process than MRI HI evidence of structural change or functional measurements of metabolic rate.

## LONGITUDINAL PERSPECTIVE

Across populations, cross-sectional studies have demonstrated that the likelihood and severity of encephalomalacia increase with age. In addition, the possibility that encephalomalacia and perfusion deficits in MDD are progressive deficits is suggested by (1) the associations with CVD risk factors, (2) the follow-up results in neurological samples indicating increased rates of future CVD, functional compromise, and death as a function of baseline encephalomalacia, and (3) the follow-up studies in MDD suggesting that encephalomalacia is associated with a poor outcome in terms of both mood disorder and cognitive status (Hickie et al., 1997; O'Brien et al., 1998a; Steffens et al., 2000), the histopathological findings in the areas containing HI, and the hypothesis of underlying ischemic CVD. Clearly, it is important to determine whether the MRI abnormalities are progressive, reflecting a degenerative disease pattern. Several groups are now conducting MRI studies examining change in encephalomalacia at long-term follow-up in patients with late-life depression. However, the data reported to date have been quite limited, although Krishnan describes new additional findings in Chapter 12.

One study examined the MRIs of MDD patients before and 6 months following ECT (Coffey et al., 1991).

Blind ratings showed strong test-retest stability in HI evaluations, with the only change being a worsening of encephalomalacia in four patients. The follow-up interval was likely too short to observe more frequent MRI changes. In this context, perfusion imaging may provide more sensitive measures of progressive effects than MRI. If ischemia in deep structures leads to encephalomalacia, it should exist prior to MRI evidence of a structural deficit and its quantification should be more sensitive to progressive change.

The findings regarding encephalomalacia in MDD are largely consistent. They suggest that an ischemic small vessel disease (CVD) leads to destruction of white matter tracts and, in some cases, subcortical nuclei. Anatomically, frontal-striatal circuits are most commonly implicated (Coffey et al., 1990; Greenwald et al., 1998).

Establishing that a progressive CVD process contributes to late-onset MDD should have important implications for our understanding of phenomenology, prevention, and treatment. There is controversial evidence that in some patients the course of affective illness becomes more virulent with aging, with shorter periods of euthymia between episodes, more abrupt onset of acute symptoms, and greater resistance to treatment. Late-onset MDD may be particularly treatment-resistant. Treatment of MDD often involves use of agents with potential cardio- and cerebrovascular effects (e.g., tricyclic antidepressants). Conceivably, some of these effects, such as hypotension or reductions in CBF or metabolism, may aggravate a CVD process, and perhaps limit efficacy or enhance side effects. Thus, there is the possibility that some treatments that are effective in suppressing the expression of the acute depressive episode in the long run contribute to disease progression. Finally, tying the functional and structural abnormalities to a CVD process may suggest alternative methods of treatment and new approaches to disease prevention.

## VOLUMETRIC BRAIN STRUCTURAL ABNORMALITIES: VENTRICULAR ENLARGEMENT AND SULCAL PROMINENCE

The earliest studies of structural brain abnormalities in psychiatric disorders concentrated on the area or volume of CSF-filled spaces, most commonly the size of the lateral ventricles and cortical sulcal widening. Particularly in the context of late-life depression, enlarged ventricles and sulcal widening have usually been interpreted as reflecting a nonspecific atrophic process resulting in the loss of brain tissue, as opposed to a developmental dysplasia, reflecting abnormal brain growth.

Scores of studies across the life span have tested whether patients with mood disorders have ventricular enlargement and increased sulcal prominence. Meta-analysis indicates that indeed both are the case, and the ventricular enlargement observed in mood disorder patients is of nearly the same magnitude as in patients with schizophrenia (Elkis et al., 1995). Thus, even outside the context of major depression in late life, there is substantial evidence for loss of brain tissue. Few studies of ventricular enlargement or sulcal prominence have focused on late-life depression. There is some evidence that ventricular enlargement may be especially prominent in late- relative to early-onset geriatric depression (Dahabra et al., 1998). This would reinforce the notion of an active atrophic process.

The possibility must be kept in mind that the evidence for an atrophic brain process in mood disorders could result from a variety of artifacts, including the effects of medications on brain structure. There is substantial evidence that lithium, tricyclic antidepressants, and perhaps monoamine oxidase inhibitors can produce fluid changes and alter cerebral microcirculation. There is a concern that antidepressant or antimanic medications may result in increased extracellular water content, which in turn may result in enlarged fluid-filled spaces, although, if anything, very recent evidence suggests that treatment with lithium may lead to an increase in cerebral gray matter content. While there is fairly compelling evidence that neuroleptic exposure is unrelated to evidence of ventricular enlargement in schizophrenia, the possible confounding effects of prior medication history may be more difficult to rule out in mood disorders. This is of greatest concern in early-onset late-life depression, where patients will have the longest history of exposure to psychotropic agents. Samples of medication-naive depressed patients may often be younger, less severely ill, and perhaps less likely to manifest the relevant brain structural phenomena. However, a variety of investigators have examined the role of medication history by correlating the type and length of previous medication exposure with imaging results. The results have been universally negative. At the same time, it must be recognized that retrospective quantification of lifetime medication exposure may have limited reliability and validity.

## Age and Age-at-Onset

Cross-sectional studies suggest that in normal individuals there appears to be little change in ventricular brain ratio (VBR), the most common measure of lateral ventricular enlargement, between approximately 20 and 60 years of age, while afterward there is a progressive increase. This pattern raises both methodological and conceptual concerns. From a methodological viewpoint, the pattern indicates that the association in normals between age and VBR is nonlinear. However, virtually all the studies across the age span that used age as a covariate in comparisons of mood disorder patients with controls or other psychiatric groups have treated this relation in

a linear manner. Not only may this have resulted in decreased sensitivity in the comparisons (and higher rates of Type II error), but some of the reported findings may be misleading. For example, Dolan et al. (1985) have been the only investigators to date to examine explicitly the interaction effects on VBR between diagnosis of unipolar or bipolar depression and age. This interaction achieved a significance level of 0.18, possibly supporting the possibility that unipolars and bipolars may manifest ventricular enlargement at different age ranges (late in unipolars and early in bipolars), and that a more sensitive data analytic strategy might have revealed a more robust effect. Similarly, the interaction between status as a mood disorder patient (unipolar or bipolar) and age achieved a significance level of 0.14. However, as the authors commented, inspection of the data indicated that it was only in the older age groups that quantitative VBR differences were evident.

Conceptually, there are other suggestions in this literature that emphasize the importance of aging effects. Jacoby and Levy (1980), in a sample 41 mood disorder patients and 50 healthy controls, all over the age of 60, failed to find a difference in average VBR. They noted, however, that nine of the patients (22%) had evidence of ventricular enlargement and that this subgroup was characterized by later onset of illness, older age, and higher mortality at 2-year follow-up than the remaining patients. In a prospective longitudinal study of the normal control community sample of Jacoby and Levy, Bird et al. (1986) found that ventricular enlargement at baseline was predictive of the development of late-onset depression.

In this light, it is conceivable that a subgroup of patients with late-onset depression, typically unipolar, may be especially likely to manifest ventricular enlargement, while ventricular enlargement may also characterize younger bipolar patients. If this were the case, cross-sectional comparison of unipolar and bipolar patients and normal controls in the younger age range would reveal that enlarged VBR is characteristic of bipolar but not unipolar disorder (e.g., Andreasen et al., 1990). At the same time, among older patients there may be no difference between bipolars and unipolars (e.g., Dolan et al., 1985). This type of specification could prove valuable in contributing to our understanding of the etiology of VBR enlargement in mood disorders. Manifestation in younger patients is compatible with the view that ventriculomegaly may reflect neurodevelopmental dysplasia, in which case it should be nonprogressive. Manifestation primarily in older late-onset patients is compatible with an atrophic process, which may or may not be progressive.

## Phenomenology

Other than the distinction between psychotic and nonpsychotic illness, few phenomenological features of depression have been found to correlate significantly with VBR or other structural measures in more than one investigation. There have been surprisingly few attempts to associate VBR with overall severity of depressive illness, as assessed by instruments such as the Hamilton Rating Scale for Depression (HRSD). In the main, such attempts have produced negative results. Schlegel et al. (1989) reported that in 44 medication-free (nonelderly) depressed patients, VBR and width of the third ventricle were associated with scores on the Brief Psychiatric Rating Scale, the Bech-Rafaelsen Melancholia Scale, Global Assessment Scale, the Rating for Emotional Blunting, and the Scale for Assessment of Negative Symptoms. At the same time, these structural measures were not associated with HRSD scores or scores on the Hamilton Rating Scale for Anxiety. Item analyses suggested that ventricular size was most closely associated with retardation-related items. They suggested that scales such as the HRSD may be too multidimensional to reveal a consistent effect, particularly since anxiety symptoms and somatic complaints may obscure relations. For the most part, patient subtyping into *endogenous* and *nonendogenous* or *melancholic* and *nonmelancholic* categories has not revealed structural differences. Several investigators have sought associations between VBR or other brain morphometric measures and a family history of psychiatric illness. No positive findings have been reported.

The significance of delusional or other psychotic symptoms in relation to ventricular enlargement is controversial. Larger VBR in psychotic mood disorder patients was reported by many but not all investigators (see Sackeim and Prohovnik, 1993, for a review). The reasons for this inconsistency are poorly understood, but it should be noted that in many cases sample size has been small. Whatever contribution is made by mood disorders to VBR and related measures, that contribution is difficult to separate from the naturally occurring variability that is substantial in normal samples. When one adds to this the possibility that effects on VBR may be dependent on age groups, gender, and/or other diagnostic subtyping (unipolar vs. bipolar), it is clear that the power to detect effects was severely compromised in much of this literature.

## Cognitive Status

Characteristically, during the acute phase of illness, the performance of patients with major depression or mania is reduced on cognitive tests heavily influenced by the adequacy of attention and concentration (e.g., immediate learning and memory) (Sackeim and Steif, 1988). Furthermore, a small subgroup of patients with major depression show more profound cognitive disturbance, with impaired orientation and global performance deficits in the range of demented patients. This

constellation in depression is usually referred to as *pseudodementia* and is seen almost exclusively in late-life depression. In depressed samples not specifically selected for cognitive impairment, there are scattered findings of inverse associations between VBR and specific cognitive measures, as well as a variety of negative findings (see Sackeim and Prohovnik, 1993, for a review). For instance, there has been a report that the degree of residual cognitive impairment following recovery from depression in an elderly sample was positively associated with VBR obtained 2 years earlier during the acute depressive phase.

Perhaps a more powerful methodology is to contrast structural findings in depressed patients with and without prominent cognitive impairment. Pearlson et al. (1989) identified 15 depressed patients who were cognitively impaired at admission and 11 patients who were unimpaired, using a cutoff of 24 on the Mini-Mental State Examination for this designation. These 26 depressed patients were all older than 60 years and were compared in CT measures to 13 patients with probable AD and 31 normal controls. Of the cognitively impaired depressed patients, 11 were reexamined at 2-year follow-up, and only 1 member of this group evidenced cognitive decline. On CT measures of VBR and brain density, the total depressed sample fell intermediate between the AD patients and controls. Specific comparisons indicated that, relative to the normal controls, VBR was larger and brain density was less in the cognitively impaired depressed group and in the AD group. The cognitively intact depressed group did not differ from the normals. Related findings indicated that VBR and brain density measures were associated with neuropsychological performance variables only in the cognitively impaired groups. This study suggested that ventricular enlargement and possibly other structural abnormalities may be particularly manifest in elderly depressed patients with concurrent, reversible, and moderate to marked cognitive impairment.

## Course of Illness

Many descriptive features regarding the course of affective illness have been correlated with VBR and other brain morphometric measures in samples unselected for age. With some important exceptions, the findings have been either negative or isolated and unreplicated. It does not appear that duration of affective illness, duration of current episode, number of previous affective episodes, or number of previous psychiatric hospitalizations are related to structural abnormalities (see Sackeim and Prohovnik, 1993, for a review). Acute to short-term response to treatment has also shown no relation to VBR. However, Jacoby and Levy (1980) originally observed that the treatment response after 3 months did not distinguish elderly patients with and without ventricular enlargement. Nonetheless, there was a higher mortality rate in patients with such enlargement at 2-year follow-up. Shima et al. (1984) reported that larger VBR was associated with a poorer clinical outcome 9 months after hospital admission in elderly depressed patients. As noted, Bird et al. (1986) suggested that baseline VBR in a community sample was predictive of the future development of late-onset depression. Therefore, ventricular enlargement may have prognostic significance in the elderly not seen in younger populations. Increased VBR in geriatric depression may be associated with late onset of illness, greater cognitive impairment (at least during the acute phase), a poorer likelihood of recovery, and a higher rate of mortality.

## BRAIN STRUCTURAL MORPHOMETRY

With the development of high-resolution MRI and computerized techniques to segment brain tissue into gray, white, and CSF regions, in recent years the focus has shifted from measurement of CSF-filled spaces (e.g., ventricular enlargement) to assessment of the volume of specific cerebral structures. Across the age span, there is suggestive evidence for abnormal brain volume (decreased or increased) in mood disorder patients in the frontal cortex, temporal cortex, amygdala, hippocampus, and an area in the medial prefrontal cortex just below the genu of the corpus callosum, striatal, and other structures. Little of this work has yet focused on late-life depression, even though all the foregoing information suggests that deficits would be most likely manifested here. Consequently, only a few relevant findings will be emphasized.

In a sample of relatively elderly depressed patients, Coffey et al. (1993) first reported volume reduction in the prefrontal cortex. The frontal lobe volume was found to be 7% smaller in inpatients with severe depression (235.88 ml) than in the normal control subjects (254.32 ml). This difference was maintained after adjusting for the effects of age, sex, education, and intracranial size. Kumar et al. (1998) compared 18 patients with late-onset minor depression, 35 patients with late-onset major depression, and 30 nondepressed controls. The elderly groups of patients with minor or major depression had volume reduction relative to controls in the prefrontal cortex. Nonetheless, normalized prefrontal lobe volumes showed a significant linear trend with severity of depression, with volumes decreasing with illness severity. These findings suggested that there may be a common neurobiological substrate in diverse forms of late-onset mood disturbance (e.g., minor and major depression). Finally, Kumar et al. (2000) recently examined both prefrontal volume and degree of encephalomalacia in 51 patients with late-life MDD and 30 nondepressed controls. The patient group

had both reduced prefrontal volume and a greater volume of HI on MRI (encephalomalacia). The extent of encephalomalacia correlated significantly among patients with the degree of medical co-morbidity. However, the prefrontal volume reduction and the degree of encephalomalacia were not associated, suggesting that these structural abnormalities may represent independent pathological processes in late-life depression.

Using PET functional brain imaging measures in nonelderly samples, Drevets (1998) has shown reduced rCBF and rCMR$_{glu}$ in a specific area of the subgenual prefrontal cortex of patients with unipolar or bipolar depression. Both MRI and subsequent neuropathological investigations suggest that there is a pronounced loss of gray matter in this region in both forms of mood disorder. Despite its theoretical importance, whether this phenomenon occurs in late-life depression, particularly late-onset MDD, is unknown.

In two studies, Sheline and colleagues showed volume reduction in the hippocampus in euthymic women with a history of MDD (Sheline, 2003; Sheline et al., 1996, 1999). The volume loss had functional significance, as it was associated with verbal memory deficits. While again this work did not focus on late-life depression, it is of special relevance. The theory guiding this work is that the atrophic effects of stress-related glucocorticoid release during episodes of MDD lead to destruction of hippocampal tissue. Sheline et al. (1999) reported that the number of lifetime days in a depressive episode correlated with the magnitude of the hippocampal volume loss, while age alone was not a predictor. In more recent work, Sheline et al. (2003) found that the number of days in an untreated depressive episode correlated with the structural measure, while there was no association with the number of days depressed but taking antidepressant medication.

Given that elderly patients with early-onset depressive illness are likely to have the longest lifetime periods of MDD, one should predict that hippocampal volume loss would be most marked in this group. This possibility is under active investigation.

## FUNCTIONAL BRAIN ABNORMALITIES

Relatively few studies have used imaging techniques to examine functional brain activity in late-life depression. Furthermore, all studies, whether prior to or following treatment, have examined elderly patients in the *resting* state. Indeed, across all age groups, there has been sparse investigation in major depression of abnormalities in functional activity in the context of an affective or cognitive challenge when specific circuits are being activated (or deactivated). It is well established in other disorders that challenge conditions can reveal or highlight dysfunctional networks.

## Baseline Deficits

Across the life span, there is now an extensive literature documenting abnormalities in resting CBF and CMR in patients during episodes of MDD. With some notable exceptions (Drevets, 1998), most studies report abnormalities in the direction of reductions in global and/or topographic activity (most commonly involving prefrontal cortex, caudate, and cingulate gyrus). Studies in late-life depression (of both early and late onset) have generally revealed more profound abnormalities than studies in younger MDD populations. Indeed, the evidence for global reductions in CBF and CMRglu in MDD comes almost exclusively from studies of late-life MDD (see Ketter et al., 2001, for an exception).

Upadhaya et al. (1990) studied with HMPAO SPECT 18 MDD patients over the age of 66, 14 AD patients, and 12 normal controls. They found a global CBF deficit in the MDD group (normalized to cerebellum), as well as regional reductions in frontal, temporal, and parietal regions. Also using HMPAO SPECT, Curran et al. (1993) studied 20 elderly MDD patients (mean age of 70) who were receiving medications. The major findings included reduced CBF in frontal and temporal cortex, as well as in anterior cingulate, thalamus, and caudate. Bench et al. (1993), using PET, found reduced CBF in dorsolateral prefrontal cortex, angular gyrus, and anterior cingulate in 40 patients with MDD (mean

age of 57), half of whom were on medications. In a sample of 39 medication-free elderly MDD patients compared to matched controls, Lesser et al. (1994) used both HMPAO SPECT to study regional CBF and the $^{133}$Xe inhalation technique to assess global CBF. Despite being younger than controls, the patients had a 13.5% reduction in global CBF. Of note, patients with late-onset MDD tended to have lower global CBF than early-onset patients. The patients also had topographic reductions in CBF in frontal, temporal, and parietal regions.

Two recent HMPAO SPECT studies have further replicated findings of regional CBF reductions in late-life MDD (Awata et al., 1998; Ebmeier et al., 1998). Of note, Ebmeier et al. (1998) also found more extensive perfusion abnormalities in late-onset compared with early-onset patients.

The only published study to measure CMR$_{glu}$, that of Kumar et al. (1993), found marked global reductions in a small sample of patients with late-life MDD. The global CMR$_{glu}$ reduction was comparable to that in patients with AD. In addition, Kumar et al. reported regional deficits in prefrontal, temporal, and parietal cortex.

In a series of studies at Columbia University, we have examined structural and functional brain abnormalities in late-life MDD. Our first report was on a relatively large sample (N = 41) of predominantly elderly (mean

**Regional Metabolic Rate for Glucose**

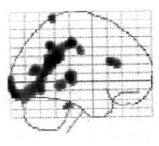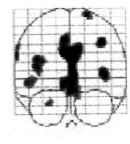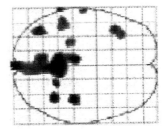

**Regional Cerebral Blood Flow**

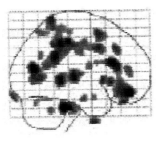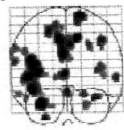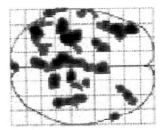

FIGURE 11.3 Preliminary findings from a positron emission tomography study of patients with late-onset major depression. The statistical parametric mapping glass brains represent the differences between patients and matched controls in resting regional cerebral blood flow (rCBF) and regional cerebral metabolic rate (rCMR) at baseline. All the signficant clusters reflected reduced functional activity in the patient sample. Note that the rCBF and rCMR maps are nearly identical for posterior brain regions, but only in rCBF measurement was their prominent abnormality in the depressed group in prefrontal cortex. This abnormality was more prominent on the right side.

age = 60.2) inpatients with MDD studied at baseline (eyes closed, at rest) with the $^{133}$Xe inhalation planar technique (32 scintillation detectors) while free of psychotropic medication (Sackeim et al., 1990). Compared to healthy controls ($N = 40$) matched for age, gender, end-tidal partial carbon dioxide pressure (pCO$_2$), blood pressure, and hemoglobin, the MDD group had a marked deficit in global cortical CBF, averaging 12% to 14% below normal values. Both traditional multivariate techniques and the Scaled Subprofile Model (SSM) (Alexander and Moeller, 1994; Moeller and Strother, 1991; Moeller et al., 1987) were applied to characterize topographic CBF deficits. Both approaches indicated that depressed patients had CBF reductions in a specific cortical pattern. The SSM characterized this pattern as involving selective frontal, superior temporal, and anterior parietal regions, a pattern we referred to as the *depression profile*. The magnitude of this topographic deficit covaried with patient age and the severity of depressive symptoms, such that older and more severely depressed patients manifested the greatest topographic abnormality.

In later work, we contrasted the global and topographic CBF deficits in elderly MDD patients with matched samples of AD patients and normal controls ($N = 30$ per group) (Sackeim et al., 1993). Relative to controls, the global cortical CBF reduction in MDD patients was of the same magnitude as in AD patients. As seen in Figure 11.3, this work also suggested that the specific topographic abnormality distinguished depressed patients from both matched controls and matched patients with AD. We have also shown that younger patients with MDD share the prefrontal CBF deficits, without the associated reductions in the superior temporal and anterior parietal cortex.

Also using the $^{133}$Xe inhalation technique, we reported a study of 20 elderly depressed outpatients who were compared to 20 matched normal controls (Nobler et al., 2000). Patients were 67.8 years of age on average, met DSM-IV criteria for MDD (unipolar, nonpsychotic), and at baseline scored at least 18 on the 24-item Hamilton Rating Scale for Depression. They were also free of medical conditions and medications known to confound CBF measurement. Patients had a minimum 14-day psychotropic medication washout prior to rCBF assessment. The depressed sample was matched to a normal control group with respect to age, sex, and systolic and diastolic blood pressure.

After omnibus testing to establish that there were group differences in regional values, three methods were used to determine topographic differences. First, given repeated observations of prefrontal CBF deficits in MDD, an a priori frontal ratio was computed. This corresponded to the mean CBF from 10 frontal detectors (5 per hemisphere) relative to CBF from the remaining 22 posterior detectors. Second, SSM was ap-

plied blind to patient or control status. Subjects were scored for the degree to which they expressed each of a set of topographic patterns, as well as for global CBF stripped of topographic contamination. Third, using SSM, scores on the topographic deficit previously obtained in depressed inpatients (Sackeim et al., 1990, 1993), reflecting CBF reductions in selective prefrontal, superior temporal, and anterior parietal regions (depression profile), were computed for this new sample.

In this study, elderly outpatients in an episode of MDD did not differ from matched normal controls in resting global cortical CBF (unlike the inpatient samples), but had significant topographic reductions in rCBF, principally involving frontal, temporal, and anterior parietal cortical regions. This topographic abnormality was expressed in reduced values for the a priori frontal ratio, in the blind SSM analysis, and when we contrasted scores on a previously obtained depression profile in patients and controls.

Overall, there is broad consensus among the studies of functional brain activity at rest in late-life depression. In several studies, typically involving inpatients with severe depression, global cortical deficits on the order of 10% to 15% were observed. Given the determinants of CBF and CMR, this could suggest a marked diminution of synaptic activity across the cortex. However, as discussed earlier, our ongoing work, assessing both CBF and CMR at rest in patients with late-onset major depression, has shown that deficits are more marked at baseline in CBF than in CMR (Fig. 11.4). This mismatch between metabolism and blood flow suggests that there is vascular compromise in addition to a deficit in functional activity.

There is also concordance in this area in characterizing the cortical areas subject to especially profound functional reduction. These extend broadly across the prefrontal cortex but also involve superior temporal and anterior parietal regions. The cortical deficits in late-life depression may have greater posterior cortical involvement than those in younger MDD samples, and the implicated cortical network is known to play a prominent role in motivation and attention (Sackeim et al., 1990).

## TREATMENT AND RECOVERY EFFECTS IN LATE-LIFE DEPRESSION

Few studies of late-life depression have focused on the changes in functional brain activity that occur following treatment. A critical question concerns the extent to which CBF and CMR disturbances seen at pretreatment baseline represent state, trait, or episode-dependent abnormalities (Sackeim and Prohovnik, 1993). Given the evidence for structural brain abnormalities, it would not be surprising if successful treatment in late-life

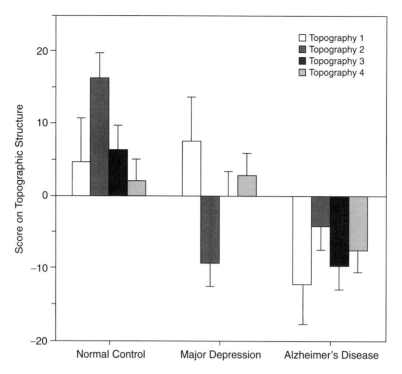

FIGURE 11.4 A representation of the findings of Sackeim et al. (1993). Scores on four topographic patterns for normal controls, elderly patients with major depression, and patients with Alzheimer's disease are shown. Depressed patients were abnormal only in the second network, involving prefrontal, temporal, and anterior parietal deficits. The third network represented the classic abnormality in Alzheimer's disease, involving cerebral blood flow (CBF) reduction in temporoparietal areas. However, compared to controls, these patients also showed dysregulation in all four cortical networks. The figure illustrates the specificity of the baseline topographic abnormality in late-life depression.

MDD did not fully reverse baseline functional deficits. Studies of patients before, during, and following treatment are vital to answer this question. However, treatments, whether pharmacological (i.e., antidepressants) or physical (i.e., ECT), may exert independent effects on CBF and/or CMR, distinct from or overlapping with those associated with clinical recovery.

Preclinical studies have shown that antidepressant medications, particularly tricyclics, have pronounced effects on capillary permeability, CBF, and CMR. Chronic antidepressant treatment often results in reduced functional activity in a regionally distributed fashion. In contrast, studies in younger adults of changes in CBF and CMR following effective pharmacological treatment of MDD have yielded inconsistent findings. Functional activity has often been reported as decreased following treatment, particularly in the ventrolateral and orbital frontal cortex (including the anterior cingulate). However, several studies have shown no change in at least some baseline cortical abnormalities, while other studies have found at least partial reversal of baseline cortical deficits, particularly in dorsolateral prefrontal cortex, or complex patterns of increases and decreases (see Drevets, 1998; Mayberg, 2003; Sackeim et al., 2000, for reviews). None of these studies concentrated on late-life depression, and in general, sample sizes have been small, with heterogeneous imaging and treatment methods.

In contrast, findings appear to be more consistent with ECT. With one exception, imaging studies have found decreased CBF or CMR in anterior cortical regions acutely and in the short term following ECT (e.g., Nobler et al., 1994).

Our group has extended the study of CBF abnormalities in geriatric depression by examining the effects of treatment and the clinical response on baseline deficits (Nobler et al., 1994, 2000). Using the $^{133}$Xe inhalation technique, rCBF was assessed prior to a course of ECT (pretreatment baseline), 30 minutes before and 50 minutes following a single treatment (*acute effects*), during the week following the ECT course, and 2 months after ECT (Nobler et al., 1994). Sixty-eight patients (mean age = 56.8 years) participated across the substudies. Patients were withdrawn from psychotropic medications (other than lorazepam) prior to ECT (mean washout = 19 days). A blind evaluation team determined number of ECT treatments and the clinical response. Patients received at least eight treatments before being classified as nonresponders. The CBF assessments were made under resting, supine conditions (eyes occluded). Overall, larger acute postictal CBF reductions at the sixth ECT, both globally and in a particular pattern of brain regions, were associated with a superior outcome following treatment (Color Fig. 11.5 in separate color insert). Similar patterns were observed during the week following ECT. Global CBF remained reduced (relative to pretreatment baseline) at 2-month follow-up in formerly depressed patients, with strong stability in a pretreatment topographic deficit. The findings suggested that baseline CBF abnormalities in MDD were not reversed by successful treatment with ECT. Rather, particularly in responders, ECT led to additional global and topographic CBF reductions, most markedly in anterior frontal regions.

In a second study, described earlier (Nobler et al., 2000), 20 elderly outpatients received treatment with antidepressant medication following baseline $^{133}$Xe inhalation rCBF. Eleven patients participated in a double-blind, randomized study of nortriptyline versus sertraline, while the remaining nine patients received nortriptyline in an open fashion. After 6–9 weeks on medication, resting rCBF and clinical assessments were repeated. Clinical response was defined as at least a 50% reduction in mean HRSD score from baseline and a final HRSD score <10. Following the medication trial, 11 patients were nonresponders (9 to nortriptyline, 2 to sertraline) and 9 were responders (6 to nortriptyline, 3 to sertraline). There were no differences at baseline or following treatment between responders and nonresponders in age, gender, blood pressure, hemoglobin, or pCO$_2$ values. Over the treatment course, the group as a whole did not change in global CBF, and responders and nonresponders did not differ in change in global CBF. In contrast, there was a significant interaction between response status and brain region, indicating that responders and nonresponders differed in the topography of CBF change.

Four topographic patterns were identified by a blind SSM analysis. Responders and nonresponders differed significantly only in the expression of the first pattern. This difference was due principally to responders manifesting CBF reductions in specific prefrontal and anterior temporal regions, a pattern of change not seen in nonresponders. To further test this association, across the sample we correlated scores for change in this topography with depression severity ratings. Greater expression of this pattern of CBF reduction in selective prefrontal and anterior temporal regions following treatment was associated with a greater percentage change in HRSD scores from baseline ($r = -0.47$) and lower posttreatment absolute HRSD scores ($r = 0.51$). It did not appear that treatment with nortriptyline or sertraline influenced this relationship. The sample as a whole did not change in expression of the depression profile, and there was no difference between responders and nonresponders in change in this measure. In sum, treatment with antidepressant medications did not result in reversal of the baseline deficit.

Instead, pharmacotherapy responders showed further selective CBF reductions in frontal and anterior temporal regions. The magnitude of change in this pattern was correlated with the extent of clinical improvement.

Strikingly, in two independent samples of patients with late-life MDD (Nobler et al., 1994, 2000), successful treatment with either antidepressants or ECT did not reverse baseline CBF reductions. Rather, a therapeutic response to both somatic therapies was associated with further deepening of perfusion deficits, suggesting that the CBF abnormalities either represent a trait phenomenon in geriatric depression or that the physiological alterations that result in symptomatic improvement are distinct from the pathophysiology of the illness.

The consistency of this pattern was further tested in our recent PET study in patients with late-onset major depression. In this work, patients underwent a PET battery after a minimum 3-week medication washout and at least 8 weeks of treatment with an antidepressant medication, which in almost all cases was sertraline. At these two time points, the fully quantified PET assessments included two resting studies of rCBF (with and without a snorkel), rCBF under hypercapnic challenge (inhalation of 5% CO$_2$), and a fully quantified measurement at rest of rCMR for glucose. After completion of the 8-week standardized medication period, patients were followed for an additional 2 years. When appropriate, they were withdrawn from psychotropics 24 months after their last set of PET measurements, and 1 month later fully quantified assessments were obtained of resting rCBF and rCBF during hypercapnic challenge.

The preliminary analyses of this study strongly corroborate the earlier claims that a clinical response to pharmacotherapy is associated with reduced functional activity in specific regions. Statistical parametric mapping (SPM) analyses indicated that the normal control group that was studied at intervals matched to the patient sample did not show clusters of consistent change over the 8-week acute treatment interval. However, in both the resting CBF and CMR studies, patients who evidenced a clinical response showed distinct changes compared to nonresponders and to themselves at baseline.

Color Figure 11.6 (in the separate color insert) represents the clusters of change in CMR that distinguished responders and nonresponders superimposed on a three-dimensional structural image. Responders differed from nonresponders by manifesting greater reductions in metabolic activity predominantly in left and right medial frontal lobes (BA 9), left sublobar insula (BA 13), left cingulate gyrus (BA 32), right temporal lobe, and transverse gyrus (BA 42). An SSM analysis conducted across the patient sample and blind to clinical outcome status identified a single network, heavily weighted by voxels in the regions noted above, as accounting for most of the change between the baseline and posttreatment assessments. Change on this metabolic topography accounted for more than 80% of the variance in change in HRSD scores.

To establish the extent to which changes within the nonresponder or responder subgroups were responsible for these effects, SPM analyses were restricted to each subgroup, and the extent and location of changes in rCBF and rCMR from baseline to the posttreatment time point were identified. Nonresponders did not show consistent change over the two time points in either CBF or CMR. Responders showed essentially the same effects for both measurements. As seen in Color Figure 11.7 (in the separate color insert), the patterns that distinguished responders and nonresponders (Color Fig. 11.6) was fully preserved in the contrast of the two time points within the responder group. Therefore, as in the previous work, prefrontal reductions in CBF and metabolism were strongly associated with a positive clinical outcome.

It was noted earlier that at baseline the sample of late-onset patients had a mismatch between CBF and CMR, with greater deficits relative to controls in CBF. In contrast, the changes observed after the acute treatment interval were virtually identical in the CBF and CMR measures. This strongly suggests that an altered metabolic demand accompanied the clinical response, resulting in parallel changes in vascular supply (CBF) and metabolic rate (CMR). Another implication is that the baseline disparity between CBF and CMR was maintained after acute treatment. In other words, the pathophysiological changes that accrued with successful treatment of the depressive symptoms involved alterations of functional activity in a specific pathway with a parallel impact on CMR and CBF. There was no evidence that pharmacological treatment altered CBF or CMR in a consistent manner independent of the clinical outcome. Furthermore, the mismatch between CBF and CMR was largely unaltered after the acute treatment period, suggesting by these data that it reflects a trait-level abnormality.

An implication of this work, in line with the imaging studies in ECT samples and some prior pharmacological studies, is that effective treatment results in physiological alterations distinct from the abnormalities that characterized patients at baseline. Consequently, it would appear that effective treatment does not reverse the baseline deficits. To the extent that there is topographical overlap, effective treatment may accentuate the baseline abnormalities. This perspective is compatible with the view that somatic treatments for depression are efficacious in suppressing symptomatic expression, but they do not ameliorate the underlying biological disturbance generating the illness.

The imaging data in this study on baseline and acute posttreatment effects derived from substantial samples involving 30 patients and 30 matched controls. At this point, 17 patients have been studied at the 2-year follow-up time point, with the group largely medication free and euthymic. The initial findings are surprising and, if sustained, will be of considerable theoretical importance. At long-term follow-up, one might expect further deterioration in CBF in the patient group and increased differentiation from normal controls. This would be compatible with the concept of a progressive CVD. Instead, the preliminary (and interim) findings suggest that the CBF deficits are strongly attenuated at the medication-free follow-up, with little differentiation from normal controls. This result was unexpected and, particularly since these are the first long-term, medication-free data in major depression, the study requires replication.

How should we interpret this reversal at long-term follow-up? The normalization of CBF deficits suggests that if an ischemic CVD process characterizes late-onset depression, it is only manifest during the period surrounding symptomatic expression. In other words, compromised CBF may be an expression of the episode of illness and may provide our first marker of the episode. This perspective assumes that the 2-year interval was sufficient for the episode to resolve in the majority of patients. In contrast, the fact that patients had been withdrawn from medication a month before PET assessments could be a major confound, with the CBF increases in patients reflecting a withdrawal phenomenon. Alternatively, the act of treating, especially in patients who achieve euthymia, may artificially suppress CBF (and CMR), obscuring a normalization that may have occurred much earlier in time. To fairly consider these different possibilities, it will be necessary to conduct physiological assessments at a variety of intervals following symptomatic remission, with and without concomitant continuation/maintenance treatment with antidepressant medications.

## CONCLUSION

There is growing evidence that at least a subgroup of patients with late-life major depression have a vascular origin of the illness. This view is reinforced by the excess of MRI HIs (encephalomalacia) suggesting small vessel disease, the association of encephalomalacia with age and cerebrovascular risk factors (e.g., hypertension), the histological evidence indicating that an arteriosclerotic process often is responsible for the HI, and the pathophysiological evidence indicating that encephalomalacia in neurological samples is associated with widespread diminution in cerebral perfusion, limited vascular reserve, and compensatory increases in oxygen extraction. Furthermore, it is evident that when studied in the depressed state, patients with late-life

MDD often have profound disturbances of CBF and CMR. These disturbances characteristically involve prefrontal, superior temporal, and anterior parietal cortical regions, but they may also reflect global reductions in functional brain activity. Finally, the limited study of late-life MDD following a response to somatic treatments suggests that baseline abnormalities do not normalize when symptomatic remission is achieved, but may become more exaggerated in patients who show substantial improvement. These findings converge in suggesting that an ischemic disease process, possibly progressive, may be responsible for some manifestations of MDD in late-life.

However, the preliminary findings in our recent work challenge central concepts of the relations of vascular disease to late-onset depression. First, an excess of MRI HIs was not found in our comparison of patients to matched controls. We suspect that careful matching for cerebrovascular risk factors may be the source of this discrepancy. Such matching has rarely been attempted in studies of major depression, and it may be that late-onset patients manifest the same degree of structural stigmata as controls with the same level of risk factors. Rather, patients with late-onset major depression may be more likely to have cerebrovascular risk factors than the general population. In other words, these risk factors may be overrepresented in late-onset major depression, but their impact on MRI HIs is not more profound in individuals who develop late-onset major depression.

More critically, the preliminary findings regarding long-term changes in rCBF suggest a major revision to the traditional view of vascular depression. The fact that CBF normalized after a 2-year period suggests that ischemic brain changes are bound by the period of symptom manifestation or, more likely, by the period of the underlying depressive episode. In essence, it is possible that deleterious cerebrovascular effects are a consequence or an expression of the depressive episode rather than a cause. If true, this perspective would underscore the importance of early and aggressive treatment of these episodes.

Undoubtedly, there are multiple etiologies to late-life MDD. Indeed, much of the evidence regarding structural and functional brain abnormalities indicates greater dysfunction in patients with late-onset illness. Commonly, these patients have a low rate of family history of mood disorders; relations with a family history of cerebrovascular or cardiovascular disease have yet to be explored. Especially in patients with late-life MDD and early onset, alternative etiologies are likely at play. These patients also show structural and functional brain abnormalities, but there is a greater likelihood in this group that these deficits reflect the consequences of a lifetime of depressive illness, as opposed to being central etiological factors.

## ACKNOWLEDGMENTS

Preparation of this chapter was supported in part by Grant MH55646 from the National Institute of Mental Health, Bethesda, MD. This chapter incorporates and updates material in Sackeim (2001). Many individuals in the Department of Biological Psychiatry, New York State Psychiatric Institute, and the Department of Radiology, Columbia University, contributed to our recent PET study of cerebrovascular abnormalities in patients with late-onset depression. These individuals include Drs. Robert DeLaPaz, Sarah H. Lisanby, Brett Mensh, Mitchell S. Nobler, Steven P. Roose, Ronald van Heertum, and Shan Yu.

## REFERENCES

Alexander, G.E. and Moeller, J.R. (1994) Application of the scaled subprofile model to functional imaging in neuropsychiatric disorders: A principal components approach to modeling brain function in disease. *Hum Brain Mapp* 2:79–94.

Andreasen, N.C., Swayze, V., 2d, Flaum, M., et al. (1990) Ventricular abnormalities in affective disorder: clinical and demographic correlates. *Am J Psychiatry* 147:893–900.

Awad, I.A., Johnson, P.C., Spetzler, R.F., et al. (1986a) Incidental subcortical lesions identified on magnetic resonance imaging in the elderly. II. Postmortem pathological correlations. *Stroke* 17:1090–1097.

Awad, I.A., Masaryk, T., and Magdinec, M. (1993) Pathogenesis of subcortical hyperintense lesions on magnetic resonance imaging of the brain. Observations in patients undergoing controlled therapeutic internal carotid artery occlusion. *Stroke* 24:1339–1346.

Awad, I.A., Modic, M., Little, J.R., et al. (1986b) Focal parenchymal lesions in transient ischemic attacks: Correlation of computed tomography and magnetic resonance imaging. *Stroke* 17:399–403.

Awad, I.A., Spetzler, R.F., Hodak, J.A., et al. (1986c) Incidental subcortical lesions identified on magnetic resonance imaging in the elderly. I. Correlation with age and cerebrovascular risk factors. *Stroke* 17:1084–1089.

Awata, S., Ito, H., Konno, M., et al. (1998) Regional cerebral blood flow abnormalities in late-life depression: Relation to refractoriness and chronification. *Psychiatry Clin Neurosci* 52:97–105.

Aylward, E.H., Roberts-Twillie, J.V., Barta, P.E., et al. (1994) Basal ganglia volumes and white matter hyperintensities in patients with bipolar disorder. *Am J Psychiatry* 151:687–693.

Bench, C.J., Friston, K.J., Brown, R.G., et al. (1993) Regional cerebral blood flow in depression measured by positron emission tomography: the relationship with clinical dimensions. *Psychol Med* 23:579–590.

Bird, J.M., Levy, R., and Jacoby, R.J. (1986) Computed tomography in the elderly: Changes over time in a normal population. *Br J Psychiatry* 148:80–85.

Boiten, J., Lodder, J., and Kessels, F. (1993) Two clinically distinct lacunar infarct entities? A hypothesis. *Stroke* 24:652–656.

Boone, K.B., Miller, B.L., Lesser, I.M., et al. (1992) Neuropsychological correlates of white-matter lesions in healthy elderly subjects. A threshold effect. *Arch Neurol* 49:549–554.

Breteler, M.M.B., van Amerongen, N.M., van Swieten, J.C., et al. (1994b) Cognitive correlates of ventricular enlargement and cerebral white matter lesions on magnetic resonance imaging: The Rotterdam Study. *Stroke* 25:1109–1115.

Breteler, M.M.B., van Swieten, J.C., Bots, M.L., et al. (1994a) Cerebral white matter lesions, vascular risk factors, and cognitive function in a population-based study: The Rotterdam Study. *Neurology* 44:1246–1252.

Brown, F.W., Lewine, R.J., Hudgins, P.A., et al. (1992) White matter hyperintensity signals in psychiatric and nonpsychiatric subjects. *Am J Psychiatry* 149:620–625.

Brown, M.M., Pelz, D.M., and Hachinski, V. (1990) Xenonenchanced CT measurement of cerebral blood flow in cerebrovascular disease (abstract). *J Neurol Neurosurg Psychiatry* 53:815.

Chimowitz, M.I., Estes, M.L., Furlan, A.J., et al. (1992) Further observations on the pathology of subcortical lesions identified on magnetic resonance imaging. *Arch Neurol* 49:747–752.

Coffey, C.E., Figiel, G.S., Djang, W.T., et al. (1990) Subcortical hyperintensity on magnetic resonance imaging: A comparison of normal and depressed elderly subjects. *Am J Psychiatry* 147:187–189.

Coffey, C.E., Weiner, R.D., Djang, W.T., et al. (1991) Brain anatomic effects of electroconvulsive therapy. A prospective magnetic resonance imaging study. *Arch Gen Psychiatry* 48:1013–1021.

Coffey, C.E., Wilkinson, W.E., Weiner, R.D., et al. (1993) Quantitative cerebral anatomy in depression. A controlled magnetic resonance imaging study. *Arch Gen Psychiatry* 50:7–16.

Curran, S.M., Murray, C.M., Van Beck, M., et al. (1993) A single photon emission computerised tomography study of regional brain function in elderly patients with major depression and with Alzheimer-type dementia. *Br J Psychiatry* 163:155–165.

Dahabra, S., Ashton, C.H., Bahrainian, M., et al. (1998). Structural and functional abnormalities in elderly patients clinically recovered from early- and late-onset depression. *Biol Psychiatry* 44:34–46.

De Reuck, J., Decoo, D., Strijckmans, K., et al. (1992) Does the severity of leukoaraiosis contribute to senile dementia? A comparative computerized and positron emission tomographic study. *Eur Neurol* 32:199–205.

Dolan, R.J., Calloway, S.P., and Mann, A.H. (1985) Cerebral ventricular size in depressed subjects. *Psychol Med* 15:873–878.

Drevets, W.C. (1998) Functional neuroimaging studies of depression: The anatomy of melancholia. *Annu Rev Med* 49:341–361.

Dupont, R.M., Butters, N., Schafer, K., et al. (1995) Diagnostic specificity of focal white matter abnormalities in bipolar and unipolar mood disorder. *Biol Psychiatry* 38:482–486.

Dupont, R.M., Jernigan, T.L., Butters, N., et al. (1990) Subcortical abnormalities detected in bipolar affective disorder using magnetic resonance imaging. Clinical and neuropsychological significance. *Arch Gen Psychiatry* 47:55–59.

Ebmeier, K.P., Cavanagh, J.T., Moffoot, A.P., et al. (1997) Cerebral perfusion correlates of depressed mood. *Br J Psychiatry* 170:77–81.

Ebmeier, K.P., Glabus, M.F., Prentice, N., et al. (1998) A voxel-based analysis of cerebral perfusion in dementia and depression of old age. *Neuroimage* 7:199–208.

Elkis, H., Friedman, L., Wise, A., et al. (1995) Meta-analyses of studies of ventricular enlargement and cortical sulcal prominence in mood disorders. Comparisons with controls or patients with schizophrenia. *Arch Gen Psychiatry* 52:735–746.

Erkinjuntti, T., Gao, F., Lee, D.H., et al. (1994) Lack of difference in brain hyperintensities between patients with early Alzheimer's disease and control subjects. *Arch Neurol* 51:260–268.

Fazekas, F., Kleinert, R., Offenbacher, H., et al. (1993) Pathologic correlates of incidental MRI white matter signal hyperintensities. *Neurology* 43:1683–1689.

Figiel, G.S., Krishnan, K.R., Breitner, J.C., and Nemeroff, C.B. (1989) Radiologic correlates of antidepressant-induced delirium: The possible significance of basal-ganglia lesions. *J Neuropsychiatry Clin Neurosci* 1:188–190.

Figiel, G.S., Krishnan, K.R., and Doraiswamy, P.M. (1990) Subcortical structural changes in ECT-induced delirium. *J Geriatr Psychiatry Neurol* 3:172–176.

Figiel, G.S., Krishnan, K.R., Doraiswamy, P.M., et al. (1991) Subcortical hyperintensities on brain magnetic resonance imaging: A comparison between late age onset and early onset elderly depressed subjects. *Neurobiol Aging* 12:245–247.

Fujikawa, T., Yamawaki, S., and Touhouda, Y. (1994) Background factors and clinical symptoms of major depression with silent cerebral infarction. *Stroke* 25:798–801.

Fujikawa, T., Yokota, N., Muraoka, M., et al. (1996) Response of patients with major depression and silent cerebral infarction to

antidepressant drug therapy, with emphasis on central nervous system adverse reactions. *Stroke* 27:2040–2042.

Greenwald, B.S., Kramer-Ginsberg, E., Krishnan, R.R., et al. (1996) MRI signal hyperintensities in geriatric depression. *Am J Psychiatry* 153:1212–1215.

Greenwald, B.S., Kramer-Ginsberg, E., Krishnan, K.R., Ashtari, M., Auerbach, C., and Patel, M. (1998) Neuroanatomic localization of magnetic resonance imaging signal hyperintensities in geriatric depression. *Stroke* 29:613–617.

Hatazawa, J., Shimosegawa, E., Satoh, T., et al. (1997) Subcortical hypoperfusion associated with asymptomatic white matter lesions on magnetic resonance imaging. *Stroke* 28:1944–1947.

Hickie, I., Scott, E., Mitchell, P., et al. (1995) Subcortical hyperintensities on magnetic resonance imaging: Clinical correlates and prognostic significance in patients with severe depression. *Biol Psychiatry* 37:151–160.

Hickie, I., Scott, E., Wilhelm, K., and Brodaty, H. (1997) Subcortical hyperintensities on magnetic resonance imaging in patients with severe depression—a longitudinal evaluation. *Biol Psychiatry* 42:367–374.

Isaka, Y., Iiji, O., Ashida, K., and Imaizumi, M. (1993) Cerebral blood flow in asymptomatic individuals—relationship with cerebrovascular risk factors and magnetic resonance imaging signal abnormalities. *Jpn Circ J* 57:283–290.

Isaka, Y., Nagano, K., Narita, M., et al. (1997) High signal intensity on T2-weighted magnetic resonance imaging and cerebral hemodynamic reserve in carotid occlusive disease. *Stroke* 28:354–357.

Jacoby, R.J. and Levy, R. (1980) Computed tomography in the elderly. 3. Affective disorder. *Br J Psychiatry* 136:270–275.

Jenkins, M., Malloy, P., Salloway, S., et al. (1998) Memory processes in depressed geriatric patients with and without subcortical hyperintensities on MRI. *J Neuroimag* 8:20–26.

Ketter, T.A., Kimbrell, T.A., George, M.S., Dunn, R.T., Speer, A.M., Benson, B.E., et al. (2001) Effects of mood and subtype on cerebral glucose metabolism in treatment-resistant bipolar disorder. *Biol Psychiatry* 49:97–109.

Krishnan, K.R., Hays, J.C., and Blazer, D.G. (1997) MRI-defined vascular depression. *Am J Psychiatry* 154:497–501.

Krishnan, K.R., McDonald, W.M., Doraiswamy, P.M., et al. (1993) Neuroanatomical substrates of depression in the elderly. *Eur Arch Psychiatry Clin Neurosci* 243:41–46.

Kumar, A., Bilker, W., Jin, Z., et al. (2000) Atrophy and high intensity lesions: complementary neurobiological mechanisms in late-life major depression. *Neuropsychopharmacology* 22:264–274.

Kumar, A., Jin, Z., Bilker, W., et al. (1998) Late-onset minor and major depression: Early evidence for common neuroanatomical substrates detected by using MRI. *Proc Natl Acad Sci USA* 95:7654–7658.

Kumar, A., Newberg, A., Alavi, A., et al. (1993) Regional cerebral glucose metabolism in late-life depression and Alzheimer disease: A preliminary positron emission tomography study. *Proc Natl Acad Sci USA* 90:7019–7023.

Lebowitz, B.D., Pearson, J.L., Schneider, L.S., et al. (1997) Diagnosis and treatment of depression in late life. Consensus statement update. *JAMA* 278:1186–1190.

Lesser, I.M., Boone, K.B., Mehringer, C.M., et al. (1996) Cognition and white matter hyperintensities in older depressed patients. *Am J Psychiatry* 153:1280–1287.

Lesser, I.M., Mena, I., Boone, K.B., et al. (1994) Reduction of cerebral blood flow in older depressed patients. *Arch Gen Psychiatry* 51:677–686.

Lesser, I.M., Miller, B.L., Boone, K.B., et al. (1991) Brain injury and cognitive function in late-onset psychotic depression. *J Neuropsychiatry Clin Neurosci* 3:33–40.

Lopez, O.L., Becker, J.T., Rezek, D., Wess, J., Boller, F., Reynolds, C.F.d., et al. (1992) Neuropsychiatric correlates of cerebral white-matter radiolucencies in probable Alzheimer's disease. *Arch Neurol* 49:828–834.

Lupien, S.J., Nair, N.P., Briere, S., Maheu, F., Tu, M.T., Lemay, M., et al. (1999) Increased cortisol levels and impaired cognition in human aging: Implication for depression and dementia in later life. *Rev Neurosci* 10:117–139.

MacQueen, G.M., Campbell, S., McEwen, B.S., Macdonald, K., Amano, S., Joffe, R.T., et al. (2003) Course of illness, hippocampal function, and hippocampal volume in major depression. *Proc Natl Acad Sci USA* 100:1387–1392.

Mayberg, H.S. (2003) Modulating dysfunctional limbic-cortical circuits in depression: towards development of brain-based algorithms for diagnosis and optimised treatment. *Br Med Bull* 65:193–207.

McEwen, B.S. (2001) Plasticity of the hippocampus: Adaptation to chronic stress and allostatic load. *Ann NY Acad Sci* 933:265–277.

McEwen, B.S., and Lasley, E.N. (2003) Allostatic load: When protection gives way to damage. *Adv Mind Body Med* 19:28–33.

Meguro, K., Hatazawa, J., Yamaguchi, T., et al. (1990) Cerebral circulation and oxygen metabolism associated with subclinical periventricular hyperintensity as shown by magnetic resonance imaging. *Ann Neurol* 28:378–383.

Miyao, S., Takano, A., Teramoto, J., et al. (1992) Leukoaraiosis in relation to prognosis for patients with lacunar infarction. *Stroke* 23:1434–1438.

Moeller, J.R., and Strother, S.C. (1991) A regional covariance approach to the analysis of functional patterns in positron emission tomographic data. *J Cereb Blood Flow Metab* 11:A121–A135.

Moeller, J.R., Strother, S.C., Sidtis, J., and Rottenberg, D. (1987) Scaled subprofile model: A statistical approach to the analysis of functional patterns in positron emission tomographic data. *J Cereb Blood Flow Metab* 7:649–658.

Moody, D.M., Brown, W.R., Challa, V.R., et al. (1995) Periventricular venous collagenosis: Association with leukoaraiosis. *Radiology* 194:469–476.

Munoz, D.G., Hastak, S.M., Harper, B., et al. (1993) Pathologic correlates of increased signals of the centrum ovale on magnetic resonance imaging. *Arch Neurol* 50:492–497.

Nobler, M.S., Oquendo, M.A., Kegeles, L.S., Malone, K.M., Campbell, C., Sackeim, H.A., et al. (2001) Decreased regional brain metabolism following electroconvulsive therapy. *Am J Psychiatry* 158:305–308.

Nobler, M.S., Roose, S.P., Prohovnik, I., Moeller, J.R., Louie, J., Van Heertum, R.L., et al. (2000) Regional cerebral blood flow in mood disorders, V.: Effects of antidepressant medication in late-life depression. *Am J Geriatr Psychiatry* 8:289–296.

Nobler, M.S., Sackeim, H.A., Prohovnik, I., et al. (1994) Regional cerebral blood flow in mood disorders: III. Effects of treatment and clinical response in depression and mania. *Arch Gen Psychiatry* 51:884–897.

O'Brien, J., Ames, D., Chiu, E., et al. (1998) Severe deep white matter lesions and outcome in elderly patients with major depressive disorder: follow up study. *BMJ* 317:982–984.

O'Brien, J., Desmond, P., Ames, D., et al. (1996) A magnetic resonance imaging study of white matter lesions in depression and Alzheimer's disease. *Br J Psychiatry* 168:477–485.

Pearlson, G.D., Rabins, P.V., Kim, W.S., et al. (1989) Structural brain CT changes and cognitive deficits in elderly depressives with and without reversible dementia ("pseudodementia"). *Psychol Med* 19:573–584.

Sackeim, H.A. (2001a) Brain structure and function in late-life depression. In: Morihisa, J.M., ed. *Review of Psychiatry*, vol. 20, *Advances in Brain Imaging*. Washington, DC: American Psychiatric Press, pp. 83–121.

Sackeim, H.A. (2001b) The definition and meaning of treatment-resistant depression. *J Clin Psychiatry* 62(Suppl 16):10–17.

Sackeim, H.A., Lisanby, S.H., Nobler, M.S., et al. (2000) MRI hyperintensities and the vascular origins of late-life depression. In: Andrade, C., ed. *Progress in Psychiatry*. New York: Oxford University Press, pp. 73–116.

Sackeim, H.A. and Prohovnik, I. (1993) Brain imaging studies in depressive disorders. In: Mann, J.J. and Kupfer, D., eds. *Biology of Depressive Disorders*. New York: Plenum, pp. 205–258.

Sackeim, H.A., Prohovnik, I., Moeller, J.R., et al. (1990) Regional cerebral blood flow in mood disorders. I. Comparison of major depressives and normal controls at rest. *Arch Gen Psychiatry* 47:60–70.

Sackeim, H.A., Prohovnik, I., Moeller, J.R., et al. (1993) Regional cerebral blood flow in mood disorders: II. Comparison of major depression and Alzheimer's disease. *J Nucl Med* 34:1090–1101.

Sackeim, H.A. and Steif, B.L. (1988) The neuropsychology of depression and mania. In: Georgotas, A. and Cancro, R., eds. *Depression and Mania*. New York: Elsevier, pp. 265–289.

Salloway, S., Malloy, P., Kohn, R., et al. (1996) MRI and neuropsychological differences in early- and late-life-onset geriatric depression. *Neurology* 46:1567–1574.

Schlegel, S., Maier, W., Philipp, M., et al. (1989) Computed tomography in depression: Association between ventricular size and psychopathology. *Psychiatry Res* 29:221–230.

Sheline, Y.I. (2003) Neuroimaging studies of mood disorder effects on the brain. *Biol Psychiatry* 54:338–352.

Sheline, Y.I., Gado, M.H., and Kraemer, H.C. (2003) Untreated depression and hippocampal volume loss. *Am J Psychiatry* 160:1516–1518.

Sheline, Y.I., Sanghavi, M., Mintun, M.A., and Gado, M.H. (1999) Depression duration but not age predicts hippocampal volume loss in medically healthy women with recurrent major depression. *J Neurosci* 19:5034–5043.

Sheline, Y.I., Wang, P.W., Gado, M.H., Csernansky, J.G., and Vannier, M.W. (1996) Hippocampal atrophy in recurrent major depression. *Proc Natl Acad Sci U S A* 93:3908–3913.

Shima, S., Shikano, T., Kitamura, T., Masuda, Y., Tsukumo, T., Kanba, S., et al. (1984) Depression and ventricular enlargement. *Acta Psychiatr Scand* 70:275–277.

Simpson, S.W., Jackson, A., Baldwin, R.C., et al. (1997) IPA/Bayer Research Awards in Psychogeriatrics. Subcortical hyperintensities in late-life depression: Acute response to treatment and neuropsychological impairment. *Int Psychogeriatr* 9:257–275.

Steffens, D.C., Conway, C.R., Dombeck, C.B., Wagner, H.R., Tupler, L.A., and Weiner, R.D. (2001) Severity of subcortical gray matter hyperintensity predicts ECT response in geriatric depression. *J ECT* 17:45–49.

Steffens, D.C., MacFall, J.R., Payne, M.E., Welsh-Bohmer, K.A., and Krishnan, K.R. (2000) Grey-matter lesions and dementia. *Lancet* 356:1686–1687.

Swayze, V.W. 2nd, Andreasen, N.C., Alliger, R.J., et al. (1990) Structural brain abnormalities in bipolar affective disorder. Ventricular enlargement and focal signal hyperintensities. *Arch Gen Psychiatry* 47:1054–1059.

Tarvonen-Schroder, S., Kurki, T., Raiha, I., et al. (1995) Leukoaraiosis and cause of death: A five year follow-up. *J Neurol Neurosurg Psychiatry* 58:586–589.

Thomas, A.J., Ferrier, I.N., Kalaria, R.N., et al. (2000) Elevation in late-life depression of intercellular adhesion molecule-1 expression in the dorsolateral prefrontal cortex. *Am J Psychiatry* 157:1682–1684.

Thomas, A.J., O'Brien, J.T., Davis, S., Ballard, C., Barber, R., Kalaria, R.N., et al. (2002) Ischemic basis for deep white matter hyperintensities in major depression: A neuropathological study. *Arch Gen Psychiatry* 59:785–792.

Upadhyaya, A.K., Abou-Saleh, M.T., Wilson, K., et al. (1990) A study of depression in old age using single-photon emission computerised tomography. *Br J Psychiatry Suppl* 9:76–81.

van Swieten, J.C., van den Hout, J.H., van Ketel, B.A., et al. (1991) Periventricular lesions in the white matter on magnetic resonance imaging in the elderly. A morphometric correlation with arteriolosclerosis and dilated perivascular spaces. *Brain* 114:761–774.

Zubenko, G.S., Sullivan, P., Nelson, J.P., et al. (1990) Brain imaging abnormalities in mental disorders of late life. *Arch Neurol* 47:1107–1111.

# 12 | Late-life depression and the vascular hypothesis

## K. RANGA R. KRISHNAN

The etiology of depression and the factors affecting the course of depression in the elderly are not well understood. A genetic etiology is generally thought to be of less importance in patients presenting with depression for the first time later in life. Maier et al. (1991) clearly established that late-onset depression (LOD) patients have a higher familial rate of depression than age-matched controls, but the rate in LOD is less than in early-onset depression (EOD). Thus, at least in LOD, other reasons may play a significant role. An issue that has to be kept in mind is that the dichotomous classification of depression in late life by age-at-onset is also a fluid concept that has significant limitations. This includes the fact that defining the age-at-onset is difficult; is it onset of first symptoms or onset of a defined syndrome? Another issue may be memory and recall of depression. A final concern is that individuals with EOD may develop in later life characteristics of LOD. However, despite these limitations and problems, the concept that patients with older age-at-onset are different from those with a younger age-at-onset has gained ground.

## DEVELOPMENT OF CONCEPTS RELATING BRAIN STRUCTURAL CHANGE AND DEPRESSION

The concept of vascular depression is not a new idea. Gaupp (1905) (as quoted by Post, 1962) described elderly patients with depression secondary to what was termed *arteriosclerosis*. Many of these patients had persistent apathy. Felix Post made a similar observation. We should emphasize here that all these early suggestions were based purely on clinical evidence of cerebral vascular damage, usually caused by strokes. What is new is the technology used to demonstrate subtle structural brain ischemic change in vivo by magnetic resonance imaging (MRI) and other imaging techniques. These changes on MRI appear as signal hyperintensities on $T_2$-weighted images (Color Fig. 12.1 in separate color insert). A variety of terms have been used to describe these changes. One of the more common terms is *leukoen-*

*cepahalopathy*. Another popular term is *silent infarcts*. Other terms used include *leukoaraiosis, unidentified bright objects*, and *hyperintensities*.

Age has been the primary factor related to these changes. The pathological correlates of these changes have been studied (Awad et al., 1986a, 1986b; Boyko et al., 1992). Sometimes these lesions appear to be lacunes. Early Duke Mental Health Clinical Research Center studies using MRI suggested that subcortical ischemic structural changes are more prevalent in LOD patients and that these changes may play a role in the pathophysiology of those depressions. In our first study of 35 depressed patients (Krishnan et al., 1988), 72% of LOD subjects had leukoaraiosis. Coffey et al. (1988, 1989, 1990) replicated these findings in 67 elderly depressed patients referred for electroconvulsive therapy (ECT). Figiel et al. (1991) compared the incidence and severity of subcortical hyperintensities in 10 LOD patients with those of 9 age- and atherosclerotic risk factor–matched EOD elderly patients. Lesions were more frequent among patients with LOD than EOD in the frontal and basal ganglia regions. Since that time, numerous studies have confirmed these findings. Because of space limitations, we will not review this large recent literature in detail, but note that Steffens and Krishnan (1998) have summarized recent findings.

## RISK FACTORS FOR HYPERINTENSITIES

These are much the same as those reported for stroke (i.e., hypertension, diabetes, hyperlipidemia, smoking, coronary artery disease, and possibly elevated plasma homocysteine levels) (Awad et al., 1986a,b; Inzitari et al., 1990). The relationship, however, has not been consistently observed (Hendrie et al., 1989; Hunt et al., 1989). The current consensus is that these changes are more severe and significant among those with risk factors. The same patterns have been reported in depressed subjects in our center (Coffey et al., 1988, 1989). Also, there is a large body of literature that, with few exceptions (Lyness et al., 1998), links depression with cerebrovascular risk factors such as hypertension, diabetes, smoking, and cardiovascular disease (Carney et al., 1988; Coulehan et al., 1990; Dalack 1990; Friedman and Bennet 1977; Glassman et al., 1990; Habib et al., 1991; Huapaya and Ananth 1990; Lyness et al., 2000; Rabkin et al., 1983; Tresch et al., 1985).

The National Institutes of Health Consensus Development Conference stated that one of the most promising lines of future research in this area is to clarify the relationship between subcortical brain abnormalities, depressive and cognitive symptomatology, and EOD versus LOD in the elderly.

It is important to keep in mind that this relationship has also been established in epidemiological studies. We have also investigated these lesions in a community sample using the Cardiovascular Health Study (CHS) database of 3660 individuals with MRI scans. Steffens et al. (1999a) reported that, when age, race, gender, hypertension, cardiovascular disease, functional status, and Modified Mini-Mental State Examination score were controlled for, the number of small (<3 mm) basal ganglia lesions was significantly associated with reported depressive symptoms, but white matter grade was not. In subsequent logistic regression models, number of basal ganglia lesions remained a significant predictor after controlling for non-MRI variables and severity of white matter lesions. The level of depression in this study was modest and may not reflect major depression. It is possible that even mild depression may be related to ischemic pathology in the elderly.

## LESION LOCATION AND GERIATRIC DEPRESSION

A large body of evidence suggests that the basal ganglia and frontal lobes, areas primarily affected by hyperintensities in LOD, are involved in the pathophysiology of depression. These studies led us to develop a model based on the basal ganglia circuits described by Alexander and Crutcher (1990). The model provides a neuroanatomical basis for the pathophysiology of depression and leads to a number of testable hypotheses (Krishnan and McDonald, 1995). Lesions of the frontal lobe probably damage the glutamatergic projections of the frontal cortex to the striatum, and lesions of the basal ganglia damage the GABAergic component of the system, including the limbic-striatal interface. The limbic-striatal interface has been implicated in motivation and psychomotor expression. Thus, based on this model, one can hypothesize that patients with these lesions would have decreased motivation and psychomotor changes, either retardation or agitation. Preliminary data suggest a trend toward a relationship between severity of anhedonia and deep white matter hyperintensities (DWMH) and subcortical gray matter hyperintensities (SGH). In addition, these brain regions

have been implicated in specific types of cognitive changes: impaired psychomotor speed, frontal initiation functions, memory encoding and retrieval, and visuospatial perception. Thus, one can hypothesize a relationship between these lesions and specific aspects of core depressive symptomatology, namely, anhedonia, lassitude, and memory and other cognitive deficiencies.

Greenwald and colleagues (1998), in collaboration with Duke investigators, have shown an association between geriatric depression and left frontal deep white matter ($p < .005$) and left putamenal ($p < .04$) hyperintensities. Recently, we have demonstrated larger numbers of left-sided lesions among elderly depressives. In addition, we found larger numbers of white matter lesions in the medial orbital frontal cortex in older depressives versus controls using the Statistical Parametric Mapping (SPM) technique. Thus, the model of vascular depression does not rest on the mere presence of lesions; rather, it is the specific location within the brain that confers validity.

In a recent study, we evaluated common areas of clustering of vascular lesions. Magnetic resonance images were acquired on 88 elderly depressed patients and 47 age- and gender-matched nondepressed controls. The MRI protocol includes a volumetric, dual-contrast, fast spin-echo pulse sequence. Imaging was performed at 1.5T on a commercial MRI system (GE Signa, GE Medical Systems, Milwaukee, WI) with the standard quadrature head coil. Pulse sequence parameters were: Tr = 3000 msec, echo time (Te) = 30, 130 msec, echo train length (ETL) = 16, field-of-view = 22 cm, slice thickness = 3 mm, slices acquired without gaps, imaging bandwidth = ±16 kHz, number of excitations (Nex) = 1, 256 × 256 matrix. This dataset was segmented on a SUN workstation using MRX (software developed by General Electric, Schenectady, New York) and a semiautomated method in which tissue classes (gray matter, white matter, cerebrospinal fluid) and lesions were identified by operator selection.

Statistical Parametric Mapping (SPM) was performed on a SUN workstation using SPM99 (Wellcome Department of Cognitive Neurology) (Friston et al., 1995). The lesion's image was extracted from the segmented image and then normalized spatially using a spatial transformation determined by normalizing the proton density image data from which the lesions were segmented to the SPM proton density (PD) template image provided in the SPM release. The transformation distorts the lesion's nominal intensity value; it was restored to a value of 128 after normalization. Each normalized image was smoothed with a low-pass three-dimensional spatial filter with a kernel value of five pixels in the $x$, $y$, and $z$ directions (Wright et al., 1995). In this way, the lesion images can be thought of as representing *lesion density* in a given voxel. A statistical parametric map was formed from a two-group $t$-test to test for differences in lesion density between depressed individuals and controls. The significance level was set at $p < .01$.

One of the pitfalls of using spatial normalization and registration is that if there are volumetric differences between the study group (depressed in this case) and controls, there will be spatial normalization differences between the groups that could cause the edges of structures to systematically misregister, potentially masquerading as group local differences. As a result, it is often better to use the study group as its own control rather than trying to compare this group with normals. This can be done with the depressed group by evaluating the correlation between lesion density and Hamilton Depression Rating Scale (HAM-D) score.

Statistical Parametric Mapping analysis of 88 elderly depressives and 47 age- and gender-matched controls showed two major regions of increased lesion density in the patients in the medial-orbital prefrontal white matter (MacFall et al., 2001). In the depressed group, SPM was used to identify regions correlated with HAM-D scores. Without considering limited regions of interest, the corrected $p$-value was found to be significant ($p < .005$) for the medial-orbital prefrontal region and for a left-sided region in the internal capsule.

## DEPRESSION OUTCOMES OF PATIENTS WITH VASCULAR BRAIN CHANGES

An important area of research involves determination of the differential treatment outcome for patients with vascular depression. Studies attempting to examine both the prognostic implications of incidental MRI lesions and the treatment response are limited and contradictory. Coffey et al. (1988) retrospectively studied the response of 67 elderly depressives referred for ECT. Of these, 44 were found to have either MRI-defined hyperintensities or computed tomography (CT) lucencies. After receiving an average of 9 ECT treatments (range, 6–14), 43 of the 44 patients were determined to have either a good (44%) or an excellent (54%) response to treatment. Other studies reached a markedly different conclusion. Hickie et al. (1995) selected patients with a history of refractory depression and risk factors for cerebrovascular disease (CVD) (hypertension, a history of stroke) and concluded that severity of white matter hyperintensities (WMH) predicted a poorer outcome of antidepressant treatment (both medications and ECT). In a 2-year longitudinal follow-up study, this group (Hickie et al., 1997) concluded that the presence of WMH predicted a probable dementia syndrome of the vascular type and residual dysfunction.

In the past few years, there have been several studies on the treatment response of patients with vascular depression. Yanai et al. (1998) retrospectively investigated the relationship between major depression and *silent cerebral infarction* (SCI). Thirty-two patients with and 32 patients without SCI were followed for 3 years. This group found a significant difference in the number of subsequent hospitalizations for the SCI-positive group. Krishnan et al. (1998) classified 57 depressed patients as having vascular depression or nonvascular depression, and found that the cohort with vascular depression showed no statistical difference in rate of recovery than the nonvascular depression group. However, older subjects with vascular depression evidenced less recovery. Simpson et al. (1998) studied 75 elderly patients (ages 65 to 85) treated with 12 weeks of monotherapy with either a selective serotonin reuptake inhibitor (SSRI), lofepramine, amitriptyline, imipramine, or dothiepin. They found greater resistance to monotherapy in patients with hyperintensities in the deep white matter, basal ganglia, and pontine reticular formation. In logistic regression analysis, the presence of more than five basal ganglia hyperintensities and hyperintensities in the pontine reticular formation was predictive of resistance to antidepressant monotherapy. O'Brien et al. (1998), in a follow-up study of 60 older depressives, demonstrated that those with severe (Fazekas grade 3) deep white matter lesions had significantly worse outcomes than those without such lesions. Furthermore, the mean survival time of subjects with severe lesions was less than that of those without such lesions.

## LESIONS AND ELECTROCONVULSIVE THERAPY OUTCOME

In 41 patients treated with ECT, we examined the association between outcome of an acute course of ECT treatment and lesion ratings (dichotomized as Fazekas rating 0–1 vs. 2–3). For SGH, 23 patients with ratings of 0–1 had significantly greater improvement in clinical global impression (CGI)-severity scores ($\Delta = -3.2$) compared with 18 patients with ratings of 2–3 ($\Delta = -2.3$), $p < .009$, F-test. The number of treatments did not differ between the groups (9.6 vs. 10.3). For (PVH) and DWMH, there were no significant differences in clinical improvement or number of ECT treatments. As another measure of severity of hyperintensities, we compared patients with hyperintensities present (score of 1, 2, or 3) in two of three of the areas (i.e., SGH, PVH, and DWMH) versus none or one hyperintensity present in one of three of the areas. The more severely affected group required a greater number of treatments (10.7) than the less severely affected group (8.6) ($Z = 1.826$, $p = .068$, Wilcoxon two-sample test). Thus, severe SGH was associated with limited improvement with ECT, and having multiple areas of involvement of hyperintensities was associated with more treatments and no difference in improvement. This was the first report of a specific treatment effect for a particular region of hyperintensities (Steffens et al., 2001).

## EXECUTIVE DYSFUNCTION AND VASCULAR DEPRESSION

Alexopoulos and colleagues at Cornell have further refined the notion of vascular depression by linking it to neuropsychological markers of fronto-striatal damage, interpreted as executive dysfunction and specifically as difficulties with initiation and perseveration on the Mattis Dementia Scale (Alexopoulos et al., 2000; Kinderman et al., 2000). We have also found an association between geriatric depression and poor performance on similar tasks. Recently, Butters et al. (2000) showed that cognitively impaired older depressives showed some improvement in cognition after acute treatment, but had residual impairment in memory and executive functions.

## COGNITIVE OUTCOMES OF GERIATRIC DEPRESSION

Previous studies (Jorm et al., 1991; Kokmen et al., 1991; Speck et al., 1995) have shown that a prior history of depression is associated with an increased risk of Alzheimer's disease (AD). The finding that individuals with LOD who also evidence cognitive impairment frequently develop dementia within a few years after the presentation of their depression (Alexopoulos, 1993; Alexopoulos et al., 1993; Kral and Emery 1989; Reding et al., 1985), implies that LOD is sometimes a prodrome of dementia. In a longitudinal prospective study, Devanand et al. (1996) followed 849 nondemented community-dwelling individuals with varying degrees of cognitive impairment (none, mild, or moderate) for 1 to 5 years to determine the risk of incident dementia. Depressed mood at baseline was associated with an increased risk of incident dementia (relative risk 2.94%, CI = 1.76–4.91). In a large meta-analysis, Jorm et al. (1991) found that a history of depression was associated with onset of AD after age 70 only if depressive symptoms had appeared within 10 years before the onset of dementia. However, depression with onset more than 10 years before the onset of dementia was associated with onset of AD at *any* age, suggesting that previous depression can sometimes represent more than an early (prodromal) symptom of dementing illness. A reanalysis (van Duijn et al., 1994) examined the studies from Jorm's meta-analysis that included information on family history of dementia. This report suggested that a lifetime history of depression increased the risk of AD, regardless of the family history, suggesting that prior occurrence of depression may influ-

ence the risk independently of any genetic diathesis toward AD. Speck et al. (1995) also recently found that depression is a risk factor for AD, even for depressive symptoms occurring more than 10 years before the onset of dementia symptoms.

In a sample of 142 elderly twins from a large study of dementia, Steffens et al. (1997) examined major depression, apolipoprotein E (APOE) genotype, and AD using time-dependent proportional hazards models. Compared with the risk of AD for those with no history of depression and no $\epsilon 4$ allele, the risk ratio for AD with two $\epsilon 4$ alleles was 2.87 (CI = 1.56–5.28), with one $\epsilon 4$ allele was 1.82 (CI = 1.09–3.04), and with LOD and no $\epsilon 4$ allele was 2.95 (CI = 1.55–5.62). There was no interaction between prior depression and APOE genotype. Risk ratios declined substantially with an increasing interval between onset of depression and AD. Our findings suggest that, for some individuals, the association of depression and AD may reflect the occurrence of prodromal depressive symptoms rather than a true risk relationship.

## COGNITIVE OUTCOMES OF VASCULAR DEPRESSION

Our data, recently published in *Lancet* (Steffens et al., 2000b), noted that the volume of gray matter lesions in later demented patients was found to be threefold higher than that of nondemented patients (hazard ratio [HR] = 2.232, CI = 1.337–3.725). In the CHS, the presence of *infarct-like lesions* predicted later cognitive decline on the modified Mini-Mental State Examination (Kuller et al., 1998).

## APOLIPOPROTEIN E AND COGNITION

Since the first studies at Duke in 1993 linking APOE and late-onset and sporadic AD (Corder et al., 1993; Saunders et al., 1993; Strittmatter et al., 1993), the importance of APOE $\epsilon 4$ and impaired cognitive functioning is becoming more firmly established (Riley et al., 2000), including a study by Steffens et al. (1999b) in an elderly female population of Cache County, Utah.

In a population study based in Cache County (Breitner et al., 1999; Steffens et al., 2000a), we examined 3297 community-dwelling elderly, 131 with late-onset (age 60 or over) major depression. All cases of depression onset had to precede onset of dementia. Controlling for age and APOE $\epsilon 4$ (both were highly significant predictors in all models), LOD was predictive of any dementia (OR = 1.935, $p$ = .027), strongly predictive of vascular dementia (OR = 3.250, $p$ = .012), and less predictive of AD (OR = 1.577, $p$ = .192).

In this latter study, we found that current depression and APOE were independent predictors of lower cognitive scores, a finding reminiscent of that of our study of veteran twins, which showed that depression and APOE were independent risk factors for later dementia (Steffens et al., 1997). These findings, along with those of the CHS, suggest that APOE is independent of lesions and depression in its effects on cognition.

## MORBIDITY AND MORTALITY OUTCOMES OF VASCULAR DEPRESSION

The existing literature on nonpsychiatric outcomes of lesions is scant, particularly in samples of depressed older individuals. In a nondepressed sample, Bracco et al. (1993) found that 1 of 12 subjects with extensive white matter disease was demented at the 3-year follow-up.

There is a literature examining vascular change and mortality in samples not assessed for depression. What is not clear is whether the effect is seen more often in patients with depression. Inzitari et al. (1997) found a higher mortality rate among neurological patients with leukoaraiosis (LA) than without it (RR = 1.64, CI = 1.15–2.34), with a nearly threefold increased risk of dying from vascular causes. The same group had found a 6-year cumulative stroke risk of 49% among cases with LA and 16% among controls (HR = 3.0, CI = 1.2–7.5); patients with lacunar infarcts had the worst prognoses. Others have found a high degree of vascular death among patients with LA (Tarvonen-Schroder et al., 1995). Briley et al. (2000) found that neurologically damaged patients with severe LA had an increased risk of death (HR = 2.91, CI = 1.5–5.6) and falls (HR = 6.8, CI = 1.5–30).

## LEUKOARAIOSIS AND LACUNAR STROKE: APPARENTLY DIFFERENT OUTCOMES

Clavier et al. (1994) found a high (80%) 4-year survival rate and a low recurrence rate among lacunar stroke patients. Salgado et al. (1996) reported a 5-year survival rate of 86% and a stroke recurrence rate of 63%. Miyao et al. (1992) found that the presence of LA among patients with lacunar infarct predicted mortality. We performed a National Death Index query on 338 patients enrolled in the previous MHCRC between 1984 and 1994. In a manuscript under review, we used Cox proportional hazards models to confirm that mortality is associated with older age and being male. We also found that males with higher on the Center for Epidemiologic Studies Depression Scale (CES-D) scores and females with more severe vascular conditions at baseline or later age of depression onset had higher mortality, a higher stroke recurrence rate, and a higher incidence of dementia. These findings highlight the importance of subcortical vascular change as an entity distinct from stroke.

Taken together, these findings strongly suggest that vascular lesions at baseline predict a poor acute response to somatic treatment and are somewhat suggestive of higher relapse.

The association of cerebrovascular changes and geriatric depression must be placed in the context of the growing evidence linking hippocampal volume changes and depression. Elderly depressives, compared with nondepressed controls, have been shown to have smaller hippocampal volumes (Steffens et al., 2000a), with later-onset depressives having smaller hippocampal volumes than depressives with an earlier onset. Cerebrovascular disease is known to increase the risk of cognitive decline and dementia (Kuller et al., 1998; Snowdon et al., 2000), so it is essential to examine it along with hippocampal changes and APOE, as all three are likely to exert independent effects on cognition and dementia. The scientific importance of this paradigm is obvious: if vascular lesions and hippocampal changes in the brains of older people lead to secondary depression that is clinically similar to primary depression, then those changes may provide important clues to brain sites involved in depression in general and to pathophysiology of later dementia. The clinical importance of cognitive outcomes in geriatric depression has aspects that are both obvious and more subtle: (1) *prevention* of LOD and cognitive decline may involve control of cerebrovascular risk factors and risk factors for AD; (2) *treatment* of LOD may need to include both adequate treatment of risk factors and, when appropriate, anticoagulation or cholinesterase inhibition; and (3) *consequences* of worsening of CVD or hippocampal atrophy among depressives may include more severe depression, as well as an increased risk of stroke and dementia. Before costly or controversial prevention or treatment trials can be undertaken, it is incumbent upon researchers to firmly establish the consequences of these changes.

## CONCEPTUAL FRAMEWORK

1. A model for depression: Based on the available data, we believe that a number of risk factors can lead to the development of fronto-striatal lesions. Once these lesions are formed, the individual is at risk for depression. Stress or aggravating life events can then precipitate depression. Social support, both real and perceived, can mitigate this effect.

2. A model linking LOD with subsequent cognitive changes.

The links between depression and cognition are complex. There is a large literature on the neuropsychology of depression that focuses on attention, speed of processing, and executive function (Alexopoulos et al., 1997). It is also possible that depression may lead to hippocampal atrophy with attendant cognitive decline (Sheline et al., 1996, 1999). In addition, depression may represent a prodrome of dementia, either AD or vascular dementia (Alexopoulos et al., 1993; Steffens et al., 1997). The neuropathology associated with these changes is likely multifactorial, with at least two major processes being salient: *neurodegenerative* and *vascular*. The neurodegenerative process involves hippocampal volume and APOE genotype. The vascular process as it relates to depression involves frontal and striatal areas, particularly prefrontal cortex and caudate. In the present application, we hypothesize that the cognitive decline and later dementia experienced by elderly depressives may be associated with two underlying pathologies that contribute uniquely and interactively to cognitive function and decline.

These relationships are shown in Figure 12.2. Not shown are the social factors (decreased social support and negative life events), medical conditions, and functional impairment that may affect the outcome of depression.

## HIPPOCAMPUS AND GERIATRIC DEPRESSION

The relationship between the hippocampus and affective disorders remains poorly understood (Steffens et al., 2000a). Clearly, the hippocampus is involved in memory and disorders of memory, that is, AD. Yet evidence is growing that the hippocampus is involved in psychiatric disorders as well. Sapolsky proposed a stress model of GC-induced neurotoxicity of hippocampal neurons (Sapolsky, 1999; Sapolsky et al., 1986). While posttraumatic stress disorder was initially examined to test this model, recent studies have made a case for studying depression and hippocampal volume. The rationale for such studies has been based in part on the

finding of hypothalamic-pituitary-adrenal dysfunction in depression.

In a series of reports, Sheline et al. (1996) found an association between degree of hippocampal volume reduction and total lifetime duration of major depression. They also found that among women aged 23–86, those with a history of depression had smaller hippocampal volumes bilaterally than controls (Sheline et al., 1999). In terms of the implication for geriatric depression, one would expect, based on these findings, that older depressed patients with EOD would have smaller hippocampal volumes. Recently, Steffens et al. (2000a) examined the hippocampal volume in geriatric depression. Given the clinical observation that many late-life depressed patients proceeded to develop dementia, we sought to test the opposite hypothesis: that patients with LOD have smaller hippocampal volumes. We found that older depressed patients (compared with elderly controls) had smaller volume of the right ($p = 0.014$) and left ($p = 0.073$) hippocampus. In addition, among depressed patients, age-at-onset was negatively but not significantly related to right hippocampal volume ($p = 0.052$) and left hippocampal volume ($p = 0.062$).

There is solid evidence linking hippocampal atrophy and dementia, especially AD, with recent studies showing diffuse hippocampal atrophy in AD (Laakso et al., 2000) and quantifying the rate of hippocampal atrophy (Jack et al., 1998). It would appear that vascular changes and changes in hippocampal volume likely contribute to both depression and cognitive outcomes.

## CONCLUSION

We initially introduced the term *arteriosclerotic depression* to describe depression that arises secondary to these brain ischemic changes. Subsequently, Alexopuolos proposed a broad clinical definition of vascular depression. This definition is simple and covers depres-

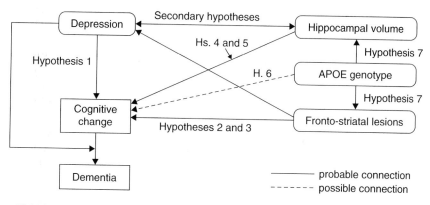

FIGURE 12.2 A representation of the contributions of a neurodegenerative process and vascular pathology to cognitive decline and depressive syndromes in the elderly. APOE, apolipoprotein E.

TABLE 12.1. *Criteria for Subcortical Ischemic Depression*

1. Criteria for major depressive episode.

2. Evidence for subcortical ischemic change on neuroimaging, such as hyperintense areas on computed tomography or $T_2$-weighted magnetic resonance imaging scans.

3. The presence of a risk factor for cerebrovascular disease is not required, but it may support the diagnosis. When present, the condition should be specified on Axis III. Examples include hypertension, coronary artery disease, and atrial fibrillation.

sion attributable to vascular disease. As Table 12.1 shows, we have developed criteria for a subtype of vascular depression defined in part by neuroimaging findings (Krishnan et al., 1997; Steffens et al., 1998).

As we try to define the boundaries of this entity, we should keep in mind that vascular disease is a common part of aging. Atherosclerotic processes start early in life. Additional literature demonstrates that depression is a risk factor for the development of arteriosclerosis. Thus, depression itself may play a role in the development of vascular disease. In addition, a common antecedent of the two conditions cannot be ruled out. Also, as noted earlier, depressive symptoms have been related to CVD. Thus, although we have defined vascular depression in the context of major depression, it may exist in other syndromes of depression, dysthymia, and so on. This highlights some of the problems in current psychiatric classification systems.

REFERENCES

Alexander, G.E., and Crutcher, M.D. (1990) Functional architecture of basal ganglia circuits: Neural substrates of parallel processing. *Trends Neurosci* 13:266–271.

Alexopoulos, G.S., Meyers, B.S., Young, R.C., et al. (2000) Executive dysfunction and long-term outcomes of geriatric depression. *Arch Gen Psychiatry* 57:285–290.

Alexopoulos, G.S., Meyers, B.S., Young, R.C., Kakuma, T., Silbersweig, D., and Charlson, M. (1997) Clinically defined vascular depression. *Am J Psychiatry* 154:562–565.

Alexopoulos, G.S., Meyers, B.S., Young, R.C., Mattis, S., and Kakuma, T. (1993) The course of geriatric depression with "reversible dementia": A controlled study. *Am J Psychiatry* 150: 1693–1699.

Alexopoulos, G., Young, R., and Meyers, B. (1993) Geriatric depression: Age-of-onset and dementia. *Biol Psychiatry* 34:141–145.

Awad, I.A., Johnson, P.C., and Spetzler, R.F. (1986a) Incidental subcortical lesions identified on magnetic resonance imaging in the elderly: II. Postmortem pathological correlations. *Stroke* 17: 1090–1097.

Awad, I.A., Spetzler, R.F., Hodak, J.A., Awad, C.A., and Carey, R. (1986b) Incidental subcortical lesions identified on magnetic resonance imaging in the elderly. I. Correlation with age and cerebrovascular risk factors. *Stroke* 17:1084–1089.

Boyko, O.B., Alston, S.R., Muellette, C., Fuller, G.N., and Burger, R.C. (1994) Clinical utility of post-mortem MR imaging in neuropathology. *Arch Pathol Lab Med* 118:219–225.

Bracco, L., Campani, D., Baratti, E., et al. (1993) Relation between MRI features and dementia in cerebrovascular disease patients with leukoaraiosis: A longitudinal study. *J Neurosci* 120(2): 131–136.

Breitner, J.C., Wyse, B.W., Anthony, J.C., et al. (1999) APOE-epsilon4 count predicts age when prevalence of AD increases, then declines: The Cache County Study. *Neurology* 53:321–331.

Briley, D.P., Haroon, S., Sergent, S.M., and Thomas, S. (2000) Does leukoaraiosis predict morbidity and mortality? *Neurology* 54(1): 90–94.

Butters, M.A., Becker, J.T., Nebes, R.D., et al. (2000) Changes in cognitive functioning following treatment of late-life depression. *Am J Psychiatry* 157:1949–1954.

Carney, I.M., Rich, M.W., teVelde, A., Saini, J., Clark, J., and Freedland, K.E. (1988) The relationship between heart rate, heart rate variability and depression in patients with coronary artery disease. *J Psychosom Res* 32:159–164.

Clavier, I., Hommel, M., Besson, G., Noelle, B., and Perrer, J.E. (1994) Long-term prognosis of symptomatic lacunar infarcts: A hospital-based study. *Stroke* 25(10):2005–2009.

Coffey, C.E., Figiel, G.S., and Djang, W.T. (1988) Leukoencephalopathy in elderly depressed patients referred for ECT. *Biol Psychiatry* 24:143–161.

Coffey, C.E., Figiel, G.S., and Djang, W.T. (1989) White matter hyperintensity on MRI clinical and neuroanatomic correlates in the depressed elderly. *J Neuropsychiatry Clin Neurosci* 1:135–144.

Coffey, C.E., Figiel, G.S., Djang, W.T., et al. (1990) Subcortical hyperintensity on MRI: A comparison of normal and depressed elderly subjects. *Am J Psychiatry* 147:187–189.

Corder, E.H., Saunders, A.M., Strittmatter, W.J., et al. (1993) Gene dose of apolipoprotein E type 4 allele and the risk of Alzheimer's disease in late onset families. *Science* 261:921–923.

Coulehan, J.L., Schulberg, H.C., Block, M.R., Janosky, J.E., and Arena, V.C. (1990) Medical co-morbidity of major depressive disorder in a primary medical practice. *Arch Intern Med* 150:2362–2367.

Dalack, W.R. (1990) Perspectives on the relationship between cardiovascular disease and affective disorder. *J Clin Psychiatry* 51:4–9.

Devanand, D.P., Sano, M., Tang, M.X., et al. (1996) Depressed mood and the incidence of Alzheimer's disease in the elderly living in the community. *Arch Gen Psychiatry* 53:175–182.

Figiel, G.S., Krishnan, K.R.R., Doraiswamy, P.M., Rao, V.P., Nemeroff, C.B., and Boyko, O.B. (1991) Subcortical hyperintensities on brain magnetic resonance imaging: A comparison between late age onset and early onset elderly depressed subjects. *Neurobiol Aging* 26:245–247.

Friedman, M., and Bennet, P. (1977) Depression and hypertension. *Psychosom Med* 39:134–140.

Friston, K.J., Ashburner, J., Frith, C.D., Poline, J.B., Heather, J.D., and Frackowiak, R.S.J. (1995) Spatial registration and normalization of Images. *Hum Brain Mapp* 2:165–189.

Glassman, A.H., Helzer, J.E., Covey, L.S., et al. (1990) Smoking, smoking cesssation, and major depression. *JAMA* 264:1546–1549.

Greenwald, B.S., Kramer-Ginsberg, E., Krishnan, K.R., Ashtari, M., Auerbach, C., and Patel, M. (1998) Neuroanatomic localization of magnetic resonance imaging: Single hyperintensities in geriatric depression. *Stroke* 29(3):613–617.

Habib, M., Royere, M.L., Habib, G., et al. (1991) Changes in personality and hypertension: The "athymhormic" syndrome. *Arch Maladies Coeur Vaisseaux* 84(84):1225–1230.

Hendrie, H.C., Farlow, M.R., Austrom, M.G., Edwards, M.K., and Williams, M.A. (1989) Foci of increased T2 signal intensity on brain MR scans of healthy elderly subjects. *Am J Neuroradiol* 10:703–707.

Hickie, I., Scott, E., Mitchell, P., Wilhelm, K., Austin, M.P., and Bennett, B. (1995) Subcortical hyperintensities on magnetic resonance imaging: Clinical correlates and prognostic significance in patients with severe depression. *Biol Psychiatry* 37:151–160.

Hickie, I., Scott, E., Wilhelm, K., and Brodaty, H. (1997) Subcortical hyperintensities on magnetic resonance imaging in patients with severe depression—a longitudinal evaluation. *Biol Psychiatry* 42:367–374.

Huapaya, L., and Ananth, J. (1990) Depression associated with hypertension: A review. *Psychiatric J Univ Ottawa* 5:58–62.

Hunt, A.L., Orrison, W.W., Yeo, R.A., et al. (1989) Clinical significance of MRI white matter lesions in the elderly. *Neurology* 39:1470–1474.

Inzitari, D., Cadelo, M., Marranci, M.L., Pracucci, G., and Pantoni, L. (1997) Vascular deaths in elderly neurological patients with leukoaraiosis. *J Neurol Neurosurg Psychiatry* 62:177–181.

Inzitari, D., Giordano, G.P., Ancona, A.L., Pracucci, G., and Mascalchi, M. (1990) Leukoaraiosis, intracerebral hemmorage, and arterial hypertension. *Stroke* 21(10):1419–1423.

Jack, C.R., Petersen, R.C., Xu, Y., et al. (1998) Rate of medial temporal lobe atrophy in typical aging and Alzheimer's disease. *Neurology* 51:993–999.

Jorm, A.F., van Duijn, C.M., Chandra, V., et al. (1991) Psychiatric history and related exposures as risk factors for Alzheimer's disease: A collaborative re-analysis of case-control studies. *Int J Epidemiol* 20(suppl 2):S43–S47.

Kinderman, S., Kalayam, B., Brown, G.G., Burdick, K.E., and Alexopoulos, G.S. (2000) Executive functions and P300 latency in elderly depressed patients and control subjects. *Am J Psychiatry* 8(1):57–65.

Kokmen, E., Beard, C.M., Chandra, V., Offord, K.P., Schoenberg, B.S., and Ballard, D.J. (1991) Clinical risk factors for Alzheimer's disease: A population-based case-control study. *Neurology* 41:1393–1397.

Kral, V.A., and Emery, O.B. (1989) Long-term follow-up of depressive pseudodementia of the aged. *Can J Psychiatry* 34:445–446.

Krishnan, K.R.R., Goli, Z., Ellinwood, E.H., Franz, R.D., Blazer, D.G., and Nemeroff, C.B. (1988) Leukoencephalopathy in patients diagnosed as major depressives. *Biol Psychiatry* 23:519–522.

Krishnan, K.R.R., Hays, J.C., and Blazer, D.G. (1997) MRI defined vascular depression. *Am J Psychiatry* 154:497–501.

Krishnan, K.R.R., Hays, J.C., George, L.K., and Blazer, D.G. (1998) Six-month outcomes for MRI-related vascular depression. *Depression Anxiety* 8(4):142–146.

Krishnan, K.R.R., and McDonald, W.M. (1995) Arteriosclerotic depression. *Med Hypotheses* 44:111–115.

Kuller, L.H., Shemanski, L., Manolio, T., et al. (1998) Relationship between ApoE, MRI findings, and cognitive function in the Cardiovascular Health Study. *Stroke* 29:388–398.

Laakso, M.P., Frisoni, G.B., Kononen, M., et al. (2000) Hippocampus and entorhinal cortex in frontotemporal dementia and Alzheimer's disease: A morphometric MRI study. *Biol Psychiatry* 47(12):1056–1063.

Lyness, J.M., Caine, E.D., Cox, C., King, D.A., Conewell, Y., and Olivares, T. (1998) Cerebrovascular risk factors and later-life major depression. Testing a small-vessel brain disease model. *Am J Geriatr Psychiatry* 6:5–13.

Lyness, J.M., King, D.A., Conwell, Y., Cox, C., and Caine, E.D. (2000) Cerebrovascular risk factors and 1-year depression outcome in older primary care patients. *Am J Psychiatry* 157:1499–1501.

MacFall, J.R., Payne, M.E., Provenzale, J.E., and Krishnan, K.R.R. (2001) Medial orbital frontal lesions in late onset depression. *Biol Psychiatry* 49:803–806.

Maier, W., Lichtermann, D., Minges, J., Heun, R., Hallmayer, J., and Klingler, T. (1991) Unipolar depression in the aged: Determinants of familial aggregation. *J Affect Disord* 23:53–61.

Miyao, S., Takano, A., Teramoto, J., and Takahashi, A. (1992) Leukoaraiosis in relation to prognosis for patients with lacunar infarction. *Stroke* 23(10):1434–1438.

O'Brien, J., Ames, D., Chiu, E., Schweitzer, I., Desmond, P., and Tress, B. (1998) Severe deep white matter lesions and outcome in elderly patients with major depressive disorder: follow up study. *Br Med J* 317(7164):982–984.

Post, F. (1962) The significance of affective symptoms in old age. *Institute of Psychiatry*. Maudsley Monographs #10. London: Oxford University Press.

Rabkin, J.F., Charles, E., and Kass, F. (1983) Hypertension and DSM-III depression in psychiatric outpatients. *Am J Psychiatry* 140:1072–1074.

Reding, M., Haycox, J., and Blass, J. (1985) Depression in patients referred to a dementia clinic: A three year prospective study. *Arch Neurol* 42:894–896.

Riley, K.P., Snowdon, D.A., Saunders, A.M., Roses, A.D., Mortimer, J.A., and Nanayakkara, N. (2000) Cognitive function and apolipoprotein E in very old adults: Findings from the Nun Study. *J Gerontol B Psychol Sci Soc Sci* 55:S69–S75.

Salgado, A.V., Ferro, J.M., and Gouveia-Oliveira, A. (1996) Long-term prognosis of first-ever lacunar strokes. A hospital-based study. *Stroke* 27(4):661–666.

Sapolsky, R.M. (1999) Glucocorticoids, stress, and their adverse neurological effects: Relevance to aging. *Exp Gerontol* 34:721–732.

Sapolsky, R.M., Krey, L.C., and McEwen, B.S. (1986) The neuroendocrinology of stress and aging: The glucocorticoid cascade hypothesis. *Endocrinol Rev* 7:284–301.

Saunders, A.M., Strittmatter, W.J., Schmechel, D., et al. (1993) Association of apolipoprotein E allele E4 with late-onset familial and sporadic Alzheimer's disease. *Neurology* 43:1467–1472.

Schulz, R., Beach, S.R., Ives, D.G., Martire, L.M., Ariyo, A.A., and Kop, W.J. (2000) Association between depression and mortality in older adults. The Cardiovascular Health Study. *Arch Intern Med* 160:1761–1768.

Sheline, Y.I., Sanghavi, M., Mintun, M.A., and Gado, M.H. (1999) Depression duration but not age predicts hippocampal volume loss in medically healthy women with recurrent major depression. *J Neurosci* 19:5034–5043.

Sheline, Y.I., Wang, P.W., Gado, M.H., Csernansky, J.G., and Vannier, M.W. (1996) Hippocampal atrophy in recurrent major depression. *Proc Natl Acad Sci USA* 93:3908–3913.

Simpson, S., Baldwin, R.C., Jackson, A., and Burns, A.S. (1998) Is subcortical disease associated with a poor response to antidepressants? Neurological, neuropsychological and neuroradiological findings in late-life depression. *Psychol Med* 28(5):1015–1026.

Snowdon, D.A., Greiner, L.H., and Markesbery, W.R. (2000) Linguistic ability in early life and the neuropathology of Alzheimer's disease and cerebrovascular disease. Findings from the Nun Study. *Ann NY Acad Sci* 903:34–38.

Speck, C.E., Kukull, W.A., Brenner, D.E., et al. (1995) History of depression as a risk factor for Alzheimer's disease. *Epidemiology* 6:366–369.

Steffens, D.C., Byrum, C.E., McQuoid, D.R., et al. (2000a) Hippocampal volume in geriatric depression. *Biol Psychiatry* 48:301–309.

Steffens, D.C., Conway, C.R., Dombeck, C.B., Wagner, H.R., Tupler, L.A., and Weiner, R.D. (2001) Severity of subcortical gray matter hyperintensity predicts ECT response in geriatric depression. *J ECT* 17(1):45–49.

Steffens, D.C., Helms, M.J., Krishnan, K.R., and Burke, G.L. (1999a) Cerebrovascular disease and depression symptoms in the cardiovascular health study. *Stroke* 30:2159–2156.

Steffens, D.C., and Krishnan, K.R.R. (1998) Structural neuroimaging and mood disorders: Recent findings, implications for classification, and future directions. *Biol Psychiatry* 43:705–712.

Steffens, D.C., MacFall, J.R., Payne, M.E., Welsh-Bohmer, K.A., and Krishnan, K.R.R. (2000b) Grey-matter lesions and dementia. *Lancet* 356:1686–1687.

Steffens, D.C., Norton, M.C., Plassman, B.L., et al. (1999b) Enhanced cognitive performance with estrogen use in nondemented community-dwelling older women. *J Am Geriatr Soc* 47:1171–1175.

Steffens, D.C., Plassman, B.L., Helms, M.J., Welsh-Bohmer, K.A., Saunders, A.M., and Breitner, J.C. (1997) A twin study of late-onset depression and apolipoprotein E epsilon 4 as risk factors for Alzheimer's disease. *Biol Psychiatry* 41:851–856.

Steffens, D.C., Skoog, I., Norton, M.C., et al. (2000c) Prevalence of depression and its treatment in an elderly population: The Cache County study. *Arch Gen Psychiatry* 57:601–607.

Strittmatter, W.J., Saunders, A.M., Schmechel, D., et al. (1993) Apolipoprotein E: High-avidity binding to B-amyloid and increased frequency of type 4 allele in late-onset familial Alzheimer disease. *Proc Natl Acad Sci USA* 90:1977–1981.

Tarvonen-Schroder, S., Kurki, T., Raiha, I., and Sourander, L. (1995) Leukoaraiosis and cause of death: A five year follow up. *J Neurol Neurosurg Psychiatry* 58(5):586–589.

Tresch, D.D., Folstein, M.F., and Rabins, P.V. (1985) Prevalence and significance of cardiovascular disease and hypertension in elderly patients with dementia and depression. *J Am Geriatr Soc* 33:530–537.

van Duijn, C.M., Clayton, D.G., Chandra, V., et al. (1994) Interaction between genetic and environmental risk factors for Alzheimer's disease: A reanalysis of case-control studies. *Genet Epidemiol* 11:539–551.

Wright, I.C., McGuire, P.K., Poline, J.B., et al. (1995) A voxel-based method for the statistical analysis of gray and white matter density applied to schizophrenia. *Neuroimage* 2:244–252.

Yanai, I., Fujikawa, T., Horiguchi, J., Yamawaki, S., and Touhouda, Y. (1998) The 3-year course and outcome of patients with major depression and silent cerebral infarction. *J Affect Disord* 47(1–3):25–30.

# 13 | Hypothalamic-pituitary-adrenal axis activity in mood and cognition in the elderly: Implications for symptoms and outcomes

JENNIFER KELLER, THERESA M. BUCKLEY, AND ALAN F. SCHATZBERG

Although major depression was once thought to be particularly common in the elderly, more recent studies have indicated otherwise. Epidemiological studies have demonstrated that major depression occurs in 4% of the general elderly population, while 10%–25% have depressive symptoms (Blazer, 2002). However, those age 65 and older have the highest rate of suicide. Depression is a disease; it is not part of the normal aging process. Depression in the elderly may be qualitatively different from depression in other age groups, with higher rates of cognitive impairment and co-morbid medical illnesses. Indeed, depression in the elderly is associated with poorer outcomes of co-morbid medical syndromes (including higher mortality rates).

In this chapter, we discuss the possible role that elevated hypothalamic-pituitary-adrenal (HPA) axis activity may play in key aspects of depression in the elderly. We begin by reviewing the regulation of the HPA axis and the actions of glucocorticoids. Then we discuss HPA axis abnormalities and changes in depression, followed by potential cognitive consequences in aging. Next, we explore specific brain structures accounting for some of the cognitive changes evident in geriatric depression. Finally, we examine depression and elevated HPA activity as a risk factor for mortality.

## REGULATION AND FUNCTION OF THE HYPOTHALAMIC-PITUITARY-ADRENAL AXIS

The HPA axis is a stress-responsive system that consists of forward-stimulating arms and feedback loops that together regulate the production of glucocorticoids (GCs). As we shall discuss, the HPA axis has been implicated in mood regulation and cognitive functioning. It consists of the hypothalamus, pituitary gland, and adrenal gland and receives information from other structures including the hippocampus and amygdala. During stress, the HPA axis is activated. The hypothalamus then secretes two hormones, corticotropin-releasing hormone (CRH) and arginine vasopressin (AVP), which act on the pituitary to increase adrenocorticotropic hormone (ACTH) release. Corticotropin-releasing hormone interacts with receptors on corticotropins in the pituitary that secrete ACTH, which is then carried to the adrenal cortex, where it stimulates the production and release of cortisol. Circulating GCs regulate the production and release of hypothalamic CRH and ACTH through negative feedback loops to the hypothalamus and pituitary. Cortisol is the adrenal GC stress hormone secreted in humans.

Cortisol then binds to GC receptors. Two key GC receptors in the brain are mineralocorticoid receptors (MRs), or Type I receptors, and glucocorticoid receptors (GRs), or Type II receptors. In the brain, MRs are found predominantly in the hippocampus and limbic structures, while GRs are more widely distributed (Joels and de Kloet, 1992; Patel et al., 2000). Mineralocorticoid receptors have a high affinity for corticosterone, cortisol, and aldosterone, while GRs have a high affinity for synthetic GC analogs such as dexamethasone and prednisone and a low affinity for corticosterone and cortisol. This bilevel system may enable the brain to distinguish between two types of GC secretion, a stress-dependent release and a circadian release (de Kloet, 1992; Orchinik et al., 1995). Additionally, GCs modulate neurotransmitter systems and regulate the circuitry of many brain regions (McEwen, 1999). Presumably, they have a role in the survival and death of neurons, dendritic branching and synapse formation, the abundance of certain structural proteins in glial cells, and the operation of various second messenger systems (Orchinik et al., 1995)

Abundant evidence suggests that disrupted GC levels result in disturbances of mood and cognition, neurophysiological changes (e.g., electroencephalographic [EEG] changes), neurotransmitter activity alteration, and a variety of neuroanatomical changes (e.g., cortical atrophy, hippocampal degeneration) (Sapolsky et al., 1985, 1986). Chronic elevations of cortisol have been associated with dysfunction of the immune system, neurodegeneration in aging, and disturbances in cognition (Chrousos and Gold, 1992; McEwen, 2000). Excessive corticosteroid levels have frequently been related to a number of clinical states, including depression, schizophrenia, and Alzheimer's disease, as well as Cushing's disease.

## HYPOTHALAMIC-PITUITARY-ADRENAL AXIS AND DEPRESSION

Clinical and preclinical studies have presented substantial evidence to suggest that alterations of the stress hormone system (HPA axis) play a major causal role in the development of depression. Some authors, however, have suggested that this is secondary to the stress accompanying depression or to the neurotransmitter imbalances causing the depressive symptoms (Gold and Chrousos, 1985; Nemeroff, 1988). At any rate, the HPA system clearly has an important role in the expression of depression. With other components of the stress hormone system, the action of corticosteroid hormones has two modes. First, corticosteroids maintain the basal activity of the HPA system and control the sensitivity or threshold of the system's response to stress. Second, corticosteroid feedback helps to terminate stress-induced HPA system activity. Thus, corticosteroids facilitate the ability to cope with, adapt to, and recover from stress (de Kloet et al., 1998). If this system is dysfunctional, the ability to react to and handle stress will be impaired.

There is abundant evidence of cortisol hypersecretion in patients with mood disorders. Approximately 40%–60% of drug-free depressed patients present with hypercortisolemia (Gold et al., 1986; Murphy, 1991). Patients with major depression have been found to have an abnormal response on the dexamethasone suppression test (DST). In the DST, patients are typically given a dose of dexamethasone, a synthetic corticosteroid, in the evening and then cortisol is measured the next day. The normal response is inhibition of cortisol secretion because of the negative feedback from the dexametha-

sone. Those who do not suppress are considered DST nonsuppressors, and nonsuppression is often associated with elevated levels of cortisol. Many depressed patients are nonsuppressors. Greden et al. (1983) found that nonsuppression in the DST typically normalizes with recovery from depression. This normalization typically precedes or coincides with (rather than follows) clinical recovery. Failure to normalize the DST response even after adequate antidepressant treatment may be a risk factor for relapse (Nemeroff and Evans, 1984; Rothschild and Schatzberg, 1982).

Cognition has also been found to be impaired in depression, and that impairment has been correlated with the cortisol level. For example, Rubinow et al. (1984) found a positive correlation between mean urinary free cortisol level and number of errors on an abstract reasoning test in nonmedicated depressed patients. In fact, all of the cortisol hypersecretors in the study were cognitively impaired. Wolkowitz et al. (1990) found that depressed patients who were DST nonsuppressors made more errors on verbal learning tests than controls. Similarly, Van Londen et al. (1998) found that in patients with major depression, better global cognitive performance was correlated negatively with baseline plasma cortisol levels.

Our group and others have suggested that major depression with psychotic features (PMD) is a distinct syndrome (Schatzberg and Rothschild, 1992). Indeed, PMD patients have more cognitive impairments than do depressed patients without psychosis (Belanoff et al., 2001; Schatzberg et al., 2000). In particular, patients with PMD have highly replicable findings of greater HPA activation: high rates of nonsuppression on the DST, elevated post–dexamethasone administration cortisol levels, and high levels of 24-hour urinary free cortisol (e.g., Anton, 1987; Nelson and Davis, 1997; Rothschild et al., 1982; Schatzberg et al., 1983). These findings are not just due to a difference in the severity of the depression (e.g., Brown et al., 1988; Evans et al., 1983). Anton (1987) found that it was the older PMD patients who had the highest cortisol levels, suggesting an interaction between age and type of depression. Furthermore, Schatzberg et al. (1983) compared cortisol levels in PMD patients to cortisol levels in those with schizophrenia. They found high afternoon cortisol levels in PMD patients but not in schizophrenia patients. They concluded that the high cortisol levels were not due to psychosis per se, but rather to the presence of psychosis in the context of an affective disorder. Hence, there appears to be even greater HPA axis activity in psychotic major depression than in nonpsychotic major depression.

Similar cognitive and mood impairments are found in Cushing's disease and have been related to the cortisol level. Cushing's disease is a disorder of the endocrine system that is characterized by hypercortisolemia.

In Cushing's disease, hypersecretion of cortisol is associated with a high incidence of depression and memory impairment, as well as hippocampal atrophy. Cushing's disease is associated with a high rate of fatigue, decreased energy, irritability, decreased memory and concentration, depressed mood, and insomnia. These symptoms are similar to those seen in major depression, and in Cushing's disease they are directly correlated with elevated circulating cortisol levels (Starkman et al., 2001).

Cognitive dysfunction in Cushing's disease includes visual and verbal memory, attention and concentration, and delayed recall (e.g., Starkman et al., 1986, 2001; Whelan et al., 1980). Direct correlations have been found between the severity of the patients' overall cognitive impairment and their levels of cortisol. Importantly, both mood and cognitive functioning improve in Cushing's patients once their plasma cortisol levels are reduced (e.g., Mauri et al., 1993; for review, see Wolkowitz and Reus, 1999). These data suggest an etiological role for cortisol elevations in this psychiatric symptomatology.

In summary, cortisol has been shown to be elevated in depression and to have even greater elevations in psychotic major depression and Cushing's disease. There is some evidence that this relationship is mediated by age, with older depressed patients having higher cortisol levels. In both Cushing's disease and depression, greater cognitive impairment has been correlated with elevated cortisol levels. Importantly, these mood, cognitive, and even structural brain changes (to a limited degree) may be reversible once elevated cortisol levels are lowered.

## GERIATRIC DEPRESSION, COGNITION, AND HYPOTHALAMIC-PITUITARY-ADRENAL ACTIVITY

Depression in the elderly is often complicated by other medical and psychosocial problems, including cognitive decline, disability, medical illness, and social isolation. A significant number of depressed older adults also have cognitive impairment. Impaired cognition and depressive symptoms double in frequency every 5 years after the age of 70 in community residents. The combination of these symptoms is present in 25% of 85-year-old subjects (Arve et al., 1999). Depressed patients have disturbances in attention, speed of processing, and executive function even when they are not demented (Lockwood et al., 2002). Even after remission of depressive symptomatology, processing speed and working memory impairments can remain (Nebes et al., 2000). Cognitive dysfunction of older depressed patients is often, but not always, due to an underlying dementing disorder. Furthermore Rubinow et al. (1984) found a robust correlation between age and number of

test errors in depressed patients. Thus, it appears that age and depression interact to produce severe cognitive impairments in the elderly.

There are probably many causes of cognitive impairment in geriatric depression. Aging and depression are both generally associated with relative hypercortisolemia, and hypercortisolemia has been shown to have negative effects on cognition (for review, see Belanoff et al., 2001). We have already noted that cognitive dysfunction is associated with elevated cortisol in Cushing's disease. Additionally, elevated levels of cortisol have been associated with numerous cognitive deficits in healthy controls including increased intrusion errors and errors of commission (Wolkowitz et al., 1990), decreased performance on the paragraph recall test (Newcomer et al., 1999), poorer performance on selective attention and explicit memory tasks (Lupien et al., 1994, 1999), and impairment on executive functioning tests (Young et al., 1999). When synthetic cortisol is administered to healthy controls, the cognitive impairments are reversible once medication is discontinued (Newcomer et al., 1999).

## AGING AND HYPOTHALAMIC-PITUITARY-ADRENAL ACTIVITY

Aging is generally associated with a relative increase in HPA activity, and HPA axis hyperactivity is often associated with a decrease in MR or GRs. Normal aging is also associated with changes in the cortisol rhythm (Kern et al., 1996; Van Cauter et al., 1996). Higher rates of dexamethasone nonsuppression have been found in elderly depressed and elderly demented patients, and age has been implicated in the higher post-dexamethasone cortisol levels in elderly depressed patients (Asnis et al., 1981; Georgotas et al., 1986).

Age-related increases in cortisol levels have been correlated with age-related memory decline, but it is unclear whether this reflects a direct effect of cortisol on memory substrates (Heffelfinger and Newcomer, 2001). Lupien and colleagues assessed cortisol levels longitudinally in the age and found considerable variation in plasma cortisol levels, with evidence of distinct subgroups of subjects. Between subgroups, there was no gender difference in cortisol history and no change in the circadian rhythm or corticosteroid-binding globulin levels. However, for the neuropsychological data, the group that had increasing cortisol levels from year to year and currently high basal cortisol levels showed significant memory impairments compared to the other two groups (Lupien et al., 2002). The authors suggest that cumulative exposure to moderately high levels of cortisol in the elderly may be a risk factor for the development of memory impairments. Thus, given that depression is associated with increased cortisol levels, older people who have experienced recurrent depression throughout their lives may be at risk for developing memory and cognitive problems. In fact, Jorm (2001) concluded that the longer one experiences depression, the higher the risk of cognitive decline or Alzheimer's disease (AD) in later life.

## DEPRESSION, DEMENTIA, AND HYPOTHALAMIC-PITUITARY-ADRENAL ACTIVITY

There is high co-morbidity between depression and dementia. An early concept of *pseudodementia* was based on the assumption that biological abnormalities of depression were the cause of cognitive impairment in the context of depression. Further evaluation of patients with pseudodementia has shown that many of these patients progress to irreversible dementia (Alexopoulos et al., 1993), suggesting that depressive pseudodementia may be a preclinical or an early-stage dementing disorder. Indeed, depressive symptoms have often been observed to precede the development of dementia (Alexopoulos et al., 2002). This finding is consistent with that of Jorm (2000), who concluded that a lengthy period of depression is a risk factor for cognitive decline. Importantly, not all cases of geriatric depression with cognitive impairment lead to irreversible dementia (Alexopoulos et al., 1993).

Recent studies have also suggested that depression may play a causal role in the structural brain abnormalities seen in patients with dementia (Alexopoulos, 2003). Although there are many different causes of dementia, most of the research that will be discussed has examined dementia of the Alzheimer's type. Excessive GCs and other stress hormones—which, as noted, play a role in depression—reduce neurotropic factors, inhibit neurogenesis, and may promote amyloid neurotoxicity, thus accelerating the pathological cascade of AD. Similarly, changes in brain stem aminergic nuclei that occur during AD have been thought to contribute to depression (Zubenko et al., 1990). Thus, Alexopoulos (2003) concluded that once depression develops as part of the brain changes of AD, it may accelerate the progression of the neuropathological changes of AD.

The presence of the apolipoprotein E4 (APOE4) allele is a risk factor for AD (Steffens et al., 1997). However, in patients without this allele (i.e., those without this risk factor), individuals with late-onset depression had a 2.95 times higher risk of developing AD than those without a history of depression. Some studies have found that a lifetime history of depression increases the risk of AD, regardless of the presence or absence of a family history of dementing disorders (Van Duijn et al., 1994). In a meta-analysis, Jorm et al. (1991) examined the history of depression and its relationship to AD. They found that a history of depression was associated with onset of AD after the age of 70 years only when depressive symptoms had appeared within 10 years before the onset of dementia. However, depression with onset more than 10 years before the diagnosis of dementia was associated with onset of AD at any age. This suggests that depression in early and middle life is a risk factor for AD, while some cases of late-onset depression are prodromal states of dementia (Alexopoulos et al., 2000a).

Elevated cortisol levels are observed in AD and may contribute to AD by lowering the threshold for neuronal degeneration. Hypothalamic-pituitary-adrenal hyperactivity in AD has been found, as evidenced by increased cortisol concentrations in plasma and urine and nonsuppression in the DST. Peskind and colleagues (2001) found that cortisol levels were higher in AD patients than in normal older control subjects. Furthermore, cerebrospinal fluid (CSF) cortisol levels differed with respect to the APOE genotype in both groups. Higher cortisol levels were associated with increased frequency of the APOE4 allele and decreased frequency of the APOE2 allele. The APOE4 allele increases the risk of AD, while APOE2 decreases the risk (Corder et al., 1994). Thus, the increased HPA activity associated with depression may interact with a genetic predisposition to AD and lead to neuronal degeneration and ultimately to the expression of AD.

## BRAIN STRUCTURES IN COGNITION AND DEPRESSION

Co-morbid depression and cognitive dysfunction have been associated with poor outcomes in depression, a longer duration of illness, and a more chronic course in community samples (Beekman et al., 2002). Studies have attempted to identify and clarify the role of specific brain structures and/or regions in cognitive and affective processes in depression. The primary structures under study have been the prefrontal cortex, hippocampus, and amygdala. The prefrontal cortex is important for executive functioning; that is, it oversees (attends, integrates, formulates, modifies, and monitors) all nervous system activity. The hippocampus and amygdala are part of the limbic system, which is the body's emotion-regulating system. The hippocampus is primarily associated with learning and memory, and the amygdala is important for the interpretation of emotional and motivational experiences.

Evidence suggests that depression in the elderly may be qualitatively different from depression in other age groups. Depression in the elderly is associated with more medical co-morbidity and more cognitive problems, particularly in executive functioning. This executive dysfunction may not completely remit after the depression clears, and continued executive dysfunction is associated with early relapse. Depression in the elderly is also associated with a number of changes in the brain including structural and functional changes. Some of these regions play a key role in the cognitive functions that are disrupted in elderly depression.

## FRONTAL LOBE

Several studies have suggested that frontal lobe dysfunction may contribute to the development of late-life depression (for review, see Alexopoulos, 2002). First, executive functioning is impaired in older depressed patients (Elliott et al., 1996; Kindermann et al., 2000; Lockwood et al., 2002). Selective and sustained attention impairments occur in both younger and older depressed patients, although tasks requiring response inhibition and sustained effort are preferentially impaired in geriatric depressed patients (Lockwood et al., 2002). A large percentage of depressed geriatric patients also have abnormal initiation/preservation errors, which is a prefrontal function (Kindermann and Brown, 1997). Much of the executive dysfunction remits with improvement of the depression, but it can persist to some degree. Furthermore, executive dysfunction predicts a poor response to therapy and early relapse (Alexopoulos et al., 2002a; Kalayam and Alexopoulos, 1999). Alexopoulos et al. (2000) found that executive dysfunction was associated with early relapse and recurrence of late-life depression but that memory impairment, disability, medical issues, social support, or number of previous episodes did not influence the course of geriatric depression. Thus, there is some evidence that frontal lobe dysfunction may be intimately tied to geriatric depression.

A number of studies have found reduced volume and activity of prefrontal cortex (PFC) structures in depression (Drevets and Price, 1997) and in aging (Coffey et al., 1992; Gunning-Dixon and Raz, 2000). The PFC mediates cortical restraint on the amygdala (Davidson, 2002), the HPA axis (Diorio et al., 1993), and brain stem noradrenergic nuclei (Gray and Bingaman, 1996). Cortisol administration to healthy controls alters processes associated with PFC functions, such as inhibition, attention, and planning (Lupien et al., 1999; Young et al., 1999). In nonhuman primates, Lyons et al. (2000) found that cortisol impairs medial PFC behavioral inhibition, and in rats it leads to reorganization of PFC dendritic fibers (Wellman, 2001). Lesioning on an area analogous to the PFC in rats leads to increased HPA axis and sympathetic nervous system activity. These prefrontal functions are intimately tied to geriatric depression, and in animals, prefrontal impairments clearly lead to HPA dysfunction.

## LIMBIC AND FRONTO-STRIATAL CONNECTIONS

Imaging studies have found a variety of structural abnormalities associated with depression, including the relationship between fronto-striatal and limbic impairment and between fronto-striatal impairment and executive dysfunction. Both imaging and neuropsychological data suggest that specific functions of the frontal, nonparietal regions decline with age (Daigneault and Braun, 1993). Diffusion tensor imaging (DTI) is a magnetic resonance imaging (MRI) technique that quantifies the integrity of white matter in selected regions. Alexopoulos et al. (2002b) found that compromised white matter lateral to the anterior cingulate and at the level of the middle frontal gyrus was associated with executive dysfunction and a poor remission rate in citalopram-treated elderly depressed patients.

Reduced volumes have been found in the anterior cingulate, caudate, putamen, hippocampus, and amygdala in depressed patients compared to controls (Sheline et al., 1999). Specifically in elderly depressed patients, researchers have reported a bilateral reduction in orbitofrontal cortex and white matter hyperintensities, particularly in the medial orbitofrontal cortex (Krishnan et al., 1993). The subcortical white matter hyperintensities have also been associated with executive dysfunction (Boone et al., 1992). Similarly, in Cushing's syndrome, researchers have found relationships between hypercortisolemia and changes in brain structures: ventricular enlargement and cortical atrophy (Momose et al., 1971), and hippocampal reductions (Starkman et al., 1992).

## HIPPOCAMPUS AND AMYGDALA

The hippocampal formation is a key receptor site for GCs in the brain and is known to have an important role in inhibiting the HPA axis in humans (Mandell et al., 1963; Wilson et al., 1980). Type I receptors are found predominantly in the hippocampus, while Type II receptors are more diffusely scattered throughout the brain. Mineralocorticoid receptors in the hippocampus are lost as part of the normal aging process, and both hippocampal damage and receptor loss are associated with learning impairments. There is strong evidence for an association between elevated cortisol levels and hippocampal and/or GR damage (for review, see Belanoff et al., 2001). Reduced hippocampal volume has been found in depressed elderly subjects (Steffens et al., 2000). This may also be a risk factor for the later development of dementia (Steffens et al., 2002). The degenerated hippocampus in the elderly may be responsible for some of the HPA axis hyperactivity observed (Dodt et al., 1994) since hippocampal damage, in general, can result in increased activity of the HPA axis (Landfield and Eldridge, 1991).

With respect to hippocampal tissue, animal studies show that excessive levels of GCs can be toxic. Issa et al. (1990) studied three groups of rats: (1) aged and cognitively impaired, (2) aged and cognitively unimpaired, and (3) young controls. The greatest amount of hippocampal pyramidal cell damage was present in the rats that were aged and cognitively impaired and in those with the highest corticosterone levels. In the rat, sustained exposure to elevated GC levels is associated with hippocampal atrophy and severe memory impairments (Landfield et al., 1981). Sapolsky et al. (1986) have also argued that in rats, elevated levels of GCs as well as high cumulative exposure to concentrations of these hormones lead to hippocampal degeneration. Similarly, cumulative exposure to high levels of GCs can be particularly detrimental for the aged hippocampus in humans (for review, see Lupien et al., 1999). Furthermore, in Cushing's syndrome, Starkman et al. (1992) found relationships with reduced hippocampal volume, poorer verbal memory, and elevated cortisol levels. Hippocampal volume was negatively correlated with mean plasma cortisol level and positively correlated with verbal memory scores. Although some researchers have suggested that hypercortisolemia itself is enough to cause hippocampal damage, others have suggested that chronically elevated GC concentrations in the absence of stress do not injure the hippocampus (Leverenz et al., 1999). Indeed, Leverenz et al. found that GCs administered to elderly rhesus monkeys did not cause hippocampal damage.

The amygdala is involved in the regulation of emotion and thus is an important structure in depression. Depressed patients (both unipolar and bipolar) demonstrated increased left amygdala metabolism, which is correlated with depression severity and plasma cortisol levels (Drevets et al., 2002). Elevated amygdala metabolism during remission has also been associated with a risk of relapse (Drevets, 2001). Additionally, the amygdala inhibits the PFC (Davidson, 2002) and activates the HPA axis (Prewitt and Herman, 1994). These data suggest that elevated amygdala activity could account for a variety of the cognitive and GC abnormalities. It may reflect either the effect of amygdala activity on CRH secretion or the effect of cortisol on amygdala function.

Although there are some inconsistencies, overall there appear to be strong links between depression, HPA activity, and cognitive performance in the elderly. Research on aging and depression has reported similar changes in structures and functions, particularly in the PFC. It is possible that these systems interact to affect the progression of neuropathological changes, and that for those who have other genetic predispositions, such as APOE4, they interact to accelerate the progression of these changes.

## DEPRESSION, AGING, AND MORTALITY

The HPA axis and the sympathoadrenal system together mediate the body's adaptive responses to stress. Dysregulation of the system is caused by a cumulative burden of repetitive or chronic environmental stress challenges. This dysregulation contributes to a variety of physical illnesses including hypertension, arteriosclerosis, insulin resistance, and sometimes disorders of the immune system (for review, see Vanitallie, 2002). There is evidence that depression and elevated cortisol are mediating factors in these illnesses.

Major depression appears to be an independent risk factor for the development of coronary heart disease and osteoporosis, and alters the prognosis of these and other disorders. Frasure-Smith and colleagues (1993, 2000) have found that depression after myocardial infarction increases the risk of cardiac mortality. Cortisol exerts many effects that contribute to coronary artery disease. It inhibits the growth hormone (GH) and gonadal axes. Inhibition of these axes leads to increased visceral fat accumulation, which can lead to dyslipidemia and, along with hypercortisolism, to insulin resistance, hyperinsulinism, and their sequelae (Gold and Chrousos, 2002). Excessive glucose has deleterious effects on the immune system, glucose metabolism, bone, hippocampal neurons, and memory (Cizza et al., 2001; Ligier and Sternberg, 1999; Sapolsky, 2001). Although not known, theoretically the increases in visceral fat may be cumulative over repeated depressive episodes and may lead to adverse metabolic effects even during remission (Gold et al., 2002). Additionally, a deficiency in GH doubles the risk of developing premature cardiovascular disease in adulthood (Erfurth et al., 1999; Hew et al., 1998).

Specific catecholamine dysfunction has also been found in depression, much of which is associated with hypercortisolism and potentially with cardiac risk. Rosenbaum et al. (1983) measured urinary free cortisol and urinary 3-methoxy-4-hydroxyphenylglycol (MHPG) levels in severely depressed patients and nonpsychiatric controls. Cortisol levels, but not MHPG levels, were significantly higher in depressed patients than in control subjects. A positive correlation between MHPG levels and cortisol levels was reported in depressed patients but not in control subjects. Similarly, Roy and colleagues (1986, 1988) have found significantly higher urinary output of norepinephrine (NE) and its metabolites in depressed patients compared to controls. Finally, Wong et al. (2000) found that depressed patients had higher cerebrospinal fluid (CSF) NE and plasma cortisol levels than nondepressed controls. Diurnal variation of these measures was normal in the depressed patients. Control subjects showed a significant correlation between plasma cortisol and CSF CRH levels, whereas the depressed patients showed no relationship between these parameters. Overall, these results suggest bidirectional links between a central hypernoradrenergic state and the hyperfunctioning of specific central CRH pathways that are driven and sustained by hypercortisolism (Wong et al., 2000). The dysregulation of the HPA system that causes the changes in cortisol and catecholamines is a likely mechanism by which further arrhythmias occur and lead to increased mortality in cardiac patients with co-morbid depression.

Patients with major depression are also at risk for loss of bone density. Activation of the HPA system, suppression of the GH and reproductive axes, and NE-mediated activation of the release of proinflammatory cytokines are all risk factors. Michelson et al. (1996) reported greater than expected bone density loss in women with major depression. A subgroup of their sample (approximately 30%) had significant bone density loss. Importantly, it is unclear how readily this bone density can be regained once it is lost.

People with major depressive disorder also demonstrate higher mortality rates than do those without a history of depression (Bruce et al., 1994; Pulska et al., 2000). This pattern holds true even after controlling for demographic variables such as age, gender, and co-morbid medical illnesses, and it is independent of suicide, smoking, and other risk factors for poor health (Wulsin et al., 1999). Mortality is also associated with an increasing number of depressive symptoms in women (Whooley and Browner, 1998) and in a cohort of Japanese-American men (Takeshita et al., 2002). Vythilingam et al. (2003) found that psychotic depression was associated with a twofold increase in mortality compared to depression without psychotic features. These findings held true after controlling for age and additional medical illnesses.

Older adults are also at risk for suicide. People age 65 and older are at higher risk for suicide than any other age group. Within this age group, those 85 years of age and older are at even greater risk, having a rate almost twice the national average (Hoyert et al., 2001). There is some evidence to suggest that HPA axis hyperactivity is associated with suicide/mortality. In postmortem studies, researchers have found that people who committed suicide, compared to those who died by other violent means, had great adrenal weights (Dorovini-Zis and Zis, 1987; Szigethy et al., 1994), fewer binding sites for corticotropin-releasing factor (CRF) in the frontal cortex (Nemeroff et al., 1988), and higher levels of CRF in CSF (Arato et al., 1989). Coryell and Schlesser (2001) followed patients with depression or schizoaffective disorder over a 15-year period. They found that patients who had abnormal DST results at baseline hospitalization were nine times more likely to commit suicide. DST nonsuppression is often related to

elevated cortisol levels. Other researchers have found similar relationships between abnormal DST and suicide attempts (e.g., Pfeffer et al., 1991; Targum et al., 1983). Roy (1992) found no relationship between CRH and cortisol levels in depressed patients who attempted suicide and those who did not. However, depressed patients who made violent suicide attempts had higher afternoon and postdexamethasone plasma cortisol levels, and significantly more of them were nonsuppressors than patients who made nonviolent suicide attempts. These findings suggest the possibility that dysregulation of the HPA axis may be a factor in violent suicidal behavior.

Depression has a definite, albeit not fully understood, connection to other physical illnesses, dementias, and mortality. The link between depression and mortality can be direct (e.g., through suicide) or indirect (e.g., as a risk factor for early cardiac mortality). The link could reflect a common biological phenomenon such as excessive HPA axis activity with increased catecholamine release. Overall results from a host of studies reviewed suggest that elevated HPA axis activity plays an integral role in the expression and outcome of depression as well as in co-morbid medical diseases in the elderly.

ACKNOWLEDGMENTS
Research and preparation of this chapter were supported by grants from the National Institute of Mental Health: MH 062131, MHMH50604, MH019938, and MH 47573. Alan F. Schatzberg is a founder of Corcept Therapeutics.

REFERENCES

Alexopoulos, G.S. (2002) Frontostriatal and limbic dysfunction in late-life depression. *Am J Geriatr Psychiatry* 10:687–695.

Alexopoulos, G.S. (2003) Clinical and biological interactions in affective and cognitive geriatric syndromes. *Am J Psychiatry* 160: 811–814.

Alexopoulos, G.S., Kiosses, D.N., Choi, S.J., Murphy, C.F., and Lim, K.O. (2002b) Frontal white matter microstructure and treatment response of late-life depression: A preliminary study. *Am J Psychiatry* 159:1929–1932.

Alexopoulos, G., Kiosses, D., Klimstra, S., Kalayam, B., and Bruce, M. (2002a) Clinical presentation of the "depression-executive dysfunction syndrome" of late life. *Am J Geriatr Psychiatry* 10: 98–106.

Alexopoulos, G., Meyers, B., Young, R., Mattis, S., and Kakuma, T. (1993) The course of geriatric depression with "reversible dementia": A controlled study. *Am J Psychiatry* 150:1693–1699.

Anton, R.F. (1987) Urinary free cortisol in psychotic depression. *Biol Psychiatry* 22:24–34.

Arato, M., Banki, C.M., Bissette, G., and Nemeroff, C.B. (1989) Elevated CSF CRF in suicide victims. *Biol Psychiatry* 25:355–359.

Arve, S., Lauri, S., Lehtonen, A., and Tilvis, R.S. (1999) Patient's and general practitioner's different views on patient's depression. *Arch Gerontol Geriatr* 28:247–257.

Asnis, G.M., Sachar, E.J., Halbreich, U., Nathan, R.S., Novacenko, H., and Ostrow, L.C. (1981) Cortisol secretion in relation to age in major depression. *Psychosom Med* 43:235–242.

Beekman, A.T.F., Geerlings, S.W., Deeg, D.J.H., Smit, J.H., Schoevers, R.S., et al. (2002) The natural history of late-life depression: A 6-year prospective study in the community. *Arch Gen Psychiatry* 59:605–611.

Belanoff, J.K., Gross, K., Yager, A., and Schatzberg, A.F. (2001) Corticosteroids and cognition. *J Psychiatr Res* 35:127–145.

Belanoff, J.K., Kalehzan, M., Sund, B., Ficek, S.K.F., and Schatzberg, A.F. (2001) Cortisol activity and cognitive changes in psychotic major depression. *Am J Psychiatry* 158:1612–1616.

Blazer, D. (2002) *Depression in Late Life.* New York: Springer.

Boone, K.B., Miller, B.L., Lesser, I.M., Mehringer, C.M., Hill-Gutierrez, E., et al. (1992) Neuropsychological correlates of white-matter lesions in healthy elderly subjects. A threshold effect. *Arch Neurol* 49:549–554.

Brown, R.P., Stoll, P.M., Stokes, P.E., Frances, A., Sweeney, J., et al. (1988) Adrenocortical hyperactivity in depression: Effects of agitation, delusions, melancholia, and other illness variables. *Psychiatry Res* 23:167–178.

Bruce, M.L., Leaf, P.J., Rozal, G.P., Florio, L., and Hoff, R.A. (1994) Psychiatric status and 9-year mortality data in the New Haven Epidemiologic Catchment Area Study. *Am J Psychiatry* 151:716–721.

Chrousos, G.P., and Gold, P.W. (1992) The concepts of stress and stress system disorders. Overview of physical and behavioral homeostasis. *JAMA* 267:1244–1252.

Cizza, G., Ravn, P., Chrousos, G.P., and Gold, P.W. (2001) Depression: A major, unrecognized risk factor for osteoporosis? *Trends Endocrinol Metab* 12:198–203.

Coffey, C.E., Wilkinson, W.E., Parashos, I.A., Soady, S.A., Sullivan, R.J., et al. (1992) Quantitative cerebral anatomy of the aging human brain: A cross-sectional study using magnetic resonance imaging. *Neurology* 42:527–536.

Corder, E.H., Saunders, A.M., Risch, N.J., Strittmatter, W.J., Schmechel, D.E., et al. (1994) Protective effect of apolipoprotein E type 2 allele for late onset Alzheimer disease. *Nat Genet* 7:180–184.

Coryell, W., and Schlesser, M. (2001) The dexamethasone suppression test and suicide prediction. *Am J Psychiatry* 158:748–753.

Daigneault, S., and Braun, C. M. (1993) Working memory and the Self-Ordered Pointing Task: Further evidence of early prefrontal decline in normal aging. *J Clin Exp Neuropsychol* 15:881–895.

Davidson, R.J. (2002) Anxiety and affective style: Role of prefrontal cortex and amygdala. *Biol Psychiatry* 51:68–80.

de Kloet, E.R. (1992) Corticosteroids, stress, and aging. *Ann NY Acad Sci* 663:357–371.

de Kloet, E.R., Vreugdenhil, E., Oitzl, M.S., and Joels, M. (1998) Brain corticosteroid receptor balance in health and disease. *Endocrine Rev* 19:269–301.

Diorio, D., Viau, V., and Meaney, M.J. (1993) The role of the medial prefrontal cortex (cingulate gyrus) in the regulation of hypothalamic-pituitary-adrenal responses to stress. *J Neurosci* 13:3839–3847.

Dodt, C., Theine, K.J., Uthgenannt, D., Born, J., and Fehm, H.L. (1994) Basal secretory activity of the hypothalamo-pituitary-adrenocortical axis is enhanced in healthy elderly. An assessment during undisturbed night-time sleep. *Eur J Endocrinol* 131:443–450.

Dorovini-Zis, K., and Zis, A.P. (1987) Increased adrenal weight in victims of violent suicide. *Am J Psychiatry* 144:1214–1215.

Drevets, W.C. (2001) Neuroimaging and neuropathological studies of depression: Implications for the cognitive-emotional features of mood disorders. *Curr Opin Neurobiol* 11:240–249.

Drevets, W.C., and Price, J.L. (1997) Subgenual prefrontal cortex abnormalities in mood disorders. *Nature* 286:824–827.

Drevets, W.C., Price, J.L., Bardgett, M.E., Reich, T., Todd, R.D., and Raichle, M.E. (2002) Glucose metabolism in the amygdala in depression: Relationship to diagnostic subtype and plasma cortisol levels. *Pharmacol Biochem Behav* 71:431–447.

Elliott, R., Sahakian, B.J., McKay, A.P., Herrod, J.J., Robbins, T.W., and Paykel, E.S. (1996) Neuropsychological impairments in unipolar depression: The influence of perceived failure on subsequent performance. *Psychol Med* 26:975–989.

Erfurth, E.M., Bulow, B., Eskilsson, J., and Hagmar, L. (1999) High incidence of cardiovascular disease and increased prevalence of cardiovascular risk factors in women with hypopituitarism not receiving growth hormone treatment: Preliminary results. *Growth Horm IGF Res* 9:21–24.

Evans, D.L., Burnett, G.B., and Nemeroff, C.B. (1983) The dexamethasone suppression test in the clinical setting. *Am J Psychiatry* 140:586–589.

Ferrari, E., Magri, F., Dori, D., Migliorati, G., Nescis, T., et al. (1995) Neuroendocrine correlates of the aging brain in humans. *Neuroendocrinology* 61:464–470.

Frasure-Smith, N., Lesperance, F., Gravel, G., Masson, A., Juneau, M., et al. (2000) Social support, depression, and mortality during the first year after myocardial infarction. *Circulation* 101:1919–1924.

Frasure-Smith, N., Lesperance, F., and Talajic, M. (1993) Depression following myocardial infarction: Impact on 6-month survival. *JAMA* 270:1819–1825.

Georgotas, A., McCue, R.E., Kim, O.M., Hapworth, W.E., Reisberg, B., et al. (1986) Dexamethasone suppression in dementia, depression, and normal aging. *Am J Psychiatry* 143:452–456.

Gold, P.W., and Chrousos, G.P. (1985) Clinical studies with corticotropin releasing factor: Implications for the diagnosis and pathophysiology of depression, Cushing's disease, and adrenal insufficiency. *Psychoneuroendocrinology* 10:401–419.

Gold, P.W., and Chrousos, G.P. (2002) Organization of the stress system and its dysregulation in melancholic and atypical depression: High vs. low CRH/NE states. *Mol Psychiatry* 7:254–275.

Gold, P.W., Drevets, W.C., and Charney, D.S. (2002) New insights into the role of cortisol and the glucocorticoid receptor in severe depression. *Biol Psychiatry* 52:381–385.

Gold, P.W., Loriaux, D.L., Roy, A., Kling, M.A., Calabrese, J.R., et al. (1986) Responses to corticotropin-releasing hormone in the hypercortisolism of depression and Cushing's disease. Pathophysiologic and diagnostic implications. *N Engl J Med* 314:1329–1335.

Gray, T.S., and Bingaman, E.W. (1996) The amygdala: Corticotropin-releasing factor, steroids, and stress. *Crit Rev Neurobiol* 10:155–168.

Greden, J.F., Gardner, R., King, D., Grunhaus, L., Carroll, B.J., and Kronfol, Z. (1983) Dexamethasone suppression tests in antidepressant treatment of melancholia. The process of normalization and test-retest reproducibility. *Arch Gen Psychiatry* 40:493–500.

Gunning-Dixon, F.M., and Raz, N. (2000) The cognitive correlates of white matter abnormalities in normal aging: A quantitative review. *Neuropsychology* 14:224–232.

Heffelfinger, A.K., and Newcomer, J.W. (2001) Glucocorticoid effects on memory function over the human life span. *Dev Psychopathol* 13:491–513.

Hew, F.L., O'Neal, D., Kamarudin, N., Alford, F.P., and Best, J.D. (1998) Growth hormone deficiency and cardiovascular risk. *Baillieres Clin Endocrinol Metab* 12:199–216.

Hoyert, D.L., Arias, E., Smith, B.L., Murphy, S.L., and Kochanek, K.D. (2001) Deaths: final data for 1999. *National Vital Statistics Report* 41(8).

Issa, A.M., Rowe, W., Gauthier, S., and Meaney, M.J. (1990) Hypothalamic-pituitary-adrenal activity in aged, cognitively impaired and cognitively unimpaired rats. *J Neurosci* 10:3247–3254.

Joels, M., and de Kloet, E.R. (1992) Control of neuronal excitability by corticosteroid hormones. *Trends Neurosci* 15:25–30.

Jorm, A.F. (2000) Is depression a risk factor for dementia or cognitive decline? A review. *Gerontology* 46:219–227.

Jorm, A.F. (2001) History of depression as a risk factor for dementia: An updated review. *Aust NZ J Psychiatry* 35:776–781.

Jorm, A.F., van Duijn, C.M., Chandra, V., Fratiglioni, L., Graves, A.B., et al. (1991) Psychiatric history and related exposures as risk factors for Alzheimer's disease: A collaborative reanalysis of case-control studies. EURODEM Risk Factors Research Group. *Int J Epidemiol* 20:S43–S47.

Kalayam, B., and Alexopoulos, G.S. (1999) Prefrontal dysfunction and treatment response in geriatric depression. *Arch Gen Psychiatry* 56:713–718.

Kern, W., Dodt, C., Born, J., and Fehm, H.L. (1996) Changes in cortisol and growth hormone secretion during nocturnal sleep in the course of aging. *J Gerontol A Biol Sci Med Sci* 51:M3–M9.

Kindermann, S.S., and Brown, G.G. (1997) Depression and memory in the elderly: A meta-analysis. *J Clin Exp Neuropsychol* 19:625–642.

Kindermann, S.S., Kalayam, B., Brown, G.G., Burdick, K.E., and Alexopoulos, G.S. (2000) Executive functions and P300 latency in elderly depressed patients and control subjects. *Am J Geriatr Psychiatry* 8:57–65.

Krishnan, K.R., McDonald, W.M., Doraiswamy, P.M., Tupler, L.A., Husain, M., et al. (1993) Neuroanatomical substrates of depression in the elderly. *Eur Arch Psychiatry Clin Neurosci* 243:41–46.

Landfield, P.W., Braun, L.D., Pitler, T.A., Lindsey, J.D., and Lynch, G. (1981) Hippocampal aging in rats: A morphometric study of multiple variables in semithin sections. *Neurobiol Aging* 2:265–275.

Landfield, P.W., and Eldridge J.C. (1991) The glucocorticoid hypothesis of brain aging and neurodegeneration: Recent modifications. *Acta Endocrinol (Copenh)* 125(suppl 1):54–64.

Leverenz, J.B., Wilkinson, C.W., Wamble, M., Corbin, S., Grabber, J.E., et al. (1999) Effect of chronic high-dose exogenous cortisol on hippocampal neuronal number in aged nonhuman primates. *J Neurosci* 19:2356–2361.

Ligier, S., and Sternberg, E.M. (1999) Neuroendocrine host factors and inflammatory disease susceptibility. *Environ Health Perspect* 107:701–707.

Lockwood, K.A., Alexopoulos, G.S., and van Gorp, W.G. (2002) Executive dysfunction in geriatric depression. *Am J Psychiatry* 159:1119–1126.

Lupien, S.J., Lecours, A.R., Lussier, I., Schwartz, G., Nair, N.P.V., and Meaney, M.J. (1994) Basal cortisol levels and cognitive deficits in human aging. *J Neurosci* 14:2893–2903.

Lupien, S.J., Nair, N.P., Briere, S., Maheu, F., Tu, M.T., et al. (1999) Increased cortisol levels and impaired cognition in human aging: Implication for depression and dementia in later life. *Rev Neurosci* 10:117–139.

Lupien, S.J., Wilkinson, C.W., Briere, S., Menard, C., Ng Ying Kin, N.M.K., and Nair, N.P.V. (2002) The modulatory effects of corticosteroids on cognition: Studies in young human populations. *Psychoneuroendocrinology* 27:401–416.

Lyons, D.M., Lopez, J.M., Yang, C., and Schatzberg, A.F. (2000) Stress-level cortisol treatment impairs inhibitory control of behavior in monkeys. *J Neurosci* 20:7816–7821.

Mandell, A., Chapman, L., Rand, R., and Walter, R. (1963) Plasma corticosteroids: Changes in concentration after stimulation of hippocampus and amygdala. *Science* 139:1212–1213.

Mauri, M., Sinforiani, E., Bono, G., Vignati, F., Berselli, M.E., et al. (1993) Memory impairment in Cushing's disease. *Acta Neurol Scand* 87:52–55.

McEwen, B.S. (1999) Stress and the aging hippocampus. *Frontiers Neuroendocrinol* 20:49–70.

McEwen, B.S. (2000) The neurobiology of stress: From serendipity to clinical relevance. *Brain Res* 886:172–189.

Michelson, D., Stratakis, C., Hill, L., Reynolds, J., Galliven, E., et al. (1996) Bone mineral density in women with depression. *N Engl J Med* 335:1176–1181.

Momose, K.J., Kjellberg, R.N., and Kliman, B. (1971) High incidence of cortical atrophy of the cerebral and cerebellar hemispheres in Cushing's disease. *Radiology* 99:341–348.

Murphy, B.E. (1991) Steroids and depression. *J Steroid Biochem Mol Biol* 38:537–559.

Nebes, R.D., Butters, M.A., Mulsant, B.H., Pollock, B.G., Zmuda, M.D., et al. (2000) Decreased working memory and processing speed mediate cognitive impairment in geriatric depression. *Psychol Med* 30:679–691.

Nelson, J.C., and Davis, J.M. (1997) DST studies in psychotic depression: A meta-analysis. *Am J Psychiatry* 154:1497–1503.

Nemeroff, C.B. (1988) The role of corticotropin-releasing factor in the pathogenesis of major depression. *Pharmacopsychiatry* 21:76–82.

Nemeroff, C.B., and Evans, D.L. (1984) Correlation between the dexamethasone suppression test in depressed patients and clinical response. *Am J Psychiatry* 141:247–249.

Nemeroff, C.B., Owens, M.J., Bissette, G., Andorn, A.C., and Stanley, M. (1988) Reduced corticotropin releasing factor binding sites in the frontal cortex of suicide victims. *Arch Gen Psychiatry* 45:577–579.

Newcomer, J.W., Selke, G., Melson, A.K., Hershey, T., Craft, S., et al. (1999) Decreased memory performance in healthy humans induced by stress-level cortisol treatment. *Arch Gen Psychiatry* 56:527–533.

Orchinik, M., Weiland, N.G., and McEwen, B.S. (1995) Chronic exposure to stress levels of corticosterone alters GABAA receptor subunit mRNA levels in rat hippocampus. *Mol Brain Res* 34:29–37.

Patel, P.D., Lopez, J.F., Lyons, D.M., Burke, S., Wallace, M., and Schatzberg, A.F. (2000) Glucocorticoid and mineralocorticoid receptor mRNA expression in squirrel monkey brain. *J Psychiatr Res* 34:383–392.

Peskind, E.R., Wilkinson, C.W., Petrie, E.C., Schellenberg, G.D., and Raskind, M.A. (2001) Increased CSF cortisol in AD is a function of APOE genotype. *Neurology* 56:1094–1098.

Pfeffer, C.R., Stokes, P., and Shindledecker, R. (1991) Suicidal behavior and hypothalamic-pituitary-adrenocortical axis indices in child psychiatric inpatients. *Biol Psychiatry* 29:909–917.

Prewitt, C.M., and Herman, J.P. (1994) Lesion of the central nucleus of the amygdala decreases basal CRH mRNA expression and stress-induced ACTH release. *Ann NY Acad Sci* 746:438–440.

Pulska, T., Pahkala, K., Laippala, P., and Kivela, S.L. (2000) Depressive symptoms predicting six-year mortality in depressed elderly finns. *Int J Geriatr Psychiatry* 15:940–946.

Rosenbaum, A., Maruta, T., Schatzberg, A., Orsulak, P., Jiang, N., et al. (1983) Toward a biochemical classification of depressive disorders, VII: Urinary free cortisol and urinary MHPG in depressions. *Am J Psychiatry* 140:314–318.

Rothschild, A.J., and Schatzberg, A.F. (1982) Fluctuating postdexamethasone cortisol levels in a patient with melancholia. *Am J Psychiatry* 139:129–130.

Rothschild, A.J., Schatzberg, A.F., Rosenbaum, A.H., Stahl, J.B., and Cole, J.O. (1982) The dexamethasone suppression test as a discriminator among subtypes of psychotic patients. *Br J Psychiatry* 141:471–474.

Roy, A. (1992) Hypothalamic-pituitary-adrenal axis function and suicidal behavior in depression. *Biol Psychiatry* 32:812–816.

Roy, A., Guthrie, S., Karoum, F., Pickar, D., and Linnoila, M. (1988) High intercorrelations among urinary outputs of norepinephrine and its major metabolites. A replication in depressed patients and controls. *Arch Gen Psychiatry* 42:158–161.

Roy, A., Pickar, D., Douillet, P., Karoum, F., and Linnoila, M. (1986) Urinary monoamines and monoamine metabolites in subtypes of unipolar depressive disorder and normal controls. *Psychol Med* 16:541–546.

Rubinow, D.R., Post, R.M., Savard, R., and Gold, P.W. (1984) Cortisol hypersecretion and cognitive impairment in depression. *Arch Gen Psychiatry* 41:279–283.

Sapolsky, R.M. (2001) Depression, antidepressants, and the shrinking hippocampus. *PNAS* 98:12320–12322.

Sapolsky, R.M., Krey, L., and McEwen, B. (1985) Prolonged glucocorticoid exposure reduces hippocampal neuron number: Implications for aging. *J Neurosci* 5:1222–1227.

Sapolsky, R.M., Krey, L.C., and McEwen, B.S. (1986) The neuroendocrinology of stress and aging: The glucocorticoid cascade hypothesis. *Endocrine Rev* 7:284–301.

Schatzberg, A.F., Posener, J.A., DeBattista, C., Kalehzan, B.M., Roths-child, A.J., and Shear, P.K. (2000) Neuropsychological deficits in psychotic versus nonpsychotic major depression and no mental illness. *Am J Psychiatry* 157:1095–1100.

Schatzberg, A.F., and Rothschild, A.J. (1992) Psychotic (delusional) major depression: Should it be included as a distinct syndrome in DSM-IV? *Am J Psychiatry* 149:733–745.

Schatzberg, A., Rothschild, A., Stahl, J., Bond, T., Rosenbaum, A., et al. (1983) The dexamethasone suppression test: Identification of subtypes of depression. *Am J Psychiatry* 140:88–91.

Sheline, Y.I., Sanghavi, M., Mintun, M.A., and Gado, M.H. (1999) Depression duration but not age predicts hippocampal volume loss in medically healthy women with recurrent major depression. *J Neurosci* 19:5034–5043.

Starkman, M.N., Gebarski, S.S., Berent, S., and Schteingart, D.E. (1992) Hippocampal formation volume, memory dysfunction, and cortisol levels in patients with Cushing's syndrome. *Biol Psychiatry* 32:756–765.

Starkman, M.N., Giordani, B., Berent, S., Schork, M.A., and Schteingart, D.E. (2001) Elevated cortisol levels in Cushing's disease are associated with cognitive decrements. *Psychosom Med* 63:985–993.

Starkman, M.N., Schteingart, D.E., and Schork, M.A. (1986) Correlation of bedside cognitive and neuropsychological tests in patients with Cushing's syndrome. *Psychosomatics* 27:508–511.

Steffens, D.C., Byrum, C.E., McQuoid, D.R., Greenberg, D.L., Payne, M.E., et al. (2000) Hippocampal volume in geriatric depression. *Biol Psychiatry* 48:301–309.

Steffens, D.C., Payne, M.E., Greenberg, D.L., Byrum, C.E., Welsh-Bohmer, K.A., et al. (2002) Hippocampal volume and incident dementia in geriatric depression. *Am J Geriatr Psychiatry* 10:62–71.

Steffens, D.C., Plassman, B.L., Helms, M.J., Welsh-Bohmer, K.A., Saunders, A.M., and Breitner, J.C.S. (1997) A twin study of late-onset depression and apolipoprotein E [epsi]4 as risk factors for Alzheimer's disease. *Biol Psychiatry* 41:851–856.

Szigethy, E., Conwell, Y., Forbes, N.T., Cox, C., and Caine, E.D. (1994) Adrenal weight and morphology in victims of completed suicide. *Biol Psychiatry* 36:374–380.

Takeshita, J., Masaki, K., Ahmed, I., Foley, D.J., Li, Y.Q., et al. (2002) Are depressive symptoms a risk factor for mortality in elderly Japanese American men? The Honolulu-Asia Aging Study. *Am J Psychiatry* 159:1127–1132.

Targum, S., Rosen, L., and Capodanno, A. (1983) The dexamethasone suppression test in suicidal patients with unipolar depression. *Am J Psychiatry* 140:877–879.

Van Cauter, E., Leproult, R., and Kupfer, D.J. (1996) Effects of gender and age on the levels and circadian rhythmicity of plasma cortisol. *J Clin Endocrinol Metab* 81:2468–2473.

Van Duijn, C.M., Clayton, D.G., Chandra, V., Fratiglioni, L., Graves, A.B., et al. (1994) Interaction between genetic and environmental risk factors for Alzheimer's disease: A reanalysis of case-control studies. EURODEM Risk Factors Research Group. *Genet Epidemiol* 11:539–551.

Van Londen, L., Goekoop, J.G., Zwinderman, A.H., Lanser, J.B., Wiegant, V.M., and De Wied, D. (1998) Neuropsychological performance and plasma cortisol, arginine vasopressin and oxytocin in patients with major depression. *Psychol Med* 28:275–284.

Vanitallie, T.B. (2002) Stress: A risk factor for serious illness. *Metabolism* 51:40–45.

Vythilingam, M., Chen, J., Bremner, J.D., Mazure, C.M., Maciejewski, P.K., and Nelson, J.C. (2003) Psychotic depression and mortality. *Am J Psychiatry* 160:574–576.

Wellman, C.L. (2001) Dendritic reorganization in pyramidal neurons in medial prefrontal cortex after chronic corticosterone administration. *J Neurobiol* 49:245–253.

Whelan, T.B., Schteingart, D.E., Starkman, M.N., and Smith, A. (1980) Neuropsychological deficits in Cushing's syndrome. *J Nerv Ment Dis* 168:753–757.

Whooley, M.A., and Browner, W.S. (1998) Association between depressive symptoms and mortality in older women. Study of Osteoporotic Fractures Research Group. *Arch Intern Med* 158:2129–2135.

Wilson, M.M., Greer, S.E., Greer, M., A., and Roberts, L. (1980) Hippocampal inhibition of pituitary-adrenocortical function in female rats. *Brain Res* 197:433–441.

Wolkowitz, O.M., and Reus, V.I. (1999) Treatment of depression with antiglucocorticoid drugs. *Psychosom Med* 61:698–711.

Wolkowitz, O., Reus, V., Weingartner, H., Thompson, K., Breier, A., et al. (1990) Cognitive effects of corticosteroids. *Am J Psychiatry* 147:1297–1303.

Wong, M.-L., Kling, M.A., Munson, P.J., Listwak, S., Licinio, J., et al. (2000) Pronounced and sustained central hypernoradrenergic function in major depression with melancholic features: Relation to hypercortisolism and corticotropin-releasing hormone. *Proc Natl Acad Sci USA* 97:325–330.

Wulsin, L.R., Vaillant, G.E., and Wells, V.E. (1999) A systematic review of the mortality of depression. *Psychosom Med* 61:6–17.

Young, A.H., Sahakian, B.J., Robbins, T.W., and Cowen, P.J. (1999) The effects of chronic administration of hydrocortisone on cognitive function in normal male volunteers. *Psychopharmacology* 145:260–266.

Zubenko, G.S., Moossy, J., and Kopp, U. (1990) Neurochemical correlates of major depression in primary dementia. *Arch Neurol* 47:209–214.

# 14 | The neuroendocrinology of aging

STUART N. SEIDMAN

A primary postulate of senescence is that the ability to regulate the internal environment in response to changes in the internal or external milieu is reduced (Hazzard, 1997). Age-related endocrinological changes are generally seen in this context. Although there develops with age a progressive reduction in homeostatic regulation of endocrine function, such changes are generally not apparent under normal circumstances. Indeed, most basal plasma hormone concentrations do not change with age. When the systems are stressed, however, as in a glucose challenge, impaired function becomes evident. The potential of such normative endocrine changes to have a negative impact on central nervous system (CNS) functioning would appear to be great. However, although data are limited, the evidence that does exist does not support any such age-related neuroendocrine effects. In this chapter, we will first consider the role of hormones in neuropsychiatry, review general age-related changes in endocrine systems, and describe the implications of these changes for late-life depressive illness. Then we will focus on the example of age-related testosterone decline in men in order to examine specific depression-related issues raised by this hormonal dysregulation.

## HORMONES AND NEUROPSYCHIATRY

Hormones help to coordinate behavior with other physiological events in the body, such as sexual behavior with fertility and food seeking with the appropriate metabolic state (McEwen, 1998). It has long been recognized that hormones exert potent behavioral and emotional effects. In the medical literature, endocrinopathies have frequently been associated with state-dependent psychiatric symptoms: male hypogonadism with loss of libido, low mood, and low energy; hypothyroidism with depression and cognitive dysfunction; hyperthyroidism with anxiety, irritability, and psychomotor agitation; acromegaly with hypersomnia and loss of libido; Cushing's syndrome and Addison's disease with dysphoric mood; hypercortisolemia with euphoria and psychosis; and hyperprolactinemia with low libido (Halbreich, 1997; Valenti, 1992). Psychoendocrine investigators have demonstrated

hormonal dysregulations associated with psychiatric conditions, particularly the hypothalamic-pituitary-adrenal (HPA) and hypothalamic-pituitary-thyroid (HPT) axes in affective disorders (Prange, 1998). Indeed, the primary goal of some of the pioneers in biological psychiatry, such as Manfred Bleuler and Edward Sachar, was to relate psychopathology to endocrine dysregulation (Holsboer, 2000). Although this approach was overshadowed by the dramatic advances in the psychopharmacological approach, important contributions continue to be made that suggest that hormone axis dysregulation is etiologically related to affective illness in some individuals (Holsboer, 2001). Yet, the relation between endocrine axis pathology and psychiatric symptoms and syndromes remains poorly elucidated, and this knowledge deficit is particularly glaring with regard to age-associated changes in these systems.

## CENTRAL NERVOUS SYSTEM MECHANISMS OF HORMONAL ACTION

The CNS and the endocrine glands interact closely via structural and functional connections. Hypothalamic peptides, pituitary hormones, and endocrine gland hormones influence a wide range of cellular actions. In recent years, new studies have illuminated at least three important mechanisms of hormonal action in the brain:

1. *Hormones as direct neurotransmitters.* This is the likely mechanism of action of hypothalamic peptides, which bind to membrane receptors and modulate the production of second messengers such as inositol triphosphate, diacylglycerol, and cyclic adenosine monophosphate (cAMP). Second messengers activate protein kinase enzymes, which play a central role in protein phosphorylation (Valenti, 1992).

2. *Hormones as neuromodulators.* Through intranuclear receptor binding, hormones modulate genomic expression, and thereby regulate protein synthesis of synthetic and metabolic enzymes for neurotransmitters, neuropeptides, neurotransmitter transporters, receptors, growth factors, and signal transduction proteins (McEwen, 1998; Schmidt and Rubinow, 1997). Neurotransmission can be influenced at multiple levels: neu-

rotransmitter synthesis and storage, presynaptic receptor activation, enzymatic neurotransmitter inactivation and reuptake, postsynaptic receptor concentration and binding, and membrane microviscosity (Valenti, 1992).

3. *Hormones as neurophic factors.* Peptides such as thyrotropin-releasing hormone (TRH) and adrenocorticotropic hormone (ACTH) influence cerebral cortex neuronal maturation and axon growth in vitro. Sex steroids and thyroid hormone influence the axoplasmic transport mechanisms that maintain neuronal structure and function (McEwen, 1998; Valenti, 1992). These are particularly important during critical developmental periods that involve structural changes of neurons and their connections, so-called organizational effects.

## AGE-RELATED CHANGES IN HORMONE AXES

Normative, age-related anatomical changes in endocrine glands include a decrease in weight, development of an atrophic appearance accompanied by vascular changes and fibrosis, and a tendency to form adenomas (Heuser and Hazzard, 1994). Basal hormone levels are generally not influenced by age. However, this minimal change under basal conditions actually reflects a balance of typically reduced secretion along with reduced clearance. In addition, unbound fractions of hormones (e.g., testosterone, insulin, adrenal androgens, and thyroid hormone) are affected by changes in the plasma concentration of binding proteins. Receptor binding does not appear to change systematically with age, but some postreceptor responses to hormone action are decreased with age, particularly carbohydrate metabolism and steroid actions. Finally, age-related changes in catecholaminergic tone—particularly dopamine and norepinephrine release—affect pituitary hormone release. For example, in elderly men, the increase in dopaminergic tone contributes to an increase in gonadotropins, a decrease in prolactin, and a decrease in thyroid-stimulating hormone (TSH). The increase in central noradrenergic tone affects TSH, luteinizing hormone (LH), and growth hormone (GH) secretion.

Although there are significant alterations in hormone production, metabolism, and action with age, a new equilibrium is typically established that is near normal at rest but less adaptable to change. Notably, the magnitude of age-related alterations is highly variable: whereas only minor changes occur in pituitary dynamics, adrenal physiology, and thyroid function, the changes in carbohydrate homeostasis, reproductive function, and calcium metabolism are more apparent. There is, however, no evidence that such regulatory changes play a role in the pathophysiology of senescence or depression.

## CARBOHYDRATE METABOLISM

Increasing age is associated with a progressive decline in carbohydrate tolerance, a slight increase in fasting blood glucose level, and a striking increase in blood glucose level following an oral glucose challenge. Approximately 40% of elderly individuals have evidence of glucose intolerance, though it remains undiagnosed in at least half (Smith et al., 2002). Mechanisms presumed to underlie these changes include age-related changes in body composition, diet, activity, insulin clearance, and insulin action. Insulin secretion appears to be unchanged by age but clearance is reduced, thereby increasing insulin levels. More importantly, insulin action is impaired; that is, it is less effective in inducing glucose metabolism in peripheral tissues due to a postreceptor defect in glucose transport into cells. Carbohydrate intolerance with increasing age appears to be an independent risk factor for stroke and for coronary artery disease (Smith et al., 2002). Preventive measures such as exercise and weight control improve glucose control (Hazzard, 1997).

## PARATHYROID

Mild hyperparathyroidism is a para-aging phenomenon: there is clear evidence of increasing parathyroid hormone levels with increasing age, with an overall 30% increase between ages 30 and 80 (Glendenning and Vasikaran, 2002). Although there is no apparent change in total calcium, there is a slight decrease in ionized calcium. The major mechanism responsible for the reduction in ionized calcium (which likely stimulates the increased parathyroid hormone) is the age-related reduction in renal mass, which leads to a reduction in 1,25-dihydroxyvitamin $D_3$ levels and, in turn, to a reduction in calcium absorption. The development of mild, normocalcemic hyperparathyroidism is variable, and the clinical implications are generally minimal; it is not typically associated with osteoporosis or hip fracture, except in extreme cases (Melin et al., 2001).

## HYPOTHALAMIC-PITUITARY-THYROID AXIS

There appear to be no clinically significant age-related changes in thyroid function, and most basal hormone levels remain in the normal range. There are, however, mild age-related increases in TSH and anti-thyroid antibodies (Hollowell et al., 2002), reductions in triiodothyronine ($T_3$) and thyroxine ($T_4$), and a slight reduction in $T_4$ clearance (Gupta et al., 2001; Magri et al., 2002). The TRH stimulation of TSH is somewhat blunted in the elderly, and elderly men appear to have greater TSH blunting than elderly women (Targum et al., 1989). Despite the lack of a strong para-aging effect on the HPT axis, a significant proportion of the elderly have thyroid dysfunction. Moreover, thyroid dysfunction in the elderly may put them at particular risk for bone loss, cognitive dysfunction, and depression (Ben-Shlomo et al., 2001; Prinz et al., 1999).

## HYPOTHALAMIC-PITUITARY-ADRENAL AXIS

Any threat or perceived threat (i.e., stressor) activates the HPA axis, which regulates the adaptive response. A cascade begins in the CNS that involves pituitary release of ACTH and culminates with adrenal release of glucocorticoids, which modulate metabolism, reproduction, inflammation, and immunity, as well as hippocampal neurogenesis and apoptosis (Plotsky et al., 1998; Thrivikraman et al., 2000). The primary regulator of ACTH release is corticotropin-releasing factor (CRF), which is secreted from the parvocellular perikarya in the hypothalamic paraventricular nuclei (PVN).

The HPA axis remains intact and little changed by age in most individuals: ACTH secretion is relatively stable, and adrenal reactivity to exogenous ACTH is well maintained. The one consistent age-related HPA change is the cortisol response to stress: following a stressful stimulus, elderly individuals develop higher cortisol levels and a slower return to baseline. In addition, the circadian pattern of cortisol secretion is blunted in elderly individuals, with an apparent increase in nocturnal cortisol secretion (a pattern that is particularly evident in patients with dementia) (Ferrari et al., 2001). Data suggest that HPA sensitivity to glucocorticoid negative feedback declines with age. It has been proposed that glucocorticoids damage hippocampal neurons that are important for this sensitivity, which may worsen the insensitivity in a vicious cycle and cause cognitive dysfunction (Sapolsky, 1999).

Overall, age-related changes in plasma cortisol are variable. In data pooled from multiple cross-sectional studies, the mean basal cortisol level in 158 subjects younger than 60 years of age from seven independent studies was $8.91 \pm 1.61$ $\mu g/dl/hr$, while the mean basal cortisol level in 123 subjects older than 60 years of age from six independent studies was $10.79 \pm 2.34$ $\mu g/dl/hr$, supporting an age-associated increase (Lupien et al., 1996). Similarly, in a study that used 24-hour sampling with 149 healthy men age 16–83, increasing age was associated with higher evening cortisol levels (19.3 nmol/L per decade), particularly in men older than age 50 (Van Cauter et al., 2000). Longitudinal studies, however, suggest a more complicated picture. For example, in a population-based study in men age 40–70 years that included an 8-year follow-up ($n$ = 1156), the morning cortisol level decreased an average 0.9% per year (Feldman et al., 2002).

In another longitudinal study, cortisol levels in 51 healthy male and female elderly subjects were assessed using 24-hour sampling methodology yearly for 3–6 years (Lupien et al., 1996). Subjects were categorized into one of three subgroups based on the change in cortisol level (i.e., increased, decreased, or unchanged). The age of the subjects was not related either to cortisol level or to the pattern of change in cortisol secretion over time, and there were no group differences with regard to weight, height, body mass index, pulse, blood pressure, or blood glucose. In a subsample of 19 subjects who completed neuropsychiatric assessments, there was a positive correlation ($r = 0.15$, $p < .05$) between the obsession-compulsion subscale of the (SCL-90) questionnaire and the cortisol slope. Moreover, there were group differences in cognitive performance. The slope of the change in cortisol level over time predicted cognitive deficits: those whose cortisol level increased were more likely to have impairments in tasks measuring explicit memory and selective attention (though normal vigilance), while those with declining cortisol levels developed impairments in vigilance (but normal memory) (Lupien et al., 1996). These findings suggest considerable heterogeneity with regard to age-related HPA axis changes and, moreover, lend some support to the hypothesis that such changes have neuropsychiatric implications.

## DEHYDROEPIANDROSTERONE

Dehydroepiandrosterone (DHEA) and its metabolite, DHEA sulfate (together abbreviated DHEA[S]), and androstenedione are the major androgenic steroids secreted by the adrenal cortex. Although not potent androgens themselves, they are converted in target organs to testosterone and dihydrotestosterone (DHT). This is likely to have significant androgenic consequences in females (Wolkowitz et al., 2000). In addition, DHEA(S) is produced in situ in brain tissue and hence is termed a *neurosteroid* (Rupprecht, 1997).

Plasma and CSF DHEA(S) levels decline with age: at age 70, DHEA(S) levels are about 20% of those at age 20 (Wolkowitz et al., 2000). In an 8-year population-based longitudinal study, DHEA(S) levels declined 5.2% per year in middle-aged men (Feldman et al., 2002). Many, but not all, studies have reported lowered levels of DHEA(S) or lowered ratios of DHEA(S) to cortisol in patients with depression, chronic fatigue syndrome, postpartum depression, and anxiety (Wolkowitz et al., 2000). Similarly, in many population-based studies of the elderly, the DHEA(S) level has been positively correlated with cognitive and general functional abilities and negatively associated with mortality. Some investigators have, therefore, proposed DHEA(S) as a marker of *successful aging* (Ravaglia et al., 1997; Wolkowitz et al., 2000). There is speculation that DHEA(S) *buffers* the deleterious effects of excessive glucocorticoid exposure. For example, it has been shown to prevent or reduce hippocampal neurotoxicity induced by the glutamate agonist N-methyl-D-aspartate (NMDA), corticosterone, and oxidative stressors. Overall, accumulating descriptive and epidemiological data suggest a relationship between DHEA(S) levels and functional abilities, memory, mood, and sense of well-being, though there are many inconsistencies in the literature.

Studies in which DHEA has been administered to those with normal and subnormal DHEA(S) levels have shown that this treatment is generally well tolerated and is not associated with significant changes in physical examination, hepatic, thyroid, hematological, and/or prostatic function. Relatively common side effects include acne, oily skin, nasal congestion, and headache. Less commonly reported side effects include insomnia, overactivation (including disinhibition, aggression, and mania), hirsutism, increased body odor, itching, irregular menstrual cycles, and voice deepening (Wolkowitz et al., 2000).

## GROWTH HORMONE

Two hypothalamic peptides—growth hormone releasing hormone (GHRH) and somatostatin—exert opposing effects on pituitary GH release. Pulsatile GH secretion occurs in response to GHRH stimulation and to reduced somatostatin tone—generally during the first few hours of sleep and after meals or exercise. With age, the pituitary pulses of GH release remain constant. However, the amplitude—and therefore the circulating GH level—declines approximately 14% per decade. This leads to reduced production (mostly hepatic) of insulin-like growth factor 1 (IGF-1), which mediates most of the actions of GH (Corpas et al., 1993; Dinan, 1998). In women, the decline in GH may be mediated by the decline in ovarian steroids: estradiol is correlated with GH secretion, though hormone replacement therapy (HRT) has been shown not to affect IGF-1 levels (Blackman et al., 2002). There is no effect of testosterone on GH or IGF-1 secretion (Blackman et al., 2002; Tenover, 1998).

The age-related decline in GH and IGF-1 has been termed *somatopause* (Corpas et al., 1993; Dinan, 1998). Some authors have suggested that the age-related GH deficiency contributes to frailty and to alterations in body composition, such as decreased muscle mass and strength, reduced bone mass, and in-

creased adiposity. Exogenous GH leads to significant increases in IGF-1 (Blackman et al., 2002; Rudman et al., 1990), an effect that is more pronounced in men. Short-term exogenous GH produces an increase in lean body mass, bone density, and skin thickness, as well as reduced adiposity; these effects may not be long-lasting (i.e., greater than 1 year) and appear to be more pronounced in men (Blackman et al., 2002; Rudman et al., 1990; Rudman and Mattson, 1994). There is no evidence that exogenous GH affects mood, though this has not been well studied.

In a well-designed clinical trial, Blackman and colleagues (2002) demonstrated that GH with or without sex steroids led to increased lean body mass (LBM) and decreased fat mass (FM). The study was a double-blind, placebo-controlled, parallel-group trial involving 57 women and 74 men age 65–88 years. Subjects were randomized to receive one of four regimens: (*1*) GH plus sex steroids (women: transdermal estradiol, 100 μg/day, plus oral medroxyprogesterone acetate, 10 mg/day, during the last 10 days of each 28-day cycle [HRT]; men: testosterone enanthate, biweekly intramuscular injections of 100 mg); (*2*) GH plus placebo sex steroids; (*3*) sex steroids plus placebo GH; or (*4*) placebo GH plus placebo sex steroids. In women, LBM increased by 0.4 kg with placebo, 1.2 kg with HRT ($p = .09$), 1.0 kg with GH ($p = .001$), and 2.1 kg with GH plus HRT ($p < .001$). Fat mass decreased significantly in both GH groups, but edema was a common side effect in these groups, affecting 11/29 (38%). In men, LBM increased by 0.1 kg with placebo, 1.4 kg with testosterone ($p = .06$), 3.1 kg with GH ($p < .001$), and 4.3 kg with GH plus testosterone ($p < .001$). Fat mass decreased significantly in the male GH and GH plus testosterone groups. Strength and maximum oxygen uptake were significantly increased only in the GH plus testosterone group, and these changes were related to changes in LBM. Carpal tunnel symptoms were common in men taking GH plus testosterone (32%), and arthralgias and glucose intolerance were significantly increased in men receiving GH.

## PROLACTIN

Many age-related hormonal axis changes are related to changes in the activity of CNS neurotransmitters and neuropeptides that regulate hypothalamic and pituitary hormones. For example, dopamine and serotonin are major regulators of prolactin release. Changes that occur in prolactin release may be a consequence of age-related changes in dopaminergic tone. Specifically, although the frequency of pulsatile prolactin release is unchanged with age, there is a blunted nocturnal rise in prolactin, a reduced amplitude of prolactin pulses, and overall an increase in basal serum level (Nicholas et al., 1998). In an 8-year population-based longitudinal study, prolactin levels increased 5.3% per year in middle-aged men (Feldman et al., 2002). The manifestations of mild hyperprolactinemia are minimal, but it can cause a secondary hypogonadism, worsen sexual dysfunction, and/or accelerate age-related bone loss.

Treatment of hyperprolactinemia consists of correction of the underlying cause, as the majority of cases are secondary to illnesses (e.g., hypothyroidism) or medications (e.g., neuroleptics, cimetidine). If the etiology is a microadenoma (defined as a pituitary tumor <10 mm), the most appropriate treatment is watchful waiting, since the majority of prolactin-secreting microadenomas are stable or involute with time. Symptomatic microadenomas (e.g., those causing sexual dysfunction or worsening osteoporosis) are treated with dopamine agonists such as bromocriptine.

## FEMALE HYPOTHALAMIC-PITUITARY-GONADAL AXIS

Menopause is a normative state of relative estrogen deficiency. The average age of onset of menopause is 50 years, and is unrelated to menarche, body composition, diet, or socioeconomic status. In the years preceding menopause, the loss of ova and their associated follicles leads to ovarian resistance to follicle-stimulating hormone (FSH) stimulation and to a reduction in the major ovarian estrogen, 12-beta-estradiol. The principal postmenopausal circulating estrogen is estrone, a weaker estrogen than estradiol, which is produced in extraglandular sites (particularly adipose) from the metabolism of androstenedione (Bancroft and Cawood, 1996). Since estrogen secretion is reduced two- to sixfold and androgen production only one and a half- to twofold, the ratio of estrogens to androgens decreases after menopause. Perimenopause describes the time period from the first hormonal and clinical signs of menopause until one year after menopause (Steiner et al., 2003).

Although normative, menopause can be considered pathological, and independent of age, this female hypogonadal state is associated with acceleration of age-related bone loss, vasomotor symptoms (e.g., hot flashes and night sweats), and urogenital dryness and atrophy (which can lead to dyspareunia). Hormone replacement therapy—particularly following the modification of estrogen therapy to include progestin—has long been advocated as a cornerstone of postmenopausal management. This was based on observational reports suggesting that HRT conferred benefits beyond the management of hot flashes and vaginal dryness. Specifically, HRT was thought to protect against cardiovascular and cerebrovascular events, protect against osteoporosis, reduce mood swings, and improve cognition (Stampfer et al., 1991).

Although substantial clinical evidence refuting such salutary effects has been available for years, recent findings from very large prospective clinical trials have lent further support to this negative view of HRT and have led to a dramatic change in clinical practice. In brief, the current clinical consensus supports the view that although HRT may provide some relief from traditional menopausal symptoms and osteoporosis, because of its negative effects on other age-related conditions (e.g., breast cancer, myocardial infarction, and the development of blood clots associated with pulmonary embolism and/or stroke), including a small but significant increase in mortality (Grady et al., 2001, 2002; Hulley et al., 2002; Yaffe et al., 2001), long-term HRT is not currently recommended. Tissue selectivity would appear to be especially important in ensuring the safety of estrogenic agents. The search, therefore, for the perfect selective estrogen receptor modifier (SERM) is especially promising. For example, raloxifene has negative receptor activity in breast cells (with an apparent reduction in the risk of breast cancer) and positive receptor activity in bone and brain. Further research is needed to establish the role of SERMs in neuropsychiatry.

## MALE HYPOTHALAMIC-PITUITARY-GONADAL AXIS

Testosterone is the most potent and abundant androgen. Secretion occurs in pulsatile bursts, and is regulated through negative feedback on the hypothalamus and pituitary. In young adult males, testosterone levels are higher in the morning and vary seasonally (Perry et al., 2001). Approximately 98% of testosterone molecules are protein bound: just over half are weakly bound to albumin, and the remainder are tightly bound to sex hormone-binding globulin (SHBG). Free testosterone diffuses into target cells, where it is converted to dihydrotestosterone (DHT) and estradiol. Testosterone and DHT bind to the androgen receptor. The steroid-receptor complex binds to specific sequences of genomic DNA, which thereby influences messenger RNA production and modulates the synthesis of a wide array of enzymatic, structural, and receptor proteins. In addition, testosterone influences cellular activity in a nongenomic manner through activation of the membrane and second messengers (Rubinow and Schmidt, 1996).

A progressive decline in LH and testosterone levels occurs in aging men: men in their 70s have mean plasma testosterone levels that are 35% lower than that of comparable young men, and more than 25% of men over age 75 appear to be testosterone-deficient (Vermeulen and Kaufman, 1995). The etiology of age-related hypogonadism is multifactorial. First, testosterone production is reduced because of a decrease in the number of Leydig cells. Although there is also a decrease in testosterone clearance, the reduced clearance does not entirely compensate for the reduced production, so there is a net decline. Second, diurnal variation—that is, the morning peak in testosterone secretion—is lost in elderly men (Vermeulen and Kaufman, 1995). Third, the concentration of SHBG increases with age. Since this is the primary testosterone-binding protein, the effect is a steeper decline in serum free testosterone (Field et al., 1994). Finally, there is some reduction in hypothalamic-pituitary function, with a blunted feedback response to low testosterone levels (despite generally high levels of gonadotropins) and to gonadotropin-releasing hormone (GnRH) stimulation. In addition, the normal pulsatile GnRH release is replaced by irregular pulses that are less effective in stimulating LH release from the pituitary (Mulligan et al., 1997).

The extent to which an age-dependent decline in androgen levels leads to health problems is being debated vigorously (Seidman and Roose, 2000). Some investigators argue that the age-associated testosterone deficiency, or *andropause*, is responsible for many of the typical signs of male aging, such as impaired hematopoiesis, sexual dysfunction, decrease in LBM, skin alterations, decrease in body hair, decrease in bone mineral density that results in osteoporosis, and increase in visceral fat and obesity, as well as for neuropsychiatric problems, such as weakness, fatigue, loss of libido, depression, anxiety, irritability, insomnia, and memory impairment (Morales et al., 2000). Yet, it has been difficult to correlate hormone levels with presumed andropausal phenomena (McKinlay et al., 1989).

Multiple clinical trials of testosterone replacement in younger men have demonstrated that replacement reverses hypogonadal sequelae: body weight, fat-free muscle mass, and muscle size and strength increase; continued bone loss is prevented; sexual function and secondary sex characteristics (e.g., facial hair) are restored and maintained; and hematocrit increases (Burris et al., 1992; Luisi and Franchi, 1980; Villareal and Morley, 1994). There are only limited controlled data on the effects of testosterone replacement in elderly men with mild and apparently age-related testosterone decline, and none that specifically addresses psychiatric symptoms. Studies in aging men are particularly important, since the age-related testosterone deficiency is generally more modest than the profound hypogonadism studied in testosterone replacement trials in younger men. In elderly men with mild hypogonadism, factors such as genetic vulnerability (e.g., androgen receptor polymorphism), changes in end-organ responsivity to testosterone, and relative change from baseline may be important modulators of hypogonadal sequelae. In the few systematic studies that do exist, testosterone replacement has been shown to enhance upper limb strength (Bakhshi et al., 2000; Sih et al., 1997) and mass (Snyder et al., 1999b), improve bone mineral density (Snyder et al., 1999a) (though this effect may occur via aromatization to estrogen), increase hematocrit (an effect that is independent of erythropoietin) (Hajjar et al., 1997), and reduce leptin levels (an effect that may improve visceral adiposity) (Sih et al., 1997). There have been no consistently demonstrated major effects of testosterone on cholesterol, cardiovascular disease, or benign prostatic hypertrophy (Hajjar et al., 1997; Sih et al., 1997).

## DEPRESSION AND NEUROENDOCRINE DYSREGULATION IN THE ELDERLY

Depression in late life is common and underrecognized. It contributes to medical morbidity and mortality, reduced quality of life, and increased health-care costs. Geriatric depression is typically a heterogeneous construct comprised of a relatively small number who meet DSM criteria for major depressive disorder (MDD), a somewhat larger group with a chronic low mood syndrome (i.e., dysthymia), and the large majority with significant dysphoria, frequently occurring in the setting of physical illness or stressful life events (Blazer, 1997, 1999). Diagnosis and treatment are, therefore, influenced and often complicated by co-morbid medical illness and adverse life events, as well as by cognitive impairment. Importantly, the prevalence of MDD in medically ill patients, hospitalized patients, and nursing home residents is much higher than in community populations (Blazer, 1997). In addition, some data suggest that late-onset MDD and dysthymia are biologically distinct from earlier-onset depressions, and in particular may be less medication-responsive (Alexopoulos et al., 2002; Devanand et al., 1994; Stek et al., 2002).

Although genetic predisposition is well supported for younger patients, it is likely that the genetic contribution is weaker in late-onset MDD. Age-related changes in CNS monoamine and neuroendocrine function may play a relatively larger role in the etiology of later-onset MDD. However, the fact that such neurotransmitter and neuroendocrine changes are common in later life and the fact that MDD does not appear to increase with age, mitigate the assumption that older persons are especially vulnerable to MDD based on these age-related CNS physiological changes.

Factors that may be relevant to this issue include the higher cardiovascular mortality of depressed individuals, protective factors that may be operative in late life, and potential vulnerabilities in subpopulations. In addition, the high prevalence of *low-grade* depression (including dysthymia) suggests that a subthreshold form of depressive illness might be etiologically related to age-related changes in neurophysiology. We will briefly review neuroendocrine factors that may be relevant to late-life depression and then focus on the specific role of the age-related testosterone decline in male depression.

## HORMONAL AXIS DYSREGULATION AND LATE-LIFE DEPRESSION

There is no known "smoking gun" in geriatric neuroendocrinology that consistently supports an etiological connection between age-associated hormonal dysregulation and late-life depression. Some of the age-related changes in hormonal axis functioning are similar to those that have been described in patients with MDD, such as blunted HPA and HPT axis reactivity. Such commonalities do not necessarily indicate an etiological association, and they are likely to reflect the homeostatic dysregulation common to both depression and aging. Importantly, they make the putative depressive markers less specific for depression in geriatric populations. The complex neuroendocrinology of depression has been well reviewed (Lebowitz et al., 1997; Prange, 1998).

## HYPOTHALAMIC-PITUITARY-ADRENAL AXIS, DEPRESSION, AND AGE

Hypothalamic-pituitary-adrenal dysregulation may contribute to depressive illness (Holsboer, 2000; Plotsky et al., 1998). Evidence supporting the link between the HPA axis and depression includes the following: (1) patients with MDD (compared to controls) have elevated cortisol in plasma, CSF, and urine; resistance to the normal suppression of cortisol and ACTH secretion by dexamethasone; and increased CSF CRH; (2) at least one-third of patients with high levels of cortisol due to Cushing's disease or to exogenous glucocorticoids develop a reversible mood syndrome (Plotsky et al., 1998); and (3) some studies suggest that adrenal gland hypertrophy is a reversible state marker of depression (Rubin et al., 1995).

The association between hypercortisolemia and depression has long been of interest to psychiatric investigators. Sachar and colleagues (1970) showed that in MDD-associated hypercortisolism, in contrast to Cushing's disease, the secretory *pattern* was dysregulated; that is, there were more secretory bursts, but between these bursts cortisol levels returned to baseline (Holsboer, 2001). This led to the introduction of the dexamethasone suppression test (DST), which detects resistance to glucocorticoid-mediated feedback as a putative diagnostic marker of melancholic depression. In the traditional test, 1 mg of dexamethasone was administered at 11 P.M., and blood was drawn for cortisol measurement the next day at 4 P.M. and 11 P.M. High plasma cortisol (generally above 5 g/dl) was associated with endogenous depression. In the original studies (Carroll et al., 1981), DST nonsuppression was 90% sensitive and 50% specific for MDD, and the degree of nonsuppression generally correlated with severity of the depression and normalized following remission. This finding generated a great deal of research interest. Further studies have tempered the early enthusiasm for the DST. Its specificity is generally less than 30% for MDD, since DST nonsuppression occurs commonly in the setting of medical illnesses, medication use, malnutrition, and infection (Copolov et al., 1989).

A significant improvement in sensitivity (i.e., more than 80%) has been achieved by combining the DST with CRH stimulation (Deuschle et al., 1998; Heuser et al., 1994; Schule et al., 2001). In this combined test, following administration of 1.5 mg dexamethasone the previous night (11:00 P.M.) and 100 $\mu$g intravenous CRH the next day (3:00 P.M.), five specimens are drawn for cortisol measurement at 3:00, 3:15, 3:30, 3:45, and 4:00 P.M. Cortisol is consistently high in patients with MDD and normalizes after remission. Importantly, those who remit and do not exhibit a normalization of this combined DST/CRH test are at high risk for relapse within the next 6 months. In addition, HPA normalization precedes clinical recovery, and a return to an abnormal HPA system precedes clinical relapse—suggesting that HPA dysregulation is not a result of depressive illness (e.g., via stress or malnutrition).

The standard DST has been extensively studied in elderly nondepressed and depressed populations. In the general population, there is a gradual increase in nonsuppression with increasing age, so that in persons older that 75, the DST is not useful in distinguishing depressed patients. Magni and colleagues (1986) compared DST results in 38 depressed elderly patients hospitalized for medical illnesses to those in 18 nondepressed, nonelderly controls hospitalized in the same ward. In the depressed elderly group, 73% of those with MDD and 11% of those with dysthymia had a positive DST; in the control group, 11% had a positive DST.

The DST has also been used to follow the clinical response to antidepressant treatment in elderly patients. For example, in a 7-week, double-blind clinical trial, 95 elderly depressed individuals were randomized to moclobemide 400 mg, nortriptyline 75 mg, or placebo (Kin et al., 1997). Sixty-one percent of the randomized patients were DST nonsuppressors. The baseline DST status was not associated with the clinical status, but it did predict the treatment outcome: DST nonsuppressors were more likely to respond to treatment with nortriptyline (48%) than with moclobemide (19%) or placebo (20%); in DST suppressors, the situation was reversed: nortriptyline 7%, moclobemide 31%, placebo 18%. In a study in which DSTs were followed in 58 patients with MDD treated with electroconvulsive therapy (ECT), plasma cortisol levels decreased significantly from the pretreatment to the immediate post-treatment period, and they declined further during the first week after the ECT course. The response to antidepressant therapy was associated with increased plasma dexamethasone levels, whereas changes in cortisol levels were independent of the clinical outcome (Devanand et al., 1991). Finally, in a study of elderly inpatients with MDD, 60% were nonsuppressors at baseline compared to 17% after intensive treatment; that is, the DST normalized in 75% of the initial non-suppressors (Meyers et al., 1993).

Some data suggest that elderly depressed patients have a greater HPA dysregulation than nondepressed controls and that HPA-serotonergic dysfunction may distinguish geriatric depression. Slotkin and colleagues (1997) measured platelet serotonin transporter binding sites and transport function, as well as administering the DST in 13 young (age <50) and 15 elderly (age >60) patients with MDD. The density and affinity of transporter molecules showed no differences between young and elderly depressed patients, regardless of DST results. However, there was an interaction between transporter function, age, and DST: elderly DST suppressors ($n = 9$) showed a deficit in [$^3$H]serotonin uptake capabilities and resistance to imipramine inhibition of uptake. No such defects were seen in the young depressed cohort, regardless of DST status, or in elderly depressed DST nonsuppressors.

Further interest in the HPA axis and depression concerns the central regulator of the HPA axis, corticotropin-releasing hormone (CRH), and its role *outside* the neuroendocrine system. There are at least two receptors for CRH, and it has been demonstrated that via one of these, CRH type 1, CRH exerts behavioral changes in rats that mimic depression—and are reversed by receptor antagonists. In humans, there is preliminary evidence supporting the antidepressant efficacy of a CRH type 1 receptor antagonist—irrespective of the patient's baseline HPA functioning, and without interfering with the patient's HPA axis feedback regulation (Arborelius et al., 1999).

## DEHYDROEPIANDROSTERONE, DEPRESSION, AND AGE

Correlational studies in humans have provided indirect evidence of an effect of DHEA on depressive illness and/or mood. Some studies have reported lowered levels of DHEA(S) or lowered ratios of DHEA(S) to cortisol in patients with MDD. For example, patients with MDD who fail to remit after robust treatment have rel-

atively low baseline DHEA-to-cortisol ratios. Based on such data, it has been speculated that in the presence of inadequate DHEA concentrations, high cortisol concentrations inhibit recovery (Young et al., 2002).

In a 12-week antidepressant treatment study, DHEA(S) and cortisol levels were assessed in elderly control subjects ($n = 16$) and in elderly depressed patients who remitted ($n = 44$) or failed to remit ($n = 16$) with pharmacological treatment (i.e., nortriptyline or paroxetine). In patients who achieved remission, DHEA(S) levels were lower at week 12 than at week 0 ($p = .0001$); levels were unchanged in controls and nonremitters (Fabian et al., 2001). The remaining literature examining DHEA(S) levels in depression is inconsistent.

Many studies have also assessed the relation between DHEA(S) level and overall well-being and cognitive functioning. In population-based studies, cognitive and general functional abilities have been shown to be positively correlated with DHEA(S) levels in the elderly, but in some studies the correlations were gender-specific, inverse, and/or negative. In a recent study in which neuropsychological evaluations and sex hormone assays were completed for 188 elderly female nursing home residents (mean age: 87.8 years; standard deviation: 7.0 years), the DHEA(S) level was inversely correlated with scores on multiple cognitive tests, including the Mini-Mental State Exam, the Test for Severe Impairment, and the Immediate Recall, Copy, and Recognition tests of the Visual Reproduction Subtest of the Wechsler Memory Scale-Revised (WMS-R; VR) (Breuer et al., 2002). Cumulatively, the descriptive and epidemiological data in humans raise the possibility of a relation between DHEA(S) levels and functional abilities, memory, mood, and sense of well-being, although many inconsistencies exist in the literature, and the reported abnormalities in patients with depression have not been uniformly replicated. Nonetheless, even if endogenous DHEA(S) levels are not decreased in depression, it is possible that pharmacological increases in their levels may have mood- and memory-enhancing effects.

Wolkowitz and colleagues (1997) administered physiological doses of DHEA to six elderly men and women with MDD and low DHEA(S) levels. Mood and aspects of memory improved significantly; moreover, such improvements were significantly related to DHEA(S) and the DHEA(S)-to-cortisol ratio. In a follow-up study (Wolkowitz et al., 1999), 12 men and 10 women with MDD (all but 7 on antidepressant medication) were randomized to receive DHEA or placebo for 6 weeks. The mean Hamilton Depression Rating Scale (HAM-D) decreased 30.5% in the DHEA-treated subjects and 5.3% in the placebo-treated subjects; about half of those receiving DHEA had a clinically meaningful response. Finally, it has been shown in a placebo-controlled trial that DHEA replacement enhances mood and libido in women with adrenal insufficiency (Arlt et al., 1999). Overall, review of the DHEA treatment literature suggests that in certain situations DHEA administration appears to enhance mood, energy, sleep, the sense of well-being, functional capabilities, and memory. However, conclusions are limited by inadequate methodologies, small study sample sizes, and discrepant results. Positive effects, if they do occur, may be more likely in elderly, depressed, or medically ill patients than in young, healthy individuals. They may also be more likely to emerge after at least 1 or more months of treatment.

## HYPOTHALAMIC-PITUITARY-THYROID AXIS, DEPRESSION, AND AGE

The classic HPT dysregulation that occurs in depressed individuals—a blunted TSH response to TRH—is also evident in many normal elderly individuals (Targum et al., 1989). The TRH stimulation test involves obtaining a baseline TSH, administering intravenous TRH, and then measuring TSH at regular intervals. A normal response is a TSH rise of $>5$ $\mu$U/ml above baseline. Serum TSH following TRH stimulation is blunted in depressed individuals and hypothyroid patients and exaggerated in hyperthyroid patients (Loosen, 1992; Targum et al., 1984). Mild hypothyroid symptoms such as cold intolerance, constipation, psychomotor slowing, and decreased exercise tolerance are common to both depression and aging, and are thus easily missed as symptoms of hypothyroidism unless the index of suspicion is high. The laboratory diagnosis of hypothyroidism is generally clear, with a low $T_4$ level and a high TSH level. A TSH level of 5–10 $\mu$U/ml is suggestive, and a level over 10 $\mu$U/ml is diagnostic of hypothyroidism; levels below $\mu$U/ml suggest hyperthyroidism. Hormone axis normalization should precede specific treatment for depression.

## HYPOTHALAMIC-PITUITARY-GONADAL AXIS, DEPRESSION, AND AGE

### Menopause, Depression, and Hormone Replacement

In early life, women have higher rates of depression than do men. Some data suggest that this gender differential ends at menopause—consistent with theories that implicate the menstrual cycle in the increased risk of depression in women (Morrison and Tweedy, 2000). The most commonly reported mood symptoms in perimenopausal women include irritability, tearfulness, anxiety, labile mood, fatigue, and lack of motivation (Steiner et al., 2003). Such symptoms are linked to the precipitous decline of high and erratic estradiol levels (Prior, 1998). Despite clinic-based reports suggesting that menopause is associated with depressive symptoms, most population-based studies do not demonstrate an increased incidence of MDD (Avis et al., 1997; Birkhauser, 2002; Maartens et al., 2002).

Surgical menopause has been the predominant clinical model for investigation of the psychiatric effects of estrogen. In multiple studies, oophorectomized premenopausal women who received supraphysiological doses of either estrogen, androgen, or a combination had a decline in depressive symptoms coincident with their higher plasma hormone levels; when hormones were withdrawn, depressive symptoms increased (Sherwin, 1988). In perimenopausal women with depression, estrogen replacement therapy (ERT) is associated with a significant decline in tearfulness, emotional numbness, mood instability, and dysphoria (Morrison and Tweedy, 2000). In a recent clinical trial, 50 depressed perimenopausal women (i.e., meeting criteria for MDD, dysthymic disorder, or minor depressive disorder) were randomized to receive ERT (100 $\mu$g 17-beta-estradiol) or placebo for 12 weeks. Remission was observed in 68% of those who received ERT and in 20% of those who received placebo ($p = .001$) (Soares et al., 2002). Finally, of particular interest is the finding from a retrospective data analysis of a clinical trial in which 127 elderly women received sertraline or placebo: ERT use was associated with a better clinical outcome in sertraline-treated women, suggesting that the selective serotonin reuptake inhibitor (SSRI)–estrogen combination may be an effective antidepressant strategy (Schneider et al., 2001).

Overall, there are no conclusive data on the effects of estrogen for the prevention or treatment of mood disorders in postmenopausal women. Current data suggest that estrogen improves mood in surgically menopausal, perimenopausal, and nondepressed postmenopausal women. There are limited data supporting the use of estrogen alone in postmenopausal MDD, and given the potential risks of this treatment, it should not be considered a first-line therapy.

## TESTOSTERONE AND MALE NEUROPSYCHIATRIC FUNCTIONING

Testosterone's influence occurs at multiple levels: metabolic processes, peripheral tissues, the spinal cord, and the brain (Schmidt and Rubinow, 1997). Nonspecific metabolic effects (e.g., increased hematocrit, anabolism) and/or stimulatory effects on genital tissue could indirectly influence neuropsychiatric functioning (e.g., via increased general arousal). Specific CNS activation occurs via binding of androgen receptors by testosterone or DHT, estrogen receptors by estradiol, and through membrane-associated actions (Schmidt and Rubinow, 1997).

Experimental evidence has demonstrated that testosterone has a direct influence on male sexual behavior, aggression, and dominance in lower mammals. These direct effects appear to be more influenced by social factors in primates. For example, in a multimale group of rhesus macaques (*Macaca mulatta*), castration leads to an immediate reduction in sexual behavior; in a single-male, multiple-female group, postcastration sexual behavior declines after one month; and in a male-female pair, reduced sexual activity does not occur until 2 months after testosterone suppression (Wallen et al., 1991). In human males, the behavioral effects of androgens are less apparent and are likely to be even more influenced by social factors. Nonetheless, consistent evidence supports an effect of testosterone on sexual behavior, aggression, and cognition.

## Sexual Behavior

The best-established testosterone–behavior relationship in human males is with sexual function: increasing plasma androgen levels at puberty are correlated with the onset of nocturnal emission, masturbation, dating, and infatuation. Males with an early onset of androgen secretion (i.e., precocious puberty) often develop in parallel an early interest in sexuality and erotic fantasies (Feder, 1984). Most striking, testosterone replacement in hypogonadal men leads to a dramatic increase in sexual desire, sexual activity and frequency of erections (Anderson et al., 1992). Suppression of testosterone secretion in eugonadal men leads to reduced sexual desire and activity and a decrease in spontaneous erections (Bagatell et al., 1994). There appears to be a threshold (which varies from person to person) below which sexual function is impaired.

## Aggression

Testosterone appears to play some role in aggression, though social factors have a strong influence. Anti-androgens are used to reduce aggressiveness in male sex offenders, and suppression of testosterone in eugonadal men consistently reduces outward-directed aggression. Numerous correlational studies have examined the relation between plasma testosterone level and measures of aggression in human males (Archer, 1991; Olweus et al., 1988). Interpretation of these studies is limited by the known increase in testosterone that occurs as a *result* of aggressive encounters and by the social context. Furthermore, studies have differed in measures of aggression used—that is, actual behavior versus aggressive traits—and subject characteristics, and cannot be easily summarized. Some investigators have reported positive correlations between testos-

terone level and some aspects of aggression, especially among subjects selected on the basis of violent behavior (i.e., male prisoners) (Archer, 1991; Dabbs et al., 1996; Olweus et al., 1988). Others have found no correlation between testosterone level and multiple aspects of aggression (Olweus et al., 1988). In a comprehensive review of the topic, Archer (1991) concluded that (*1*) consistent evidence suggests that violent male offenders have significantly higher testosterone levels than less violent individuals and (*2*) there is a small but statistically significant correlation between testosterone level and hostility in a variety of male populations, which is stronger when aggressiveness is rated by others in the person's social environment compared to self-assessment.

## Cognitive Functioning

Spatial cognition—tasks that include visual perception, spatial attention, object identification, or visual memory processes—is a sexually dimorphic cognitive function. Women excel at tasks requiring fine motor dexterity and verbal fluency, and men excel on block rotation tasks and on embedded-figures tests. In studies assessing the relation between testosterone level and cognitive performance in young adult men with normal testosterone levels, multiple studies have demonstrated a positive correlation between spatial ability and testosterone level (Christiansen and Knussmann, 1987; Gordon and Lee, 1986; Gouchie and Kimura, 1991; Hannan et al., 1991), and in one study (Christiansen and Knussmann, 1987) a negative correlation between testosterone level and verbal ability.

Two well-designed correlational studies have been done in elderly men. In a small study, 30 healthy men (mean age 69 years) completed five cognitive tests measuring verbal memory, spatial memory, verbal fluency, mental rotation, and susceptibility to interference. The only significant association demonstrated was a negative correlation between total testosterone level and verbal fluency ($r = -0.38$, $p < .05$) (Wolf and Kirschbaum, 2002). In a more comprehensive study, cognitive function was carefully assessed in 310 men (mean age 73 years). Men with higher bioavailable (but not total) testosterone levels had better scores on the Mini-Mental State Examination (MMSE), Trails B, and Digit Symbol ($p < .001$) (Yaffe et al., 2002).

Some evidence about the impact of testosterone on cognitive functioning can be derived from interventional studies using exogenous androgens and anti-androgens. In a placebo-controlled study in which testosterone levels were exogenously manipulated in 32 eugonadal young men, Cherrier and colleagues (2002) demonstrated that an experimentally induced low testosterone level was associated with a significant decrease in verbal memory. O'Connor and colleagues (2001) demonstrated that an experimentally induced increase in testosterone level in 30 eugonadal young men was associated with a decrease in spatial ability (i.e., the Block design subtest of the Wechsler Adult Intelligence Scale–Revised [WAIS–R]) and an increase in verbal fluency.

Elderly hypogonadal men have also been studied in clinical intervention trials. In a placebo-controlled testosterone replacement study with 32 elderly hypogonadal men followed for 1 year, Sih and colleagues (1997) failed to demonstrate an effect of testosterone on cognition. Kenny and colleagues (2002) randomized 67 elderly hypogonadal men to receive transdermal testosterone patches or placebo patches for 1 year; 44 men completed the trial, with the following results: scores on the Digit Symbol test improved in both the testosterone and placebo groups; scores on Trails B improved in men treated with testosterone ($p < .005$), although the changes were not statistically different from those seen in the placebo group; and end-of-study scores on Trails B for the entire group were correlated with testosterone levels ($p = .016$).

Finally, in two clinical trials of testosterone in elderly men, hypogonadism was not an entry criterion. In one, Cherrier and colleagues (2001) randomized 25 elderly men to testosterone, 100 mg/week, or placebo for 6 weeks. Significant improvements in cognition were observed for spatial memory (recall of a walking route), spatial ability (block construction), and verbal memory (recall of a short story) in the testosterone group compared to the placebo group and compared to baseline. In the second trial, Janowsky and colleagues (1994) randomized 56 men (mean age 67 years) to receive testosterone or placebo patches for 3 months. Compared to men who received placebo, men who received testosterone had enhanced spatial cognition (especially visual perception and spatial constructional processes), as measured by the Block Design subtest of the WAIS-R. Of note, the decrease in estrogen level among men receiving testosterone appeared to be a better predictor of Block Design performance than the increase in testosterone level. This trial was limited by the relatively low testosterone dose employed and the limited sensitivity of the cognitive tests. Cumulatively, these data support a role for gonadal steroids in cognitive processsing, and the area warrants further investigation.

## MALE DEPRESSIVE ILLNESS, HYPOTHALAMIC-PITUITARY-GONADAL AXIS FUNCTIONING, AND AGE

The psychiatric symptoms of hypogonadism overlap with symptoms of depressive disorders and include low libido, fatigue, loss of confidence, and irritability (Wang et al., 2000). Initial interest in this relation has focused on MDD: first, on whether men with MDD have HPG abnormalities and, second, on whether hypogonadal men develop a distinct *secondary* MDD that might be reversible with testosterone replacement

Overall, there is no consistent evidence that men with MDD—at any age—have significant HPG dysfunction, though evidence does support a blunting of early morning LH and testosterone release in men with melancholic MDD (Rupprecht et al., 1988; Schweiger et al., 1999). Anecdotal reports suggest that in some hypogonadal men, co-morbid MDD remits with testosterone replacement (Ehrenreich et al., 1999; Heuser et al., 1999; Rinieris et al., 1979) or augmentation to antidepressant medication (Seidman and Rabkin, 1998), and that in hypogonadal human immunodeficiency virus (HIV)–infected men, testosterone replacement is associated with improved mood, libido, and energy (Grinspoon et al., 2000; Rabkin et al., 2000). It had been assumed that testosterone replacement in hypogonadal men with MDD would conform to the *hypothyroid* model, that is, hormone axis normalization as an effective antidepressant. However, in a double-blind, randomized clinical trial of testosterone replacement versus placebo in 30 men with MDD and mild hypogonadism, we found that testosterone replacement was indistinguishable from placebo in antidepressant efficacy (Seidman et al., 2001). A recent randomized, placebo-controlled clinical trial suggests that testosterone replacement may be effective as an antidepressant augmentation (Pope et al., 2003).

A second area of interest has been population-based studies in which the relation between markers of HPG axis functioning (e.g., testosterone level) and depressive symptoms can be assessed. In multiple large epidemiological studies, both testosterone level and depressive symptoms were assessed in middle-aged and elderly men. The largest and most methodologically rigorous one was the Massachusetts Male Aging Study (MMAS) (Araujo et al., 1998), a population-based survey of 1709 men age 40–70 that included a morning testosterone level assessment and a self-report depression instrument, the Center for Epidemiologic Studies Depression Scale (CES-D). There was no correlation between CES-D-diagnosed depression (using the standard cutoff of 16) and the total testosterone level (OR 0.9, 95% CI = 0.75–1.1) (Araujo et al., 1998).

The Rancho Bernardo Study was a population-based study of most adult residents of a southern California community (Barrett-Connor et al., 1999). In a 10- to 15-year follow-up study that included 82% of surviving community residents, 856 men age 50–89 (mean age, 70 years, SD = 9.2) completed the Beck Depression Inventory (BDI) and had a morning testosterone level measured. Free testosterone level was inversely correlated with BDI score (B = $-0.302$, adjusted SE = 0.11, $p = .007$), signifying more depressive symptoms with lower free testosterone levels.

Morley and colleagues (2000) developed a forced yes-or-no 10-item symptom checklist for a presumed hypogonadal syndrome termed *androgen deficiency of the aging male* (ADAM). In a validation study with 316 Canadian physicians, sensitivity was 88% and specificity was 60%, and when administered on repeated occasions, it had a coefficient of variation of 11.5%. Mean scores in 21 men treated with testosterone replacement decreased from 5.8 to 2.1. Two findings were particularly striking. First, using a bioavailable testosterone threshold for hypogonadism of 60 ng/dl, the prevalence of hypogonadism increased steadily from 5% at age 40 to 70% at age 70. Second, the largest area of overlap, that is, false positives, occurred in men with depression.

In a recent study completed in Belgium, Delhez and colleagues (2003) evaluated morning hormone levels and self-reported psychiatric symptoms in 153 men age 50–70 years. Using a threshold level of free testosterone $<70$ ng/dl to diagnose hypogonadism, they found that 70% of the screened men were hypogonadal. Using a Carroll rating scale (CRS) for depression, they found that free testosterone was negatively correlated with CRS score ($r = -0.17$); moreover, when 25 frankly depressed subjects (CRS $> 14$) were removed from the analysis, the association was stronger ($r = -0.33$, $p < .01$). Nonetheless, overall psychiatric morbidity among hypogonadal men was not high, leading the authors to speculate that low testosterone was associated with mild or *minor* depression.

Supporting this view, our group assessed testosterone levels in three groups of elderly men, and observed that those with dysthymia (295 ng/dl, range 180–520 ng/dl; $n = 32$) had median total testosterone levels significantly lower than those of age-matched men with MDD (425 ng/dl, range 248–657 ng/dl; $n = 12$) or age-matched nondepressed men (defined by CES-D $\leq 5$) from the MMAS sample (423 ng/dl, range 9–1021 ng/dl; $n = 175$). Notably, among elderly dysthymic men, the testosterone level was in the hypogonadal range (i.e., $\leq 300$ ng/dl) in 56.3% (Seidman et al., 2002).

## CONCLUSION

With age, there is a progressive reduction in homeostatic regulation of endocrine function. In this chapter, we considered the role of hormones in neuropsychiatry, reviewed general age-related changes in endocrine systems, and assessed the potential implications of these changes for late-life depressive illness, with a focus on age-related testosterone decline in men. Overall, although data are limited, there is no clear pathophysiological association between normative, age-related endocrine hypofunctioning and depressive illness.

It has been suggested that subclinical endocrinopathies (e.g., mild testosterone deficiency) are etiologically important in the development of subthreshold neuropsychiatric problems (e.g., dysthymia) (Prange, 1998; Seidman et al., 2002). In aging populations, both of these conditions are common—even normative—and an association between the two is particularly difficult to detect. In this regard, a better delineation of the role of age-related hormonal changes in the psychiatric problems of aging could be of substantial public health importance.

REFERENCES

Alexopoulos, G.S., Borson, S., Cuthbert, B.N., et al. (2002) Assessment of late-life depression. *Biol Psychiatry* 52:164–174.

Anderson, R.A., Bancroft, J., and Wu, F.C. (1992) The effects of exogenous testosterone on sexuality and mood of normal men. *J Clin Endocrinol Metab* 75:1503–1507.

Araujo, A.B., Durante, R., Feldman, H.A., et al. (1998) The relationship between depressive symptoms and male erectile dysfunction: Cross-sectional results from the Massachusetts Male Aging Study. *Psychosom Med* 60:458–465.

Arborelius, L., Owens, M.J., Plotsky, P.M., and Nemeroff, C.B. (1999) The role of corticotropin-releasing factor in depression and anxiety disorders. *J Endocrinol* 160:1–12.

Archer, J. (1991) The influence of testosterone on human aggression. *Br J Psychol* 82, 1–28.

Arlt, W., Callies, F., Van Vlijmen, J.C., et al. (1999) Dehydroepiandrosterone replacement in women with adrenal insufficiency. *N Engl J Med* 341:1013–1020.

Avis, N.E., Crawford, S.L., and McKinlay, S.M. (1997) Psychosocial, behavioral, and health factors related to menopause symptomatology. *Women's Health* 3:103–120.

Bagatell, C.J., Heiman, J.R., Rivier, J.E., and Bremner, W.J. (1994) Effects of endogenous testosterone and estradiol on sexual behavior in normal young men. *J Clin Endocrinol Metab* 78:711–716.

Bakhshi, V., Elliott, M., Gentili, A., et al. (2000) Testosterone improves rehabilitation outcomes in ill older men. *J Am Geriatr Soc* 48:550–553.

Bancroft, J., and Cawood, E.H.H. (1996) Androgens and the menopause: A study of 40–60 year old women. *Clin Endocrinol* 45:577–587.

Barrett-Connor, E., Von Muhlen, D.G., and Kritz-Silverstein, D. (1999) Bioavailable testosterone and depressed mood in older men: The Rancho Bernardo Study. *J Clin Endocrinol Metab* 84:573–577.

Ben-Shlomo, A., Hagag, P., Evans, S., and Weiss, M. (2001) Early postmenopausal bone loss in hyperthyroidism. *Maturitas* 39:19–27.

Birkhauser, M. (2002) Depression, menopause and estrogens: Is there a correlation? *Maturitas* 41(suppl 1):S3–S8.

Blackman, M.R., Sorkin, J.D., Munzer, T., et al. (2002) Growth hormone and sex steroid administration in healthy aged women and men: A randomized controlled trial. *JAMA* 288:2282–2292.

Blazer, D.G. (1997) Depression in the elderly. Myths and misconceptions. *Psychiatr Clin North Am* 20:111–119.

Blazer, D. (1999) EURODEP Consortium and late-life depression [editorial]. *Br J Psychiatry* 174:284–285.

Breuer, B., Martucci, C., Wallenstein, S., et al. (2002) Relationship of endogenous levels of sex hormones to cognition and depression in frail, elderly women. *Am J Geriatr Psychiatry* 10:311–320.

Burris, A.S., Banks, S.M., Carter, C.S., et al. (1992) A long-term, prospective study of the physiologic and behavioral effects of hormone replacement in untreated hypogonadal men. *J Andrology* 13:297–304.

Carroll, B.J., Feinberg, M., Greden, J.F., et al. (1981) A specific laboratory test for the diagnosis of melancholia. Standardization, validation, and clinical utility. *Arch Gen Psychiatry* 38:15–22.

Cherrier, M.M., Anawalt, B.D., Herbst, K.L., et al. (2002) Cognitive effects of short-term manipulation of serum sex steroids in healthy young men. *J Clin Endocrinol Metab* 87:3090–3096.

Cherrier, M.M., Asthana, S., Plymate, S., et al. (2001) Testosterone supplementation improves spatial and verbal memory in healthy older men. *Neurology* 57:80–88.

Christiansen, K., and Knussmann, R. (1987) Sex hormones and cognitive functioning in men. *Neuropsychobiology* 18:27–36.

Copolov, D.L., Rubin, R.T., Stuart, G.W., et al. (1989) Specificity of the salivary cortisol dexamethasone suppression test across psychiatric diagnoses. *Biol Psychiatry* 25:879–893.

Corpas, E., Harman, S.M., and Blackman, M.R. (1993) Human growth hormone and human aging. *Endocrinol Rev* 14:20–39.

Dabbs, J.M., Hargrove, M.F., and Heusel, C. (1996) Testosterone differences among college fraternities: Well-behaved vs. rambunctious. *Person individ Diff* 20:157–161.

Delhez, M., Hansenne, M., and Legros, J. (2003) Andropause and psychopathology: Minor symptoms rather than pathological ones. *Psychoneuroendocrinology* 28:863–874.

Deuschle, M., Schweiger, U., Gotthardt, U., et al. (1998) The combined dexamethasone/corticotropin-releasing hormone stimulation test is more closely associated with features of diurnal activity of the hypothalamo-pituitary-adrenocortical system than the dexamethasone suppression test. *Biol Psychiatry* 43:762–766.

Devanand, D.P., Nobler, M.S., Singer, T., et al. (1994) Is dysthymia a different disorder in the elderly? *Am J Psychiatry* 151:1592–1599.

Devanand, D.P., Sackeim, H.A., Lo, E.S., et al. (1991) Serial dexamethasone suppression tests and plasma dexamethasone levels. Effects of clinical response to electroconvulsive therapy in major depression. *Arch Gen Psychiatry* 48:525–533.

Dinan, T.G. (1998) Psychoneuroendocrinology of depression. Growth hormone. *Psychiatr Clin North Am* 21:325–339.

Ehrenreich, H., Halaris, A., Ruether, E., et al. (1999) Psychoendocrine sequelae of chronic testosterone deficiency. *J Psychiatr Res* 33:379–387.

Fabian, T.J., Dew, M.A., Pollock, B.G., et al. (2001) Endogenous concentrations of DHEA and DHEA-S decrease with remission of depression in older adults. *Biol Psychiatry* 50:767–774.

Feder, H.H. (1984) Hormones and sexual behavior. *Annu Rev Psychol* 35:165–200.

Feldman, H.A., Longcope, C., Derby, C.A., et al. (2002) Age trends in the level of serum testosterone and other hormones in middle-aged men: Longitudinal results from the Massachusetts male aging study. *J Clin Endocrinol Metab* 87:589–598.

Ferrari, E., Casarotti, D., Muzzoni, B., et al. (2001) Age-related changes of the adrenal secretory pattern: Possible role in pathological brain aging. *Brain Res Brain Res Rev* 37:294–300.

Field, A.E., Colditz, G.A., Willett, W.C., et al. (1994) The relation of smoking, age, relative weight, and dietary intake to serum adrenal steroids, sex hormones, and sex hormone-binding globulin in middle-aged men. *J Clin Endocrinol Metab* 79:1310–1316.

Glendenning, P., and Vasikaran, S.D. (2002) Vitamin D status and redefining serum PTH reference range in the elderly. *J Clin Endocrinol Metab* 87:946–947.

Gordon, H.W., and Lee, P.A. (1986) A relationship between gonadotropins and visuospatial function. *Neuropsychologia* 24:563–576.

Gouchie, C., and Kimura, D. (1991) The relationship between testosterone levels and cognitive ability patterns. *Psychoneuroendocrinology* 16:323–334.

Grady, D., Brown, J.S., Vittinghoff, E., et al. (2001) Postmenopausal hormones and incontinence: The Heart and Estrogen/Progestin Replacement Study. *Obstet Gynecol* 97:116–120.

Grady, D., Herrington, D., Bittner, V., et al. (2002) Cardiovascular disease outcomes during 6.8 years of hormone therapy: Heart and Estrogen/Progestin Replacement Study follow-up (HERS II). *JAMA* 288:49–57.

Grinspoon, S., Corcoran, C., Stanley, T., et al. (2000) Effects of hypogonadism and testosterone administration on depression indices in HIV-infected men. *J Clin Endocrinol Metab* 85:60–65.

Gupta, A., Habubi, N., and Thomas, P. (2001) Abnormalities of thyroid hormonal function tests in hospitalised elderly patients: A prospective study. *Int J Clin Pract* 55:582–583.

Hajjar, R.R., Kaiser, F.E., and Morley, J.E. (1997) Outcomes of long-term testosterone replacement in older hypogonadal males: A retrospective analysis. *J Clin Endocrinol Metab* 82:3793–3796.

Halbreich, U. (1997) Hormonal interventions with psychopharmacological potential: An overview. *Psychopharmacol Bull* 33:281–286.

Hannan, C.J.J., Friedl, K.E., Zold, A., et al. (1991) Psychological and serum homovanillic acid changes in men administered androgenic steroids. *Psychoneuroendocrinology* 16:335–343.

Hazzard, W.R. (1997) Ways to make "usual" and "successful" aging synonymous. Preventive gerontology. *West J Med* 167:206–215.

Heuser, M.D., and Hazzard, W.R. (1994) Geriatric medicine. *JAMA* 271:1675–1677.

Heuser, I., Hartmann, A., and Oertel, H. (1999) Androgen replacement in a 48, XXYY-male patient [letter]. *Arch Gen Psychiatry* 56:194–195.

Heuser, I., Yassouridis, A., and Holsboer, F. (1994) The combined dexamethasone/CRH test: A refined laboratory test for psychiatric disorders. *J Psychiatr Res* 28:341–356.

Hollowell, J.G., Staehling, N.W., Flanders, W.D., et al. (2002) Serum TSH, T(4), and thyroid antibodies in the United States population (1988 to 1994): National Health and Nutrition Examination Survey (NHANES III). *J Clin Endocrinol Metab* 87:489–499.

Holsboer, F. (2000) The stress hormone system is back on the map. *Curr Psychiatry Rep* 2:454–456.

Holsboer, F. (2001) Stress, hypercortisolism and corticosteroid receptors in depression: Implications for therapy. *J Affect Disord* 62:77–91.

Hulley, S., Furberg, C., Barrett-Connor, E., et al. (2002) Noncardiovascular disease outcomes during 6.8 years of hormone therapy: Heart and Estrogen/progestin Replacement Study follow-up (HERS II). *JAMA* 288:58–66.

Janowsky, J.S., Oviatt, S.K., and Orwoll, E.S. (1994) Testosterone influences spatial cognition in older men. *Behav Neurosci* 108:325–332.

Kenny, A.M., Bellantonio, S., Gruman, C.A., et al. (2002) Effects of transdermal testosterone on cognitive function and health perception in older men with low bioavailable testosterone levels. *J Gerontol A Biol Sci Med Sci* 57:M321–M325.

Kin, N.M., Nair, N.P., Amin, M., et al. (1997) The dexamethasone suppression test and treatment outcome in elderly depressed patients participating in a placebo-controlled multicenter trial involving moclobemide and nortriptyline. *Biol Psychiatry* 42:925–931.

Lebowitz, B.D., Pearson, J.L., Schneider, L.S., et al. (1997) Diagnosis and treatment of depression in late life. Consensus statement update. *JAMA* 278:1186–1190.

Loosen, P.T. (1992) The thyroid state of depressed patients. *Clin Neuropharmacol* 15(suppl 1, pt A):382A–383A.

Luisi, M., and Franchi, F. (1980) Double-blind group comparative study of testosterone undecanoate and mesterolone in hypogonadal male patients. *J Endocrinol Invest* 3:305–308.

Lupien, S., Lecours, A.R., Schwartz, G., et al. (1996) Longitudinal study of basal cortisol levels in healthy elderly subjects: Evidence for subgroups. *Neurobiol Aging* 17:95–105.

Maartens, L., Knottnerus, J., and Pop V. (2002) Menopausal transition and increased depressive symptomatology. A community based prospective study. *Maturitas* 42:195–200.

Magni, G., Schifano, F., De Leo, D., et al. (1986) The dexamethasone suppression test in depressed and non-depressed geriatric medical inpatients. *Acta Psychiatr Scand* 73:511–514.

Magri, F., Muzzoni, B., Cravello, L., et al. (2002) Thyroid function in physiological aging and in centenarians: Possible relationships with some nutritional markers. *Metabolism* 51:105–109.

McEwen, B.S. (1998) Gonadal and adrenal steroids and the brain: Implications for depression. In: Halbreich, U. ed. *Hormones and Depression*. New York: Raven Press, pp. 239–253.

McKinlay, J.B., Longcope, C., and Gray, A. (1989) The questionable physiologic and epidemiologic basis for a male climacteric syndrome: Preliminary results from the Massachusetts Male Aging Study. *Maturitas* 11:103–115.

Melin, A., Wilske, J., Ringertz, H., and Saaf, M. (2001) Seasonal variations in serum levels of 25-hydroxyvitamin D and parathyroid hormone but no detectable change in femoral neck bone density in an older population with regular outdoor exposure. *J Am Geriatr Soc* 49:1190–1196.

Meyers, B.S., Alpert, S., Gabriele, M., et al. (1993) State specificity of DST abnormalities in geriatric depression. *Biol Psychiatry* 34:108–114.

Morales, A., Heaton, J.P., and Carson, C.C. (2000) Andropause: A misnomer for a true clinical entity. *J Urol* 163:705–712.

Morley, J.E., Charlton, E., Patrick, P., et al. (2000) Validation of a screening questionnaire for androgen deficiency in aging males. *Metabolism* 49:1239–1242.

Morrison, M.F., and Tweedy, K. (2000) Effects of estrogen on mood and cognition in aging women. *Psychiatr Ann* 30:113–119.

Mulligan, T., Iranmanesh, A., Johnson, M.L., et al. (1997) Aging alters feed-forward and feedback linkages between LH and testosterone in healthy men. *Am J Physiol* 273:R1407–R1413.

Nicholas, L., Dawkins, K., and Golden, R.N. (1998) Psychoneuroendocrinology of depression. Prolactin. *Psychiatr Clin North Am* 21:341–358.

O'Connor, D.B., Archer, J., Hair, W.M., and Wu, F.C. (2001) Activational effects of testosterone on cognitive function in men. *Neuropsychologia* 39:1385–1394.

Olweus, D., Mattsson, A., Schalling, D., and Low, H. (1988) Circulating testosterone levels and aggression in adolescent males: A causal analysis. *Psychosom Med* 50:261–272.

Perry, P.J., Lund, B.C., Arndt, S., et al. (2001) Bioavailable testosterone as a correlate of cognition, psychological status, quality of life, and sexual function in aging males: Implications for testosterone replacement therapy. *Ann Clin Psychiatry* 13:75–80.

Plotsky, P.M., Owens, M.J., and Nemeroff, C.B. (1998) Psychoneuroendocrinology of depression. Hypothalamic-pituitary-adrenal axis. *Psychiatr Clin North Am* 21:293–307.

Pope, H.G.J., Cohane, G.H., Kanayama, G., et al. (2003) Testosterone gel supplementation for men with refractory depression: A randomized, placebo-controlled trial. *Am J Psychiatry* 160:105–111.

Prange, A.J., Jr. (1998) Psychoendocrinology: A commentary. *Psychiatr Clin North Am* 21:491–505.

Prinz, P.N., Scanlan, J.M., Vitaliano, P.P., et al. (1999) Thyroid hormones: Positive relationships with cognition in healthy, euthyroid older men. *J Gerontol A Biol Sci Med Sci* 54:M111–M116.

Prior, J.C. (1998) Perimenopause: The complex endocrinology of the menopausal transition. *Endocrinol Rev* 19:397–428.

Rabkin, J.G., Wagner, G., and Rabkin, R. (2000) A double-blind, placebo-controlled trial of testosterone therapy for HIV-positive men with hypogonadal symptoms. *Arch Gen Psychiatry* 57:141–147.

Ravaglia, G., Forti, P., Maioli, F., and et al. (1997) Determinants of functional status in healthy Italian nonagenarians and centenarians: A comprehensive functional assessment by the instruments of geriatric practice. *J Am Geriatr Soc* 45:1196–1202.

Rinieris, P.M., Malliaras, D.E., Batrinos, M.L., and Stefanis, C.N. (1979) Testosterone treatment of depression in two patients with Klinefelter's syndrome. *Am J Psychiatry* 136:986–988.

Rubin, R.T., Phillips, J.J., Sadow, T.F., and McCracken, J.T. (1995) Adrenal gland volume in major depression. Increase during the depressive episode and decrease with successful treatment. *Arch Gen Psychiatry* 52:213–218.

Rubinow, D.R., and Schmidt, P.J. (1996) Androgens, brain, and behavior. *Am J Psychiatry* 153:974–984.

Rudman, D., Feller A.G., Nagraj H.S., et al. (1990) Effects of human growth hormone in men over 60 years old. *N Engl J Med* 323:1–6.

Rudman, D., and Mattson, D.E. (1994) Serum insulin-like growth factor I in healthy older men in relation to physical activity. *J Am Geriatr Soc* 42:71–76.

Rupprecht, R. (1997) The neuropsychopharmacological potential of neuroactive steroids. *J Psychiatr Res* 31:314–315.

Rupprecht, R., Rupprecht, C., Rupprecht, M., et al. (1988) Different reactivity of the hypothalamo-pituitary-gonadal-axis in depression and normal controls. *Pharmacopsychiatry* 21:438–439.

Sachar, E.J., Hellman, L., Fukushima, D.K., and Gallagher, T.F. (1970) Cortisol production in depressive illness. A clinical and biochemical clarification. *Arch Gen Psychiatry* 23:289–298.

Sapolsky, R.M. (1999) Glucocorticoids, stress, and their adverse neurological effects: Relevance to aging. *Exp Gerontol* 34:721–732.

Schmidt, P.J., and Rubinow, D.R. (1997) Neuroregulatory role of gonadal steroids in humans. *Psychopharmacol Bull* 33:219–220.

Schneider, L.S., Small, G.W., and Clary, C.M. (2001) Estrogen replacement therapy and antidepressant response to sertraline in older depressed women. *Am J Geriatr Psychiatry* 9:393–399.

Schule, C., Baghai, T., Zwanzger, P., et al. (2001) Sleep deprivation and hypothalamic-pituitary-adrenal (HPA) axis activity in depressed patients. *J Psychiatr Res* 35:239–247.

Schweiger, U., Deuschle, M., Weber, B., et al. (1999) Testosterone, gonadotropin, and cortisol secretion in male patients with major depression. *Psychosom Med* 61:292–296.

Seidman, S.N., Araujo, A.B., Roose, S.P., et al. (2002) Low testosterone levels in elderly men with dysthymic disorder. *Am J Psychiatry* 159:456–459.

Seidman, S.N., and Rabkin, J.G. (1998) Testosterone replacement therapy for hypogonadal men with SSRI-refractory depression. *J Affect Disord* 48:157–161.

Seidman, S.N., and Roose, S.P. (2000) The male hypothalamic-pituitary-gonadal axis: Pathogenic and therapeutic implications in psychiatry. *Psychiatr Ann* 30:102–112.

Seidman, S.N., Spatz, E., Rizzo, C., and Roose, S.P. (2001) Testosterone replacement therapy for hypogonadal men with major depressive disorder: A randomized, placebo-controlled clinical trial. *J Clin Psychiatry* 62:406–412.

Sherwin, B.B. (1988) Affective changes with estrogen and androgen replacement therapy in surgically menopausal women. *J Affect Disord* 14:177–187.

Sih, R., Morley, J.E., Kaiser, F.E., et al. (1997) Testosterone replacement in older hypogonadal men: A 12-month randomized controlled trial. *J Clin Endocrinol Metab* 82:1661–1667.

Slotkin, T.A., Hays, J.C., Nemeroff, C.B., and Carroll, B.J. (1997) Dexamethasone suppression test identifies a subset of elderly depressed patients with reduced platelet serotonin transport and resistance to imipramine inhibition of transport. *Depress Anxiety* 6:19–25.

Smith, N.L., Barzilay, J.I., Shaffer, D., et al. (2002) Fasting and 2-hour postchallenge serum glucose measures and risk of incident cardiovascular events in the elderly: The Cardiovascular Health Study. *Arch Intern Med* 162:209–216.

Snyder, P.J., Peachey, H., Hannoush, P., et al. (1999a) Effect of testosterone treatment on bone mineral density in men over 65 years of age. *J Clin Endocrinol Metab* 84:1966–1972.

Snyder, P.J., Peachey, H., Hannoush, P., et al. (1999b) Effect of testosterone treatment on body composition and muscle strength in men over 65 years of age. *J Clin Endocrinol Metab* 84:2647–2653.

Soares, C.N., Joffe, H., Cohen, L.S., and Almeida, O.P. (2002) Efficacy of 17beta-estradiol on depression: Is estrogen deficiency really necessary? *J Clin Psychiatry* 63:451–452.

Stampfer, M.J., Colditz, G.A., Willett, W.C., et al. (1991) Postmenopausal estrogen therapy and cardiovascular disease. Ten-year follow-up from the nurses' health study. *N Engl J Med* 325:756–762.

Steiner, M., Dunn, E., and Born, L. (2003) Hormones and mood: From menarche to menopause and beyond. *J Affect Disord* 74:67–83.

Stek, M.L., Van Exel, E., Van Tilburg, W., et al. (2002) The prognosis of depression in old age: Outcome six to eight years after clinical treatment. *Aging Ment Health* 6:282–285.

Targum, S.D., Greenberg, R.D., Harmon, R.L., et al. (1984) The TRH test and thyroid hormone in refractory depression. *Am J Psychiatry* 141:463–469.

Targum, S.D., Marshall, L.E., Magac-Harris, K., and Martin, D. (1989) TRH tests in a healthy elderly population. Demonstration of gender differences. *J Am Geriat Soc* 37:533–536.

Tenover, J.L. (1998) Male hormone replacement therapy including "andropause." *Endocrinol Metab Clin North Am* 27:969–987.

Thrivikraman, K.V., Nemeroff, C.B., and Plotsky, P.M. (2000) Sensitivity to glucocorticoid-mediated fast-feedback regulation of the hypothalamic-pituitary-adrenal axis is dependent upon stressor specific neurocircuitry. *Brain Res* 870:87–101.

Valenti, G. (1992) Psychoneuroendocrinology of aging: The brain as target organ of hormones. *Psychoneuroendocrinology* 17:279–282.

Van Cauter, E., Leproult, R., and Plat, L. (2000) Age-related changes in slow wave sleep and REM sleep and relationship with growth hormone and cortisol levels in healthy men. *JAMA* 284:861–868.

Vermeulen, A., and Kaufman, J.M. (1995) Ageing of the hypothalamo-pituitary-testicular axis in men. *Horm Res* 43:25–28.

Villareal, D.T., and Morley, J.E. (1994) Trophic factors in aging. *Drugs Aging* 4:492–509.

Wallen, K., Eisler, J.A., Tannenbaum, P.L., et al. (1991) Antide (Nal-Lys GnRH antagonist) suppression of pituitary-testicular function and sexual behavior in group-living rhesus monkeys. *Physiol Behav* 50:429–435.

Wang, C., Swerdloff, R.S., Iranmanesh, A., et al. (2000) Transdermal testosterone gel improves sexual function, mood, muscle strength, and body composition parameters in hypogonadal men. Testosterone Gel Study Group. *J Clin Endocrinol Metab* 85:2839–2853.

Wolf, O.T., and Kirschbaum, C. (2002) Endogenous estradiol and testosterone levels are associated with cognitive performance in older women and men. *Horm Behav* 41:259–266 41:259–266.

Wolkowitz, O.M., Brizendine, L., and Reus, V.I. (2000) The role of dehydroepiandrosterone (DHEA) in psychiatry. *Psychiatr Ann* 30:123–128.

Wolkowitz, O.M., Reus, V.I., Keebler, A., et.al. (1999) Double-blind treatment of major depression with dehydroepiandrosterone (DHEA). *Am J Psychiatry* 156:646–649.

Wolkowitz, O.M., Reus, V.I., Roberts, E., et al. (1997) Dehydroepiandrosterone (DHEA) treatment of depression. *Biol Psychiatry* 41:311–318.

Yaffe, K., Krueger, K., Sarkar, S., et al. (2001) Cognitive function in postmenopausal women treated with raloxifene. *N Engl J Med* 344:1207–1213.

Yaffe, K., Lui, L.Y., Zmuda, J., and Cauley, J. (2002) Sex hormones and cognitive function in older men. *J Am Geriatr Soc* 50:707–712.

Young, A.H., Gallagher, P., and Porter, R.J. (2002) Elevation of the cortisol-dehydroepiandrosterone ratio in drug-free depressed patients. *Am J Psychiatry* 159:1237–1239.

# IV | TREATMENT

DESPITE the devastating impact of late-life depression, the clinician must often make critical treatment decisions based on inadequate information. There is a paucity of rigorously designed, adequately powered, randomized, controlled trials (comparator or placebo) of antidepressant interventions. The scant information that is available about the treatment of late-life depression comes primarily from antidepressant medication trials or studies of other somatic therapies; psychotherapy has been particularly neglected. The state of our knowledge is so underdeveloped that, for example, the critical question of whether age itself is a moderator of the treatment outcome has not been definitively answered.

There are several reasons why knowledge in this area is so limited. To receive Food and Drug Administration (FDA) approval, the clinical trials that demonstrate the efficacy and safety of new antidepressant medications are invariably conducted in young and otherwise healthy depressed patient samples. There is no incentive for the pharmaceutical industry to risk testing a new treatment in a late-life population that, by virtue of age, has a greater number of co-morbid medical conditions and an increased use of concomitant medications. (On average, a person over the age of 65 takes five prescription medications per day.) A medication that is well tolerated and safe in a younger population may have a direct deleterious effect on common co-morbid conditions in older patients (e.g., tricyclics and ischemic heart disease) or an indirect deleterious effect through an increased risk of drug–drug interactions (e.g., a selective serotonin reuptake inhibitor that has significant inhibitory effects on cytochrome P-450 isoenzymes.

Though such considerations make the need for efficacy and safety studies in a late-life population even more compelling, they have had an inhibitory effect on the pharmaceutical industry. Of note, FDA regulations have recently changed. For a new treatment to be approved, pharmacokinetic data must be obtained in a late-life population. However, this requirement only applies to new drug applications; efficacy and safety testing are still not required in the elderly. Nonetheless, perhaps because of the increasing size of the late-life population, a few well-designed industry-sponsored studies of antidepressant medications in the treatment of late-life depression have recently been completed.

Ageism is one reason that psychological treatments have been inadequately studied in older patients. The belief that psychotherapeutic treatments are inappropriate for geriatric patients is widespread. This bias was evident from the inception of psychotherapy. Freud commented that older patients (he meant those over the age of 40) were unlikely to benefit from psychotherapeutic interventions due to the character rigidity that comes with age. The demographics of use support the notion that there is a widespread belief that psychotherapy is for the young and troubled. Nonetheless, the limited number of psychotherapy studies in older patients have produced positive findings, and as in younger patients, there may be a subgroup of older patients for whom combination treatment with medication and psychotherapy is especially effective.

With the ethics of research receiving increasing attention, special protections have been afforded to vulnerable populations, including patients in late life. Since some degree of cognitive impairment is common in older depressed patients, institutional review boards (IRBs) have paid special attention to this issue. As a result, recruitment and consent procedures for research studies have become more restrictive. However, ageism can also influence IRBs, and regulations intended to protect older patients may, in fact, discriminate against them. For example, in a recent treatment study comparing an established antidepressant medication to placebo in depressed patients over the age of 75, one IRB required that, by virtue of age alone, all patients should be considered cognitively impaired and stipulated that special procedures be followed for recruitment and assessment. This type of blanket policy is the essence of prejudice; patients are considered to have a liability or deficiency based solely on their membership in a group, in this case people over the age of 75, rather than based on an evaluation of the individual.

Some of the chapters in this part review the available data, regardless of study design, particularly for treatments already in widespread clinical use despite the limited evidence supporting their efficacy and safety. Especially in the late-life population, the clinician must calculate the risk-benefit ratio of a treatment intervention by considering not only potential adverse effects, but also the increased risk of mortality due to co-morbid conditions were the depression not treated. This is cogently illustrated in depressed patients with symptomatic ischemic heart disease, either angina or myocardial infarction, who have an increased risk of cardiac death compared to nondepressed patients with comparable cardiac illness.

Clinical judgment is always an important component of the decision-making process when making treatment recommendations. Unfortunately, clinicians must rely disproportionately on their clinical experience and judgment when treating late-life depression, since relevant and reliable information is so limited.

# 15 | Pharmacokinetics and pharmacodynamics in late life

BRUCE G. POLLOCK

Older patients are a pharmacologically sensitive population. They frequently bear a high burden of medical illness, consume more drugs than younger patients, are subject to more extensive multiple medication regimens, and account for more adverse drug events. Complications from pharmacotherapy represent a major health problem for elders. For those in their 80s, adverse drug reactions are seven times higher than for those in their 20s (Beard, 1992). Psychoactive medications continue to rank with anticoagulants as the most common medications associated with preventable adverse drug events in nursing homes (Gurwitz et al., 2000). There is also a high prevalence of psychotropic medication use among homebound elders, a group that is at even higher risk of adverse drug experiences and is not subject to oversight by regulatory agencies (Golden et al., 1999).

Although patients over the age of 65 (representing 13% of the U.S. population) account for 25% to 39% of prescription drug costs, the old are often excluded from clinical and regulatory trials of drugs intended for their consumption (Atkin et al., 1999). While this policy is well intentioned, the U.S. Food and Drug Administration's *Guidance for Industry: Content and Format for Geriatric Labeling* (2001) is voluntary, without any financial incentives and therefore is expected to result in only modest benefit. In contrast, the Pediatric Provisions of the Food and Drug Modernization Act of 1997 (continued as the Best Pharmaceuticals for Children Act 2001, PL 107–109), which grants additional patent exclusivity for conducting studies, has resulted in a meaningful increase in the clinical pharmacological knowledge base for children.

The premise guiding this chapter is that if a drug has physiological activity, a threshold of medication exposure is necessary for therapeutic effect; conversely, excessive exposure to a drug or its active metabolites may lead to adverse effects. In addition to concerns regarding excessive drug concentrations, nonadherence or partial adherence to a pharmacotherapy regimen is a major problem in both treatment and interpretation of clinical trials. The elderly may be more sensitive to

lower concentrations of an antidepressant because of age- or illness-associated neurotransmitter and receptor changes. Nonetheless, the first requirement for rational therapeutics in an older population is to control for the immense variability in drug concentration.

A drug's dose seldom has an unambiguous relationship to its plasma concentration. Pharmacokinetics provides a way of describing and predicting drug concentrations in plasma and various tissues over time. Diversity in concentration is especially marked in older patients due to poor treatment adherence and/or pharmacokinetic differences among patients. With age, liver volume and blood flow diminish, while drug-metabolizing isoenzymes are differentially affected by age, genetics, and, most important, multiple interacting medications (Schmucker, 2001). Moreover, the age-associated reduction in renal clearance results in the accumulation of active drug metabolites.

Throughout the 1970s and 1980s, efforts were made to establish concentration–effect relationships for the tricyclic antidepressants. This research drew attention to doses that were frequently too low to be therapeutically effective, as well as to individuals with atypically high drug concentrations. For newer antidepressants and antipsychotics, it is often part of a deliberate marketing strategy to avoid explorations of drug concentration variability, let alone possible concentration relationships to adverse events, in Phase IV trials. Failure to address this issue resulted in notable difficulties with the introduction of bupropion and clozapine (which produce seizures at high doses) and, for older patients, the introduction of fluoxetine and risperidone (which produce agitation, akathisia, and extrapyramidal syndromes). Although the selective serotonin reuptake inhibitors (SSRIs), which have relatively flat dose-response curves, have become first-line treatments for depression in the elderly, unnecessarily high SSRI drug concentrations may result in unnecessary side effects and high costs. Recently, high plasma paroxetine and sertraline concentrations were associated with adverse cognitive and psychomotor effects in healthy older subjects (Furlan et al., 2001). Moreover, assessment of drug concentrations may have a role in evaluating treatment adherence for these drugs with delayed onset and variable therapeutics (Foglia and Pollock, 1997). This is especially important for the elderly with hepatic or renal impairment or with polypharmacy regimens, with an increased risk of drug–drug interactions. Controlling the immense variability in drug concentration in an older population is one step toward optimizing drug therapy to achieve advantageous outcomes and avoid detrimental ones.

Finally, controlling for antidepressant drug exposures permits the study of possible genetic differences, which may influence the response. Recently, older depressed patients with the *ll* serotonin transporter promoter genotype have been found to have a more robust initial response to paroxetine (Pollock et al., 2000a). In contrast to results obtained with other SSRIs, this polymorphism did not influence the overall antidepressant response at 12 weeks (Lotrich et al., 2001). In these older patients, plasma paroxetine levels were over 100 ng/ml, a concentration believed to be sufficient for noradrenergic involvement (Owens et al., 2000).

## AGE-ASSOCIATED PHYSIOLOGICAL CHANGES

Age-associated pharmacokinetic differences may be due to changes in absorption, distribution, metabolism, or elimination of a drug (Table 15.1). The multidimensional changes associated with aging are, of course, highly complex and variable, and only the most superficial generalizations can be made (Pollock, 1998).

### Absorption

The absorption of nutrients that require active transport, such as iron, thiamine, and calcium, is often impaired in the elderly. Nonetheless, the rate and extent of passive drug absorption do not appear to be affected by normal aging. Antacids, high-fiber supplements, and the cholesterol binding resin, cholestyramine, may significantly diminish the absorption of medications. Food may have a modest and variable effect on some antidepressants, such as sertraline.

### Distribution

For the majority of psychotropics that are lipid-soluble, the loss of lean body mass with aging leads to increases in their volume of distribution, resulting in longer half-lives and drug accumulation. This is because a drug's half-life is directly proportional to its apparent volume of distribution. Conversely, for water-soluble drugs such as lithium and digoxin, the volume of distribution is diminished in older patients, reducing the margin of safety after acute increases in plasma drug concentration.

Reductions in serum albumin with age and possible increases in alpha-1-acid glycoprotein with illness may affect the amount of drug bound to plasma proteins. However, it is now recognized that changes in plasma protein binding are of clinical significance only when therapeutic drug monitoring is used to adjust dosing, since total drug concentrations (free plus protein bound) are usually reported (Benet and Hoener, 2002). The total drug level may be considered too low if a drug's free fraction is increased by diminished plasma proteins or drug displacement. Free drug levels in older patients have been found to be useful for lidocaine, theophylline, phenytoin, and digoxin. More data on the use of therapeutic plasma levels are needed for elders treated with valproate, given its increased use in dementia and its increased age-associated potential to produce thrombocytopenia and hepatotoxicity (Conley et al., 2001).

### Metabolism

In the past decade, cytochrome P450 (CYP) metabolism-based drug–drug interactions have become a major concern in drug development and clinical practice. Available evidence suggests that there is no uniform age-associated decline in liver metabolism by CYP enzymes (Schmucker, 2001). Nonetheless, reductions in hepatic mass and blood flow with aging place greater emphasis on interindividual differences in drug metabolic capacity. These metabolic differences may be either genetic or the result of interactions of multiple medications. Isoenzyme specificity suggests that inhibi-

TABLE 15.1. *Physiological Changes in the Elderly Associated with Altered Pharmacokinetics*

| Organ System | Change | Pharmacokinetic Consequence |
|---|---|---|
| Gastrointestinal tract | Decreased intestinal and splanchnic blood flow | Decreased rate of drug absorption |
| Circulatory system | Decreased concentration of plasma albumin and increased concentration of alpha-1-acid glycoprotein | Increased or decreased free concentration of drugs in plasma |
| Kidney | Decreased glomerular filtration rate | Decreased renal clearance of active metabolites |
| Muscle | Decreased lean body mass and increased adipose tissue | Altered volume of distribution of ipid-soluble drugs, leading to increased elimination half-life |
| Liver | Decreased liver size; decreased hepatic blood; variable effects on CYP450 isozyme activity | Decreased hepatic clearance |

tion or induction of a given P450 isoenzyme will affect all drugs metabolized by that specific enzyme (Pollock, 1998).

CYP2D6 is the isozyme responsible for hydroxylation of tricyclic antidepressants and venlafaxine, as well as several older neuroleptics and risperidone. Approximately 7% of the Caucasian population are genetically poor 2D6 metabolizers, which has been shown to impact nortriptyline doses (Murphy et al., 2001) and to cause adverse effects of perphenazine in older patients (Pollock et al., 1995). Concern has also been raised about potential cardiotoxicity in poor 2D6 metabolizers treated with venlafaxine or with concomitant diphenhydramine (a CYP2D6 inhibitor) (Lessard et al., 1999, 2001). Studies conducted in older unmedicated volunteers have not found an age-associated decline in CYP2D6 activity (Pollock et al., 1992b). Nevertheless, many drugs commonly used by older patients inhibit this enzyme, leading to potential interactions.

CYP3A4 is the most prevalent drug-metabolizing enzyme and is responsible for metabolizing the largest number of medications. Because it is normally a high-capacity enzyme, serious and surprising toxicity occurs when the 3A4-mediated clearance of terfenadine, astemizole, cisapride, cerivastatin, midazolam, and triazolam is inhibited. Also, because hepatic metabolism of CYP3A4 drugs is typically very rapid, many of these drugs are perfusion-limited—that is, dependent on hepatic blood flow—which may decline by 40% between ages 25 and 65. Therefore, it often appears that clearance of drugs specifically metabolized by CYP3A4 declines with age; for example, alprazolam and triazolam clearances in the elderly are only 50% to 80% of those in young adults. In particular, gender- and age-related pharmacokinetic differences have been demonstrated for several 3A4-type drugs such as sertraline, mirtazapine, and nefazodone. CYP3A4 activity may be inhibited by grapefruit juice, protease inhibitors, *mycin* antibiotics, and *azole* antifungals. Among antidepressants, nefazodone and fluvoxamine are the most potent inhibitors, followed by fluoxetine through its demethylated metabolite. The very long half-life of norfluoxetine may result in interactions many weeks after initiation of therapy. Similarly, the inhibition of the CYP3A4-mediated clearance of *statins*, resulting in muscle weakness, may be misattributed in depressed patients. The 3A4 enzyme may also be induced by other drugs, such as carbamazepine, phenytoin, topiramate, modafinil, barbiturates, steroids, and St. John's wort, increasing the risk of therapeutic failure for CYP3A4 drugs. Many CYP3A4 inhibitors (e.g., verapamil) and inducers (St. John's wort) have also been found to interact at the P-glycoprotein drug transporter, amplifying their effects on CYP3A4.

CYP1A2 metabolizes clozapine, olanzapine, fluvoxamine, and theophylline and contributes to the demethyl-

ation of some tertiary tricyclic antidepressants. This isoenzyme readily undergoes induction by cigarette smoking, cruciferous vegetables, and charcoal-broiled meats, as well as by certain medications such as omeprazole and phenobarbital. Estrogen replacement therapy in postmenopausal women has been found to inhibit CYP1A2 metabolism (Pollock et al., 1999). CYP2B6 substantially metabolizes bupropion, and there is in vitro evidence that fluoxetine, paroxetine, and sertraline may cause inhibition (Hesse et al., 2000).

## Excretion

The well-established age-associated decline in renal clearance may affect excretion of psychotropic drug metabolites and lithium in older patients. The magnitude of this decline varies greatly among the aged (Pollock et al., 1992b) and is exacerbated by physical conditions (e.g., diabetes and hypertension) and medications (e.g., nonsteroidal anti-inflammatories). Since the production of creatinine is reduced by declining muscle mass, serum creatinine is not a reliable indicator of renal function in the elderly. Accumulation of active hydroxylated metabolites of the tricyclic antidepressants in older patients was previously a subject of concern (Pollock et al., 1992a). Higher concentrations of bupropion and venlafaxine metabolites have been observed in older patients and in those with renal impairment, with uncertain clinical consequences (Sweet et al., 1995).

## PHARMACOKINETICS

It is important to appreciate the critical lack of pharmacokinetic (PK) information relevant to the majority of elders encountered in clinical practice (Table 15.2). The limited information that does exist for older subjects is largely derived from *classical* or *two-stage* PK modeling. For example, regarding fluoxetine, which has a geriatric indication, the only published data on disposition in older subjects are limited to a study of single doses in 11 healthy subjects

Traditional PK methodology requires an intensive sampling regimen (i.e., a large number of samples) usually obtained from a small number (i.e., 6–12) of volunteers. The PK parameters are determined for each individual separately, and average PK parameters are calculated as the mean of the individually determined parameters. It should also be noted that single-dose PK studies are usually not adequate to rule out the possibility of nonlinear kinetics. Results of these traditional PK studies are limited in generalizability because of the small number of patients studied, the virtual absence of the old-old and oldest-old, and the absence of those with the illnesses and concurrent medications typical of this age group (DeVane and Pollock, 1999).

TABLE 15.2. *Published and Unpublished Reports of Pharmacokinetics of Newer Antidepressants in the Elderly*

| Drug | Study Population and Design | Findings and Recommendations | Reference |
|------|---------------------------|------------------------------|-----------|
| Fluvoxamine | 13 patients 63–77 years old; 50 mg bid for 28 days | AUC and half-life were similar to those of young patients. | DeVries et al. (1993) |
| | 50 and 100 mg administered to compare elderly (ages 66–73) and young subjects (ages 19–35) | Mean maximum plasma concentrations in the elderly were 40% higher. Clearance of fluvoxamine was reduced by about 50% and, therefore, LUVOX tablets should be slowly titrated during initiation of therapy in older patients. | *Physicians' Desk Reference* (2002) |
| Fluoxetine | 11 volunteers 65–77 years old; single dose of 40 mg | Minimal differences were found. | Bergstrom et al. (1988) |
| | | Given the long half-life and nonlinear disposition of this drug, a single-dose study is not adequate to rule out the possibility of altered pharmacokinetics in the elderly, particularly if they have systemic illness or are receiving multiple drugs for concomitant diseases. A lower or less frequent dosage should also be considered for the elderly. | *Physicians' Desk Reference* (2002) |
| Sertraline | 22 volunteers >65 years old; 50 mg/day increasing to 200 mg/day for 21 days | The concentration was higher in elderly men and women compared with young men but was similar to the concentration in young women. | Ronfeld et al. (1997) |
| | 16 (8 male, 8 female) elderly patients treated for 14 days at a dose of 100 mg/day | The plasma clearance was approximately 40% lower than that in a similarly studied group of younger (25- to 32-year-old) individuals. A steady state, therefore, should be achieved after 2 to 3 weeks in older patients. | *Physicians' Desk Reference* (2002) |
| Paroxetine | 14 elderly and 16 young volunteers; single and multiple doses of 20–40 mg/day | Increased steady-state variability; 20% higher in the elderly; the half-life increases to 30 vs. 21 hr at 20 mg/day (38 hr at 30 mg/day) | Hebenstreit et al. (1989) Lundmark et al. (1989) |
| | Multiple-dose study in the elderly at doses of 20, 30, and 40 mg/day | Minimum concentrations were about 70% to 80% greater than the respective in nonelderly subjects. The initial dosage in the elderly should be reduced. | *Physicians' Desk Reference* (2002) |
| Citalopram | 10 patients 77 ± 8 years old; 20 mg/day for 14 days | The plasma level-to-dose ratio of 3.50 was higher than the ratio (1.96) reported by Overo (1982) for 55 younger patients. | Foglia et al. (1997) |
| | 24 elderly patients (69 ± 3.7 years) vs. 8 young patients (24 ± 4 years) | Only the half-life was statistically different between the groups—30% longer in the elderly; 20 mg is the recommended dose for most elderly patients | Gutierrez and Abramowitz (2000) *Physicians' Desk Reference* (2002) |
| Nefazodone | 13 volunteers 63–76 years old; single doses of 50, 100, and 200 mg | AUC is higher in the elderly than in the young; there is a gender difference; the half-life is similar among the groups. | Barbhaiya et al. (1996) |
| | | Treatment with *serzone* should be initiated at half the usual dose in elderly patients, especially women, but the therapeutic dose range is similar in younger and older patients. | *Physicians' Desk Reference* (2002) |
| Bupropion | 6 patients 63–76 years old; single dose of 100 mg, chronic dosing with 100 mg tid | There is a 20% reduction in clearance, an extended half-life (mean, 32 hr), and increased concern about metabolites. | Sweet et al. (1995) |
| | Exploration of steady-state bupropion concentrations from several depression efficacy studies involving patients given 300 to 750 mg/day divided into 3 doses | No relationship between age (18 to 83 years) and plasma concentration of bupropion was revealed. The risk of a toxic reaction may be greater in patients with impaired renal function. | *Physician's Desk Reference* (2002) |

*(continued)*

TABLE 15.2. *Published and Unpublished Reports of Pharmacokinetics of Newer Antidepressants in the Elderly (Continued)*

| Drug | Study Population and Design | Findings and Recommendations | Reference |
|---|---|---|---|
| Venlafaxine | 18 volunteers 60–80 years old; single dose of 50 mg and chronic dosing with 50 mg tid | There was a 24% increase in the steady-state half-life in the elderly and a 14% increase in metabolites. | Klamerus et al. (1996) |
| | Population pharmacokinetic analysis of 404 patients from two studies involving both bid and tid regimens | Dose-normalized trough plasma levels of either venlafaxine or O-desmethylvenlafaxine were unaltered by age or gender differences. Dosage adjustment based on the age or gender of a patient is generally not necessary. | *Physicians' Desk Reference* (2002) |
| Mirtazapine | 16 volunteers 68 ± 3 years old; single and multiple 20 mg doses | The half-life was lowest in young males (22 hr) and was similar in young and older women and older men (35 hr). | Timmer et al. (1996) |
| | 20 mg/day for 7 days in subjects of varying ages (range, 25–74 years) | Clearance was 40% lower in elderly males than in younger males; clearance in elderly females was only 10% lower than that of younger females. Caution is indicated in administering mirtazapine, orally disintegrating tablets, to elderly patients. | *Physicians' Desk Reference* (2002) |

AUC, area under the curve.

An alternative approach is population PK using mixed-effects modeling (MEM) (FDA, 1999). This statistical approach permits identification of both individual and overall population PK parameters based on only a few samples per subject and using each data point to inform the entire analysis (Sheiner and Ludden, 1992). Because a greater number of typical patients are evaluated, the results are much more applicable to clinical practice than those of traditional PK.

The MEM approach has yet to be exploited with antidepressants in geriatric clinical studies, but it has been successfully used to evaluate sparse data on other classes of compounds. Although manufacturers may have conducted population PK studies, there has been only one publication of the use of population PK with an antidepressant (Grasela et al., 1987). In this study, MEM detected an interaction between imipramine and alprazolam that was dependent on the simultaneous concentration of alprazolam, a finding that would not be possible under the study design typically used for traditional PK studies.

Population PK analyses can be incorporated into routine assessments of patients in clinical trials of antidepressants and may prove to be a significant addition to our ability to determine sources of variability in antidepressant plasma concentrations and response in older patients, particularly those with medical co-morbidity.

## PHARMACODYNAMICS

Interindividual differences in pharmacodynamics become evident when patients with similar plasma drug concentrations experience different responses. In general, older patients are more sensitive than younger ones to adverse effects of antidepressants at lower concentrations and require similar concentrations to initiate a therapeutic response (Pollock, 1999). Homeostatic mechanisms, such as postural control, water balance, orthostatic circulatory responses, and thermoregulation, are frequently less robust in the aged. This may interfere with the ability to adapt physiologically to medication. For instance, all psychotropics (including SSRIs) may increase the risk of falls and hip fracture (Liu, 1998). Similarly, the syndrome of inappropriate antidiuretic hormone secretion (SIADH) has been reported as an age-associated adverse effect of all SSRIs and venlafaxine (Kirby and Ames, 2001).

Reductions in dopamine or acetylcholine function with age may increase sensitivity to SSRIs (which indirectly reduce dopamine outflow) and antimuscarinic agents. Parkinsonism induced by SSRIs continues to require vigilant assessment in elders, and we have found that even low serum anticholinergic levels may be associated with cognitive impairment in depressed and nondepressed elders (Mulsant et al., 2003; Nebes et al., 1997). Unfortunately, anticholinergic drugs continue to be widely prescribed in older patients, including those with cognitive impairment (Roe et al., 2002).

Anticoagulants figure prominently in drug-related morbidity and mortality. Anticoagulant–antidepressant interactions may be both PK and pharmacodynamic. Among antidepressants, fluvoxamine poses the greatest risk of a PK interaction through inhibition of CYP2C9, reducing the clearance of warfarin's active S-enantiomer. In addition, fluvoxamine's inhibition of CYPs1A2 and 3A4 causes R-warfarin to accumulate, which also contributes to reduced S-warfarin clearance.

However, increased bleeding times with SSRIs alone, or in combination with anticoagulants, may also be possible due to depleting platelets of serotonin and attenuating their aggregation (Pollock et al., 2000b). Recently, both concerns (increased risk of gastrointestinal bleeding in elders) and potential benefits (protective effects against myocardial infarction in smokers) have been raised by epidemiological studies of SSRIs (Sauer et al., 2001; van Walravan et al. 2001).

## CONCLUSIONS

Because most of the data on a new drug's effects have been obtained in younger patients, unexpected side effects are not infrequent in elders. Similarly, adverse drug interactions are underdetected and underreported. Misattribution of drug-related adverse events is a particular risk in medically burdened patients, and those with complications are frequently lost to follow-up. Elders have many medical illnesses and are subject to extensive medication regimens, often with erratic adherence.

In general, age-associated PK changes result in higher and more variable drug concentrations. Nonetheless, specific information on the PK of antidepressants is inadequate, particularly with regard to medical subgroups and potential drug interactions. Although pharmacodynamic changes appear to make older patients more sensitive to the side effects of antidepressants, pharmacodynamic differences are not interpretable in the absence of drug concentration data. Population PK provides a means of assessing antidepressant drug exposure with relative ease and precision in clinical trials. This may permit detection of clinically relevant subgroups and unanticipated drug interactions. Nevertheless, without regulatory direction and/or fiscal incentives, it is unlikely that these data will become available to improve the care of depressed elders.

ACKNOWLEDGMENTS
This work was supported by USPHS Grants MH65416, MH64173, MH59666, MH52247, and MH30915.

REFERENCES

Atkin, P.A., Veitch, P.C., Veitch, E.M., and Ogle, S.J. (1999) The epidemiology of serious adverse drug reactions among the elderly. *Drugs Aging* 14:141–152.

Barbhaiya, R.H., Buch, A.B., and Greene, D.S. (1996) A study of the effect of age and gender on the pharmacokinetics of nefazodone after single and multiple doses. *J Clin Psychopharmacol* 16:19–25.

Beard, K. (1992) Adverse reactions as a cause of hospital admission in the aged. *Drugs Aging* 2:356–367.

Benet, L.Z., and Hoener, B. (2002) Changes in plasma protein binding have little clinical relevance. *Clin Pharmacol Ther* 71:115–121.

Bergstrom, R.F., Lemberger, L., Farid, N.A., et al. (1988) Clinical pharmacology and pharmacokinetics of fluoxetine: A review. *Br J Psychiatry* 153(suppl 3):47–50.

Conley, E.L., Coley, K.C., Pollock, B.G., et al. (2001) Prevalence and risk of thrombocytopenia with valproic acid: Experience at a psychiatric teaching hospital. *Pharmacotherapy* 21:1325–1330.

DeVane, C.L., and Pollock, B.G. (1999) Pharmacokinetic considerations of antidepressant use in the elderly. *J Clin Psychiatry* 60(suppl 20):38–44.

De Vries, M.H., Van Harten, J., Van Bemmel, P., and Raghoebar, M. (1993) Pharmacokinetics of fluvoxamine maleate after increasing single oral doses in healthy subjects. *Biopharm Drug Dispos* 14:291–296.

Foglia, J.P., and Pollock, B.G. (1997) Medication compliance in the elderly. *Essential Psychopharmacol* 1:243–253.

Foglia, J.P., Pollock, B.G., Kirshner, M.A., et al. (1997) Plasma levels of citalopram enantiomers and metabolites in elderly patients. *Psychopharmacol Bull* 33:109–112.

Food and Drug Administration. (1999) *Guidance for Industry: Population Pharmacokinetics*. Rockville, MD:

Food and Drug Administration (2001) Guidance for industry: Content and format for geriatric labeling. Rockville, MD.

Furlan, P.M., Kallan, M.J., Ten Have, T., Pollock, B.G., Katz, I., and Lucki, I. (2001) The cognitive and psychomotor effects of paroxetine and sertraline on healthy volunteers. *Am J Geriatr Psychiatry* 9:429–438.

Golden, A.J., Preston, R.A., Barnette, S.D., et al. (1999) Inappropriate medication prescribing in homebound older adults. *J Am Geriatr Soc* 47:948–953.

Grasela, T.H., Antal, E.J., Ereshefsky, L., et al. (1987) An evaluation of methods for estimation of population pharmacokinetics in therapeutic trials. Part II. Detection of a drug–drug interaction. *Clin Pharmacol Ther* 42:433–441.

Gurwitz, J.H., Field, T.S., Avorn, J., et al. (2000) Incidence and preventability of adverse drug events in nursing homes. *Am J Med* 109:87–94.

Gutierrez, M., and Abramowitz, W. (2000) Steady-state pharmacokinetics of citalopram in young and elderly subjects. *Pharmacotherapy* 20(12):1441–1447.

Hebenstreit, G.F., Fellerer, K., Zochling, R., et al. (1989) A pharmacokinetic dose titration study in adult and elderly depressed patients. *Acta Psychiatr Scand* 80(suppl 350):81–84.

Hesse, L.M., Venkatakrishnan, K., Court, M.H., et al. (2000) CYP2B6 mediates the in vitro hydroxylation of bupropion: Potential drug interactions with other antidepressants. *Drug Metab Dispos* 28:1176–1183.

Kirby, D., and Ames, D. (2001) Hyponatraemia and selective serotonin re-uptake inhibitors in elderly patients. *Int J Geriatr Psychiatry* 16:484–493.

Klamerus, K.J., Parker, V.D., Rudolph, R.L., et al. (1996) Effects of age and gender on venlafaxine and O-desmethylvenlafaxine pharmacokinetics. *Pharmacotherapy* 16:915–923.

Lessard, E., Yessine, M.A., Hamelin, B.A., et al. (1999) Influence of CYP2D6 activity on the disposition and cardiovascular toxicity of the antidepressant agent venlafaxine in humans. *Pharmacogenetics* 4:453–443

Lessard, E., Yessine, M.A., Hamelin, B.A., et al. (2001) Diphenhydramine alters the disposition of venlafaxine through inhibition of CYP2D6 activity in humans. *J Clin Psychopharmacol* 21:175–184.

Liu, B., Anderson, G., Mittmann, N., et al. (1998) Use of selective serotonin-reuptake inhibitors or tricyclic antidepressants and risk of hip fractures in elderly people. *Lancet* 351(9112):1303–1307.

Lotrich, F., Pollock, B.G., and Ferrell, R.E. (2001) Polymorphism of the serotonin transporter: Implications for the use of selective serotonin reuptake inhibitors. *Am J PharmacoGenomics* 1:153–164.

Lundmark, J., Scheel-Thomsen, I., Fjord-Larsen, T., et al. (1989)

Paroxetine: Pharmacokinetic and antidepressant effect in the elderly. *Acta Psychiatr Scand* 80(suppl 350):76–80.

Mulsant, B.H., Pollock, B.G., Kirshner, M., et al. (2003) Serum anticholinergic activity in a community-based geriatric sample: Relationship with cognitive performance. *Arch Gen Psychiatry* 60:198–203.

Murphy, G.M., Pollock, B.G., Kirshner, M., et al. (2001) CYP 2D6 genotyping with oligonucleotide microarrays predicts nortriptyline levels in geriatric depression. *Neuropsychopharmacology* 25:737–743.

Nebes, R.D., Pollock, B.G., Mulsant, B.H., et al. (1997) Low-level serum anticholinergicity as a source of baseline cognitive heterogeneity in geriatric depressed patients. *Psychopharmacol Bull* 33:715–719.

Owens, M.J., Knight, D.L., and Nemeroff, C.B. (2000) Paroxetine binding to the rat norepinephrine transporter in vivo. *Biol Psychiatry* 47:842–845.

Physicians' Desk Reference (2002) 56th edition. Montvale, NJ, Thomson PDR.

Pollock, B.G. (1998) Drug interactions. In: Nelson, J.C., ed. *Geriatric Psychopharmacology*. New York: Marcel Dekker, pp. 43–60.

Pollock, B.G. (1999) Adverse reactions of antidepressants in elderly patients. *J Clin Psychiatry* 60(suppl 20):4–8.

Pollock, B.G., Everett, G., and Perel, J.M. (1992a) Comparative cardiotoxicity of nortriptyline and its isomeric 10-hydroxymetabolites. *Neuropsychopharmacology* 6:1–10.

Pollock, B.G., Ferrell, R.E., Mulsant, B.H., et al. (2000a) Allelic variation in the serotonin transporter promoter affects onset of paroxetine treatment response in late-life depression. *Neuropsychopharmacology* 23:587–590.

Pollock, B.G., Laghrissi-Thode, F., Wagner, W.R., et al. (2000b) Evaluation of platelet activation in depressed patients with ischemic heart disease after paroxetine or nortriptyline treatment. *J Clin Psychopharmacol* 20:137–140.

Pollock, B.G., Mulsant, B.H., Sweet, R.A., et al. (1995) Prospective cytochrome P450 2D6 phenotyping for neuroleptic treatment in dementia. *Psychopharmacol Bull* 31:327–331.

Pollock, B.G., Perel, J., Altieri, L., et al. (1992b) Debrisoquine hydroxylation phenotyping in geriatric psychopharmacology. *Psychopharmacol Bull* 28:163–168.

Pollock, B.G., Wylie, M., Stack, J.A., et al. (1999) Inhibition of CYP1A2 mediated metabolism by estrogen replacement therapy in post-menopausal women. *J Clin Pharmacol* 39:936–940.

Roe, C.M., Anderson, M.J., and Spivack, B. (2002) Use of anticholinergic medications by older adults with dementia. *J Am Geriatr Soc* 50:836–842.

Ronfeld, R.A., Tremaine, L.M., and Wilner, K.D. (1997) Pharmacokinetics of sertraline and its N-demethyl metabolite in elderly and young male and female volunteers. *Clin Pharmacokinet* 32(suppl 1):22–30.

Sauer, W.H., Berlin, J.A., and Kimmel, S.E. (2001) Selective serotonin reuptake inhibitors and myocardial infarction. *Circulation* 104:1894–1898.

Sheiner, L.B., and Ludden, T.M. (1992) Population pharmacokinetics/dynamics. *Annu Rev Pharmacol Toxicol* 32:185–209.

Schmucker, D.L. (2001) Liver function and phase 1 drug metabolism in the elderly. *Drugs Aging* 18:837–851.

Sweet, R.A., Pollock, B.G., Wright, B., et al. (1995) Single and multiple dose bupropion pharmacokinetics in elderly patients with depression. *J Clin Pharmacol* 35:876–884.

Timmer, C.J., Paanakker J.E., and Van Hal, H.J.M. (1996) Pharmacokinetics of mirtazapine from orally administered tablets: Influence of gender, age and treatment regimen. *Hum Psychopharmacol* 11:497–509.

van Walraven, C., Mamdani, M.M., Wells, P.S., et al. (2001) Inhibition of serotonin reuptake by antidepressants and upper gastrointestinal bleeding in elderly patients: Retrospective cohort study. *Br Med J* 325:655–658.

# 16 | Antidepressant medication for the treatment of late-life depression

STEVEN P. ROOSE AND HAROLD A. SACKEIM

The pharmacological treatment of late-life depression has been strongly influenced by three principles that are based primarily, if not exclusively, on clinical observation: (1) older patients do not respond at the same rate or as robustly as younger patients, (2) older patients take longer to respond to antidepressant medication and consequently require extended treatment trials, and (3) older patients have a higher rate of side effects and adverse events than younger adults. Despite the prevalence and clinical significance of late-life depression, there is still a relative paucity of data from randomized, controlled trials (RCT) to serve as the basis for conclusions about antidepressant medication efficacy and safety in late-life samples. Consequently, the principles that inform the use of antidepressants for late-life depression in the clinical situation have largely gone untested. Recently, a number of well-designed RCTs of antidepressant treatment in late-life depression have been completed. Results of these studies, as well as new analyses of extant data, allow evidence-based conclusions about the efficacy and optimal duration of acute treatment with antidepressant medications.

## MODERATORS AND MEDIATORS OF THE ANTIDEPRESSANT RESPONSE

The response to antidepressant medication is influenced by the characteristics of the patient population (moderators) and the parameters of the treatment, including the dose and duration (mediators) (Kraemer et al., 2002). Even if there is diagnostic homogeneity—for example, all patients have unipolar major depressive disorder (MDD)—variability in the response to antidepressant medication can result from heterogeneity in the characteristics of the patient population or other features of the depressive illness itself, such as the depressive subtype. There are a number of treatment moderators, some specific to late-life depression, that have been consistently reported, albeit primarily identified by retrospective or planned secondary analyses of RCT data. Perhaps the most often replicated finding in adult

samples is that more severely depressed patients demonstrate a greater drug–placebo difference in response rate (Klein and Ross, 1993). However, there is no consensual agreement on the definition of *severity*. At times, severity is defined as a certain minimum score on a rating scale such as the Hamilton Rating Scale for Depression (HRSD); for example, patients with HRSD scores ≥26 are considered severely depressed. However, because there are different versions of the HRSD and variations in scoring conventions, the applicability of this approach across RCTs is limited. An alternative definition of severe depression is a score above the mean HRSD score of that trial. In addition to the baseline HRSD score, another dimension that is sometimes used to define severity is whether the patient has had previous episodes of depression. Thus, the interpretation of the repeated finding that severely depressed patients are more likely to respond to antidepressant medication is complicated by the lack of a consensus definition of severity.

Another moderator that impacts the treatment response is the phenomenological subtype of the depressive illness. Clinical trials data strongly suggest a differential response to antidepressant medication for three specific subtypes of unipolar major depression: delusional (Chan et al., 1982; Glassman and Roose, 1981), melancholic (Danish University Antidepressant Group, 1990, 1986; Roose et al., 1994), and atypical (Liebowitz et al., 1988). The first evidence that the phenomenological subtype could impact the response to antidepressant treatment came from a study that established the therapeutic plasma level of imipramine; patients with delusional depression responded at a significantly lower rate to tricyclic antidepressant (TCA) therapy than patients with nondelusional depression. Data from RCTs have also documented that patients with the atypical depression syndrome respond at a higher rate to monoamine oxidase inhibitors (MAOIs) compared to TCAs, and evidence from RCTs, historical comparison studies, and secondary analyses suggests that selective serotonin reuptake inhibitors (SSRIs) are not as effective as TCAs in the treatment of the

192

melancholic subtype. Delusional depression and melancholia are syndromes that occur more frequently in older patients. Thus, the moderating effects of the subtype on the treatment response are particularly relevant in a late-life sample.

Age itself may moderate the response to antidepressants. There is a long-standing clinical belief that older patients do not respond at the same rate or as robustly as younger patients (Reynolds, 1994). Though age may have an independent effect on the treatment response, age is also associated with an increased medical burden as measured by the cumulative illness rating scale—geriatric version (CIRS-G), and decreased social support, factors that may be independent moderators of the treatment response in the elderly (Caine et al., 1994; George et al., 1989). More recently, it has been suggested that late-onset depression, defined as a first episode at age 50 or 60, is a predictor of a low response rate to antidepressants and a deteriorating course of illness. Late onset is also associated with structural abnormalities evident on magnetic resonance imaging (MRI) scans and cognitive dysfunction, both of which have independently been associated with a poor treatment response (Figiel et al., 1991; Hickie et al., 1995). Five of the seven suggested treatment moderators—severity, depressive subtype, age-at-onset, medical burden, social support—are easily determined as part of an initial evaluation, and only structural abnormalities on the MRI scan and neuropsychological assessment require special procedures. Nonetheless, most studies of late-life depression have not collected these data or analyzed outcome results while controlling for moderators of treatment response.

With respect to treatment mediators, one of the most important is the definition of outcome. For many years, the standard definition of response in clinical trials of antidepressants was a 50% reduction from the baseline HRSD score. Though a 50% reduction represents significant symptomatic improvement, patients who begin treatment with high baseline HRSD scores can be classified as responders and yet can still be quite symptomatic. An increasing body of data indicates that depressed patients who remain symptomatic, albeit improved, after treatment have a high rate of relapse and can develop a chronic course of illness (American Psychiatric Association, 2000). Consequently, the field has moved to a more rigorous outcome criterion of remission, defined as a final HRSD or other scale score less than an a priori determined number irrespective of the initial baseline score—for example, in late-life depression trials, often a final HRSD score of ≤10. Patients meeting this remission criterion are believed to have better long-term outcomes. However, though current practice is to treat patients until they achieve remission, the definition of remission has yet to be empirically determined.

Other important mediators of response in antidepressant trials are dose and duration of treatment. With respect to dose, there are sufficient data to establish the minimally effective dose for the SSRIs and other antidepressants, although the optimum dose, defined as a therapeutic plasma level for TCAs, is more elusive for all other classes of antidepressant medications.

With respect to the necessary duration of antidepressant treatment, it is a long-standing adage that elderly patients with major depression respond more slowly to antidepressant medications than younger patients (Reynolds et al., 1996). This difference in the speed of antidepressant response has been attributed to pharmacodynamic changes associated with aging and/or an increase in the degree of treatment resistance with repeated episodes or with age. The longer time required to achieve remission may also result from the common practice of using slower dose escalation schedules with the elderly. Many clinicians maintain that a lower starting dose coupled with a slower dose escalation schedule improves tolerability in older patients. This is considered particularly important because older patients may be more sensitive to antidepressant medications, due to age-associated pharmacokinetic changes that result in higher plasma and brain concentrations or pharmacodynamic changes such as increased receptor sensitivity.

The *start low, go slow* approach to antidepressant medication treatment in late-life depression was first promulgated in the era when TCAs were the primary treatment for major depression and when the tertiary TCAs, such as amitriptyline and imipramine, were more widely used than the secondary TCAs, which have fewer anticholinergic or orthostatic side effects. However, there is scant evidence to support the view that side effects, such as orthostatic hypotension or anticholinergic phenomena, are minimized by slow dose escalation of secondary TCAs (e.g., nortriptyline) (Roose, 1990). Furthermore, the necessity of the start low, go slow strategy for treatment of geriatric major depression with SSRIs is essentially untested.

Whether due to a lower starting dose and a slowed dose escalation and/or other contributing factors, the belief that older patients with depression respond more slowly than younger patients has resulted in the dictum that for the elderly, 12 weeks are necessary for an antidepressant trial to be considered adequate (Young and Meyers, 1992). This stipulation entails that even patients who have shown minimal or no benefit after 6, 8, or 10 weeks must continue for a full 12 weeks before being classified as nonresponders. However, the evidence supporting the belief that the elderly with major depression respond slowly and therefore require a long acute trial duration is sparse and contradictory. Georgotas et al. (1989) reported that extending a nortriptyline trial from 7 to 9 weeks resulted in a significantly higher response rate. At the end of 7 weeks, 26 of 48 (54%) patients treated with nortriptyline had met response criteria; only 4 additional patients responded during the 2-week extension, raising the total response rate to 62%. The number of slow responders was small, and Georgotas et al. noted that these patients had low plasma levels of nortriptyline in the early weeks of the study and required a dose increase. Despite these limitations, this work is cited frequently as demonstrating the need for longer treatment trials in late-life depression.

Other studies suggest that the time course of improvement is not slowed in older patients. There have been several studies of patients over the age of 60 years in whom a therapeutic level of TCA (either imipramine, nortriptyline, or desipramine) was reached by week 2 of treatment (Halpern and Glassman, 1990). These studies found that 90% of patients who met response criteria did so by the end of week 4. Flint and Rifat (1996) reported on 101 depressed patients, with an average age of 74 years, treated with nortriptyline in a 6-week open trial. Seventeen patients (17%) did not complete the trial due to intolerance or noncompliance. Among the patients who completed the treatment trial, 73% met criteria for remission, defined as a final HRSD score >10. Of the patients who remitted, 12% met criteria by the end of week 2, 44% by the end of week 3, 70% by the end of week 4, 88% by the end of week 5, and 100% by the end of week 6. The average time to remission was 3.87 weeks.

In contrast to these studies with TCAs, in which a response occurred early and there was no pattern of late responders, an increase in response rate from week 8 to week 12 was reported in two randomized trials of SSRIs in patients with late-life depression. One study involved randomization to sertraline or fluoxetine, and the other study compared outcomes with sertraline and nortriptyline (Bondareff et al., 2000; Newhouse et al., 2000). Hypothetically, the increased response rate at 12 weeks could be due to at least two different patterns of clinical improvement. One set of patients who responded only at the trial end point may have improved substantially earlier but met response criteria only at week 12. Alternatively, there may have been a group of elderly patients who showed little or no symptom reduction at week 8 but then improved dramatically over the next 4 weeks, meeting response criteria at week 12. If the increase in response rate at the trial end point was due to improvement mostly between weeks 8 and 12, this would imply that all patients deserve a 12-week trial, even those who have no significant improvement after 8 weeks. However, if the responders at week 12 had shown significant improvement by week 8, this would imply that the additional weeks of treatment only benefit patients with significant improvement and that lack of response at the trial end point can be predicted by the degree of symptom change at earlier time points.

Recently, these two trials in late-life depression and a 12-week RCT comparing sertraline to fluoxetine in young adults with depression were reanalyzed, comparing the time to onset of response and remission and prediction of the outcome at the end of the trial based on the degree of symptomatic improvement at an earlier time point (Roose and Sackeim, 2002). The first geriatric study enrolled 236 outpatients over the age of 60 with unipolar MMD and a score of $\geq 18$ on the HRSD. Patients were randomized to fluoxetine (20 mg/day for 4 weeks, with the option thereafter to increase the dose to 40 mg/day) or sertraline (50 mg/day for 4 weeks, with the option thereafter to increase the dose to 100 mg/day). The HRSD scores were obtained at baseline, following 1 week of placebo administration, and at least every 2 weeks during the 12-week trial. The second geriatric trial enrolled 210 outpatients 60 years of age or older and used a trial design similar to that of the first trial. Patients were randomized to clinician-determined, flexible dose treatment with nortriptyline (50–100 mg/day) or sertraline (50–150 mg/day). The third study enrolled outpatients 18 to 60 years of age and was similar in design to the geriatric trials. Patients were randomized to fluoxetine (20 mg/day for 4 weeks with the option thereafter to increase the dose to 80 mg/day) or sertraline (50 mg/day for 4 weeks with the option thereafter to increase the dose to 150 mg/day). Studies were compared with respect to response rate, a 50% reduction from baseline HRSD, and two remission classifications, a final HRSD score $\leq 10$ and $\leq 6$. Onset of a sustained response or remission, defined as beginning at the trial week when the patient first met the specific response or remission criterion and continued to meet that criterion for the remainder of the trial, was compared across the studies.

There were no differences in the studies or in the treatments with respect to completion rates or outcomes. For the geriatric trials, the three response and remission rates were 68%, 58%, and 38%, respectively, and for the younger patients they were 72%, 54%, and 34%. Across the three 12-week trials, the median times to onset of a sustained response and the two remission outcomes were 6, 8, and 9 weeks, respectively. Onset of response was faster in the midlife patients, but the difference compared to late-life patients was less than 1 week. A substantial proportion of the patients in each study met the onset criteria only at the final visit (response: 19.7%; remission$_{10}$: 22.2%; and remission$_6$: 36.0%); therefore, it could not be determined whether the outcome was sustained. Thus, in this subgroup, the optimal trial duration is unknown but it is at least 12 weeks.

As outcome criteria become more stringent, treatment trials lengthen, and since most patients do not attain remission in a single antidepressant trial, early identification of patients who will not respond becomes increasingly important in order to minimize exposure to ineffective treatments. Regardless of medication condition, study, or remission criteria, by week 6 at least 60% of eventual nonremitters could be detected, with at most 20% false positives—that is, eventual remitters at week 12 wrongly classified as eventual nonremitters at week 6.

The results of these RCTs in mid-age and late-life samples do not support the long-held belief that younger patients respond more robustly and quickly to antidepressant medication than older patients. Furthermore, extended trials (e.g., 12 weeks) only benefit patients who have demonstrated symptomatic improvement before 6 weeks and thus are not mandatory for all patients.

## ANTIDEPRESSANT MEDICATIONS

Though the antidepressant literature is vast, including case reports, open trials, and randomized comparator and placebo-controlled trials, this chapter will focus on comparator and placebo-randomized trials that had the most rigorous methodology and adequate presentation of results.

## TRICYCLIC ANTIDEPRESSANTS

There are scores of randomized, placebo-controlled, and comparator (usually an SSRI) trials of TCA treatment for late-life depression. However, most placebo-controlled trials involving TCAs were done before the routine use of plasma level measurements to ensure optimal TCA treatment. Randomized, controlled trials comparing TCAs to SSRIs have invariably been supported by the pharmaceutical industry and consequently do not compare an SSRI to optimal TCA treatment. Consequently, most comparator trials of TCA treatment in late-life depression involve inadequate doses of tertiary amine TCAs, amytriptyline or imipramine. Nonetheless, the results of these studies establish that TCAs are effective for the treatment of older depressed patients. With respect to optimal TCA treatment for late-life depression, nortriptyline has been demonstrated to induce the least orthostatic hypotension and has a documented *therapeutic window* that guides dosing (Roose et al., 1981). Consequently, nortriptyline has emerged as the TCA of choice to treat late-life depression. However, there are no rigorous placebo-controlled trials of nortriptyline in late-life depression, so conclusions on the efficacy of this medication are based on the results of three open and three randomized comparator trials.

In one study, 101 patients meeting DSM-III-R criteria for MDD were treated openly with nortriptyline

(Flint and Rifat, 1996). All patients reached a dose of 75 mg. At the end of week 1, the dose was adjusted, if necessary, to achieve a plasma level within the therapeutic window of 50 to 150 ng/ml. The treatment duration was 6 weeks, and the remission criterion was a final HRSD (17-item) score ≤10; 60% of the intent-to-treat sample and 75% of patients who completed the trial met the remission criterion. To establish the speed of response, the authors determined the week of treatment at which the 61 patients who met the criterion for remission at the end of the study first achieved a sustained remission. Not surprisingly, at the end of week 1, no patient met the criterion for remission, so the cumulative response rate was 0. At week 2, 11% of the sample met the remission criterion; at week 3, 33% (so the cumulative rate at the end of week 3 was 11% plus 33%, or 44%); at week 4, 25%; and at week 5, 20%. Thus, the accumulated remission rate at the end of week 5 was 89%. With respect to TCAs, it may be that the slower dose escalation often used with older patients, rather than an intrinsic difference in the rapidity of response between young and old, is a critical factor in the delayed response.

A second, open 6-week trial of nortriptyline with the dose adjusted to achieve a therapeutic plasma level of the drug, reported on 42 inpatients, mean age 70, with cardiac disease and melancholic depression (Roose et al., 1994). The remission criterion was a final HRSD (21-item) score of ≤8; the intent-to-treat remission rate was 67%, the completer remission rate was 82%, and the dropout rate was 19%.

Three RCTs compared nortriptyline to an SSRI; two studies compared a therapeutic plasma level of nortriptyline to that of paroxetine, and one study compared flexible-dose nortriptyline to sertraline. Mulsant et al. (2001) compared nortriptyline to paroxetine in 116 inpatients and outpatients, mean age 72, in a 12-week trial. The remission criterion was a final HRSD (17-item) score of ≤10; the intent-to-treat remission rate was 57% for the nortriptyline group and 55% for the paroxetine group. The dropout rate due to side effects in the nortriptyline group was significantly higher than that of the paroxetine group (33% vs. 16%, $p = .04$). A second RCT comparing a therapeutic plasma level of nortriptyline to paroxetine is included in this review, although technically it should not be considered a geriatric study because the mean age of the patients was 58 (Nelson et al., 1999). However, it is the only other study comparing a therapeutic plasma level of a TCA to that of an SSRI, and the results are consistent with the Mulsant et al. (2001) study. In this trial, 81 outpatients with ischemic heart disease were treated with medication for 6 weeks. The remission criterion was a final HRSD (17-item) score of ≤8; in the intent-to-treat analysis, 63% of the nortriptyline group and 61% of the paroxetine group were remitters. The dropout rate for the nortriptyline group (35%) was significantly higher than that of the paroxetine group (10%). The rate of remission in patients who completed the study was 85% for nortriptyline and 68% for paroxetine. This was not a statistically significant difference, although the power of this comparison was limited by the small size of the completer group. Note that the paroxetine remission rate was the same in the 6-week and 12-week trials. The RCT comparing sertraline to nortriptyline included 210 patients, mean age 68, randomized to 12 weeks of medication treatment (Bondareff et al., 2000). This study did not report remission rates but only response rates defined as a 50% reduction from baseline HRSD (24 items); the intent-to-treat response rate was 41% for the nortripyline group and 52% for the sertraline group.

## Tricyclic Side Effects and Safety

Unfortunately, despite their great effectiveness, the clinical utility of TCAs in the late-life population is limited by their side effect and safety profiles. The TCAs have significant anticholinergic effects, and although the total anticholinergic load is lower for desipramine and nortriptyline than for the tertiary TCAs, the anticholinergic side effects can be problematic. The anticholinergic effects of TCAs include dry mouth, constipation, and blurred vision. More important, the geriatric population is particularly susceptible to anticholinergic induced urinary retention and cognitive impairment (Pollock, 1999).

The major safety problem with respect to the TCAs is their cardiovascular effects. Tricyclic overdosage involves a high mortality rate; as little as three times the daily dose can result in death from heart block or arrhythmias (Roose and Glassman, 1989). The TCAs have type 1A antiarrhythmic activity and consequently are presumed to confer an increased risk of sudden cardiovascular death if given to patients with ischemic heart disease (Glassman et al., 1993). Given the prevalence of occult and manifest ischemic heart disease in both men and women over the age of 60, the decision to prescribe TCAs in this population must reflect a careful consideration of the risk-benefit ratio.

## SELECTIVE SEROTONIN REUPTAKE INHIBITORS

As in younger depressed patients, the SSRIs are the most often prescribed class of antidepressants for the treatment of late-life depression. However, the number of rigorous placebo or comparator RCTs reporting response and remission data is still strikingly small. The SSRIs appear to have equivalent efficacy and side effect profiles. There are differences in pharmacokinetics, and the potential for drug–drug interactions are of special importance in the geriatric population.

## FLUOXETINE

There are four large studies of fluoxetine in late-life depression; one placebo-controlled; one a three-cell study comparing venlafaxine, placebo, and fluoxetine; one an RCT with fluoxetine as the comparator drug; and one an open treatment trial. In the first study, fluoxetine was compared to placebo in 671 patients (Tollefson et al., 1995). The dosing schedule was 20 mg/day for 6 weeks, and the remission criterion was a final HRSD (17-item) score of ≤7. The intent-to-treat remission rate was 23% for fluoxetine and 13% for placebo; in the completer analysis, the remission rate was 27% for fluoxetine and 16% for placebo. Although fluoxetine was significantly more effective than placebo in both the intent-to-treat and completor analyses, compared to years of clinical experience with therapeutic plasma levels of TCAs, the remission rates in this study were disappointingly low. However, this was the first geriatric study using an SSRI, and the fixed dose of 20 mg and the relatively short trial duration were considered possible contributors to the disappointing outcome. In the comparator RCT, 225 patients, mean age 68, were randomized to either fluoxetine, 20–40 mg/day, or sertraline, 50–100 mg/day, for 12 weeks (Newhouse et al., 2000). The intent-to-treat remission rate was 46% for fluoxetine and 45% for sertraline; the completor remission rate was 60% for fluoxetine and 59% for sertraline; the dropout rate was 33% for the fluoxetine group and 32% for the sertraline group. This study also reported an intriguing analysis of the response pattern of a subsample of patients (42 treated with sertraline, 33 treated with fluoxetine) over the age of 75. Even in this group of the oldest patients, for both sertraline and fluoxetine, 95% of patients who achieved a 50% reduction in baseline HRSD did so by the end of week 8. As with the studies of therapeutic plasma levels of nortriptyline, these data challenge the clinical observation that the older the patient, the lower the response to antidepressant medication, and the belief that antidepressant trials in late-life depression must be extended to 12 weeks for all patients. Finally, 308 patients meeting DSM-III criteria for MDD, mean age 66, were treated openly with 20 mg/day fluoxetine for 8 weeks (Mesters et al., 1992). The remission criterion was a final HRSD (24-item) score of ≤10; the intent-to-treat remission rate was 35%, the completer remission rate was 50%, and the dropout rate was 29%.

## SERTRALINE

In addition to the two randomized, controlled comparator trials previously described—nortriptyline versus sertraline and fluoxetine versus sertraline, in which the intent-to-treat remission rate was 51% for sertraline and 45% for sertraline, respectively, there is a recently completed rigorous, large, placebo-controlled trial of sertraline in late-life depression (Schneider et al., 2003). In this study, 716 patients, mean age 70, were randomized to flexible-dose sertraline, 50–100 mg/day, or placebo in an 8-week trial. The criterion for remission was a final HRSD (17-item) score of ≤10; the intent-to-treat remission rate was 29% in the sertraline group compared to 23% in the placebo group ($p < .05$).

## PAROXETINE

In addition to the two previously described trials that compared a therapeutic plasma level of nortriptyline to paroxetine, in which the intent-to-treat remission rates, defined as a final HRSD (24-item) score of ≤10), were 61% and 58%, respectively, there is a third completed trial that compared mirtazapine to paroxetine (Schatzberg et al., 2002). In this study, 255 patients, mean age 72, were randomized to mirtazapine, 30–45 mg/day, or paroxetine, 30–40 mg/day, in an 8-week clinical trial. The remission criterion was a final HRSD (17-item) score of ≤7; the intent-to-treat remission rates, 38% for mirtazapine and 28% for paroxetine, were not statistically different.

## CITALOPRAM

Many of the treatment studies of citalopram in late-life depression included patients with both depression and dementia or significant cognitive impairment; therefore, the results of these studies are not comparable to those of the other antidepressant trials previously discussed. (Gottfries, 1996; Nyth et al., 1992). However, there are two studies that do provide comparable information on citalopram in this population; the first is a single-blind comparison between citalopram and a therapeutic plasma level of nortriptyline (Navarro et al., 2001), and the second is a recently completed comparison of citalopram to placebo in depressed patients over the age of 75 (Roose et al., 2002). In the first study, 58 patients, mean age 71, were randomized to treatment with 30–40 mg/day of citalopram versus a therapeutic plasma level of nortriptyline in a 12-week clinical trial. The intent-to-treat remission rate, defined as a final HRSD (17-item) score of <7, was 69% for citalopram and 93% for nortriptyline. The remission rates for both medications were strikingly high in comparison to those in other trials. Whether this resulted from differences in patient populations or study designs is not obviously apparent.

The second trial is unique in the literature because it is the only study to focus on treatment of depression in the old-old. In this study 174 patients, 75 years of age or older, were randomized to treatment with citalopram, 20–40 mg/day, or placebo in an 8-week clinical trial. The patient cohort was 58% female, mean age 80, and with a mean baseline HRSD (24-item) score of 24. The intent-to-treat remission rate, defined as a final HRSD (24-item) score of ≤10, was 35% for citalopram and 33% for placebo. The sample was divided into patients with "severe" versus "not severe" depression, defined as patients with HRSD scores either above or below the mean score of 24, respectively. The not-severe group had a baseline HRSD of 22 and included 47 patients randomized to citalopram and 59 to placebo. In this group, the remission rates, defined as a final HRSD score of ≤10, were not statistically different, 34% for citalopram and 41% for placebo. The severe patient group (mean baseline HRSD score of 28) included 37 patients randomized to citalopram and 31 to placebo. In this group, the intent-to-treat remission rate was 36% for citalopram versus 19% for placebo ($p < .05$). Thus, citalopram was significantly more effective than placebo in the severe but not in the not-severe patients. This difference did not reflect an increased efficacy of citalopram in the severe compared to the not-severe patients, but rather a decreased efficacy of placebo in the severe group.

## SELECTIVE SEROTONIN REUPTAKE INHIBITOR SIDE EFFECT PROFILE IN GERIATRIC PATIENTS

As a group, the SSRIs have the same side effect profile in older patients as in younger patients—nausea, agitation, insomnia, and sexual dysfunction. Discontinuation rates for SSRIs are not statistically different from those reported for a therapeutic plasma level of nortriptyline in the geriatric samples (Roose and Suthers, 1998).

With respect to safety, the SSRIs offer a significant advantage over the TCAs. The SSRIs are relatively benign in overdosage (Barbey and Roose, 1998) and have been extensively tested in patients with ischemic heart disease, congestive heart failure, and immediately post-myocardial infarction (Glassman et al., 2002; Roose et al., 1997, 1998). In contrast to the TCAs, the SSRIs have a relatively benign cardiovascular profile and have no deleterious effect on blood pressure, heart rate, cardiac conduction, or cardiac rhythm.

## OTHER ANTIDEPRESSANTS

### Venlafaxine

In the one rigorous study of venlafaxine in late-life depression, 204 patients, mean age 71, were randomized to treatment with either venlafaxine 75–225 mg/day, fluoxetine 20–60 mg/day, or placebo in an 8-week clinical trial (Schatzberg and Cantillon, 2000). The intent-to-treat remission rate, defined as a final HRSD (24-item) score of <8, was 42% for venlafaxine, 29% for fluoxetine, and 38% for placebo (no statistically significant differences). Significantly more patients treated with venlafaxine (27%) and fluoxetine (19%) dropped out of the study due to side effects compared to the placebo group (9%) (p < .05).

## Mirtazapine

As previously discussed, there is one study of mirtazapine in late-life depression, an RCT trial comparing it with paroxetine (Schatzberg et al., 2002). The intent-to-treat remission rate, defined as a final HRSD score of ≤10, was 38% for mirtazapine compared to 28% for paroxetine, but the difference was not statistically different. Treatment discontinuation due to adverse events was similar in both groups, 33% for mirtazapine and 29% for paroxetine.

## Bupropion

There is one RCT comparator trial of bupropion versus paroxetine in late-life depression; this provides the only data available on bupropion in this population. In

this study 100 patients, mean age 70, with a baseline HRSD (24-item) score of 27, were randomized to treatment with either bupropion, 100–300 mg/day, or paroxetine, 10–40 mg/day, in a 6-week clinical trial (Weihs et al., 2000). The response rate, defined as a 50% reduction from the baseline HRSD, was 71% in the bupropion group and 77% in the paroxetine group. Remission data were not reported. Discontinuation due to adverse events was 17% in the bupropion group and 15% in the paroxetine group.

## PLACEBO VERSUS COMPARATOR CONTROLLED TRIALS

In summary, there have been only four placebo-controlled trials of antidepressant treatment in patients with late-life depression, with just one trial conducted in the old-old (Table 16.1). Two of these trials were negative; that is, the response to medication was not statistically different from the response to placebo, although across the four studies the response rates to medication were similar. However, the active treatments in these trials are not only placebo and medication; in RCTs there are a variety of nonspecific psychosocial supports that accompany the administration of placebo and medication. For example, relative to clinical care in the community, RCTs differ in the frequency and du-

TABLE 16.1. *Placebo-Controlled Trials*

| | Drug | N | Age | Sex (% F) | Dose (mg/day) | Length | HRSD Baseline | Delta HRSD | % Response | % Remission |
|---|---|---|---|---|---|---|---|---|---|---|
| Tollefson et al. (1995) | Fluoxetine | 335 | 67 | 54 | 20 | 6 wk | 22.2 | | 42* | 28** |
| | Placebo | 336 | 68 | 55 | | | 22.1 | | 30 | 18 |
| | | | | | | | 17 items | | | ≤7 criterion |
| Schatzberg and Cantillon (2000) | Venlafaxine | 104 | 71 | 56 | 150–225 | 8 wk | 24 | | 57 | 42 |
| | Fluoxetine | 100 | 71 | 45 | 20–60 | | 24 | | 48 | 29 |
| | Placebo | 96 | 71 | 46 | | | 24 | | 52 | 38 |
| | | | | | | | 20 items | | | ≤8 criterion |
| Schneider et al. (2003) | Sertraline | 350 | 70 | 58 | 50–100 | 8 wk | 21 | | 35†† | 29† |
| | Placebo | 366 | 70 | 60 | | | 21 | | 26 | 23 |
| | | | | | | | 17 items | | | ≤10 criterion |
| | Sertraline (severe) | 66 | 70 | 57 | | | 24 | | | |
| | Placebo (severe) | 71 | 70 | 62 | | | 23 | | | |
| | Sertraline (not severe) | 284 | 70 | 57 | | | 21 | | | |
| | Placebo (not severe) | 295 | 70 | 57 | | | 21 | | | |
| Roose et al. (2002) | Citalopram | 84 | 80 | 54 | 20–40 | 8 wk | 24 | | 41 | 35 |
| | Placebo | 90 | 79 | 62 | | | 24 | | 38 | 33 |
| | | | | | | | 24 items | | | ≤10 criterion |
| | Citalopram | 47 | | | | | 22 | | 36 | 34 |
| | Placebo (not severe) | 59 | | | | | 22 | | 46 | 41 |
| | Citalopram | 37 | | | | | 28 | | 46†† | 35† |
| | Placebo (severe) | 31 | | | | | 28 | | 23 | 19 |

†p < .05; *p < .01; ††p < .007; **p < .001.
HRSD, Hamilton Rating Scale for Depression.

TABLE 16.2. *Trials Comparing Two Antidepressant Medications*

| Study | Drug | N | Age | Sex (% F) | Dose (mg/day) | Length | HRSD Baseline | Delta HRSD | % Response | % Remission |
|---|---|---|---|---|---|---|---|---|---|---|
| Navarro et al. (2001) | Citalopram* | 29 | 72 | 62 | 30–40 | 12 wk | 27 | 17 | | 69 |
| | Nortriptyline | 29 | 70 | 65 | Plasma level | | 26 | 21 | | 93 |
| | | | | | | | 17 items | | | ≤7 criterion |
| Nelson et al. (1999) | Paroxetine** | 41 | 58 | 12 | 20–30 | 6 wk | 23 | 12.7 | 66 | 61 |
| | Nortriptyline | 40 | 58 | 22 | Plasma level | | 22 | 13.1 | 73 | 63 |
| | | | | | | | 17 items | | | ≤8 criterion |
| Mulsant et al. (2001) | Paroxetine*** | 62 | 71 | 77 | 20–40 | 12 wk | 22 | 11 | | 55/32 |
| | Nortriptyline | 54 | 73 | 65 | Plasma level | | 23 | 12.8 | | 57/35 |
| | | | | | | | 17 items | | | ≤10/≤6 criterion |
| Newhouse et al. (2000) | Sertraline | 117 | 63 | 68 | 50–100 | 12 wk | 25 | 11.3 | 73 | 60 |
| | Fluoxetine | 119 | 51 | 67 | 20–40 | | 25 | 11.3 | 71 | 60 |
| | | | | | | | 24 items | | | ≤10 criterion |
| Bondareff et al. (2000) | Sertraline | 105 | 68 | 60 | 50–150 | 12 wk | 25 | 14 | 52 | |
| | Nortriptyline | 105 | 68 | 58 | 25–100 | | 25 | 12.5 | 41 | |
| | | | | | | | 24 items | | | |
| Schatzberg et al. (2002) | Mirtazapine | 126 | 72 | 50 | 15–45 | 8 wk | 22 | 11 | 58 | 38 |
| | Paroxetine | 120 | 72 | 53 | 20–40 | | 22 | 10 | 50 | 29 |
| | | | | | | | 17 items | | | ≤8 criterion |

*Single-blind study conducted in Spain; inpatients comprised 15% of the sample.
**Outpatients with ischemic heart disease.
***Inpatients comprised 50% of the sample; 55% of the sample was melancholic.
HRSD, Hamilton Rating Scale for Depression.

ration of physician visits, provision of free medication and medical workup, intensive interaction with study staff during and between visits, social service support, and so on. Few RCTs or naturalistic studies have systematically assessed the extent and nature of *extra-study* psychosocial support. It may well be that the extensive, but overlooked, psychosocial supports in an RCT have a significant impact on therapeutic outcomes, especially in the elderly, who are often socially isolated and have limited financial resources. Indeed, variation in the provision of such social supports may be a critical variable contributing to the marked differences in rates of response among groups participating in multicenter studies (Roose and Schatzberg, in press).

In order to obtain more clinically relevant data, future trials comparing medication to placebo should mirror standard clinical practice in as many respects as possible, including the frequency and duration of visits and the type and extent of psychosocial support provided. This may diminish placebo remission rates and increase detection of an antidepressant effect attributable to medication.

Another concern is whether results of placebo-controlled trials delimit the response and remission rates that may be obtained in clinical practice (Roose et al., 2002). In comparison to placebo-controlled trials, the comparator trials reviewed consistently reported greater effect sizes and higher response and remission rates (Tables 16.2, 16.3, 16.4) (Roose et al., 2002). The greater

TABLE 16.3. *Percentage Response in Comparison Trials*

| Placebo | Fluoxetine | Sertraline | NT | Paroxetine | Citalopram | Venlafaxine | Mirtazapine |
|---|---|---|---|---|---|---|---|
| 26 | | 35 | | | | | |
| 52 | 48 | | | | | 57 | |
| 38 | 42 | | | | | | |
| 38 | | | | | 41 | | |
| | | | 93 | | 69 | | |
| | 71 | 73 | | | | | |
| | | 52 | 41 | | | | |
| | | | 73 | 66 | | | |
| | | | 67 | 65 | | | |
| | | | 50 | | | | |
| | | | | | | | 58 |

NT, nortriptyline.

TABLE 16.4. *Change in the Hamilton Rating Scale for Depression in Comparison Trials*

| Placebo | Fluoxetine | Sertraline | NT | Paroxetine | Citalopram | Venlafaxine | Mirtazapine |
|---|---|---|---|---|---|---|---|
| 6.4 | 8.1 | | | | | | |
| 6.6 | | 7.4 | | | | | |
| 9.2 | | | | | 10.0 | | |
| | | | 21.0 | | 17.0 | | |
| | | | 13.1 | 12.7 | | | |
| | | | 12.8 | 11.0 | | | |
| | | 14.0 | 12.5 | | | | |
| | 11.3 | 11.3 | | | | | |
| | | | | | | 10.0 | 11.0 |

NT, nortriptyline.

antidepressant effect in comparator trials has often been understood as exclusively the product of physician and patient bias; that is, all parties know that the patient is receiving an active treatment, and consequently there are increased expectations that improvement will occur. These expectations result in higher rates of response and remission due to a combination of rater bias in outcome assessment and greater actual improvement due to the effects of patient expectancies.

However the results of placebo-controlled trials may also be influenced by patient bias. Many older patients find it disconcerting, or even humiliating, to respond to a placebo, fearing that such an outcome would result in their being labeled a hypochondriac or worse. Since it may be more acceptable to some patients to be a medication nonresponder than a placebo responder, late-life patients participating in placebo-controlled trials may report minimal improvement to protect against an undesired outcome.

In summary, placebo-controlled trials involve the most radical departures from standard practice. The results of such trials are not unbiased, and due to a variety of factors, including selection bias in enrollment, the outcomes of placebo-controlled trials may be the least applicable to the clinical situation. In contrast, it can be argued that comparator, or even open, trials of antidepressants, though uninformative with respect to efficacy, may nonetheless more truly reflect the response and remission rates that can be expected in clinical practice.

## CONCLUSION

The traditional, widely held beliefs that older patients respond differently to antidepressant medications than younger patients—specifically, that older patients take longer to respond and respond at a lower rate—were derived primarily from clinical observation. However, data from RCTs do not support these beliefs, and dif-

ferences in antidepressant treatment in the young versus the old primarily reflect safety issues secondary to the frequency of serious co-morbid illness in the elderly.

All classes of antidepressant are used for the treatment of late-life depression, and, as in younger adults, the SSRIs are the most frequently prescribed. Data from placebo-controlled trials to establish the efficacy of medication for the treatment of depression in this age group are scant. Evidence supporting the effectiveness of these treatments comes primarily from trials comparing two active treatments or from open studies. Though it can be argued that in the absence of placebo control a clinical trial cannot establish efficacy, comparator and open trials more closely replicate the clinical situation. Consequently, the results of such studies may be a good predictor of the effectiveness that clinicians can anticipate when they prescribe antidepressant medication for the treatment of late-life depression.

REFERENCES

American Psychiatric Association. (2000) *Practice Guideline for the Treatment of Patients with Major Depression*, 2nd ed. Washington, DC: American Psychiatric Press.

Barbey, J.T., and Roose, S.P. (1998) SSRI safety in overdose. *J Clin Psychiatry* 59(15):41–48.

Bondareff, W., Alpert, M., Friedhoff, A.J., Richter, E.M., Clary, C.M., and Batzar, E. (2000) Comparison of sertraline and nortriptyline in the treatment of major depressive disorder in late-life. *Am J Psychiatry* 157:729–736.

Caine, E.D., Lyness, J.M., King, D.A., and Connors, L. (1994) Clinical and etiological heterogeneity of mood disorders in elderly patients. In: Schneider, L.S., Reynolds, C.F., III, Lebowitz, B.D., and Friedhoff, A.J., eds. *Diagnosis and Treatment of Depression in Late Life*. Washington, DC: American Psychiatric Press, pp. 21–54.

Chan, C.H., Janicak, P.G., Davis, J.M., et al. (1982) Response of psychotic and non-psychotic depressed patients to tricyclic antidepressants. *J Clin Psychiatry* 48:197–200.

Danish University Antidepressant Group. (1986) Citalopram: Clinical effect profile in comparison with clomipramine. A controlled multicenter study. *Psychopharmacology* 90:131–138.

Danish University Antidepressant Group. (1990) Paroxetine: A selective serotonin reuptake inhibitor showing better tolerance, but

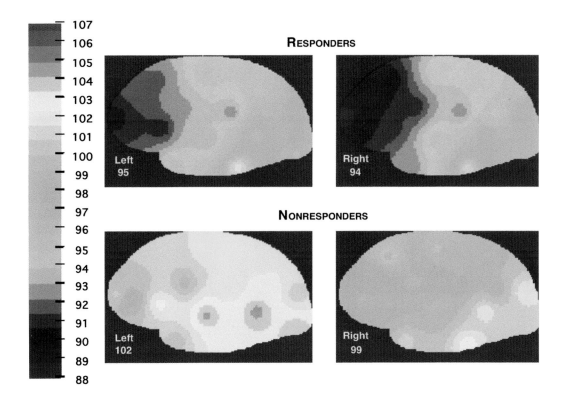

COLOR FIGURE 11.5 A representation of the findings of Nobler et al. (1994). Fifty-four patients with major depression were studied 30 minutes before and 1 hour after a single treatment with electroconvulsive therapy. The measurements were typically taken at the sixth treatment, and regional cerebral blood flow (rCBF) was fully quantified in 32 cortical regions using the xenon-133 inhalation technique. The color scale refers to the ratio of CBF following the treatment compared to prior to the treatment. A value of 100 indicates no change. Responders showed a marked decrease of CBF in bilateral prefrontal regions, while nonresponders showed no change.

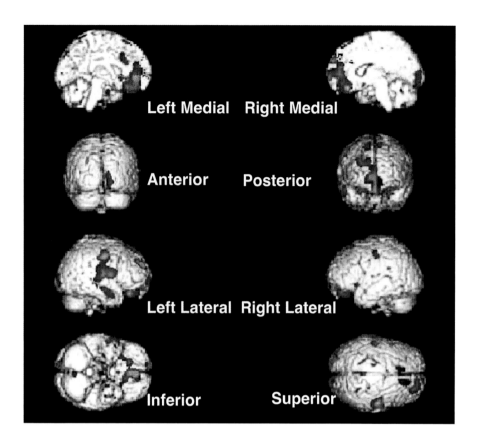

COLOR FIGURE 11.6 Comparison of responders and nonresponders in glucose metabolism change over an 8-week medication trial. These initial results derive from a longitudinal imaging study of late-onset major depression at the New York State Psychiatric Institute. The colored areas superimposed on the three-dimensional brain represent clusters of significant difference between responders and nonresponders in the magnitude of cerebral metabolic rate (CMR) change. All significant effects reflected greater CMR reductions in the responders. The area of greatest differences was medial frontal lobe.

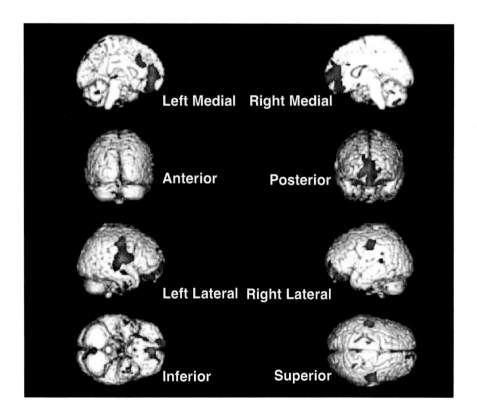

COLOR FIGURE 11.7 Areas of significant change in brain glucose metabolism over an 8-week medication trial in treatment responders. In visual comparison of Color Figures 11.6 and 11.7, it is evident that the topographic changes that distinguished responders and nonresponders were present in the analysis restricted to the responder group. In fact, a separate statistical parametric mapping analysis indicated that there were no significant changes among nonresponders. Thus, an acute response at the end of the medication trial was associated with reductions in a specific pattern of regions, with medial prefrontal changes being the most critical.

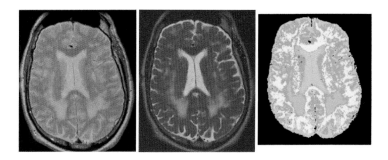

COLOR FIGURE 12.1 Proton density and T$_2$-weighted images (left, center) used in multispectral analysis to produce the segmented image (right). White matter (yellow), gray matter (gray), cerebrospinal fluid (blue), white matter lesion (green).

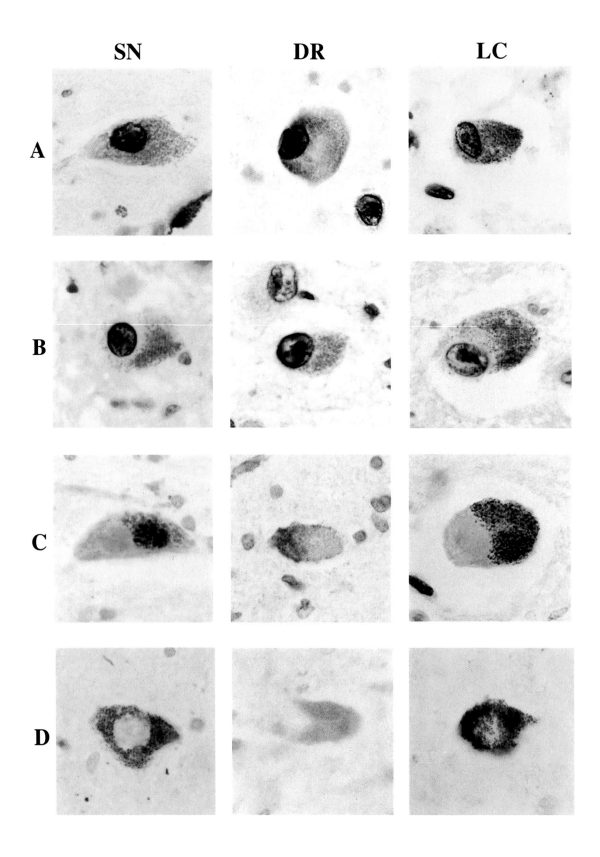

COLOR FIGURE 29.1 Apoptotic features of neurons from the substantia nigra (SN), dorsal raphe (DR), and locus ceruleus (LC) visualized by immunochemical staining of paraffin-embedded 10-$\mu$m-thick sections of fixed brain stem tissue from autopsied case with histopathologically confirmed Alzheimer's disease. Neurons with condensed nuclear chromatin containing fragmented DNA (FragEL positive) have darkly stained nuclei. Neurons expressing the ant-apoptotic protein Bcl-2 (Bcl-2 positive) have blue cytoplasm. A; neurons are FragEL-positive and Bcl-2 positive. B; neurons are FragEL positive and Bcl-2 negative. C; neurons are FragEL negative and Bcl-2 positive. D; neurons are FragEL negative and Bcl-2 negative.

weaker antidepressant effect than clomipramine in a controlled multicenter study. *J Affect Disord* 18:289–299.

Figiel, G.S., Krishnan, K.R.R., Doraiswamy, P.M., Rao, V.P., Nemeroff, C.B., and Boyko, O.B. (1991) Subcortical hyperintensities on brain magnetic resonance imaging: A comparison between late age onset and early onset elderly depressed subjects. *Neurobiol Aging* 26:245–247.

Flint, A., and Rifat, S. (1996) The effect of sequential antidepressant treatment on geriatric depression. *J Affect Disord* 36:95–105.

George, L.K., Blazer, D.G., Hughes, D.C., and Fowler, N. (1989) Social support and the outcomes of major depression. *Br J Psychiatry* 154:478–485.

Georgotas, A., McCue, R.E., Cooper, T.B.N., Nagachandran, N., and Friedhoff, A. (1989) Factors affecting the delay of antidepressant effect in responders to nortriptyline and phenelzine. *Psychiatry Res* 28:1–9.

Glassman, A.H., O'Connor, C.M., Califf, R.M., Swedberg, J., Schwartz, P., Bigger, J.T., Jr., et al. (2002) Sertraline treatment of major depression in patients with acute MI or unstable angina. *JAMA* 288:701–709.

Glassman, A.H., and Roose, S.P. (1981) Delusional depression: A distinct clinical entity? *Arch Gen Psychiatry* 38:424–427.

Glassman, A.H., Roose, S.P., and Bigger, J.T., Jr. (1993) The safety of tricyclic antidepressants in cardiac patients—risk/benefit reconsidered. *JAMA* 269:2673–2675.

Gottfries, C.G. (1996) Scandinavian experience with citalopram in the elderly. *Int Clin Psychopharmacol* 11:41–44.

Halpern, J.K., and Glassman, A.H. (1990) Defining the tricyclic non-responder. In: Roose, S.P. and Glassman, A.H., eds. *Treatment Strategies for Refractory Depression*. Washington, DC: American Psychiatric Press, pp. 13–32.

Hickie, I. Scott, E., Mitchell, P. Wilheim, K., Austin, M.P., and Bennett, B. (1995) Subcortical hyperintensities on magnetic resonance imaging: Clinical correlates and prognostic significance in patients with severe depression. *Biol Psychiatry* 37:151–160.

Klein, D.F., and Ross, D.C. (1993) Reanalysis of the National Institute of Mental Health treatment of depression collaborative research program general effectiveness report. *Neuropsychopharmacology* 8:241–251.

Kraemer, H.C., Wilson, G.T., Fairburn, C.G., and Agras, W.S. (2002) Mediators and moderators of treatment effects in randomized clinical trials. *Arch Gen Psychiatry* 59:877–883.

Liebowitz, M.R., Quitkin, F.M., Stewart, J.W., McGrath, P.J., Harrison, W.M., Markowitz, J.S., Rabkin, J.G., Tricamo, E., Goetz, D.M., and Klein, D.F. (1988) Antidepressant specificity in atypical depression. *Arch Gen Psychiatry* 45:129–137.

Mesters, P., Ansseau, M., Brasseur, R., Bussios, G., Cosyns, P., Czarka, M., De Buck, R., De Frenne, A., Dierick, M., Linkowski, P. et al. (1992) An open multicentre study to evaluate the efficacy and tolerance of fluoxetine 20 mg in depressed ambulatory patients. *Acta Psychiatrica Belgica* 92(4):232–245.

Mulsant, B.H., Pollock B.G., Nebes, R., Miller, M.D., Sweet, R.A., Stack, J., Houck, P.R., Bensasi, S., Mazumdar, S., and Reynolds, C.F. 3rd (2001) A twelve-week, double-blind randomized comparison of nortriptyline and paroxetine in older depressed patients and outpatients. *Am J Geriatr Psychiatry* 9:406–414.

Navarro, V., Gasto, C., Torres, X., Marcos, C., and Pintor, L. (2001) Citalopram versus nortriptyline in late-life depression: A 12-week randomized single-blind study. *Acta Psychiatr Scand* 103:435–440.

Nelson, J.C., Kennedy, J.S., Pollock, B.G., Laghrissi-Thode, F., Narayan, J.M., Nobler, M.S., Robin, D.W., Gergel, I., McCafferty, J., and Roose, S. (1999) Treatment of major depression with nortriptyline and paroxetine in patients with ischemic heart disease. *Am J Psychiatry* 156:1024–1028.

Newhouse, P.A., Krishnan, K.R.R., Doraiswami, P.M., Richter, E.M., Batzar, E.D., and Clary, C.M. (2000) A double-blind comparison of sertraline and fluoxetine in depressed elderly outpatients. *J Clin Psychiatry* 61:559–568.

Nyth, A.L., Gottfries, C.G., Lyby, K., Smedegaard-Andersen, L., Gylding-Sabroe, J., Kristensen, M., Refsum, H.E., Ofsti, E., Eriksson, S., and Syversen, S. (1992) A controlled multicenter clinical study of citalopram and placebo in elderly depressed patients with and without concomitant dementia. *Acta Psychiatr Scand* 86(2):138–145.

Pollock, G.G. (1999) Adverse reactions of antidepressants in elderly patients. *J Clin Psychiatry* 60:4–8.

Reynolds, C.F., III. (1994) Treatment of depression in late life. *Am J Med* 97(suppl 6A):39S–46S.

Reynolds, C.F., III, Frank, E., Kupfer, D.J., Thase, M.E., Perel, J.M., Mazumdar, S., and Houck, P.R. (1996) Treatment outcome in recurrent major depression: A post hoc comparison of elderly ("young old") and midlife patients. *Am J Psychiatry* 153:1288–1292.

Roose, S.P. (1990) Methodological issues in the diagnosis, treatment and study of refractory depression. In: Roose, S.P. and Glassman, A.H., eds. *Treatment Strategies for Refractory Depression*. Washington, DC: American Psychiatric Press, pp. 3–9.

Roose, S.P., Alexopoulos, G., Burke, W., Grossberg, G., Hakkarainen, H., Hassman, H., Jacobsen, A., Katz, I., et al. (2002). Treatment of depression in the "old-old": A randomized, double-blind, placebo-controlled trial of citalopram in patients at least 75 years of age. New Research Meeting of the American Association of Geriatric Psychiatry, Orlando, Florida.

Roose, S.P., and Glassman, A.H. (1989) Cardiovascular effects of tricyclic antidepressants in depressed patients with and without heart disease. *J Clin Psychiatry* 7:1–19.

Roose, S.P., Glassman, A.H., Attia, E., and Woodring, S. (1994) Comparative efficacy of the selective serotonin reuptake inhibitors and the tricyclics in the treatment of melancholia. *Am J Psychiatry* 151:1735–1739.

Roose, S.P., Glassman, A.H., Attia, E., Woodring, S., Giardina, E.G.V., and Bigger, J., Jr. (1998) Cardiovascular effects of fluoxetine in depressed patients with heart disease. *Am J Psychiatry* 155:660–665.

Roose, S.P., Glassman, A.H., Siris, S.G., Walsh, B.T., Bruno, R.L., and Wright, L.B. (1981) Comparison of imipramine and nortriptyline induced orthostatic hypotension: A meaningful difference. *J Clin Psychopharmacol* 1:316–319.

Roose, S.P., Laghrissi-Thode, F., Kennedy, J.S., Nelson, J.C., Bigger, J.T., Pollock, B.G., Gaffney, A., Narayan, M., Finkel, M.S., McCafferty, J., and Gergel, I. (1997) A comparison of paroxetine to nortriptyline in depressed patients with ischemic heart disease. *JAMA* 279:287–291.

Roose, S.P., and Sackeim, H.A. (2002) Clinical trials in late-life depression: Revisited. *Am J Geriatr Psychiatry* 10:503–505.

Roose, S.P., and Schatzberg, A. (2004) The efficacy of antidepressants in the treatment of late-life depression: Evidence-based conclusions. *J Clin Psychopharmacol*, In press.

Roose, S.P., and Suthers K.M. (1998) Antidepressant response in late-life depression. *J Clin Psychiatry* 59:4–8.

Schatzberg, A.F., and Cantillon, M. (2000) Antidepressant early response and remission of venlafaxine and fluoxetine in geriatric outpatients. *European Neuropsychopharmacol* 10(Suppl):S225–S226.

Schatzberg, A.F., Kremer, C., Rodrigues, H.E., Murphy, G.M., Jr., and the Mirtazapine vs. Paroxetine Study Group. (2002) Double-blind, randomized comparison of mirtazapine and paroxetine in elderly depressed patients. *Am J Geriatric Psychiatry* 10(5):541–550.

Schneider, L.S., Nelson, J.C., Clary, C.M., Newhouse, P., Krishnan,

K.R., Shiovitz, T., Weihs, K., and Sertraline Elderly Depression Study Group. (2003) An 8-week multicenter, parallel-group, double-blind, placebo-controlled study of sertraline in elderly outpatients with major depression. *Am J Psychiatry* 160:1277–1285.

Tollefson, G.D., Bosomworth, J.C., Heligeenstein, J.H., Potvin, J.H., Holman, S., et al. (1995) A double-blind, placebo-controlled clinical trial of fluoxetine in geriatric patients with major depression. *Int Psychogeriatr* 7:89–104.

Weihs, K.L., Settle, E.C., Jr., Batey, S.R., Houser, T.L., Donahue, R.M., and Ascher, J.A. (2000) Bupropion sustained release versus paroxetine for the treatment of depression in the elderly. *J Clin Psychiatry* 61:196–202.

Young, R.C., and Meyers, B.S. (1992) Psychopharmacology. In: Sadavoy, J., Lazarus, L.W., and Jarvik, L.F., eds. *Comprehensive Review of Geriatric Psychiatry*. Washington, DC: American Psychiatric Press, pp. 435–467.

# 17 | Antidepressant side effects

CARL SALZMAN

Individuals over age 65 receive one-third of all prescription medications, a disproportionate share of drugs, and fill, on average, 13 prescriptions a year (Baum et al., 1988; Chrischillis et al., 1992). In some surveys, 87%–92% of patients over the age of 65 took medication on a regular basis (Gryfe and Gryfe, 1984; Helling et al., 1987; Shaw, 1976). One risk of this abundant medication use in elderly patients is an increased risk of side effects, as illustrated by a sevenfold increase in drug side effects in 70- to 79-year-olds compared with those age 20–29. Furthermore, one-sixth of all hospital admissions of patients over the age of 70 have been attributed to side effects (Beard, 1992; Pollock, 1999).

Side effects are more common in the elderly due to an interaction of several age-related factors. Not only do older individuals take more medications, but they are likely to be physiologically more sensitive to these medications due to age-related structural and functional changes in the central nervous system (CNS). As individuals age, there is a general reduction in the body's ability to adapt to changes caused by medications such as postural control, orthostatic circulatory responses, thermoregulation, visceral muscle function, laryngeal reflexes, hypoxic responses, and cognitive function (Pollock, 1999). In addition to these age-related changes, polypharmacy predisposes to adverse drug interactions, as well as poor compliance with drug regimens, which often lead to under- or overdosing. It appears, therefore, that the increased risk of side effects is not simply due to age-related vulnerability but is a function of complex interactions between medical frailty, the increased use of medications with potentially toxic side effects, and the prescription of multiple medications (Avorn, 1998; Gurwitz and Avorn, 1991; Salzman, 1999, 2000).

This chapter will focus on categories of common antidepressant side effects in the elderly. The following factors will be considered:

1. Evidence demonstrating a higher incidence of antidepressant side effects in the elderly compared with young and middle-aged adults.

2. The relationship of altered CNS receptor sensitivity of the elderly to specific antidepressant side effects and the neurophysiologic causes of this sensitivity.

3. Altered peripheral neurotransmitter function as a predisposition to antidepressant side effects.

4. Age-associated alterations in the function of specific physiological systems throughout the body that may predispose the elderly patient to an increased risk of antidepressant side effects.

5. The role of pharmacokinetic changes and drug interactions in increasing the likelihood of antidepressant side effects.

6. The consequences of poor compliance with drug regimens and its contribution to antidepressant side effects.

7. Common side effects of antidepressants in the elderly.

## THE INCREASED LIKELIHOOD OF AN ELDERLY PERSON DEVELOPING SIDE EFFECTS

Older patients are assumed to be more sensitive to antidepressants and therefore more likely to develop side effects. It is not clear, however, whether the increased incidence of adverse antidepressant events is due to greater susceptibility to the pharmacological effects of these medications, or whether elderly depressed individuals are more likely to experience adverse events simply due to advanced age and the large number of drugs they take. An examination of the prevalence and types of side effects that elderly placebo recipients experience in controlled clinical trials can help determine whether increased adverse antidepressant reactions in the elderly are simply characteristic of the aging process. Mittmann et al. (1997) reported that 39.6% of elderly research subjects who took placebo had side effects (compared with 60.3% of tricyclic antidepressant [TCA] recipients and 59.1% of selective serotonin reuptake inhibitor [SSRI] recipients).

This meta-analytical placebo side effect rate is somewhat higher than reported in individual studies. For example, in a study comparing nefazodone and imipramine, headache, asthenia, and sweating were reported in 4% of the elderly placebo recipients, about half the rate of the active medication recipients (van Laar et al., 1995). When fluoxetine was compared with placebo on body weight, there was virtually no change in weight with placebo, with significant weight loss with fluoxetine; no placebo-treated patients discontinued therapy due to weight loss (Goldstein et al., 1997). In a study comparing placebo with moclobemide in elderly depressed subjects, all adverse events were equal in both populations with the exception of dizziness and nausea, which were twice as common in the active drug recipients. Nearly 5% of all subjects become agitated, with similar percentages experiencing fatigue and dry mouth. Sleep disturbances were equally frequent in both groups (Roth et al., 1996).

In another study of moclobemide, there was a 17% incidence of anticholinergic side effects for the placebo recipients compared with only 13% for those who took moclobemide (and 28% for those who took nortriptyline). The median number of days that these anticholinergic side effects lasted was longer for placebo than moclobemide (20 vs. 14), but was half as long as for nortriptyline. The severity of these anticholinergic effects was greater for placebo than for moclobemide, and almost as strong as the severity for nortriptyline. The same study showed that orthostatic hypotension was greater in incidence, duration, and severity for placebo than for moclobemide as well, but was considerably less intense than for nortriptyline (Nair et al., 1995).

Data from a study of clomipramine versus placebo suggested that serious side effects were unlikely among the placebo recipients, but mild side effects were frequent and approximated the number of side effects experienced by active drug takers. Seven of 10 patients who were started on placebo developed side effects; constipation and headaches were more common among the placebo recipients than among the active drug takers. By contrast, serious side effects such as dizziness, sleep disturbance, and tremor were significantly more common among the clomipramine recipients (Petracca et al., 1996).

In addition to the increased prevalence of placebo side effects, Mittmann et al. (1997) reported a 26% dropout rate due to these side effects. This meta-analytic placebo dropout rate is also higher than that reported by Gerson et al. (1999), who noted that 6.8% of elderly individuals receiving placebo dropped out due to side effects compared with 19.4% of TCA recipients and 18% of those who took SSRIs. Nonelderly subjects in antidepressant trials had a 5%–10% dropout rate due to an adverse event among placebo recipients compared with 10%–20% for SSRI recipients and 30%–35% for those who received TCAs (Tollefson and Rosenbaum, 1998).

Thus, side effects from placebo are not uncommon in depressed elderly research subjects, although in most studies, their incidence is about half that of medication. When the incidence of side effects and dropout due to placebo in elderly versus nonelderly participants in an-

tidepressant studies are compared, it appears that adverse events are more likely to occur with placebo in older than in younger individuals, but not nearly at the rate due to comparative active medications. It is difficult to compare these data with those from studies of nonelderly depressed subjects, since most clinical trials include some elderly drug recipients and data are usually presented as percentage of side effects rather than percentage of individuals experiencing the side effects. However, in reviewing new antidepressant studies, Preskorn (1995) reported a rate of side effects from 0.9% (palpitations) to 21.8% (headache) experienced by nonelderly placebo recipients who participated in double-blind, placebo-controlled trials.

It appears, therefore, that the elderly are more likely to experience side effects from placebo, especially headache and sedation, although these effects are rarely as frequent or severe as those produced by active medications. Even taking into account more frequent adverse events with placebo, side effects of active medication appear to be more frequent in the elderly participants in antidepressant clinical trials compared with younger adult and mixed-age research populations. These data support the clinical perspective that elderly patients (especially the old-old) are usually considered to be more sensitive to the effects of antidepressants than are younger adults, although there is wide interindividual variability (Salzman, 1999, 2000).

Some investigators have reported an interesting predictive relationship between side effects and therapeutic efficacy. Kin et al. (1996), for example, demonstrated that elderly patients who experienced anticholinergic side effects showed greater improvement on several measures of clinical antidepressant efficacy than those who did not experience these effects. Pretreatment systolic orthostatic hypotension was also shown to have predictive power in two separate studies. Jarvik et al. (1983) demonstrated a better outcome for elderly patients with high pretreatment systolic orthostatic blood pressure; this result was later confirmed by Stack et al. (1988). In other studies, Ackerman et al. (2000) showed that headache was associated with a good response to fluoxetine and somnolence with a good response to placebo.

## RECEPTOR MECHANISMS OF ANTIDEPRESSANT SIDE EFFECTS IN THE ELDERLY

Altered neurotransmitter synthesis and turnover, or age-related changes in receptor sensitivity and signal transduction, probably account for a significant proportion of antidepressant side effects in the elderly. The most common of these include anticholinergic side effects due to diminished CNS and peripheral acetylcholine, sedation due to reduced histamine receptor

TABLE 17.1. *Increased Sensitivity of Older Individuals to Antidepressant Side Effects*

| Age-Related Change | Relationship to ADR | Clinical Consequence |
|---|---|---|
| Increased $H_1$ receptor sensitivity | Increased sedation | Decreased daytime function; decreased cognition |
| Decreased CNS acetylcholine | Increased peripheral and central anticholinergic side effects | Dry mouth, constipation, blurred vision; disorientation, impaired memory, impaired cognition, paranoia |
| Decreased $\alpha_1$ receptor function | Orthostatic hypotension | Increased falls, hip fracture, unsteady gait |
| Decreased DA synthesis and turnover | Increased EPS with serotonergic antidepressants | Parkinsonian symptoms appearing as depression, decreased motivation, decreased physical activity |

ADR, adverse drug reaction; CNS, central nervous system; DA, dopamine; EPS, extrapyramidal side effects.
*Source*: Adapted in part from Avorn (1998) and Sunderland (1998).

function, and movement disorders due to age-related decrements in CNS dopamine. The association between altered receptor function by age or medication and the clinical consequences are shown in Table 17.1.

## Anticholinergic Effects

Cholinergic neurons in the basal forebrain decrease in size with age, with a resultant decline in cholinergic innovation throughout the brain (Mesulam et al., 1987; Sunderland, 1998). The reduction in acetylcholine is probably related to the decline in memory (Bartus et al., 1982; Coyle et al., 1983) and is markedly disturbed in Alzheimer's disease. The net result of diminished CNS cholinergic function, whether caused by decline in synthesis or impaired receptor function, is that the elderly individual becomes sensitized to medications that have cholinergic blocking properties. Anticholinergic effects of antidepressant drugs superimposed upon age-related decrements in cholinergic function produce common anticholinergic side effects in the elderly (Feinberg, 1993). These include further memory impairment, disorientation, and restlessness. As the syndrome becomes more severe, assaultiveness, paranoia, and visual hallucinations may occur. The most extreme manifestations are delirium, stupor, and coma; the delirium is often mistaken for a naturally occurring dementia.

Peripheral anticholinergic side effects of antidepressant medications are also more common in the elderly due to reduced cholinergic functioning throughout the body. Older individuals are often mildly to moderately constipated, and the peripheral anticholinergic side effects of some antidepressants (especially the TCAs) may produce severe constipation. Dry mouth, the most frequent peripheral anticholinergic side effect, may cause loss of porcelain dental fillings and lead to malfitting dentures; it may also contribute to the development of *Candida* infection or parotitis (Alexopoulos and Salzman, 1998). Urinary retention, another peripheral anticholinergic side effect in older persons, may make it difficult to urinate. In serious cases, urine retention can predispose to bladder infections that may ascend to the kidney. The anticholinergic mydriatic action of heterocyclic antidepressants can precipitate or exacerbate narrow angle glaucoma. Although this is an unusual side effect, blurred vision is quite common among older individuals who take TCAs.

Among antidepressants, TCAs have the most distinct and potent anticholinergic properties. Tertiary amines as well as secondary amines block the $M_1$ muscarinic cholinergic receptor and, depending on the dose, can produce significant anticholinergic side effects. However, anticholinergic effects are not unknown with other antidepressants. Paroxetine, an SSRI, has been the subject of clinical reports describing its anticholinergic adverse effects. Compared with other SSRIs, paroxetine is a more potent inhibitor of the $M_1$ receptor (Richelson, 1993). However, several studies have failed to find significant serum anticholinergic levels in elderly patients taking paroxetine, even those who reported anticholinergic side effects (Burrows et al., 2002; Pollack, 1999). Dry mouth has also been reported with bupropion, venlafaxine, and mirtazapine. Monoamine oxidase inhibitors can also produce an anticholinergic-like syndrome, although it is weaker than that produced by TCAs. Dry mouth, urinary retention, and constipation are the most common symptoms (Alexopoulos and Salzman, 1998).

## Dopamine

Dopaminergic neurons and $D_2$ receptors are decreased in the CNS with age. Except in pathological states such as Parkinson's disease, this diminution does not produce significant clinical consequences. However, when medications that block $D_2$ receptor function are taken by the elderly, there may be a significant further decrease in dopaminergic function within the extrapyramidal system. Adverse events that signal a decline in dopaminergic functioning include rigidity, tremor, mask-like facies, and unsteadiness, that is, extrapyramidal symptoms. In most cases these are only mildly or moderately severe, but occasionally they may produce significant functional impairment in the older person and even mask recovery from depression.

The SSRIs are the class of antidepressants most likely to reduce CNS dopaminergic function. Serotonin and dopamine exist in a reciprocal relationship in the basal ganglia (Kapur and Remington, 1996). As serotonergic function is enhanced by SSRI antidepressants, $D_2$-mediated dopamine function can diminish (Salzman et al., 1993). Parkinsonism, dystonic reactions, and akathisia, as well as worsening of motor disability in patients suffering from Parkinson's disease, have been reported in older patients treated with SSRIs (Caley and Friedman, 1992; Pollack, 1999; Steur, 1993).

### Histamine

Most of the sedating effects of antidepressants are due to their antihistaminic ($H_1$-blocking) properties, and histamine-related sedation is one of the more common side effects of various psychotropic medications in the elderly. These are particularly strong in tertiary amine TCAs, in some SSRI antidepressants (especially paroxetine), and in some of the newer antidepressants (nefazodone, mirtazapine). Central nervous system $H_1$ receptors are decreased in the frontal, parietal, and temporal cortices with the aging process (Yanai et al., 1992). The binding of $H_1$ receptors is significantly further decreased in the frontal and temporal areas in Alzheimer's disease (Higuchi et al., 2000). It is not clear whether it is the age-related reduction in the number or sensitivity of histamine ($H_1$) receptors that increases sedation, or whether older individuals are more likely to be sedated because of age-related impairment of nighttime sleep. However, since many medications and over-the-counter preparations have antihistaminic properties, the likelihood of increased sedation from polypharmacy is particularly high in older individuals. The decline in $H_1$ receptors, particularly in Alzheimer's disease patients, would account for the increased sensitivity to the sedating effects of antidepressants that have antihistaminic qualities in these demented individuals.

### CARDIOVASCULAR SIDE EFFECTS

Antidepressants, especially the TCAs, may cause alteration of cardiovascular function in the elderly. Virtually all of the newer antidepressants (SSRIs, bupropion, venlafaxine, nefazodone, mirtazapine) lack cardiotoxic effects, which gives them a distinct advantage over the TCAs. Tricyclic cardiotoxicity is caused by the quinidine-like effects of these drugs on cardiac conduction. At low plasma levels, these drugs stabilize abnormal cardiac rhythms; at higher doses, all TCAs (and their hydroxymetabolites) delay cardiac conduction and increase the heart rate. In the presence of overt heart disease, the cardiotoxicity of TCAs increases. Since TCAs are Class I antiarrhythmic drugs (Bigger et al., 1977), they may increase rather than decrease mortality in patients with ischemic heart disease (Glassman et al., 1993). The frequency of orthostatic hypotension increases, especially in patients with left ventricular impairment; falls due to orthostatic hypotension may occur in as many as 50% of these patients (Glassman et al., 1983; Roose et al., 1986). In patients who already have conduction disease, especially bundle branch block, TCA-induced delay may produce symptomatic rhythm disturbance and even death (Roose et al., 1986, 1987). Thus, it appears that TCAs may be especially dangerous for elderly patients with ischemic heart disease or preexisting abnormal conduction. Given the availability of noncardiotoxic antidepressants, these drugs are usually avoided in elderly patients with a recent myocardial infarction (MI). However, Roose et al. (1986) demonstrated both the efficacy and safety of nortriptyline in post-MI patients when the dosage and plasma levels of the drug are closely monitored and the treatment is also monitored by electrocardiograph (EKG).

The SSRI antidepressants appear to be considerably safer for cardiovascular function. In healthy (nonelderly) adults, their use may be associated with a very modest slowing of the pulse rate, without affecting either resting or postural blood pressure or EKG (Glassman 1998). In elderly patients with ischemic heart disease after MI, there were almost no cardiovascular effects of an SSRI and no evidence of cardiac harm (Roose et al., 1998a). Studies of fluoxetine as well as paroxetine (Roose et al., 1998b) demonstrated no intracardiac conduction delays and no evidence of orthostatic hypotension; both drugs were associated with a lower incidence of cardiovascular effects than nortriptyline. It appears, therefore, that the SSRI antidepressants are safe in depressed patients with heart disease. Bupropion has also been examined in depressed patients with stable but significant heart disease; no alterations in conduction, contractility, or orthostatic hypotension were observed (Roose et al., 1991).

Venlafaxine also has a low incidence of cardiotoxicity (Feighner, 1995). However, a dose-related increase in mean diastolic blood pressure has been observed in 5.5% of nonelderly patients at doses above 200 mg daily (Feighner, 1995). There is no evidence to suggest that older individuals are more susceptible to this side effect. Orthostatic hypotension due to blockade of peripheral $\alpha_1$ receptors is most often associated with TCAs, especially tertiary amines.

Orthostasis may result from age-related changes in baroreflex sensitivity that increase or decrease the heart rate in response to a physiological stress or medication (Rowe and Lipsitz, 1988). As many as 20%–30% of older individuals living in the community may have orthostatic hypotension (Caird et al., 1973). Symptomatic orthostatic hypotension may be secondary to a large number of diseases commonly found in the elderly or secondary to drugs used by elderly patients. As noted, the frequency of orthostatic hypotension increases in patients with left ventricular impairment (Glassman et al., 1983; Roose et al., 1986).

Control of blood pressure is also related to norepinephrine neurotransmission, which is diminished by the aging process peripherally as well as in the CNS (Marchi et al., 1982; Sunderland, 1998). The orthostatic hypotensive effects of the TCAs are most likely produced by blockade of peripheral $\alpha_1$ adreno receptors, predisposing the older individual to an increased risk of orthostatic hypotension when drugs with $\alpha_1$-blocking properties are administered. All TCAs are strong $\alpha_1$ blockers in the elderly, although earlier research suggests that the blood pressure decline produced by nortriptyline is less than that caused by imipramine (Alexopoulos and Salzman, 1998; Thaysse et al., 1981). Orthostatic hypotension can cause falls, fractures, strokes, or heart attacks (Glassman and Preud'Homme, 1993). Approximately 50% of depressed patients with heart failure develop significant orthostatic hypotension when treated with imipramine (Glassman, 1988; Glassman et al., 1983), suggesting that elderly patients with heart failure may be at special risk for TCA-induced orthostatic hypotension.

Although there is no evidence of altered $\alpha_1$ adreno receptor sensitivity due to age (Swift, 1990), it is possible that increased platelet $\alpha_2$ receptor binding may identify elderly individuals who possess noradrenergic defects associated with depression (Schneider, 1992). The reduction in norepinephrine neurotransmission, like the reduction in dopamine, predisposes the elderly individual to unwanted effects of further neurotransmitter blockade.

## VASCULAR SIDE EFFECTS

In addition to affecting cardiac conduction and blood pressure, some antidepressants may have hematological side effects. The SSRIs, in particular, are associated with decreased platelet aggregation (Pollock et al., 1995). Platelet factor 4 and thromboglobulin levels rise in depressed patients (compared with nondepressed cardiac patients) (Laghrissi-Thode et al., 1997). These increases are associated with an increased *sticky* state and a predisposition to thrombosis. An SSRI (paroxetine) reduced platelet stickiness, whereas a TCA (nortriptyline) did not. This decrease in platelet aggregation may also explain the ecchymosis and occasional episode of bleeding that has been associated with SSRIs (Glassman, 1998). However, there are no data to suggest that the elderly are at greater risk for this bleeding or more sensitive to the antiaggregation properties of SSRIs than younger adults.

## FALLS

As previously noted, an increased propensity toward TCA-induced orthostatic hypotension predisposes elderly patients to falls and concomitant fractures, especially of the hip. The orthostatic hypotensive effects of monoamine oxidase inhibitors also predispose elderly patients to these falls (Ray et al., 1987). However, it is not clear that orthostatic hypotension is the sole cause of the increased risk for falls. An increased prevalence of falls among the elderly in nursing homes has also been documented with SSRI use (Liu et al., 1998; Ruthazer and Lipsitz, 1993), although these drugs do not cause orthostatic hypotension. Sertraline, however, was reported to significantly increase body sway after 1 week of therapy (but not during the second week) (Laghrissi-Thode et al., 1995a); a second study using paroxetine found no significant effect on body sway (Laghrissi-Thode et al., 1995b). Nortriptyline was associated with increased body sway in the second study as well.

Unsteadiness and falls with other psychotropic drugs that do not cause orthostatic hypotension have been reported in elderly individuals. The rate of falls following the use of TCAs and SSRIs is the same in elderly individuals (Thapa et al., 1998). Benzodiazepines are also well known to increase the risk of falls in nursing home residents (Salzman, 1998); these anxiolytics do not cause orthostatic hypotension. It may be, therefore, that in addition to the obvious adverse effect of orthostatic hypotension from $\alpha$-blocking antidepressants, elderly individuals, especially the frail elderly residing in nursing homes, may be at increased risk for falls from other mechanisms, including diminished balance.

## INAPPROPRIATE ANTIDIURETIC HORMONE SECRETION

The SSRIs, and to a lesser extent the TCAs, have been associated with an increased production of inappropriate antidiuretic hormone (SIADH) (Pollock, 1999). Although rare, SIADH has been reported with the use of venlafaxine and nefazodone as well (John et al., 1998; Masood et al., 1998; Spigset and Adielsson, 1997). The hyponatremia that results from this inappropriate hormone secretion usually occurs within 2 weeks of treatment onset (Liu et al., 1996). The result of SIADH is water retention, which, in turn, causes weakness, lethargy, and weight gain. In severe cases, delirium may develop, associated with low serum sodium levels. Early warning signs include lethargy, disorientation, and muscle cramps (Pollock, 1999); discontinuing the antidepressant is essential. The mechanisms increasing the likelihood of SIADH with antidepressant therapy in the elderly have not been established. It is possible that increased fluid intake, which results from the anticholinergic effects of TCAs, might explain some of the increased water retention. Enhanced catecholamine activity may increase the release of antidiuretic hormone. A rapid increase in water intake is associated with more severe SIADH (Woo and Smith, 1997). With long half-life medications such as fluoxetine, it may take several weeks for the syndrome to disappear after drug discontinuation (Druckenbrod and Mulsant, 1994).

## WEIGHT ALTERATIONS

Weight loss is often reported in the early stages of treatment with SSRIs (Sussman, 1998). Weight gain is commonly associated with TCAs (Salzman, 1995) and with some newer antidepressants such as mirtazapine. There are no systematic studies of weight alteration with antidepressant use in elderly individuals. Weber et al., (2000), however, reported that weight gain following treatment with nortriptyline and paroxetine was equivalent during the first 12 weeks of therapy. With either drug, posttreatment weight and basal metabolic index (BMI) approximated the premorbid weight and BMI. Weight loss during antidepressant treatment, however, may seriously affect the health of a depressed, frail, elderly patient who has already lost weight due to depression. Weight gain, on the other hand, may be a serious adverse event for a depressed older individual who is already obese or who has cardiovascular illness, hyperlipidemia, or diabetes. Further research is necessary to establish the mechanisms and predictive correlates of weight alteration with antidepressant therapy in older patients.

## MEDICATION NONCOMPLIANCE AS A RISK FOR ANTIDEPRESSANT ADVERSE EVENTS

Estimates of drug regimen noncompliance in the elderly range from 40% to 80% and have clearly been associated with adverse drug effects (Salzman, 1995). The primary causes of noncompliance with antidepressant regimens include side effects, cost of medications, complicated dosing schedules, forgetfulness, and difficulty opening bottles and reading labels. Mixing drugs with similar side effects obviously enhances the possibility of an adverse event, which often increases noncompliance. This is especially true of mixtures of medications with sedating, orthostatic, or anticholinergic side effects. Given the increasing probability of polypharmacy in the elderly (especially those with chronic serious medical illnesses), the risk of adverse drug interactions leading to noncompliance is high. Noncompliance, in turn, may lead to lack of a therapeutic response when the antidepressant is not taken as prescribed or to even

more side effects when side effects of different medications are additive.

## CONCLUSION

It appears that elderly individuals are more likely than younger ones to experience adverse events from antidepressant medications. The causes of these unwanted side effects include increased sensitivity to medications, altered pharmacokinetics, and polypharmacy drug interactions. In order to ensure the maximum therapeutic benefit with as little risk as possible, clinicians must monitor very closely the use of antidepressants in the elderly and be ready to make dosage adjustments or medication changes when necessary. Elderly patients (and their families) must be advised of medication side effects as well as common drug interactions (Salzman, 2001).

REFERENCES

Ackerman, D.L., Greenland, S., Bystritsky, A., et al. (2000) Side effects and time course of response in a placebo-controlled trial of fluoxetine for the treatment of geriatric depression. *J Clin Psychopharmacol* 20:658–665.

Alexopoulos, G.S., and Salzman, C. (1998) Treatment of depression with heterocyclic antidepressants, monoamine oxidase inhibitors, and psychomotor stimulants. In: Salzman, C., ed. *Clinical Geriatric Psychopharmacology*, 3rd ed. Baltimore: Williams & Wilkins, pp. 184–244.

Avorn, J. (1998) Drug prescribing, drug taking, adverse reactions, and compliance in elderly patients. In: Salzman, C., ed. *Clinical Geriatric Psychopharmacology*, 3rd ed. Baltimore: Williams & Wilkins, pp. 21–50.

Bartus, R.T., Dean, R.L., Beer, B., et al. (1982) The cholinergic hypothesis of geriatric memory dysfunction. *Science* 217:408–417.

Baum, C., Kennedy, D.L., Knapp, D.E., et al. (1988) Prescription drug use in 1984 and changes over time. *Med Care* 26:105–114.

Beard, K. (1992) Adverse reactions as a cause of hospital admission in the aged. *Drugs Aging* 2:356–367.

Bigger, J.T., Jr., Giardina, E.G.V., Perel, J.M., et al. (1977) Cardiac antiarrhythmic effect of imipramine hydrochloride. *N Engl J Med* 296:206–208.

Burrows, A.B., Salzman, C., Satlin, A., Noble, K., Pollock, B.G., and Gersh, T. (2002) A randomized, placebo-controlled trial of paroxetine in nursing home residents with non-major depression. *Depress Anxiety* 15:102–110.

Caird, F.I., Andrews, G.R., and Kennedy, R.D. (1973) Effect of posture on blood pressure in the elderly. *Br Heart J* 35:527.

Caley, C.F., and Friedman, J.H. (1992) Does fluoxetine exacerbate Parkinson's disease? *J Clin Psychiatry* 53:278–282.

Chrischillis, E.A., Foley, D.J., and Wallace, R.B. (1992) Use of medications by persons 65 and over: Data from the established populations for epidemiologic studies of the elderly. *J Gerontol* 47:M137–M144.

Coyle, J.T., Price, D.L., and DeLong, M.R. (1983) Alzheimer's disease: A disorder of cortical cholinergic innervation. *Science* 219:1184–1190.

Druckenbrod, R., and Mulsant, B.H. (1994) Fluoxetine-induced syndrome of inappropriate antidiuretic hormone secretion. *J Geriatr Psychiatry Neurol* 7:255–258.

Feighner, J.P. (1995) Cardiovascular safety in depressed patients: Focus on venlafaxine. *J Clin Psychiatry* 56:574–579.

Feinberg, M. (1993) The problems of anticholinergic adverse effects in older patients. *Drugs Aging* 3:335–348.

Glassman, A.H. (1998) Cardiovascular effects of antidepressant drugs: Updated. *J Clin Psychiatry* 59(suppl 15):13–18.

Glassman, A.H., Johnson, L.L., Giardina, E.G.V., et al. (1983) The use of imipramine in depressed patients with congestive heart failure. *JAMA* 250:1997–2001.

Glassman, A.H., and Preud'Homme, X.A. (1993) Review of the cardiovascular effects of heterocyclic antidepressants. *J Clin Psychiatry* 54(suppl 2):16–22.

Glassman, A.H., Roose, S.P., and Bigger, J.T., Jr. (1993) The safety of tricyclic antidepressants in cardiac patients: Risk/benefit reconsidered. *JAMA* 269:2673–2675.

Goldstein, D.J., Hamilton, S.H., Mascia, D.N., et al. (1997) Fluoxetine in medically stable, depressed geriatric patients: Effects on weight. *J Clin Psychopharmacol* 17:365–369.

Gryfe, C.I., and Gryfe, B.M. (1984) Drug therapy of the aged: The problem of compliance and the roles of physicians and pharmacists. *J Am Geriatr Soc* 32:301–307.

Gurwitz, J.H., and Avorn, K. (1991) The ambiguous relation between aging and adverse drugs reactions. *Ann Intern Med* 114:956–966.

Helling, D.R., Lemke, J.H., Semla, T.P., et al. (1987) Medication use characteristics in the elderly: The Iowa 65+ rural health study. *J Am Geriatr Soc* 35:4–12.

Higuchi, M., Yanai, K., Okamura, N., et al. (2000) Histamine H(1) receptors in patients with Alzheimer's disease assessed by positron emission tomography. *Neuroscience* 99:721–729.

Jarvik, L.F., Read, S.L., Mintz, J., et al. (1983) Pretreatment orthostatic hypotension in geriatric depression: Predictor of response to imipramine and doxepin. *J Clin Psychopharmacol* 3:368–371.

John, L., Perreault, M.M., Tao, T., et al. (1998) Serotonin syndrome associated with nefazodone and paroxetine. *Ann Emerg Med* 29:287–289.

Kapur, S., and Remington, G. (1996) Serotonin–dopamine interaction and its relevance to schizophrenia. *Am J Psychiatry* 153:466–476.

Kin, N.M.K., Klitgaard, N., Nair, N.P.V., et al. (1996) Clinical relevance of serum nortriptyline and 10-hydroxy-nortriptyline measurements in the depressed elderly: A multicenter pharmacokinetic and pharmacodynamic study. *Neuropsychopharmacology* 15:1–6.

Laghrissi-Thode, F., Pollock, B.G., Miller, M.C., et al. (1995a) Comparative effects of sertraline and nortriptyline on body sway in elderly depressed patients. *Am J Geriatr Psychiatry* 3:217–228.

Laghrissi-Thode, F., Pollock, B.G., Miller, M.C., et al. (1995b) Double-blind comparison of paroxetine and nortriptyline on the postural stability of late-life depressed patients. *Psychopharmacol Bull* 31:659–663.

Laghrissi-Thode, F., Wagner, W.R., Pollock, B.G., et al. (1997) Elevated platelet factor 4 and beta-thromboglobulin plasma levels in depressed patients with ischemic heart disease. *Biol Psychiatry* 42:290–295.

Liu, B.A., Anderson, G., Mittman, N., et al. (1998) Use of selective serotonin-reuptake inhibitors of tricyclic antidepressants and risk of hip fractures in elderly people. *Lancet* 351:1303–1307.

Liu, B.A., Mittman, N., Knoweles, S.R., et al. (1996) Hyponatremia and the syndrome of inappropriate secretion on antidiuretic hormone associated with the use of selective serotonin reuptake inhibitors: A review of spontaneous reports. *Can Med Assoc J* 155:519–527.

Marchi, M., Yurkewitz, L., Giacobini, E., et al. (1982) Peripheral and central adrenergic neurons: Differences during the aging process. In: Giacobini, E., Filogamo, G., Giacobini, G., Vernadakis, A., eds. *Aging,* Vol. 20. New York: Raven Press, pp. 93–101.

Masood, G.R., Karki, S.D., and Patterson, W.R. (1998) Hyponatremia with venlafaxine. *Ann Pharmacother* 32:49–51.

Mesulam, M.-M., Mufson, E.J., and Rogers, J. (1987) Age-related shrinkage of cortically projecting cholinergic neurons: A selective effect. *Ann Neurol* 22:31–36.

Mittmann, N., Herrmann, N., Einarson, T.R., et al. (1997) The efficacy, safety and tolerability of antidepressants in late-life depression: A meta-analysis. *J Affect Disord* 46:191–217.

Nair, N.P.V., Amin, M., Holm, P., et al. (1995) Moclobemide and nortriptyline in elderly depressed patients. A randomized, multi-center trial against placebo. *J Affect Disord* 33:1–9.

Petracca, G., Tesón, A., Chemerinski, E., et al. (1996) A double-blind placebo-controlled study of clomipramine in depressed patients with Alzheimer's disease. *J Neuropsychiatry* 8:270–275.

Pollock, B.G. (1999) Adverse reactions of antidepressants in elderly patients. *J Clin Psychiatry* 60(suppl 20):4–8.

Pollock, B.G., Laghrissi-Thode, F., Wagner, W.R., et al. (1995) Increased PF4 and beta-TG in depressed patients with ischemic heart disease. Presented at the 34th annual meeting of the American College of Neuropsychopharmacology, San Juan, Puerto Rico, December 11–14.

Preskorn, S.H. (1995) Comparison of the tolerability of bupropion, fluoxetine, imipramine, nefazodone, paroxetine, sertraline, and venlafaxine. *J Clin Psychiatry* 56(suppl 6):12–21.

Ray, W.A., Griffin, M.R., and Schaffner, W. (1987) Psychotropic drug use and the risk of hip fracture. *N Engl J Med* 316:363–369.

Richelson, E. (1993) Review of antidepressants in the treatment of mood disorders. In: Dunner, D.L., ed. *Current Psychiatric Therapy.* Philadelphia: W.B. Saunders, pp. 232–239.

Roose, S.P., Dalack, G.W., Glassman, A.H., et al. (1991) Cardiovascular effects of bupropion in depressed patients with heart disease. *Am J Psychiatry* 148:512–516.

Roose, S.P., Glassman, A.H., Attia, E., et al. (1998a) Cardiovascular effects of fluoxetine in depressed patients with heart disease. *Am J Psychiatry* 155:660–665.

Roose, S.P., Glassman, A.H., Giardina, E.G.V., et al. (1986) Nortriptyline in depressed patients with left ventricular impairment. *JAMA* 256:3253–3257.

Roose, S.P., Glassman, A.H., Giardina, E.G.V., et al. (1987) Tricyclic antidepressants in depressed patients with cardiac conduction disease. *Arch Gen Psychiatry* 44:273–275.

Roose, S.P., Laghrissi-Thode, F., Kennedy, J.S., et al. (1998b) Comparison of paroxetine and nortriptyline in depressed patients with ischemic heart disease. *JAMA* 279:287–291.

Roth, M., Mountjoy C.Q., Amrien, R., et al. (1996) Moclobemide in elderly patients with cognitive decline and depression. *Br J Psychiatry* 168:149–157.

Rowe, J.W., and Lipsitz, L.A. (1988) Altered blood pressure. In: Rowe, J.W., and Besdine, R.W., eds. *Geriatric Medicine* 2nd ed. Boston: Little, Brown, pp. 193–207.

Ruthauser, R., and Lipsitz, L.A. (1993) Antidepressants and falls among elderly people in long-term care. *Am J Public Health* 83: 746–769.

Salzman, C. (1995) Medication compliance in the elderly. *J Clin Psychiatry* 56(suppl 1):18–23.

Salzman, C. (1998) Treatment of anxiety and anxiety-related disorders. In: Salzman, C., ed. *Clinical Geriatric Psychopharmacology* 3rd ed. Baltimore: Williams & Wilkins, pp. 343–370.

Salzman, C. (1999) Practical considerations for treatment of depression in elderly and very elderly long-term care patients. *J Clin Psychiatry* 60(suppl 20):30–33.

Salzman, C. (2000) Management considerations for late-life depression. *J Clin Psychiatry* 2(suppl 5):33–36.

Salzman, C. (2001) *Psychiatric Medications for Older Adults.* New York: Guilford Press.

Salzman, C., Jimerson, D., Vasile, R., et al. (1993) Response to SSRI antidepressants correlates with reduction in plasma HVA: Pilot study. *Biol Psychiatry* 34:569–571.

Schneider, L.S. (1992) Psychobiologic features of geriatric affective disorder. *Clin Geriatr Med* 8:253–265.

Shaw, S.M., and Opit, L.J. (1976) Need for supervision in the elderly receiving long-term prescribed medication. *Br Med J* 1:505–507.

Spigset, O., and Adielsson, G. (1997) Combined serotonin syndrome and hyponatremia caused by a citalopram-buspirone interaction. *Int J Psychopharmacol* 12:61–63.

Stack, J.A., Reynolds, C.F., III, Perel, J.M., et al. (1988) Pretreatment systolic orthostatic blood pressure (PSOP) and treatment response in elderly depressed inpatients. *J Clin Psychopharmacol* 8:116–120.

Steur, E. (1993) Increase of Parkinson disability after fluoxetine medication. *Neurology* 43:211–213.

Sunderland, T. (1998) Neurotransmission in the aging central nervous system. In: Salzman, C., ed. *Clinical Geriatric Psychopharmacology*, 3rd ed. Baltimore: Williams & Wilkins, pp. 51–69.

Sussman, N. (1998) Rethinking side effects of the selective serotonin-reuptake inhibitors: Sexual dysfunction and weight gain. *Psychiatr Ann* 28:89–97.

Swift, C.G. (1990) Pharmacodynamics: Changes in homeostatic mechanisms, receptor and target organ sensitivity in the elderly. *Br Med Bull* 46:36–52.

Thapa, P.B., Gideon, P., Cost, T.W., et al. (1998) Antidepressants and the risk of falls among nursing home residents. *N Engl J Med* 339:875–882.

Thaysse, P., Bjerre, M., Kragh-Sørensen, P., et al. (1981) Cardiovascular effects of imipramine and nortriptyline in elderly patients. *Psychopharmacology* 74:360–364.

Tollefson, G.D., and Rosenbaum, J.F. (1998) Selective serotonin re-uptake inhibitors. In: Schatzberg, A.F., and Nemeroff, C.B., eds. *The American Psychiatric Press Textbook of Psychopharmacology*, 2nd ed. Washington, DC: American Psychiatric Press, pp. 219–237.

van Laar, M.W., van Willigenburg, A.P.P., and Volkerts, E.R. (1995) Acute and subchronic effects of nefazodone and imipramine on highway driving, cognitive functions, and daytime sleepiness in healthy adult and elderly subjects. *J Clin Psychopharmacol* 15:30–40.

Weber, E., Stack, J., Pollock, B.G., et al. (2000) Weight change in older depressed patients during acute pharmacotherapy with paroxetine and nortriptyline. *Am J Geriatr Psychiatry* 8:245–250.

Woo, M.H., and Smithe, M.A. (1997) Association of SIADS with selective serotonin reuptake inhibitors. *Ann Pharmacother* 31:108–109.

Yanai, K., Watanabe T., Meguro, K., et al. (1992) Age-dependent decrease in histamine $H_1$ receptor in human brains revealed by PET. *NeuroReport* 3:433–436.

# 18 | Mood stabilizers

CHARLES L. BOWDEN

Use of mood stabilizers in the elderly focuses on bipolar disorders. Recognition and treatment of bipolar spectrum disorders in the elderly deal with three overlapping patient groups. Early-onset bipolar disorder almost always continues into the late years of life, with a largely unchanged illness course in terms of overall severity. A smaller but important group of patients develops bipolar disorder in old age, often secondary to general medical disorders, with mixed manic symptoms predominating. Elderly persons with dementias often have symptoms that are within the extended bipolar spectrum.

The characteristics of elderly bipolar patients are not strictly a function of age, since they differ from age-matched patients with major depressive disorder. These differences (Table 18.1) indicate more than a fourfold greater frequency of neurological disorders and more than double the mortality rate of major depressive disorder. Bipolar patients with neurological disorders are more likely to be hospitalized for their illness. Neurologically impaired patients are less likely than all manic patients to have a family history of affective disorder in first-degree relatives (33% vs. 52%). Neurologically impaired patients are much more likely to have their illness commence with a manic episode than nonneurologically impaired bipolar patients. Compared with nonelderly bipolar patients, elderly patients with bipolar disorder are more likely to have manic and mixed presentations, co-morbid neurological disorders, and other general medical disorders for which long-term use of lithium is often poorly tolerated.

The increased use of mood stabilizers in patients with dementias has been influenced by a somewhat more symptom-based than syndrome-based consideration in treatment planning. This stems from broad evidence that behavioral disturbances common to several differing disorders often respond to a single agent. Among elderly patients, an additional factor in symptom-based treatment decisions is that multiple medical problems and complex effects of several medications often stymie efforts at unequivocal diagnosis of a single syndrome. Impulsivity and aggression are the most common behavioral disturbances triggering prescription of mood stabilizers in patients with dementia. One reason is that physical aggression and verbal outbursts are the major precipitants of nursing home admission for patients with dementia. The degree of linkage between impulsive aggression and bipolar disorder is not well characterized. Dementia is present in the majority of nursing home patients. Behavioral aggression, which is largely synonymous with the term *impulsive aggression*, is the most common management problem in these patients and is present in approximately one-half of all patients with a diagnosis of dementia in two independent studies (Swearer et al., 1988). Impulsivity and aggression, though often linked, are not synonymous or always linked. Indirect evidence suggests that mood stabilizers may have more specific effects on impulsive, unpremeditated, and generally inappropriate behaviors than directly on aggression (Bowden et al., 2000; Swann et al., 2002). Examples of impulsive behaviors that are not linked with aggression, irritability, or hostility include wandering into off-limits areas and undue familiarity with strangers.

The term *mood stabilizer* has been used with increased frequency since around 1990. No single definition of this term has been developed. The definition one author has most recently suggested is: a drug that is effective in acute depression, mania, or both; is efficacious in both acute and maintenance treatment; and does not worsen any fundamental component of the disorder (e.g., depression, mania, psychosis, or cycling frequency) (Bowden, 2002b). An additional reason that the term *mood stabilizer* is often used is that mood instability is generally viewed as one of the fundamental characteristics of bipolar disorders.

Drugs that are generally viewed as meeting the above criteria as mood stabilizers are lithium, valproate, lamotrigine, and carbamazepine. Among mood stabilizers, most recent studies in the elderly have been conducted with divalproex, with open and controlled trials indicating efficacy with generally good tolerability. One reason for the interest in divalproex is the relatively greater prevalence of mixed manic symptomatology in the elderly, which is associated with a relatively better response to divalproex, and possibly to carbamazepine, than to lithium. Lamotrigine has recently demonstrated efficacy that would qualify it as a mood stabilizer. These four drugs are reviewed in detail in a subsequent section.

Other drugs have partial characteristics of mood stabilizers. Oxcarbazepine, a drug available for over 20

TABLE 18.1. *Comparison of Elderly Manic and Major Depressed Patients*

| Variable | Manic (N = 50) | Major Depressed (N = 50) | Adjusted Odds Ratio |
|---|---|---|---|
| Neurological disorder | 36% | 8% | 8.0 |
| Mortality rate | 50% | 20% | 2.4 |

years in Europe, has recently been approved in the United States for the treatment of epilepsy. Its efficacy is probably similar to that of carbamazepine; however, it has been little studied in adults with bipolar disorder and not at all in elderly patients. Its side effect profile is similar to that of carbamazepine on cognition, motor slowing, and propensity to cause hyponatremia, which is greater in elderly patients. It has fewer enzyme-inducing effects through the 3A4 oxidative pathway than does carbamazepine.

All tested antipsychotics have some antimanic properties. Olanzapine is approved for the treatment of mania (Tohen et al., 2000). Risperidone, ziprasidone, and haloperidol have also been demonstrated to be superior to placebo in placebo-controlled studies of acute mania (Keck and Ice, 2000; Sachs et al., 2001). However, evidence of maintenance phase efficacy is lacking in the published placebo-controlled monotherapy trials. The atypical antipsychotic appears not to cause or worsen depression, which has been observed with standard antipsychotic drugs (Ahlfors et al., 1981). The role and use of the antipsychotics is covered in detail in Chapter 20.

Anticonvulsants used for their mood-stabilizing properties now occupy an important position in treatments for bipolar elderly. Several additional drugs with antiepileptic properties have been studied in adult but not elderly patients with mania. These include gabapentin, topiramate, and gabatril. At least two placebo-controlled studies of both gabapentin and topiramate have not found superiority over placebo (Frye et al., 2000; Pande et al., 2000). No placebo-controlled reports suggesting efficacy in depression, mania, or maintenance treatment for these three anticonvulsants have been published. Therefore, these drugs would not qualify as mood stabilizers. It is possible that other aspects of these drugs may be of adjunctive benefit in the management of patients within the bipolar spectrum. Gabapentin has been of benefit in social phobia and appears to have anxiety-reducing properties (Davidson et al., 1982). However, no systematic studies for this use in bipolar disorder have been conducted. Topiramate has been effective in reducing binge eating symptomatology and alcohol consumption in alcoholics in blinded, placebo-controlled studies (Johnson et al., 2003). No placebo-controlled data have been published for gabatril. Open studies report low or negligible rates of response, with high rates of sedative adverse effects (Grunze et al., 1999).

## THE PREVENTION OF DEPRESSION IN ELDERLY BIPOLAR PATIENTS

In the largest study of bipolar disorder across the life span, conducted prior to the availability of any specific treatments used today, Kraepelin (1921) observed that whereas manic episodes were more frequent than depressive episodes early in the course of bipolar disorder, from the age of 50, depressive episodes constituted over 60% of all episodes. Persistent depressive episodes were predictive of worse depression 15 years later in the longitudinal National Institute of Mental Health Collaborative Clinical Study. In contrast, early, persisting manic episodes were not predictive of later manic or depressive episodes (Coryell et al., 1998). In a 1-year study of maintenance treatment of bipolar disorder, a higher lifetime number of manic and depressive episodes predicted depressive relapse, with an increase in the odds ratio of 1.24 for every category increase, $p = .002$ (Gyulai et al., 2003). These data indicate that psychiatrists caring for elderly persons with bipolar disorder are likely to observe more depressive than manic symptomatology in their patients. Therefore it is important to review what is known about the effectiveness of mood stabilizers in preventing depressive relapse.

## DIFFICULTIES IN CONDUCTING STUDIES OF MOOD STABILIZERS IN ELDERLY PATIENTS

Studies of mood stabilizers over the past decade provide a reasonably good indication of where benefit can be expected, of their tolerability, and of dosing guidelines. Difficulties in conducting research on elderly patients with bipolar disorder, or with target symptoms related to bipolar disorder, especially impulsivity and/or aggression associated with dementia, complicate the conduct of studies in the elderly and the interpretation of studies for maximum relevance to clinical practitioners. These differences are found in two general categories. First, older patients are more likely to have compromised function in one or more organ systems, and to have more concurrent diseases, than younger patients. Even though psychiatric investigators recognize the importance of endeavoring to enroll samples representative of the full spectrum of the condition of interest, this is rarely possible. Other essential drugs that a patient is taking may interfere with or, in the case of carbamazepine/oxcarbazepine, may be interfered with by the anticonvulsant. If dementia is present, the condition per se reduces assessments to those observed, rather than what the patient can reliably report. Therefore, sensitivity of the measurement of change suffers.

Additionally, elderly patients with behavioral disturbances are studied with treatments by a range of physician specialists: psychiatrists, internists, neurologists, and family practitioners. In particular, psychiatrists and neurologists apply differing terminology to similar phenomenology.

## EVIDENCE OF SPECTRUM OF EFFICACY, TOLERABILITY, AND DOSING

### Lithium Guidelines

In nonelderly patients, lithium has been demonstrated to have antimanic properties. Lithium also has some antidepressant properties, but these are slow in onset, probably not sooner than 4 weeks, and are only modestly superior to placebo treatment. Lithium has been established as effective in extending the time to intervention for manic symptoms in two recent placebo-controlled, double-blind studies (Bowden et al., 2003a, 2003b). Conversely, lithium did not extend the time to intervention for depression. For acutely manic patients, those with classical, or pure, manic symptoms are more likely to respond to lithium than are those with mixed states, rapid cycling, associated substance abuse, mania associated with any neurological disorder, or a history of numerous episodes (Bowden, 1995). Even three depressive episodes place lithium-treated patients in a group with no greater improvement than seen with placebo (Swann et al., 2000).

### Usage Guidelines

For the patient who has benefited from lithium prophylaxis, a reasonable approach to treatment as the patient ages is to recognize new complexities and manage them appropriately. Much of this can be accomplished by closer attention to the patient's general medical status and by coordination of care with other physicians. Lithium treatment of acutely depressed bipolar patients has yielded improvement in approximately 70% of patients. However, all of the early studies had methodological limitations, and only approximately 30% of patients treated were unequivocal responders (Zornberg and Pope, 1993).

Based on the three recent blinded, randomized, placebo-controlled studies of lithium in maintenance therapy employing time-to-event analyses, lithium appears to have few specific preventive effects against breakthrough depression, in contrast to its efficacy for breakthrough manic symptoms. In a 1-year study, the time to depressive relapse and the mean number of days in the study were shorter for lithium-treated than placebo-treated patients (Bowden et al., 2000b).

In two 18-month studies with similar designs, one enrolling patients recently manic and the other patients recently depressed, lithium did not differ significantly from placebo in time to intervention for depressive symptoms (Bowden et al., 2003; Calabrese et al., 2003). In a planned combined analysis of the two datasets, the larger sample size again did not indicate a significant difference between lithium and placebo.

These predictors of response can be extrapolated to elderly patients. Since elderly bipolar patients are more likely to have mania associated with other neurological conditions, and are likely to have had many episodes, they are relatively unlikely to respond well to lithium when manic. Among elderly patients treated with lithium, those with no neurological disease had an 89% response rate. Conversely, those with either dementia or extrapyramidal dysfunction had only a 4% response rate (Himmelhoch and Garfinkel, 1986). The difficulties with the use of lithium are consequent to two additive factors. First, increased age is often associated with factors that impede lithium clearance (see Table 18.2) and/or increase lithium serum levels, such as poor hydration. Second, lithium causes substantial neurological impairment, especially but not solely neu-

TABLE 18.2. *Drugs and Physiologic States with Clinically Important Renal Interactions with Lithium*

| Drug or Physiological State | Interaction |
|---|---|
| Angiotensin converting enzyme inhibitors (e.g., Lotensin, Vasote) | Increased plasma lithium consequent to decreased lithium clearance; increases may be to levels causing neurotoxicity (Ace inhibitors, 1988; Finley PR et al., 1996) |
| Thiazide diuretics | Increased plasma lithium consequent to decreased lithium clearance; may be effective in treatment of lithium-induced polyuria (Jefferson et al., 1979) |
| Nonsteroidal anti-inflammatory drugs) | Increased plasma lithium consequent to decreased lithium clearance; exceptions: aspirin, sulindac (Ragheb, 1990) |
| Aminophylline, theophylline | Decreased plasma lithium due to increased renal lithium clearance |
| Increased glomerular filtration rate (e.g., pregnancy, manic states) | Decreased plasma lithium level due to increased renal lithium clearance |
| Decreased glomerular filtration rate (e.g. renal disease, aging) | Increased plasma lithium level due to decreased renal lithium clearance |
| Increased renal tubular resorption of sodium (e.g., dehydration, decreased sodium intake, extrarenal sodium loss) | Increased plasma lithium level due to decreased renal lithium clearance |

rocognitive deficits, at serum levels that are within the same range needed for efficacy. Older patients are more sensitive to neurological side effects, particularly if they have specific neurological deficits such as mild dementia.

Lithium use in elderly patients requires actively cautious oversight. For the patient with bipolar disorder who has benefited and tolerated lithium well for many years, the dosage may need reduction with increasing age due to both reduced clearance and increased sensitivity to adverse effects. Because side effects may develop gradually, it is easy to misinterpret them as components of the aging process rather than secondary to lithium or other mood-stabilizing drugs. Peak serum levels are associated with worsening side effects in the areas of gastrointestinal upset, altered cognition, and tremor. Use of extended-release forms of lithium reduces peak-to-trough variance in serum levels and is preferable to the use of immediate-release lithium. Lithium's effects on several other organ systems require regular monitoring of renal function, thyroid function, and serum sodium level. If neurotoxicity develops from lithium use, discontinuation of the lithium will result in a gradual return to baseline cognitive function. However, cognition may remain impaired up to several weeks after elimination of lithium from serum. Patients taking lithium should generally see their physician at least bimonthly, both because symptoms can change relatively rapidly and because elderly patients may have greater difficulty summarizing their experiences over longer intervals between appointments. When possible, family members should accompany patients, or staff from assisted living facilities should either accompany or provide reports on patients.

### Drug Interactions

Lithium clearance can be reduced by nonsteroidal anti-inflammatory drugs, angiotensin converting enzyme (ACE) inhibitors, and thiazide diuretics, which though used in all age groups are more likely to be used and employed at higher doses in the elderly (ACE inhibitors, 1988; Jefferson and Kalin, 1979; Ragheb, 1990). Patients over the age of 50 are at greater risk of having lithium clearance impeded by an ACE inhibitor (Finley et al., 1996). These drugs are difficult to track, because several are incorporated into combination drug formulations, so the actual drug ingredients require some extra effort to ascertain. Reduction of lithium clearance is directly related to the sodium-losing properties of the diuretic. A substitution with a loop diuretic such as amiloride or furosemide will not usually result in a change in the serum lithium level (Batle et al., 1985; Jefferson et al., 1979).

## EFFECTS OF OTHER DISORDERS ON LITHIUM EFFICACY AND TOLERABILITY

Any disorder that results in reduced renal clearance poses risks with lithium usage. Although this may occur with acute infections, most such conditions are likely to be chronic and often develop insidiously. Lithium may lead directly to reduced renal clearance over time. A reasonable approach to management is to determine whether continuation of lithium is compatible with the medical condition. If so, the dosage of lithium should be reduced to compensate for the diminished clearance. A selected number of drugs and medical states that may be associated with increased or decreased lithium clearance is provided in Table 18.2.

Hypothyroidism, regardless of the cause, may reduce the adequacy of mood stabilization. Lithium and carbamazepine may cause hypothyroidism. If the hypothyroidism can be brought under control, lithium may be continued. However, if direct lithium effects appear to be contributing to reduced thyroid function, one should consider discontinuing lithium and switching to divalproex or carbamazepine.

## EFFECTS OF LITHIUM ON ORGAN SYSTEMS

Lithium has broad effects on organ systems because, unlike other mood-stabilizing drugs that are lipophilic, its concentration is relatively similar throughout the body. The consequent abnormalities principally affect the kidneys, thyroid gland, and nervous system. Nephrotoxicity from lithium is more likely to develop in patients who have taken the drug for more than 10 years (Gitlin, 1993; Markowitz et al., 2000). Attention to renal effects is not appreciably different from that needed for nonelderly patients. Renal function should be assessed periodically, but not less than annually, by serum creatinine testing, with more specific clearance tests employed if there is evidence of increasing creatinine levels.

For thyroid function, the current highly sensitive measurement of thyroid-stimulating hormone (TSH) is sufficient to monitor lithium effects. However, some psychiatrists believe, largely on an observational basis, that the range of TSH viewed as acceptable for patients with bipolar disorder, independent of lithium use, should differ from that used as normal by most laboratories. Specifically, psychiatrists, including this author, view levels of TSH greater than approximately 4 $\mu$I U/L as predisposing to depression and suboptimal control of mood, and therefore as requiring specific intervention for such patients.

Effects on the nervous system include cognitive impairment, reduction in psychomotor activity, and reduction in speed of nerve signal transmission in extremities. The effects of lithium on cognition have been thoroughly assessed over the past decade. The results allow a greater discrimination of functions impaired by lithium from those that are unimpaired. Understanding these differences should be useful to the psychiatrist in distinguishing between cognitive impairment due to lithium and impairment more likely due to other disease or drug factors. Lithium reduces psychomotor processing speed and verbal memory (Kocsis et al., 2002; Mitchell and Mackenzie, 1982). These effects appear to be independent of bipolar disorder and to be present with both acute and chronic use, and also have been reported in studies of healthy control subjects (Judd, 1979). Conversely, lithium appears not to interfere with attention or concentration (Loo et al., 1981). These effects are accentuated if patients have other neurological conditions, including mild dementia (Van Gerpen et al., 1999). Given the alternative treatments with somewhat better adverse effect profiles for cognitive functions in elderly patients with any dementia, lithium generally should not be used in such patients.

The cardiovascular adverse effects of lithium, commonly referred to as *sick sinus syndrome*, are principally seen in the elderly (Mitchell et al., 1982).

Lithium reduces activity levels in healthy controls and patients with bipolar disorder. The change from baseline in key symptoms and affects in hospitalized manic patients who were good responders to lithium over a 4-week period of treatment, using standard dosing and serum level ranges, was compared with the scores on the same factors for a group of healthy controls. Scores on irritability, impulsivity, and elation were all improved from baseline in the patients. However, whereas end-of-treatment scores for irritability, impulsivity, agitation, and elation remained higher than healthy control scores, the mean score for psychomotor activity of the responding manic patients was significantly below that of the healthy controls (Bowden, 1999). Clinicians and patients may interpret such subnormal activity levels as indicative of depression.

## VALPROATE USE IN ELDERLY PATIENTS

### Divalproex

Porsteinsson and associates (Porsteinsson et al., 2001; Tariot et al., 1998) studied divalproex compared with placebo in elderly patients with dementia and manic symptoms who were 65 years of age and older. Divalproex was superior to placebo in reducing agitation. A nonsignificant trend for greater improvement in manic symptoms was present. Divalproex was started at a dose of 500 mg/day and increased to 20 mg/kg/day. It was generally well tolerated; however, doses above 15 mg/kg/day were associated with increased rates of sedation. These blinded, placebo-controlled data are generally consistent with open reports.

Divalproex is effective in mania and in patients with clinical factors associated with a favorable response, with more than 10 lifetime mood episodes (Swann et al., 1999), mixed manic states (Bowden, 1995; Freeman et al., 1992; Rosa, 1991), and irritable mania (Swann et al., 2002).

Divalproex has been less well studied in acute bipolar depression, but reports indicate that acute antidepressant effects are at best mild (McElroy et al., 1988; Winsberg et al., 2001).

Divalproex has been studied in one recent randomized, placebo-controlled maintenance trial that included 26 patients over the age of 60 among the 570 enrolled. We conducted a Cox proportional hazards analysis, with age and treatment as linear or quadratic covariates. Every year of increased age at study entry reduced the hazard of developing a mood episode over the year by approximately 1%; however, the difference was not significant (patient age estimate: .00894, error .00525, chi square = 2.90, pr > chi sq = 0.09). Divalproex was superior to lithium with linear or quadratic adjustment for patient age (Wald chi square 5.68, pr > chi sq = 0.017) (Gyulai et al., 2003). The proportion of patients who discontinued early because of depression was lower for divalproex than for placebo (6.4% vs. 16%) (Bowden et al., 2002a). Similarly, among patients treated with selective serotonin reuptake inhibitors (SSRIs) for breakthrough depression, the proportion discontinued among those randomized to divalproex was significantly smaller than the proportion among those randomized to placebo (9.8% vs. 45%) (Gyulai et al., 2003). The lithium plus SSRI outcome was intermediate and did not differ significantly from that of the other two groups. The time to discontinuation for depression was nonsignificantly greater for divalproex- than for lithium-treated patients ($p = .08$). Among patients who were treated with divalproex during the open phase and then randomized, those treated with divalproex had a longer mean time to discontinuation than those randomized to lithium ($p = .03$). Among randomized patients who required addition of an SSRI, the time to SSRI addition was significantly longer among those receiving divalproex than lithium (102.6 + 81.1 vs. 59.2 + 62.9 days, $p = .03$). Among patients with previous psychiatric hospitalization, time to depressive relapse was longer in the divalproex group ($n = 100$) than in the lithium group ($n = 57$, Wilcoxon $c^2 = 5.93$, $df = 1$, $p = .01$).

Niedermier and Nasrallah (1998) reviewed factors associated with the response to valproate in 39 patients over age 60. They reported that a full or partial response was associated with a diagnosis of bipolar disorder, female gender, and manic symptoms but fewer psychotic symptoms. Valproate serum levels tended to be higher in better-responding patients, although the differences were not statistically significant (serum level in nonresponders = 57 mg/L; in marked responders = 79 mg/L).

Valproate has been consistently reported to be effective in a diverse group of patients with mood lability, agitation, or irritability in the context of mental retardation (Kastner et al., 1990) and other neurological conditions (Stoll et al., 1994), including traumatic brain injury, infections, and multiple sclerosis (Kahn et al., 1988; McElroy et al., 1987). Most such manic states have mixed features, which may be a factor in the relatively better response of such patients to valproate than to lithium (Freeman et al., 1992; Swann et al., 2000).

Compared with lithium, valproate is of further interest in bipolar elderly because of its superior effectiveness in patients with mixed manic episodes, which are more common in elderly patients. Open studies indicate that the high degree of effectiveness is maintained both with monotherapy and when combined with lithium for up to the 1-year period of study.

### Usage guidelines

The above reports indicate that dose and serum level ranges for divalproex in the elderly are variable, with some patients requiring the same ranges employed for younger persons with bipolar disorder and others obtaining most benefit with somewhat lower doses. In large placebo-controlled studies that included a small proportion of elderly patients, serum levels of 45–110 $\mu$g/ml were associated with efficacious outcomes in acutely manic patients (Bowden et al., 1994). In the 1-year maintenance study of divalproex, serum levels of 70–100 $\mu$g/ml were associated with greater relapse prevention than higher or lower valproate levels, and with greater relapse prevention than occurred with any serum level range of lithium (Keck et al., 2002). The results of Porsteinsson et al. (2001) suggest that dosage at 15 mg/kg body weight may be associated with increased rates of sedation, and should be either avoided or used cautiously.

### Organ system–related adverse effects

Valproate has few specific organ system–related adverse effects. Pancreatitis can occur rarely on an idiosyncratic basis, (Buzan et al., 1995). Valproate can increase hepatic enzyme levels; however, in the largest maintenance study, hepatic function measures did not change with treatment for 1 year (Bowden et al., 2002a).

### Other adverse effects

Valproate serum levels are associated with an increase in appetite that can result in significant weight gain.

Serum levels above 110 $\mu$g/ml were associated with increased appetite, whereas lower levels were not (Bowden et al., 2002a). It is possible, although no reports have so indicated, that somewhat lower serum levels might be associated with increased appetite in older patients, since the active free valproate moiety is a higher percentage of the total serum level in persons with lower serum albumin concentrations, which is common in the elderly. In the face of increased appetite and weight gain, unless a lower dosage can maintain benefits, one should consider discontinuing this drug.

Valproate has a relatively benign effect on cognitive function compared to other anticonvulsants. (Beghi et al., 1986; Prevey et al., 1996; Vining 1987). Elderly psychiatric patients treated with valproate had no changes in Mini Mental Status Examination scores, or side effect scores (Puryear et al., 1995). A change to divalproex alleviated cognitive side effects or motivational deficits associated with lithium use (Stoll et al., 1994). However, some patients will experience obtundation or memory impairment. Efforts to lower the dosage sufficiently to eliminate the side effects are warranted.

Valproate is metabolized principally by glucuronidation. Lamotrigine is almost solely metabolized by glucuronidation. Valproate significantly slows the metabolic disposition of lamotrigine, in general doubling its half-life (Guberman et al., 1999). When valproate is added to lamotrigine, the dose of lamotrigine should be reduced somewhat and then adjusted as clinically indicated. The serum level of valproate is minimally affected by concurrent lamotrigine use.

Valproate has gastrointestinal side effects. These are significantly reduced by the use of sustained-release preparations (Zarate et al., 2000). The extended-release form of divalproex has a substantially flatter peak-to-trough serum level ratio. This is associated with lower rates of peak level–related adverse effects such as gastrointestinal upset when compared to regular-release divalproex (Freitag et al., 2002).

### Lamotrigine

Lamotrigine has been studied in acute and maintenance treatment of bipolar disorder in general adult samples that included patients up to age 75. In one 7-week randomized, placebo-controlled trial of bipolar I depressed patients, lamotrigine was superior to placebo on most outcome measures; however, the primary outcome measure, a change in the Hamilton Rating Scale for Depression (HRSD), did not indicate a significant difference (Calabrese et al., 1999). The lesser sensitivity of the HRSD appeared to be related to its inclusion of a substantial proportion of items dealing with somatic complaints, which are relatively infrequent among patients with bipolar depression. A smaller placebo-controlled study with both crossover and randomized, parallel-group components also reported lamotrigine to be superior to placebo, and to gabapentin in the treatment of depression (Frye et al., 2000). Lamotrigine was not superior to placebo in acutely manic patients (Ascher et al., 2001). Three randomized maintenance phase studies indicate that lamotrigine is superior to placebo for management of depressive symptomatology and relapse in bipolar disorder. The superiority over placebo was found in rapidly cycling patients, particularly those with bipolar II illness subtypes, patients who had experienced a recent manic episode, and patients who had experienced a recent depressive episode (Bowden et al., 2003; Calabrese, 2000, 2003; Calabrese et al., 1999). Lamotrigine was not statistically superior to placebo in delaying the time to intervention for mania in either of the two 18-month maintenance studies. However, a significant difference in the time to intervention was present in the combined analysis of the two studies (Goodwin et al., 2004). Similarly, control of depressive and manic symptomatology over the course of the study, which enrolled manic patients, was positively correlated (Bowden et al., 2003).

Lamotrigine was significantly better tolerated than lithium in the two 18-month studies, with a side effect profile very similar to that of placebo-treated patients (Bowden et al., 2003). Lamotrigine appears to have no mood-destabilizing properties, based on aggregate results from more than 1600 patients studied in placebo-controlled, blinded trials (Bowden, 2003).

### Usage guidelines

Lamotrigine has recently been approved by the Food and Drug Administration for maintenance treatment of bipolar disorder. However, on the basis of the above evidence, the revised practice guidelines on treatment of bipolar disorder published by the American Psychiatric Association in 1992 recommend lamotrigine as a treatment for delaying depression in bipolar disorder, with the highest degree of confidence level used in their rating system (Hirschfeld et al., 2002).

No studies of lamotrigine limited to elderly bipolar patients have been published. As with valproate and carbamazepine, the extensive experience gleaned from the use of lamotrigine in treatment of epilepsies can be extrapolated to most usage and adverse effect recommendations.

Lamotrigine as monotherapy, or as combined therapy in the absence of concurrent divalproex or carbamazepine therapy, is generally started at 25 mg/day, increased to 50 mg/day after 1 week, to 75 mg/day after 2 weeks, and then increased in 50–100 mg/week increments as clinically indicated. Two studies suggest that a steady-state dosage of about 200 mg/day is more effective than a 50 mg/day dosage, both acutely and prophylactically. Lamotrigine is cleared through the liver by glucuronidation. This is the major metabolic pathway for valproate as well. When lamotrigine is started in patients taking valproate, a starting dosage of 25 mg every other day for 2 weeks, followed by 25 mg/day for 2 weeks, then 50 mg/day for 2 weeks, then increased by 50–100 mg/day as indicated, is recommended. Lamotrigine has been reported to be effective in improving the response when added to valproate in patients with bipolar disorder, with good tolerability of the combined regimen (Balfour and Bryson, 1994; Narayan and Nelson, 1997; Patterson, 1987; Smith and Perry, 1992; Walden et al., 1996). When lamotrigine is started in the presence of carbamazepine, some degree of enzyme induction causes increased clearance rates. Therefore, it should be started at 50 mg/day, and increased with the frequency of the monotherapy dosing changes. No specific recommendations for dosage alteration in elderly patients have been published.

If patients stabilized on lamotrigine stop taking the drug for a week or more, tolerance to factors contributing to the hypersensitivity response leading to severe skin and mucous membrane adverse effects is lost. The lamotrigine dosage should be retitrated in such instances.

The half-life of lamotrigine is approximately 30 hours, with a peak concentration at approximately 2.5 hours. Once-daily dosing is therefore effective. The time of dosing can be set at the time most convenient to the patient. Lamotrigine has no effects on hepatic oxidation and has full bioavailability. Lamotrigine is moderately protein bound (around 55%) and therefore has a slight tendency to displace other drugs from plasma proteins.

### Adverse effects

Headache is the only consistent adverse effect that has occurred at higher rates among lamotrigine-treated than placebo-treated patients. At very high dosages, patients may experience some obtundation and concentration impairment.

Lamotrigine can cause a severe rash, which has pathophysiological characteristics of an immune system–activated hemorrhagic vasculitis. The rash has no pathognomonic characteristics but is often present on palmar surfaces and mucous membranes, is painful, is associated with fever, and can be life-threatening. The rates of both benign rash and serious rash have been essentially similar in lamotrigine- and placebo-treated patients in recent studies employing the treatment initiation guidelines summarized above. Early clinical trials in epilepsy employed much higher initial dosing and more rapid dosing escalation, and were associated with rates of serious rash more than 10 times higher than those reported over the past decade (Messenheimer, 2002). Patients need to be informed about the risks and characteristics of serious rashes from lamotrigine and asked to report promptly any rash. This may pose problems in elderly patients who have any cognitive impairment or even severe depression. Therefore, other significant individuals in the daily life of the patient should be made aware of these issues and asked to act on the patient's behalf should they occur.

Unlike approved antidepressant drugs, all of which appear to pose an increased risk of mood instability in bipolar disorder—as indicated by increased cycling frequency or precipitation of manic or hypomanic states—placebo-controlled studies of lamotrigine have not indicated the risk of such mood destabilization. Although some potential for mood destabilization cannot be ruled out, it appears to be either absent or quite infrequent.

The data discussed earlier suggest that prophylaxis of depression in elderly bipolar patients may be more effectively handled by lamotrigine or, based on somewhat more limited data, divalproex. No placebo-controlled maintenance studies of combination regimens with two mood stabilizers in elderly or nonelderly patients have been published.

## Carbamazepine

Carbamazepine was compared with placebo in elderly patients with behavioral disturbances accompanying dementia. The global improvement was greater among the carbamazepine-treated patients (Tariot et al., 1998). No other placebo-controlled studies of carbamazepine in elderly patients have been published. Some evidence suggests that bipolar patients with associated organic disorders are more responsive to carbamazepine than to lithium. Some evidence suggests that patients with frequently recurrent severe major depression may be pathophysiologically bipolar. Mitchell and associates (Mitchell et al., 1991) reported on the effectiveness of carbamazepine in the treatment of 16 depressed patients with a mean age of 64 years (Goodnick and Schorr-Cain, 1991). Three had bipolar disorder and 13 had unipolar disorder. Fourteen had failed treatment with electroconvulsive therapy, as had 11 with lithium. Four patients had moderate responses and three had marked responses. Carbamazepine had to be discontinued in seven patients; the reasons for discontinuation were rash (two patients), hyponatremia (two patients), and gastrointestinal upset or liver failure (three patients). Two patients who relapsed subsequently responded to valproate; only 3 of 16 patients benefited long-term from carbamazepine.

Smith and Perry (1992) reviewed studies of carbamazepine in patients with aggression or agitation as the target behavioral problem. The review included studies of patients with dementia and organic mental disorders, but also studies of younger patients with mental retardation and autism. The carbamazepine studies were considered inconclusive, in contrast to a more positive outcome with beta blockers. The authors recommended that carbamazepine be reserved for patients who have failed to respond to other regimens. They noted that most studies of carbamazepine had been poorly designed.

Patterson (1988) reported on eight assaultive patients with organic mental disorders treated with carbamazepine, but did not say whether other drugs were used. The medication was generally effective, but two of the patients had to discontinue therapy because of diplopia and ataxia. An earlier report by Patterson (1987) of 13 patients also indicated a favorable response to carbamazepine. It is unclear whether these patients included the eight previously reported. Leibovici and Tariot (1988) reported two demented patients whose agitation improved with carbamazepine treatment and who tolerated the drug well. Lemke (1995) studied 15 severely demented patients with aggression who had not responded to neuroleptic treatment for agitation and hostility. Carbamazepine was started at 100 $\mu$g/day and increased as needed. Carbamazepine serum levels at the end of the trial ranged from 2.4 to 5.2 $\mu$g/ml. Haloperidol, which could also be added if clinically indicated, was used in 10 patients at an average dose of 3.4 mg/day. Activation and hostility factors from the Brief Psychiatric Rating Scale improved significantly over the 4-week trial. Carbamazepine had to be discontinued in two subjects due to leukopenia and rash, respectively.

## Usage guidelines

Assessment prior to starting carbamazepine should include a complete blood count with differential and platelet count, hepatic function measures, serum sodium, thyroid function assessment, and an electrocardiogram. Serum levels should be determined for any drugs metabolized by the 3A4 isoenzyme for which therapeutic drug monitoring is indicated (e.g., bupropion). Because of the autoinduction by carbamazepine of its own metabolism, relatively frequent serum-level monitoring needs to be continued for the first 4 to 6 months.

Carbamazepine should be initiated with 200 mg/day and slowly increased as tolerated. Even younger adults often develop neuromuscular adverse effects from carbamazepine (ataxia, diplopia, asthenia, sedation). These complications may be more common in the elderly. Gleason reported that three of nine patients treated with 200 to 1000 mg/day carbamazepine became ataxic (Kruglyak and Lander, 1995). Similarly, Patterson (1988) reported diplopia and ataxia in 2 of 8 patients, and Lemke (1995) reported that 3 of 15 patients had to discontinue therapy due to adverse effects over a 4-week period. These relatively high rates of discontinuance are consistent with reports in young subjects (Denicoff et al., 1995).

Plasma-level relationships of carbamazepine to response have not been found in either bipolar or epileptic patients. Therefore dosing is to the point of clinical response or tolerability. In young adults, responses are generally observed between 6 and 12 $\mu$g/ml. It seems prudent to aim initially for levels at the lower end of that range, especially in patients with concurrent neurological disorders.

Several adverse effects of carbamazepine are more frequent and/or more problematic in the elderly. Hyponatremia is more likely to be clinically significant, causing weakness in the elderly. Bradycardia and atrioventricular block occur principally in the elderly, with evidence of greater risk in women. A review of such complications in 26 patients found the average age of patients with these reported complications to be 65 years and 81% female. Only 5 of the 26 cases occurred in patients less than 50 years of age. Seventy-three percent of the patients developed the various bradyarrhythmias at normal doses and levels. Therefore it is important to obtain an electrocardiogram prior to starting treatment with carbamazepine in patients over 50 years of age and to consider any existing atrioventricular block as a relative contraindication (Kasarskis et al., 1992).

Both leukopenia and thrombocytopenia are relatively common in elderly patients treated with carbamazepine (Tohen et al., 1995). A somewhat more conservative threshold of concern seems warranted in the elderly because of their greater propensity to infections and bleeding problems. However, as with valproate, if the white blood count does not fall below 3000/mm$^3$, only increased vigilance in monitoring is indicated.

Carbamazepine actively induces the 3A4 isoenzyme of the CYP450 family of oxidative liver enzymes. Since many psychotropic and general medical drugs are solely or largely metabolized through 3A4, combined drug use should be undertaken only if no other regimen is effective. A partial list of such drugs is shown in Table 18.3. If it is necessary to use carbamazepine with one of these drugs, when possible, drug levels should be monitored to determine whether they are within the effective range.

## CONCLUSIONS

Mood stabilizers have several useful roles in elderly patients with psychiatric conditions. Clearly, the evidence is best established for treatment of bipolar disorder. However, symptoms characteristic of bipolar disorder occur in a wide range of dementiaform disorders and appear to be responsive to mood stabilizer treatment. Mood stabilizers vary substantially in their profile of

TABLE 18.3. *Drugs Metabolized by the 3A4 Oxidative Isoenzyme That Interact with Carbamazepine*

| | |
|---|---|
| Alprazolam | Itraconazole |
| Astemizole | Ketoconazole |
| Birth control pills | Nefazadone |
| Bupropion | Terfenadine |
| Claritin | Triazolam |

actions. Lamotrigine is the only mood stabilizer that acts primarily on depressive symptomatology. Mood stabilizers also vary greatly in tolerability. As in younger patients, the difficulties with lithium are generally greater, especially in chronic use, than are the difficulties with the other drugs reviewed here. Most importantly, given the substantial number of mood-stabilizing drugs now available, if one drug is not well tolerated, one of the others warrants a trial. By extension, it is important to have trials combining two drugs, with efforts to lower the dose of the first drug to a level well tolerated.

## REFERENCES

ACE inhibitors and lithium toxicity. (1988) Biological Therapies in Psychiatry.

Ahlfors, U.G., Baastrup, P.C., and Dencker, S.J. (1981) Flupenthixol decanoate in recurrent manic-depressive illness: A comparison with lithium. *Acta Psychiatr Scand* 64:226–237.

Ascher, J., Barnett, S., and Batey, S. (2001) Safety and tolerability of lamotrigine in controlled mood disorder trials (abstract). Presented at the annual meeting of the American Psychiatric Association, New Orleans, LA, May 2001.

Balfour, J.A., and Bryson, H.M. (1994) Valproic acid: A review of its pharmacology and therapeutic potential in indications other than epilepsy. *CNS Drugs* 2:144–173.

Batle, D.C., von Riotte, A.B., Gaviria, M., and Grupp, M. (1985) Amelioration of polyuria by amiloride in patients receiving long-term lithium therapy. *N Engl J Med* 312:408–414.

Beghi, E., DiMascio, R., and Sasanelli, F. (1986) Adverse reactions to antiepileptic drugs: A multicenter survey of clincial practice. *Epilepsia* 27:323–330.

Bowden, C.L. (1995) Predictors of response to divalproex and lithium. *J Clin Psychiatry* 56(S4):25–30.

Bowden, C.L. (2000) Valproate in mania. In Manji H.K., Bowden C.L., Belmaker R.H., eds. *Bipolar Medications–Mechanisms of Action*. Washington, DC: pp. 357–365.

Bowden, C.L. (2002a) Lamotrigine in the treatment of bipolar disorder. *Pharmacotherapy* 10:1513–1519.

Bowden, C.L. (2002b) Pharmacological treatment of bipolar disorder. In: Maj, M., Akiskal, S.H., Lopez-Ibor, J., and Sartorium, N., eds. *Bipolar Disorder*. Chichester, West Sussex, England: Wiley, pp. 191–277.

Bowden, C.L., Brugger, A.M., Swann, A.C., Calabrese, J.R., Janicak, P.G., Petty, F., Dilsaver, S.C., Davis, J.M., Rush, A.J., Small, J.G., Garza-Trevino, E.S., Risch, S.C., Goodnick, P.J., and Morris, D.D. (1994) Efficacy of divalproex vs lithium and placebo in the treatment of mania. *JAMA* 271:918–924.

Bowden, C.L., Calabrese, J.R., McElroy, S.L., Gyulai, L., Wassef, A., Petty, F., Pope, H.G., Jr., Chou, J.C.-Y., Keck, P.E., Jr., Rhodes, L.J., Swann, A.C., Hirschfeld, R.M.A., and Wozniak, P.J. (2000b) A randomized, placebo-controlled 12-month trial of divalproex and lithium in treatment of outpatients with bipolar I disorder. *Arch Gen Psychiatry* 57:481–489.

Bowden, C.L., Calabrese, J.R., Sachs, G., Yatham, L.N., Asghar, S.A., Hompland, M., Montgomery, P., Earl, N., Smoot, T.M., and De-Veaugh-Geiss, J. (2003) A placebo-controlled 18-month trial of lamotrigine and lithium maintenance treatment in recently manic or hypomanic patients with bipolar I disorder. *Arch Gen Psychiatry* 60:392–400.

Bowden, C.L., et al. (1999) Lamotrigine in rapid cycling bipolar disorder (abstract). Presented at the annual meeting of the American College of Neuropsychopharmacology, Acapulco, Mexico, December 14.

Buzan, R.D., Firestone, D., Thomas, M., and Dubovsky, S.L. (1995) Valproate-associated pancreatitis and cholecystitis in six mentally retarded adults. *J Clin Psychiatry* 56(11):529–532.

Calabrese, J.R., Bowden, C.L., Sachs, G.S., Ascher, J.A., Monaghan, E., and Rudd, D.G. (1999) A double-blind placebo-controlled study of lamotrigine monotherapy in outpatients with bipolar I depression. *J Clin Psychiatry* 60:79–88.

Calabrese, J.R., Suppes, T., Bowden, C.L., Sachs, G.S., Swann, A.C., McElroy, S.L., Kusumakar, V., Ascher, J.A., Earl, N.L., Greene, P.L., and Monaghan, F.T. (2000) A double-blind, placebo-controlled, prophylaxis study of lamotrigine in rapid-cycling bipolar disorder. *J Clin Psychiatry* 61(11):841–850.

Calabrese, J.R., Bowden, C.L., Sachs, G., Yatham, L.N., Behnke, K., Mehtonen, O.P., Montgomery, P., Ascher, J., Paska, W., Earl, N., and DeVeaugh-Geiss, J. (2003) A Placebo-controlled 18-month trial of lamotrigine and lithium maintenance treatment in recently depressed patients with bipolar I disorder. *J Clin Psychiatry* 64: 1013–1024.

Coryell, W., Turvey, C., Endicott, J., Leon, A.C., Mueller, T., Solomon, D., and Keller, M. (1998) Bipolar I affective disorder: Predictors of outcome after 15 years. *J Affect Disord* 50:109–116.

Davidson, J.R.T., Miller, R.D., Turnbull, C.D., and Sullivan, J.L. (1982) Atypical depression. *Arch Gen Psychiatry* 39:527–534.

Denicoff, K.D., Smith-Jackson, E.E., Disney, E.R., Ali, S.O., Leverich, G.S., and Post, R.M. (1997) Comparative prophylactic efficacy of lithium, carbamazepine, and the combination in bipolar disorder. *J Clin Psychiatry* 58(11):470–478.

Finley, P.R., O'Brien, J.G., and Coleman, R.W. (1996) Lithium and angiotensin-converting enzyme inhibitors: Evaluation of a potential interaction. *J Clin Psychopharmacol* 16:68–71.

Freeman, T.W., Clothier, J.L., Pazzaglia, P., Lesem, M.D., and Swann, A.C. (1992) A double-blind comparison of valproate and lithium in the treatment of acute mania. *Am J Psychiatry* 149:108–111.

Freitag, F.G., Collins, S.D., Carlson, H.A., Goldstein, J., Saper, J., Silberstein, S., Mathew, N., Winner, P.K., Deaton, R., and Sommerville, K. (2002) A randomized trial of divalproex sodium extended-release tablets in migraine prophylaxis. *Neurology* 58: 1652–1659.

Frye, M.A., Ketter, T.A., Kimbrell, T.A., Dunn, R.T., Speer, A.M., Osuch, E.A., Luckenbaugh, D.A., Cora-Locatelli, G., Leverich, G.S., and Post, R.M. (2000) A placebo-controlled study of lamotrigine and gabapentin monotherapy in refractory mood disorders. *J Clin Psychopharmacol* 20:607–614.

Gitlin, M. (1993) Lithium-induced renal insufficiency. *J Clin Psychopharmacol* 13:276–279.

Goodnick, P.J., and Schorr-Cain, C.B. (1991) Lithium pharmacokinetics. *Psychopharmacol Bull* 27:475–491.

Grunze, H., Erfurth, A., Amann, B., Giupponi, G., Kammerer, C., and Walden, J. (1999) Intravenous valproate loading in acutely manic and depressed bipolar I patients. *Clin Psychopharmacol* 19(4):303–309.

Guberman, A.H., Besag, F.M.C, Brodie, M.J., Dooley, J.M., Duchowny, M.S., Pellock, J.M., Richens, A., Stern, R.S., and Trevathan, E. (1999) Lamotrigine-associated rash: Risk/benefit considerations in adults and children. *Epilepsia* 40(7):985–991.

Gyulai, L., Bowden, C.L., McElroy, S.L., Calabrese, J.R., Petty, F., Swann, A.C., Chou, J.C.Y., Wassef, A., Risch, C.S., Hirschfeld, R.M.A., Nemeroff, C., Keck, P.E., Jr., and Wozniak, P.J. (2003) Maintenance efficacy of divalproex in the prevention of bipolar depression. *Neuropsychopharmacology* 28(7):1374–1382.

Himmelhoch, J.M., and Garfinkel, M.E. (1986) Sources of lithium resistance in mixed mania. *Psychopharmacol Bull* 22:613–620.

Hirschfeld, R.M.A., Bowden, C.L., Gitlin, M.J., Keck, P.E., Suppes, T., and Thase, M.E. (2002) Practice guideline for the treatment of patients with bipolar disorder (revision). *Am J Psychiatry* 159(4S):1–50.

Jefferson, J.W., and Kalin, N.H. (1979) Serum lithium levels and long-term diuretic use. *JAMA* 241:1134–1136.

Johnson, B.A., Ait-Daoud, N., Bowden, C.L., DiClemente, C.C., Roache, J.D., Lawson, K., Javors, M.A., and Ma, J.Z. (2003) Oral topiramate for treatment of alcohol dependence: a randomised controlled trial. *Lancet* 9370(361):1677–1685.

Judd, L. (1979) Effect of lithium on mood, cognition and personality function in normal subjects. *Arch Gen Psychiatry* 36:860–865.

Kahn, D., Stevenson, E., and Douglas, C.J. (1988) Effect of sodium valproate in three patients with organic brain syndromes. *Am J Psychiatry* 145:1010–1011.

Kasarskis, E.J., Kuo, C.S., Berger, R., and Nelson, K.R. (1992) Carbamazepine-induced cardiac dysfunction. *Arch Intern Med* 152:186–191.

Kastner, T., Friedman, D.L., Plummer, A.T., Ruiz, M.Q., and Henning, D. (1990) Valproic acid for the treatment of children with mental retardation and mood symptomatology. *Pediatrics* 86:467–472.

Keck, P.E., Jr., and Ice, K. (2000) A 3-week, double-blind, randomized trial of ziprasidone in the acute treatment of mania (abstract). *Eur Neuropsychopharmacol* 10(suppl 3):S297.

Keck, P.E., Jr., Meinhold, J.M., Prihoda, T.J., Baker, J.D., Wozniak, P.J., and Bowden, C.L. (2002, December) Relation of serum valproate and lithium concentrations to efficacy and tolerability in maintenance therapy for bipolar disorder (abstract). Presented at the 41st annual meeting of the American College of Neuropsychopharmacology, San Juan, Puerto Rico.

Kocsis, J.H., Shaw, E.D., Stokes, P.E., Wilner, P., Elliot, A.S., Sikes, C., Myers, B., Manevitz, A., and Parides, M. (2002) Neuropsychologic effects of lithium discontinuation. *J Clin Psychopharmacol* 13(4):268–275.

Kraepelin, E. (1921) *Manic-Depressive Insanity and Paranoia.* Edinburgh: E&S Livingstone.

Kruglyak, L., and Lander, E.S. (1995) Complete multipoint sib-pair analysis of qualitative and quantitative traits. *Am J Hum Genet* 57:439–454.

Leibovici, A., and Tariot, P.N. (1988) Carbamazepine treatment of agitation associated with dementia. *J Geriatr Psychiatry Neurol* 1:110–112.

Lemke, M.R. (1995) Effects of carbamazepine on agitation in Alzheimer's inpatients refractory to neuroleptics. *J Clin Psychiatry* 56:354–357.

Loo, H., Bonnel, J., Etevenon, P., Benyacoub, J., and Slowen, P. (1981) Intellectual efficiency in manic-depressive patients treated with lithium: A control study. *Acta Psychiatr Scand* 64:423–430.

Markowitz, G.S., Radhakrishnan, J., Kambham, N., Valeri, A.M., Hines, W.H., and D'Agati, V.D. (2000) Lithium nephrotoxicity: A progressive combined glomerular and tubulointerstitial nephropathy. *J Am Soc Nephrol* 11:1439–1448.

McElroy, S.L., Keck, P.E., Jr., and Pope, H.G., Jr. (1987) Sodium valproate: Its use in primary psychiatric disorders. *J Clin Psychopharmacol* 7(1):16–24.

McElroy, S.L., Pope, H.G., Jr., and Keck, P.E., Jr. (1988) Treatment of psychiatric disorders with valproate: A series of 73 cases. *Psychiatr Psychobiol* 3:81–85.

Messenheimer, J.A. (2002) Stevens-Johnson syndrome and toxic epidermal necrolysis with antiepileptic drugs commonly used in Germany: Adult and pediatric incidence estimates from registry and prescription data. Poster presented at the annual meeting of the American Association of Neurology, Denver.

Mitchell, J.E., and Mackenzie, T.B. (1982) Cardiac effects of lithium therapy in man: A review. *J Clin Psychiatry* 43:47–51.

Mitchell, P. (1991) Valproate for rapid-cycling unipolar affective disorder. *J Nerv Ment Dis* 179:503–504.

Narayan, N., and Nelson, J. (1997) Treatment of dementia with behavioral disturbance using divalproex or a combination of divalproex and a neuroleptic. *J Clin Psychiatry* 58(8):351–354.

Niedermier, J.A., and Nasrallah, H.A. (1998) Clinical correlates of response to valproate in geriatric inpatients. *Ann Clin Psychiatry* 10(4):165–168.

Pande, A.C., Crockatt, J.G., Janney, C.A., Werth, J.L., Tsaroucha, G., and the Gabapentin Bipolar Disorder Study Group. (2000) Gabapentin in bipolar disorder: A placebo-controlled trial of adjunctive therapy. *Bipolar Disord* 2(3):249–255.

Patterson, J.F. (1987) Carbamazepine for assaultive patients with organic brain disorders. *Psychosomatics* 28:79–81.

Patterson, J.F. (1988) A preliminary study of carbamazepine in the treatment of assaultive patients with dementia. *J Geriatr Psychiatry Neurol* 1:21–23.

Porsteinsson, A.P., Tariot, P.N., Erb, R., Cox, C., Smith, E., Jakimovich, L., Noviasky, J., Kowalski, N., Holt, C.J., and Irvine, C. (2001) Placebo-controlled study of divalproex sodium for agitation in dementia. *Am J Geriatr Psychiatry* 9(1):58–66.

Prevey, M.L., Delaney, R.C., Cramer, J.A., Cattanach, L., Collins, J.F., and Mattson, R.H. (1996) Effect of valproate on cognition functioning. Comparison with carbamazepine. *Arch Neurol* 53(10):1008–1016.

Puryear, L.J., Kunik, M.E., and Workman, R., Jr. (1995) Tolerability of divalproex sodium in elderly psychiatric patients with mixed diagnoses. *J Geriatr Psychiatry Neurol* 8(4):234–237.

Ragheb, M. (1990) The clinical significance of lithium-nonsteroidal anti-inflammatory drug interactions. *J Clin Psychopharmacol* 10:350–354.

Rosa, F.W. (1991) Spina bifida in infants of women treated with carbamazepine in pregnancy. *N Engl J Med* 324:674–677.

Sachs, G., Grossman, F., Okamoto, A., Ghaemi, S.N., and Bowden, C.L. (2002) Risperidone plus mood stabilizer versus placebo plus mood stabilizer for acute mania of bipolar disorder: a double-blind comparison of efficacy and safety. *Am J Psychiatry* 159:1146–1154.

Smith, D.A., and Perry, P.J. (1992) Nonneuroleptic treatment of disruptive behavior in organic mental syndromes. *Ann Pharmacother* 26:1400–1408.

Stoll, A.L., Banov, M., Kolbrener, M., Mayer, P.V., Tohen, M., Strakowski, S.M., Castillo, J., Suppes, T., and Cohen, B.M. (1994) Neurologic factors predict a favorable valproate response in bipolar and schizoaffective disorders. *J Clin Psychopharmacol* 14:311–313.

Swann, A.C., Bowden, C.L., Calabrese, J.R., Dilsaver, S.C., and Morris, D.D. (1999) Differential effect of number of previous episodes

of affective disorder on response to lithium or divalproex in acute mania. *Am J Psychiatry* 156(8):1264–1266.

Swann, A.C., Bowden, C.L., Calabrese, J.R., Dilsaver, S.C., and Morris, D.D. (2000) Mania: Differential effects of previous depressive and manic episodes on response to treatment. *Acta Psychiatr Scand* 101(6):444–451.

Swann, A.C., Bowden, C.L., Calabrese, J.R., Dilsaver, S.C., and Morris, D.D. (2002) Pattern of response to divalproex, lithium, or placebo in four naturalistic subtypes of mania. *Neuropsychopharmacology* 26(4):530–536.

Swann, A.C., Janicak, P.L., Calabrese, J.R., Bowden, C.L., Dilsaver, S.C., Morris, D.D., Petty, F., and Davis, J.M. (2001) Structure of mania: Depressive, irritable, and psychotic clusters with distinct course of illness in randomized clinical trial participants. *J Affect Disord.* 67(1–3):123–132.

Swearer, J.M., Drachman, D.A., O'Donnell, B.F., and Mitchell, A.L. (1988) Troublesome and disruptive behaviors in dementia. Relationship to diagnosis and disease severity. *J Am Geriatr Soc* 36:784–790.

Tariot, P.N., Erb, R., Podgorski, C.A., Cox, C., Patel, S., Jakimovich, L., and Irvine, C. (1998) Efficacy and tolerability of carbamazepine for agitation and aggression in dementia. *Am J Psychiatry* 155(1):54–61.

Tohen, M., Castillo-Ruiz, J., Baldessarini, R.J., Kando, K.C., and Zarate, C.A. (1995) Blood dyscrasias with carbamazepine and valproate: A pharmacoepidemiological study of 2,228 cases at risk. *Am J Psychiatry* 152:413–418.

Tohen, M., Jacobs, T.G., Grundy, S.L., McElroy, S.L., Banov, M.C., Janicak, P.G., Sanger, T., Risser, R., Zhang, F., Toma, V., Francis, J., Tollefson, G.D., and Breier, A. (2000) Efficacy of olanzapine in acute bipolar mania: A double-blind, placebo-controlled study. *Arch Gen Psychiatry* 57:841–849.

Van Gerpen, M.W., Johnson, J.E., and Winstead, D.K. (1999) Mania in the geriatric patient population: A review of the literature. *Am J Geriatr Psychiatry* 7(3):188–202.

Vining, E.P.G. (1987) Cognitive dysfunction associated with antiepileptic drug therapy. *Epilepsia* 28:18S–22S.

Walden, J., Hesslinger, B., van Calker, D., and Berger, M. (1996) Addition of lamotrigine to valproate may enhance efficacy in the treatment of bipolar affective disorder. *Pharmacopsychiatry* 29(5):193–195.

Winsberg, M.E., DeGolia, S.G., Strong, C.M., and Ketter, T.A. (in press) Divalproex therapy in medication-naive and mood stabilizer-naive bipolar II depression. *J Affect Disord.* Dec 67(1–3): 207–212.

Zarate, C.A., Jr., Tohen, M., Narendran, R., Tomassini, E.C., McDonald, J., Sederer, M., and Madrid, A.R. (2000) The adverse effect profile and efficacy of divalproex sodium compared with valproic acid: A pharmacoepidemiology study. *J Clin Psychiatry*, 60(4):232–236.

Zornberg, G.L., and Pope, H.G. (1993) Treatment of depression in bipolar disorder: New directions for research. *J Clin Psychopharmacol* 13:397–408.

# 19 | **Stimulants**

### J. CRAIG NELSON

The use of stimulants in psychiatry has a long history. In fact, amphetamine has been in continuous use for a longer period than any other Food and Drug Administration–approved psychotropic agent. Although the stimulants currently have a limited role in the treatment of depression, it has been suggested that they may be particularly useful in older depressed patients (Murray and Cassem, 1998; Wittenborn, 1982). In part, the utility of these drugs in late life may relate to their potential value in depressed patients with medical illness. This chapter will review the historical development of these agents, their mechanism of action, their pharmacokinetics, the evidence base for their efficacy, their side effects, and finally, issues related to their clinical use.

## HISTORY

The early history of the stimulant drugs has been reviewed by previous authors (Chiarello and Cole 1987; Murray and Cassem, 1998; Nelson, 1995; Satel and Nelson, 1989). Briefly, amphetamine, or phenylisopropylamine, was first synthesized by a German pharmacologist, Edelean, in 1887 (Grinspoon and Bakalar, 1977). In 1910, Barger and Dale described the physiological actions of these agents, noting that they had potent central nervous system (CNS) effects. The dextro-isomer of amphetamine, dextroamphetamine, was found to have more potent CNS effects, including euphoria, alertness, and increased energy, than the *l*-isomer (Monroe and Drell, 1947). It was thought that use of the *d*-isomer might help to reduce the cardiovascular effects of the racemic mixture, and dextroamphetamine soon became the more commonly used form.

The clinical use of amphetamine accelerated in the 1930s. In 1935, Myron Prinzmetal and Wilfred Bloomberg reported its value for the treatment of narcolepsy. In 1936, A. Myerson noted beneficial effects in depressed patients, and in 1937–1938, Charles Bradley described its "paradoxical" value in reducing hyperactivity in children. In 1938, its anorectic properties were identified. Initially, these drugs were quite popular. Only later was tolerance to some effects recognized, as well as the potential for abuse.

Other amphetamine analogs were synthesized, including methamphetamine, that were not used clinically but found a market as drugs of abuse. In 1954, Meier and others described methylphenidate (Ritalin). Once marketed, methylphenidate became the most widely used drug in child psychiatry.

## PHARMACOLOGY

Amphetamine and methylphenidate bear structural similarity to dopamine (Fig. 19.1). Thus, it is not surprising that these agents appear to act primarily through the dopamine system. Amphetamine is a racemic mixture. D-Amphetamine has more potent CNS effects, while its racemate appears to play a relatively more important role in producing cardiac effects. Methylphenidate has generally been viewed as less potent although more CNS selective. It is unclear to what extent the lesser potency of methylphenidate may be related to underdosing and its short half-life. Pemoline has often been described along with the other stimulants; however, it is structurally dissimilar and has not been extensively studied in depression. Most important, it has a delayed onset of action, so that it lacks one of the major advantages of amphetamine and methylphenidate. It will not be reviewed further.

Both amphetamine and methylphenidate are administered orally, are rapidly absorbed, and cross the blood–brain barrier. Amphetamine reaches peak levels in 2 to 3 hours. Its elimination half-life varies considerably but averages 6 hours. Dextroamphetamine is partly metabolized by the liver, but 30% to 50% is excreted unchanged. Renal excretion increases with acidification of the urine, an important facet of management of amphetamine poisoning.

Methylphenidate reaches peak levels in 1–2 hours and has a very short half-life of only 2 to 3 hours. Brain concentrations exceed those in plasma. It is almost completely metabolized.

## MECHANISM OF ACTION

The stimulant agents are indirectly acting sympathomimetic agents. That is, they do not act directly on receptors in the catecholamine system; rather, they en-

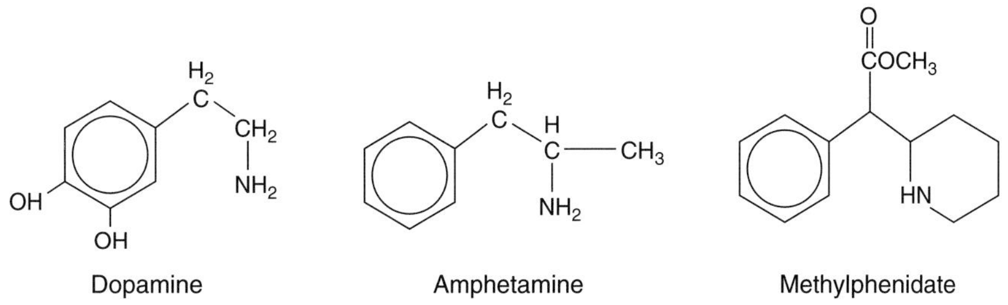

FIGURE 19.1 Structural similarity of dopamine, amphetamine, and methylphenidate.

hance transmission of dopamine and norepinephrine. Dextroamphetamine acts to release newly synthesized presynaptic catecholamines, inhibits catecholamine reuptake, and weakly inhibits monoamine oxidase (MAO) activity. Methylphenidate releases catecholamines from reserpine-sensitive presynaptic vesicles, decreases dopamine uptake, and inhibits MAO activity. Dextroamphetamine appears to be somewhat more potent in enhancing the effects of norepinephrine; however, the importance of this is unclear. The stimulants also have indirect effects on serotonin (Kuczenski et al., 1987; Rebec and Curis, 1981). The psychostimulant properties of these agents appear to be mediated primarily by dopamine, since these actions are blocked by dopamine receptor blockers but not by adrenergic receptor blockers (Jacobs and Silverstone, 1988; Nurnberger et al., 1982, 1984). Alternatively, it is possible that in depression, the noradrenergic effects are additive.

While these agents enhance catecholamine transmission, it is less clear how they act in depression. In depression the role of dopamine has received relatively less attention than serotonin and norepinephrine, although several reviews suggest that dopamine may play an important role (Randrup et al., 1975; Willner, 1983; 1995). Many of the studies that suggest a role for norepinephrine in depression also implicate dopamine. For example, reserpine, which may induce depression in some vulnerable individuals, depletes presynaptic dopamine as well as norepinephrine. In addition, just as some depressed individuals have decreased cerebrospinal fluid (CSF) levels of the metabolites of norepinephrine or serotonin, some depressed individuals have decreased CSF levels of homovanillic acid (HVA), the metabolite of dopamine. In fact, Willner (1983) concluded that the decreased HVA concentration in depressed patients, especially those with psychomotor retardation, is one of the most firmly established neurochemical findings in depression. Finally, just as it has been argued that facilitation of norepinephrine and serotonin transmission by the tricyclics and the selective serotonin reuptake inhibitors (SSRIs) suggests a role for these neurotransmitters in depression, the finding that drugs that enhance dopamine—dextroam-

phetamine and methylphenidate, the monoamine oxidase inhibitors (MAOIs), bupropion, and the dopamine agonists, piribedil and bromocriptine—have beneficial effects in depression suggests a possible role for dopamine (Willner, 1983).

Dopamine has also been implicated as mediating two important symptoms of depression—anhedonia and motor retardation. For example, Wise (1982) proposed that rewarding events activate the mesocorticolimbic dopamine pathway and, alternatively, that interruption of this activity could lead to an inability to experience pleasure. Willner et al. (1992) suggest that the chronic mild stress animal model of depression leads to decreased responsiveness to rewards and simulates anhedonia in depression. These changes are associated with a decrease in $D_2/D_3$ receptor binding in the nucleus acumens (Papp et al., 1994). Chronic antidepressant treatment reverses these changes, but this reversal is blocked by administration of $D_2/D_3$ antagonists. Willner (1991) concludes that the mesocorticolimbic dopamine system mediates the effects of antidepressants on the ability to experience pleasure, a core feature of depression.

Motor behavior also appears to be mediated in part by dopamine. Motor retardation may be associated with low dopamine activity, while dopaminergic drugs increase locomotor activity in animals (Costall and Naylor, 1979; Ungerstedt, 1979).

Certainly agents that influence the ability to experience pleasure or reverse motor retardation might be beneficial in depression; however, in many patients who show an acute response to stimulants, all symptoms of depression respond, not just anhedonia or motor retardation. Further, other effective antidepressants appear to increase interest in pleasurable activity, even if their primary effect is on serotonin or norepinephrine. Thus, while a role for dopamine in depression seems plausible, if not important, and while it would appear likely that the effects of stimulants are mediated by dopamine, it is not clear how this action of the stimulant drugs interacts with the neuropathology of depression. The same questions pertain to other selective antidepressants and reflect our lack of knowledge about the etiology of depression.

## EVIDENCE FOR THE EFFICACY OF STIMULANTS IN DEPRESSION

Subsequent to Myerson's report of the benefits of amphetamine in depressed patients in 1936, many positive open trials were reported and have been previously reviewed (Chiarello and Cole, 1987; Murray and Cassem, 1998; Nelson, 1995; Satel and Nelson, 1989). Several reports specifically noted the beneficial value of these agents in older patients. Nevertheless, the findings overall were inconsistent and sometimes contradictory. In part, this may reflect differences in the timing of effects (acute vs. chronic) or their efficacy in different types of depression. The following groups of studies are reviewed to try to make sense of these findings.

### Controlled Studies of Acute Administration

In 1971 Fawcett and Siomopoulos described the use of dextroamphetamine as a *stimulant challenge test*. Their aim was to develop a predictor of the response to tricyclic antidepressants. Several subsequent placebo-controlled studies of dextroamphetamine or methylphenidate confirmed the observation of an acute response (Brown et al. 1978; Ettigi et al., 1983; Sabelli et al., 1983; Silberman et al., 1981; Van Kammen and Murphy, 1978; Van Kammen et al., 1981). Usually beneficial effects were observed within 24 to 48 hours, although effects were observed as soon as 20 minutes after intravenous administration. The magnitude and timing of these effects appeared to be dependent on the dose and the route of administration. The usual test dose was 5 mg dextroamphetamine given orally tid, and even in severely depressed patients, about 50% showed a clinically meaningful change. Although the predictive value of this test has been debated (Gwirtsman and Guze, 1989; Little, 1988), and it was never widely used, these studies did provide placebo-controlled evidence of the acute effects of dextroamphetamine and methylphenidate.*

### Controlled Studies for Treatment of Major Depression

Ten placebo-controlled studies and one double-blind comparison study have been performed with amphetamine or methylphenidate and have been previously reviewed (Satel and Nelson, 1989). With one exception, these studies were performed between 1958 and 1972.

---

*The controversy about the value of the stimulant challenge test centered on whether the drugs used for treatment were specific for norepinephrine or whether they were mixed serotonin/norepinephrine agents. In fact, if the effects of the stimulants are mediated primarily by dopamine, the challenge test might have been better used to predict the response to a dopaminergic drug. At the time of the challenge studies, these agents were not available. Recent data indicate that bupropion binds to the dopamine transporter and inhibits uptake (Learned-Coughlin et al., 2003). In retrospect, this challenge test might have been better used to predict response to bupropion.

It appeared that the intended sample was comprised of patients with *primary* depression, although most of these studies were performed before current diagnostic criteria were employed. Seven studies were performed in outpatients and three in inpatients. The duration of treatment varied from 4 to 12 weeks.

Eight of these studies found no advantage of the stimulant over placebo. One study did demonstrate an advantage for methylphenidate over placebo (Rickels et al., 1970). The tenth found that the patients' reports favored methylphenidate but the physicians' reports did not (Rickels et al., 1972).

The largest controlled study was performed in 204 depressed veterans (Overall et al., 1962). These patients, mostly male, were randomly assigned to dextroamphetamine, 30 mg/day, with amobarbital, isocarboxizid, imipramine, or placebo for up to 12 weeks. Dextroamphetamine was not superior to placebo at 3 weeks or 12 weeks but imipramine, 225 mg/day, was more effective than placebo at 3 weeks.

Alternatively, Rickels et al. (1970) compared methylphenidate at 15 mg/day, pemoline at 75 mg/day, and placebo in 120 outpatients with mild to moderate depression. Patients were treated for 4 weeks in three different settings—general practice, a psychiatric clinic, and a private practice setting. The patients selected were those who complained of fatigue or apathy. Methylphenidate and pemoline were superior to placebo overall in the general practice and psychiatric clinic setting, but not in private practice.

These studies can be criticized for a number of design shortcomings—lack of diagnostic criteria, inclusion of psychotic depressives, and use of crossover designs; nevertheless, as noted previously (Satel and Nelson, 1989), during the same time period and using similar methods, 23 studies of imipramine were performed (Klerman and Cole, 1965). Fourteen found clear evidence of efficacy and another four found marginal advantages over placebo. Certainly the efficacy of the stimulants falls well short of the track record for imipramine. The tricyclic studies were performed in all types of depressed patients. The positive studies of stimulants were limited to those with fatigue or apathy; anxious and agitated patients were excluded.

### Efficacy in Older Patients

At least 10 studies have been performed in older patients. Five open studies reported positive results (Askinazi et al., 1986; Bachrach, 1959; Bare and Lin, 1962; Clark and Mankikar, 1979; Ferguson and Funderbunk, 1956); however, without a placebo control, these studies were difficult to evaluate. Most of these patients had chronic medical illness.

Five studies in older patients included a placebo control (Darvill and Woolley, 1959; Dube et al., 1956; Holliday and Joffe, 1965; Kaplitz, 1975; Landman et al., 1958). Four of the five found some evidence of superiority of the stimulant over placebo. For example, one study in 61 older, institutionalized, medically ill patients compared methylphenidate 30 mg with placebo (Landman et al., 1958). This was a crossover study with two 4-day treatment periods. Depressed patients were identified who demonstrated depressed mood, lethargy, or fatigue. In this study, methylphenidate was superior to placebo. In another positive study, methylphenidate was compared with placebo in 44 institutionalized elderly patients who were withdrawn and apathetic (Kaplitz, 1975). Patients received methylphenidate 20 mg or placebo for 6 weeks. Significant improvement was seen in interest, competence, and psychomotor retardation.

Although four of the five studies found evidence of drug effect, these findings were difficult to interpret. It was not clear if the target symptoms were depressive symptoms or symptoms of dementia such as apathy. These samples of older, often institutionalized, patients were often described as *senile*. Apparently some of the patients had brain disease, yet diagnostic criteria for dementia were not employed. One of the outcomes described was mental alertness, not a usual depressive symptom. In addition, the principal outcome was symptomatic improvement rather than a rating of response or remission that might be expected in more typical depression.

## Efficacy in Medically Ill Patients

A number of studies, previously reviewed, have suggested that stimulants might be of value in medically ill, depressed patients (Murray and Cassem, 1998; Satel and Nelson, 1989). Most of these were open label studies. The value of stimulants has been noted in depression with various medical disorders and conditions such as cancer (Olin and Masand, 1996), as well as in gravely ill or terminally ill patients (Burns and Eisendrath, 1994; Homes et al., 1994). Murphy and his colleagues on the consultation service at Massachusetts General Hospital (MGH) have contributed several articles on this topic and have published two of the largest series of patients in the literature (Masand et al., 1991; Woods et al., 1986).

In the first series, Woods et al. (1986) reviewed 66 patients treated with methylphenidate or dextroamphetamine on the consultation service at MGH from 1979 to 1983. All patients, who received stimulants for depression and whose charts were available, were reviewed. The choice of a stimulant was based on the judgment of the consulting physician. All patients were depressed. Of the 66 patients, 25 had major depression, 23 adjustment disorder with depressed mood, 2 organic affective syndrome, and 16 dementia and de-

pressive features. All but three met the Washington University criteria for depression secondary to medical illness in that the onset of depression coincided with or followed the onset of the medical illness (Feighner et al., 1972). The mean dose of dextroamphetamine (35 trials) was 12 mg/day (range, 2.5–30 mg/day). The mean dose of methylphenidate (36 trials) was 13.5 mg/day (range, 5–30 mg/day). The mean duration of treatment was 8.9 days.

Marked or moderate improvement occurred in 34 of the 71 trials (48%). Of the responding patients, 93% achieved their peak response within 48 hours. During the period of observation, five patients lost their initial improvement. Only 5 of the 71 trials were discontinued because of side effects. Two of these patients became more confused, but only one cardiovascular side effect was reported—sinus tachycardia. The authors noted that often the patient's medical condition was failing to progress, but that after the depression improved, the patient made further medical progress.

In the most recent of these reports, Masand and his associates (1991) described a chart review of 198 patients treated at MGH during a nonoverlapping 5-year period (from 1983 to 1988). The patients selected were those for whom the consulting psychiatrist recommended treatment with a stimulant, the patients in fact received the stimulant, and records were available for review. The average age of the patients treated was 65 years. One-hundred-fifty-four patients received dextroamphetamine, mean dose 9 mg/day (range, 2.5–30 mg/day), and 44 patients were treated with methylphenidate, mean dose 11 mg/day (range, 5–30 mg/day). Of the 198 patients, 58% had been diagnosed with major depression; the others had adjustment disorder with depressed mood, organic mood disorder, or dementia with depression. The primary medical disorders included a wide array of conditions. All but two patients met the Washington University (Feighner et al., 1972) criteria for secondary depression.

Of the 198 patients treated, 59 (30%) were judged to have a marked response and 80 (40%) had a moderate response. Fifty-nine had minimal or no change. Both men and women responded. Response rates with methylphenidate and dextroamphetamine were similar. Among the responders, 85% responded within 48 hours. The authors noted that this rapid response was particularly helpful, both because of the severity of the medical illness and because of the brief treatment period available on the medical service.

Twenty-nine patients had noteworthy side effects, and 10% of the group discontinued treatment because of side effects. Central nervous system effects were most common, with confusion, agitation, nervousness, hypomania, or delusions noted. Six patients had cardiovascular side effects including sinus tachycardia (three), elevated systolic blood pressure (two), and atrial fibrillation (one). There were no differences between the stimulants in terms of rate of side effects. All adverse events reversed quickly on dose reduction or drug discontinuation. No appetite suppression was observed, and many patients' appetite improved. Three patients relapsed after initial improvement. Most patients were not followed after discharge from the hospital.

In 1995 Wallace et al. reported one of two placebo-controlled, double-blind, crossover studies of a stimulant, methylphenidate, in medically ill depressed patients. Sixteen patients, with a mean age of 72 years, who met criteria for major depression and had serious medical illness, entered this study and 13 completed it. Patients received methylphenidate (5 mg bid for 2 days, then 10 mg bid for 2 days) or placebo for 4 days and were then crossed over to the other agent. After this period, patients received open treatment and some were followed for 6 weeks. The authors found a treatment effect and an order effect. Methylphenidate was superior to placebo, but the order of treatment was also important. During the first 4 days, both placebo and methylphenidate were effective and showed a similar rate of decline in Hamilton Rating Depression Scale (HAMD) scores. After the crossover, the methylphenidate group continued to decline, but those patients who switched to placebo showed no further change. Unfortunately, during the second 4-day period when drug–placebo differences were observed, only 3 patients were assigned to methylphenidate (10 crossed to placebo). In this small sample, side effects were minimal. No vital sign changes were observed. After 6 weeks of open treatment, the five patients who continued on methylphenidate maintained greater than 50% improvement and the four who discontinued treatment all relapsed to within 35% of the baseline HAMD rating. Because of the paucity of controlled trials in this patient group, the study is important; however, the very small sample size limits the findings.

One other placebo-controlled study has been reported in medically ill depressed patients. Wagner and Rabkin (2000) conducted a 2-week double-blind, randomized trial of dextroamphetamine in 23 men aged 18–65 with depression, fatigue and advanced human immunodeficiency virus (HIV) illness. Half of the sample had DSM-IV major depression and the other half dysthymia, subthreshold major depression, or minor depression. The mean HAMD score was 14.9. Patients with a history of substance abuse were excluded. Patients were randomized to dextroamphetamine 2.5 mg bid or placebo. Dextroamphetamine was increased by 2.5 mg/day every 2 days, with a maximum daily dose of 40 mg/day. Responders continued blind treatment for 8 weeks unless relapse or side effects occurred and then were followed with open treatment for 24 weeks. All but one patient completed the initial 2-week trial.

One patient on placebo dropped out because of anxiety. Of the 11 patients assigned to dextroamphetamine, 8 responded. Of the 12 patients assigned to placebo, 3 responded and 1 dropped out. The intention-to-treat (ITT) analysis was significant (Fisher exact test, $p < .05$), although the analysis in completers was not, $p < .10$. The average dose of dextroamphetamine was 22.9 mg/day; the most common dose was 30 mg/day. The authors found little evidence of tolerance. Of 15 patients who either responded to dextroamphetamine during the acute trial or were later switched, 10 maintained their response for 6 months. Four discontinued later because of side effects. Only one patient noted the return of depressive symptoms. The most common side effects—overstimulation, insomnia, and loss of appetite—were transient and responded to dose reduction. No serious side effects occurred. Although the numbers were low, it was suggested that patients with more severe major depression did less well and that the value of stimulants was most notable in less severely depressed patients.

## STIMULANTS FOR AUGMENTATION

In addition to their use in monotherapy, reports of the use of stimulants for augmentation of other antidepressants appeared as early as 1971 (Wharton et al., 1971). Five open studies, reviewed elsewhere (Ayd and Zohar, 1987; Nelson, 1997), reported the value of adding dextroamphetamine or methylphenidate to a tricyclic antidepressant (TCA) or MAOI. Although these studies included 67 cases, none of them was placebo-controlled. In the largest study, Fawcett et al. (1991) found that 25 of 32 patients with refractory depression responded to the addition of a stimulant to a MAOI. Many of the patients had failed to respond to other treatments, and the authors noted that their response was often sustained for several months. None of these studies specifically addressed augmentation in late-life depression, although some of the patients reported were older. And most of these studies were performed during the tricyclic era.

A single case report (Gupta et al., 1992) and two open series of cases (Masand et al., 1998; Stoll et al., 1996) described the addition of stimulants to an SSRI or a second-generation antidepressant. Stoll et al. (1996) added methylphenidate to an SSRI for five consecutive patients, and all five responded. Doses of methylphenidate varied widely (from 2.5 to 40 mg/day), but the usual doses were 15 to 20 mg/day. One of the five patients was over 65 years of age. Masand et al. (1998) treated seven patients who were partial responders to a second-generation antidepressant with a stimulant. All seven responded. A decrease in apathy and fatigue was particularly noteworthy.

An interesting question is whether stimulants given with a conventional antidepressant at the beginning of treatment might speed up the response. This had been previously described for the combination of methylphenidate and a TCA (Gwirtsman et al., 1994). Lavretsky and Kumar (2001) reported open treatment of 10 elderly depressed patients with a mean age of 79.8 years. Eight of the 10 patients responded to treatment with citalopram and methylphenidate by week 8. Four of the seven patients who started on the combination met criteria for rapid response by week 2. Although this study looked promising, it was not placebo-controlled.

Disappointing placebo-controlled study results were reported by Postolache et al. (1999). They added methylphenidate to sertraline at the beginning of treatment to speed up the response. They terminated this double-blind study early because in the first nine patients treated, none showed an early response and, in fact, none of the combined treatment patients met the criteria for a full response at 9 weeks. Dosing of methylphenidate started at 5 mg bid and was raised to 10 mg bid at 10 days. Sertraline was started at 50 mg and was raised to 100 mg. The dosing schedule for methylphenidate was rather cautious and may have contributed to the negative findings. It is also surprising that none of the five patients on combined treatment responded to sertraline, suggesting these patients might be refractory.

## DEXTROAMPHETAMINE VERSUS METHYLPHENIDATE

In large studies in which both stimulants were used, there was little evidence that one agent was more effective than another. A related question is whether these agents treat the same patients. One study (Little, 1993) explored this question in 18 depressed inpatients. The sample included men and women aged 24 to 46 years. The mean HAMD score was 22.8. Patients were treated for 1 day with dextroamphetamine 20 mg and then crossed over for 1 day to methylphenidate 40 mg. Because the HAMD is relatively insensitive to change during a 24-hour period, visual analog scales were employed. Five of the 18 patients responded to both agents. Seven responded to dextroamphetamine only, and five responded to methylphenidate only. One responded to neither. Plasma levels of methylphenidate were obtained but did not appear to explain the behavioral changes observed. The order of treatment had no effect on the outcome. The authors noted that while both agents affect dopamine, their actual mechanisms are somewhat different and might explain the difference in the response observed. Of course, it is easy to criticize this study. A 1-day treatment period may be too brief, and if more patients responded by day 2, there might have been more overlap in response. In ad-

dition, crossover designs are complicated in depression because once changes occur, they may persist into the next period. But in this case, the crossover might work against finding the differences observed. While the sample is small, the results are intriguing and suggest that depressed individuals may respond to the two agents differently. Clinically, the results suggest that a patient failing with one agent might respond to another. Similar results have been reported in children with attention deficit hyperactivity disorder (ADHD) by Elia et al. (1991), who observed that in 48 children treated in a blind crossover study, 36 responded to both methylphenidate and dextroamphetamine, but 10 responded to one drug and not the other. Only two failed to respond to both drugs. And in some patients who responded to both, side effects differed.

## DEVELOPMENT OF TOLERANCE DURING DEPRESSION TREATMENT

Although it is generally assumed that tolerance develops to the antidepressant effects of stimulants, this has not been well documented. It is worth noting that patients with ADHD do not show tolerance to the beneficial effects of the stimulants on attention and concentration, although different domains may vary with respect to tolerance. Wilbur and colleagues first described tolerance to the antidepressant effects of amphetamine in 1937. However, several open studies have reported that tolerance was not observed in responding patients even after years of treatment. Nevertheless, it is hard to reconcile the clear effects of acute administration with the disappointing results from 4- to 12-week trials without invoking tolerance as an explanation. It is possible that tolerance is less of an issue in patients who are less likely to relapse. Perhaps medically ill patients having their first episode of depression are less prone to relapse. In this situation, acute effects of stimulants might be more likely to persist. Alternatively, in patients with recurrent major depression, for whom the risk of relapse and recurrence may be high, the transient effects of stimulants might be insufficient.

## ABUSE POTENTIAL

Amphetamine and its congeners were widely used as drugs of abuse, although more recently their abuse may have diminished, in part because of the popularity of cocaine. Alternatively, among depressed patients or those with ADHD, there is very little evidence of treatment use leading to abuse (Nelson, 1995). It is not clear if the disorder protects against abuse, although clinicians may have wondered about this.

## SIDE EFFECTS

For three decades after the discovery of the antidepressant properties of imipramine, the TCAs were the primary treatment for depression. Numerous accounts indicate that in part, the choice of a stimulant, especially in medically ill patients, was based on the concern that the patient could not tolerate a TCA and the belief that the stimulants were much safer.

The most common side effects are CNS effects. Confusion has been reported, especially in demented patients (Clark and Mankikar, 1979; Woods et al., 1986). Irritability and hypomania have been reported. Suspiciousness and paranoid delusions can occur. In fact, early in the history of these drugs, *amphetamine psychosis* was described (Connell, 1958; Young and Scoville, 1938).

Another issue is whether the stimulants exacerbate preexisting anxiety. Early in the use of these drugs, it was noted that anxiety or agitation might worsen. In one study of older patients Davidoff et al. (1957) observed that 13 of 67 patients became jittery and noted that patients with preexisting agitation did poorly. These kinds of observations were made in several uncontrolled studies and then repeated in other reviews and textbooks. Some subsequent studies excluded patients who were very anxious or agitated (Rickels et al., 1970, 1972). Yet, these findings may be overstated. Controlled studies noted hyperarousal in the placebo groups. Two of these studies reported rates of agitation to be as high as 17% or 25% in both the drug and placebo groups (Overall et al., 1966; Rickels et al., 1972). These latter findings may be more consistent with a recent study finding that levels of pretreatment anxiety did not predict the response to an SSRI, sertraline, or to a dopamine-norepinephrine reuptake inhibitor, bupropion (Rush et al., 2001).

Possible induction of psychosis seems more firmly established. As noted above, amphetamine psychosis has been described with higher doses of amphetamine (Connell, 1958; Young and Scoville, 1938). In addition, elevated levels of HVA have been reported in psychotic depression (Mazure et al., 1987), suggesting increased dopamine activity in this subtype of depression. Near-psychotic depressed patients or those vulnerable to psychotic depression may be poor candidates for a stimulant.

Of particular concern is whether these agents have cardiovascular effects. This concern may relate in part to the effects of these drugs if taken intravenously. At the usual oral doses, however, cardiovascular effects are uncommon. We reviewed this issue extensively and found little evidence of consistent cardiovascular effects (Satel and Nelson, 1989). Effects on blood pressure were variable, with reports of no effects, lower blood pressure, and higher blood pressure. Having attempted to use stimulants to increase blood pressure in TCA-induced hypotension, I was impressed and disappointed that dextroamphetamine was not effective in raising blood pressure at the usual doses in these patients. A few reports describe the use of stimulants in patients with cardiac disease, finding little evidence of common serious problems (Dube et al., 1956; Ferguson and Funkerbunk, 1956). Of particular interest was the finding of Rickels et al. (1972), in a controlled trial of methylphenidate, that the rate of tachycardia observed was virtually the same in the control group as the methylphenidate group (8 of 46 vs. 9 of 46). There have been isolated reports of changes, possibly associated with medication, that were more serious. Askinazi et al. (1986) reported a case of increased ventricular ectopy, Clark and Mankikar (1979) reported acceleration of multifocal atrial tachycardia, and Masand et al. (1991) noted one case of atrial fibrillation. Usually these problems quickly disappeared on drug discontinuation.

## CONCLUSION

The stimulant drugs are certainly novel agents. While there has been great interest in the development of more rapidly acting antidepressants, the stimulants are the only currently available agents that can substantially improve depression within hours or days. Concern about possible abuse potential has limited the use of these agents, and the pharmaceutical industry has not had much interest in developing them for depression; nevertheless, skepticism about these medications runs deeper than those issues would explain. The minimal positive findings in the 10 placebo-controlled studies cited in primary major depression do not rule out their efficacy, but they suggest a more limited role for these agents than for conventional antidepressant drugs.

The literature on the use of stimulants in older patients with depression secondary to medical illness is more intriguing. Although empirically based medicine requires placebo-controlled studies to establish antidepressant efficacy, the very large studies of Murray and his associates at MGH cannot be easily ignored (Masand et al., 1991; Woods et al., 1986). The two controlled studies of Wallace et al. (1995) and Wagner and Rabkin (2000) are supportive but have very small samples. An interesting question, raised by others, is whether older medically ill patients have a different type of depression. Patients with primary unipolar major depression that is recurrent presumably have the same illness later in life that they had before. And recent studies suggest typical drug–placebo differences in recurrent depressives even in late life (Roose et al., 2002) or in the presence of medical illness (Glassman et al., 2002). Alternatively, recent studies suggest that patients whose first depressive episode occurs in late life (Finkel, 1996; Roose et al., 2002) or following serious medical illness (Glassman et al., 2002) do not show typical drug–placebo differences with SSRI treatment. Perhaps depression with initial onset in late life is a different type of depression. Possibly the acute effects of the stimulants in this group are sufficient for symptomatic improvement, and without a history of recurrent depression, the risk of relapse and recurrence is low enough that these early gains are maintained even if tolerance develops.

The literature is in agreement that if a response occurs, it is rapid, usually within 48 hours once an adequate dose is given. This has very important clinical consequences. In patients with very severe depression or medical illness, stimulants may help to avoid a crisis, hospitalization, or electroconvulsive therapy. Depressed patients who have stopped eating or stopped taking their medications for medical illness, may improve quickly with stimulants, and more serious problems may be avoided. Because of the rapid onset of effects, it is usually possible to determine quickly whether or not treatment will be effective.

Methylphenidate and dextroamphetamine appear to be equally effective. Some authors have suggested that amphetamine may be slightly more potent (even adjusting for the dose), but this has not been clearly demonstrated. There is suggestive evidence that some patients may respond to one drug but not the other.

Clinical predictors of response have not been demonstrated. Psychosis and paranoid thinking can occur, and patients vulnerable to the development of those symptoms are usually not candidates for these agents. Clinical lore suggests that anxious patients are not good candidates for these agents; however, controlled studies raise questions about this observation. As noted above, Rickels et al. (1972) found similar emergent anxiety with placebo. And the field is more sophisticated about emergent anxiety during conventional antidepressant treatment. The relative risk of treatment-emergent anxiety with the stimulants and the SSRIs has not been tested. Alternatively, it is suggested that fatigue and apathy might be better indications for the use of stimulants, but these symptoms respond to conventional antidepressants, and to date it has been very difficult to show that individual symptoms of depression predict the response to specific agents or classes of drugs.

There are considerable data indicating that the stimulants have relatively benign side effects. The most common adverse effects are behavioral. Vital sign changes and cardiac effects are relatively uncommon. The stimulants are better tolerated than the TCAs, although this advantage may be lost relative to the second-generation antidepressants, especially with regard to cardiovascular effects. If side effects occur with the stimulants, they are usually manifest early and are usually reversible.

The stimulants have been used for augmentation of other antidepressants. Several small open studies support this use, but controlled studies are lacking. The possibility of early augmentation to improve the speed of response is especially intriguing.

It is generally assumed that tolerance can develop to the antidepressant effects of stimulants, but there are few data from studies following responders systematically to document this phenomenon. And there are many reports from open studies questioning whether tolerance occurs. As noted above, tolerance may be most important in patients who are at higher risk for relapse.

The stimulants remain a unique group of agents. Unfortunately, despite their long history, they have not been well studied. Many important questions remain. For example, how can we understand their mechanism for rapid onset of effects, and might this mechanism guide us in future drug development? Are these drugs really uniquely effective in late-life depression, and what does that suggest about this disorder? The effects of these drugs appear to be mediated by dopamine, but the role of dopamine in depression remains more intriguing than well understood.

REFERENCES

Askinazi, C., Weintraub, R.J., and Karamouz, N. (1986) Elderly depressed females as a possible subgroup of patients responsive to methylphenidate. *J Clin Psychiatry* 47:467–469.

Ayd, F., and Zohar, J. (1987) Psychostimulant (amphetamine or methylphenidate) therapy for chronic and treatment-resistant depression. In: Zohar, J., and Belmaker, R.H., eds. *Treating Resistant Depression*. New York: PMA Publishing, pp. 343–355.

Bachrach, S. (1959) A new supplement for the geriatric patient. *J Am Geriatr Soc* 7:408–409.

Bare, W.W., and Lin, D.Y.P. (1962) Stimulant for the aged—long term observation with methylphenidate-vitamin-hormone combination. *J Am Geriatr Soc* 10:539–544.

Barger, G., and Dale, H.H. (1910) Chemical structure and sympathomimetic action of amines. *J Physiol* 41:19–59.

Bradley, C. (1937–1938) The behavior of children receiving Benzedrine. *Am J Psychiatry* 94:577–585.

Brown, W.A., Corriveau, D.P., and Ebert, M.H. (1978) Acute psychologic and neuroendocrine effects of dextroamphetamine and methylphenidate. *Psychopharmacology* 58:189–195.

Burns, M.M., and Eisendrath, S.J. (1994) Dextroamphetamine treatment for depression in terminally ill patients. *Psychosomatics* 35:80–83.

Chiarello, R.J., and Cole, J. (1987) The use of psychostimulants in general psychiatry. *Arch Gen Psychiatry* 44:286–295.

Clark, A.N.G., and Mankikar, G.D. (1979) *d*-Amphetamine in elderly patients refractory to rehabilitation procedures. *J Am Geriatr Soc* 27:174–177.

Connell, P.H. (1958) Amphetamine psychosis. *Maudsley Monograph, No. 5*. London: Chapman and Hall.

Costall, B., and Naylor, R.J. (1979) Behavioral aspects of dopamine agonists and antagonists. In: Horn, A.S., Korf, J., and Westerink, B.H.C., eds. *The Neurobiology of Dopamine*. New York: Academic Press, pp. 555–576.

Darvill, F.T., and Woolley, S. (1959) Double-blind evaluation of methylphenidate hydrochloride. *JAMA* 169:1739–1741.

Davidoff, E., Best, J.L., and McPheeters, H.L. (1957) The effect of Ritalin in mildly depressed ambulatory patients. *NY State J Med* 57:1753–1757.

Dube, A.H., Osgood, C.K., and Notkin, H. (1956) The effects of an analeptic (Ritalin), an ataraxic (reserpine) and a placebo in senile states. *J Chronic Dis* 5:220–234.

Elia, J., Borcherding, B.G., Rapoport, J.L., et al. (1991) Methylphenidate and dextroamphetamine treatments of hyperactivity: Are there true nonresponders? *Psychiatry Res* 36:141–155.

Ettigi, P.G., Hayes, P.E., Narasimhachari, N., et al. (1983) *d*-Amphetamine response and dexamethasone suppression test as predictors of treatment outcome in unipolar depression. *Biol Psychiatry* 18:499–504.

Fawcett, J., Kravitz, H.M., Zajecka, J.M., et al. (1991) CNS stimulant potentiation of monoamine oxidase inhibitors in treatment-refractory depression. *J Clin Psychopharmacol* 11:127–132.

Fawcett, J., and Siomopoulos, V. (1971) Dextroamphetamine response as a possible predictor of improvement with tricyclic therapy in depression. *Arch Gen Psychiatry* 25:247–255.

Feighner, J.P., Robins, E., Guze, S.B., et al. (1972) Diagnostic criteria for use in psychiatric research. *Arch Gen Psychiatry* 26:57–63.

Ferguson, J.T., and Funderbunk, W.H. (1956) Improving senile behavior with reserpine and Ritalin. *JAMA* 160:259–263.

Finkel, S.I. (1996) Efficacy and tolerability of antidepressant therapy in the old-old. *J Clin Psychiatry* 57(suppl 5):23–28.

Glassman, A.H., O'Connor, C.M., Califf, R.M., et al. (2002) Sertraline treatment of major depression in patients with acute MI or unstable angina. *JAMA* 288:701–709.

Grinspoon, L., and Bakalar, J. (1977) The amphetamines: Medical uses and health hazards. *Psychiatr Ann* 7–8:381–390.

Gupta, S., Ghaly, N., and Dewan, M. (1992) Augmenting fluoxetine with dextroamphetamine to treat refractory depression. *Hosp Commun Psychiatry* 43:281–283.

Gwirtsman, H.E., and Guze, B.H. (1989) Amphetamine, but not methylphenidate, predicts antidepressant response. *J Clin Psychopharmacol* 9:453–454.

Gwirtsman, H.E., Szuba, M.P., Toren, L., et al. (1994) The antidepressant response to tricyclics in major depression is accelerated with adjunctive use of methylphenidate. *Psychopharmacol Bull* 30:157–164.

Holliday, A.R., and Joffe, J.R. (1965) A controlled evaluation of protriptyline compared to placebo and to methylphenidate (abstract). *J New Drugs* 5:257–258.

Holmes, T.F., Sabaawi, M., and Fragala, M.R. (1994) Psychostimulant suppository treatment for depression in the gravely ill. *J Clin Psychiatry* 55:265–266.

Jacobs, D., and Silverstone, T. (1988) Dextroamphetamine-induced arousal in human subjects as a model for mania. *Psychol Med* 16:323–329.

Kaplitz, S. (1975) Withdrawn, apathetic geriatric patients responsive to methylphenidate. *J Am Geriatr Soc* 23:271–276.

Klerman, G.L., and Cole, J.O. (1965) Clinical pharmacology of imipramine and related antidepressant compounds. *Pharmacol Rev* 17:101–141.

Kuczenski, R., Segal, D.S., Leith, N.J., et al. (1987) Effects of amphetamine, methylphenidate, apomorphine on regional brain serotonin and 5-hydroxyindole acetic acid. *Psychopharmacology* 93:329–335.

Landman, M.E., Preisig, R., and Perlmann, M. (1958) A practical mood stimulant. *J Med Soc NJ* 55:55–58.

Lavretsky, H., and Kumar, A. (2001) Methylphenidate augmentation of citalopram in elderly depressed patients. *Am J Geriatr Psychiatry* 9:298–303.

Learned-Coughlin, S.M., Bergstrom, M., Savitcheva, I., et al. (2003) In vivo activity of bupropion at the human dopamine transporter as measured by positron emission tomography. *Biol Psychiatry* 54:800–805.

Little, K.Y. (1988) Amphetamine, but not methylphenidate, predicts antidepressant response. *J Clin Psychopharmacol* 8:177–183

Little, K.Y. (1993) *d*-Amphetamine versus methylphenidate effects in depressed inpatients. *J Clin Psychiatry* 54:349–355.

Masand, P., Anand, V.S., and Tanquary, J.F. (1998) Psychostimulant augmentation of second generation antidepressants: A case series. *Depress Anxiety* 7:89–91.

Masand, P., Pickett, P., and Murray, G.B. (1991) Psychostimulants for secondary depression in medical illness. *Psychosomatics* 32:203–208.

Mazure, C., Bowers, M.B., Hoffman, F., et al. (1987) Plasma catecholamine metabolites in subtypes of major depression. *Biol Psychiatry* 22:1469–1472.

Meier, R. (1954) Ritalin, eine neuartige synthetishe verbindung mit spezfischer zentraler-regender wirkungss-komponete. *Klin Wochenschr* 32:445–450.

Monroe, R.R., and Drell, H.J. (1947) Oral use of stimulants obtained from inhalers. *JAMA* 135:909–914.

Murray, G.B., and Cassem, E. (1998) Use of stimulants in depressed patients with medical illness. In: Nelson, J.C., ed. *Geriatric Psychopharmacology*. New York: Marcel Dekker, pp. 245–257.

Myerson, A. (1936) Effect of benzedrine sulfate on mood and fatigue in normal and in neurotic persons. *Arch Neurol Psychiatry* 36:816–822.

Nelson, J.C. (1995) Sympathomimetics. In: Kaplan, H.I., and Sadock, B.J., eds. *Comprehensive Textbook of Psychiatry VI*. Baltimore: Williams & Wilkins, pp. 2073–2079.

Nelson, J.C. (1997) Augmentation strategies for treatment of unipolar major depression. In: Rush, A.J., ed. *Mood Disorders, Systematic Medication Management, Modern Problems of Pharmacopsychiatry*, vol. 25. Basel: Karger, pp. 34–55.

Nurnberger, J.J., Jr., Gershon, E.S., Simmons, S., et al. (1982) Behavioral, biochemical and neurochemical responses to amphetamine in normal twins and "well-state" bipolar patients. *Psychoneuroendocrinology* 7:163–176.

Nurnberger, J.J., Jr., Simmons-Alling, S., Kessler, L., et al. (1984) Separate mechanisms for behavioral, cardiovascular and hormonal responses to dextroamphetamine in man. *Psychopharmacology* 84:200–204.

Olin, J., and Masand, P. (1996) Psychostimulants for depression in hospitalized cancer patients. *Psychosomatics* 37:57–62.

Overall, J.E., Hollister, L.E., Pokorny, A.D., et al. (1962) Drug therapy in depression. *Clin Pharmacol Ther* 3:16–22.

Overall, J.E., Hollister, L.E., Shelton, J., et al. (1966) Tranylcypromine compared with dextroamphetamine in hospitalized depressed patients. *Dis Nerv Syst* 27:653–659.

Papp, M., Klimek, V., and Willner, P. (1994) Parallel changes in dopamine D2 receptor binding in limbic forebrain associated with chronic mild stress-induced anhedonia and its reversal by imipramine. *Psychopharmacology* 115:441–446.

Postolache, T.T., Rosenthal, R.N., Hellerstein, D.J., et al. (1999) Early augmentation of sertraline with methylphenidate. *J Clin Psychiatry* 60:123–124.

Prinzmetal, M., and Bloomberg, W. (1935) The use of benzedrine for the treatment of narcolepsy. *JAMA* 105:2051–2054.

Randrup, A., Munkvad, I., Fog, R., et al. (1975) Mania, depression and brain dopamine. In: Essman, W.B., and Valzelli, L., eds. *Current Developments in Psychopharmacology*, vol. 2. New York: Spectrum Press, pp. 206–248.

Rebec, G.V., and Curis, S.D. (1981) Reciprocal changes in the firing rate of neostriatal and dorsal raphe neurons following local infusions or systemic injections of *d*-amphetamine: Evidence for neostriatal heterogeneity. *J Neurosci* 3:2240–2250.

Rickels, K., Gingrich, R., McLaughlin, F.W., et al. (1972) Methylphenidate in mildly depressed outpatients. *Clin Pharmacol Ther* 13:595–601.

Rickels, K., Gordon, P.E., Gansman, D.H., et al. (1970) Pemoline and methylphenidate in mildly depressed outpatients. *Clin Pharmacol Ther* 11:698–709.

Roose, S. (2002) Treatment of depressed patients over 75. Presented at the 15th annual meeting of the American Association of Geriatric Psychiatry, February 24–27, Orlando, FL.

Rush, A.J., Batey, S.R., Donahue, R.M., et al. (2001) Does pretreatment anxiety predict response to either bupropion SR or sertraline? *J Affect Disord* 64:81–87.

Sabelli, H.C., Fawcett, J., Javaid, J.I., et al. (1983) The methylphenidate test for differentiating desipramine–responsive from nortriptyline-responsive depression *Am J Psychiatry* 140:212–214.

Satel, S.L., and Nelson, J.C. (1989) Stimulants in the treatment of depression: a critical overview. *J Clin Psychiatry* 50:241–249.

Silberman, E.K., Reus, V.I., Jimerson, D.C., et al. (1981) Acute amphetamine response in depressed patients. *Am J Psychiatry* 138:1302–1307.

Stoll, A.L., Srinvasan, S.P., Diamond, L., et al. (1996) Methylphenidate augmentation of serotonin selective reuptake inhibitors: A case series. *J Clin Psychiatry* 57:72–76.

Ungerstedt, U. (1979) Central dopamine mechanisms and behavior. In: Horn, A.S., Korf, J., and Westerink, B.H.C., eds. *The Neurobiology of Dopamine*. New York: Academic Press, pp. 577–596.

Van Kammen, D.P., Docherty, J.P., Marder, S.R., et al. (1981) Acute amphetamine response predicts antidepressant and antipsychotic responses to lithium carbonate in schizophrenic patients. *Psychiatry Res* 4:313–325.

Van Kammen, D.P., and Murphy, D.L. (1978) Prediction of antidepressant response by a one day *d*-amphetamine trail. *Am J Psychiatry* 135:1179–1184.

Wagner, G.J., and Rabkin, R. (2000) Effects of dextroamphetamine on depression and fatigue in men with HIV: A double-blind, placebo-controlled trial. *J Clin Psychiatry* 61:436–440.

Wallace, A.E., Kofoed, L.L., and West, A.N. (1995) Double-blind, placebo-controlled trial of methylphenidate in older, depressed, medically ill patients. *Am J Psychiatry* 152:929–931.

Wharton, R.N., Perel, J.M., Dayton, P.G., et al. (1971) A potential clinical use of methylphenidate with tricyclic antidepressants. *Am J Psychiatry* 27:55–61.

Wilbur, D.L., MacLean, A.R., and Allen, E.V. (1937) Clinical observations on the effect of benzedrine sulfate. *JAMA* 109:549–554.

Willner, P. (1983) Dopamine and depression: A review of recent evidence. *Brain Res Rev* 6:211–246.

Willner, P. (1995) Dopaminergic mechanisms in depression and mania. In: Bloom, F.E. and Kupfer, D.J., eds. *Psychopharmacology: The Fourth Generation of Progress*, New York: Raven Press, Ltd., pp. 921–931.

Willner, P., Muscat, R., and Papp, M. (1992) Chronic mild stress-induced anhedonia: A realistic animal model of depression. *Neurosci Biobehav Rev* 16:525–534.

Willner, P., and Scheel-Kruger, J. (Eds.). (1991), *The Mesolimbic Dopamine System: From Motivation to Action*. Chichester: Wiley.

Wise, R.A. (1982) Neuroleptics and operant behavior: The anhedonia hypothesis. *Behav Brain Sci* 5:39–88.

Wittenborn, J.R. (1982) Antidepressant use of amphetamines and other psychostimulants. *Mod Probl Pharmacopsychiatry* 18:178–195.

Woods, S.W., Tesar, G.E., Murray, G.B., et al. (1986) Psychostimulant treatment of depressive disorders secondary to medical illness. *J Clin Psychiatry* 47:12–15.

Young, D., and Scoville, W.B. (1938) Paranoid psychoses in narcolepsy and possible danger of benzedrine treatment. *Med Clin North Am* 22:637–645.

# 20 | Antipsychotics

CHRISTIAN R. DOLDER, JONATHAN P. LACRO, AND DILIP V. JESTE

The use of antipsychotics in older adults presents many interesting and challenging therapeutic issues. Frequent concomitant medication use in the elderly, pharmacokinetic and pharmacodynamic changes with aging, and older adults' sensitivity to antipsychotic side effects such as tardive dyskinesia and anticholinergic effects make appropriate use of antipsychotic treatment in this population important and sometimes challenging. In recent years, the development of atypical antipsychotics has provided therapeutic options with improvements over conventional antipsychotics, including a reduced risk of side effects such as tardive dyskinesia and extrapyramidal symptoms, a possible potential for greater improvement in negative symptoms and some cognitive functions in schizophrenia, and reportedly, a more beneficial thymoleptic profile.

In this chapter, we discuss basic principles of antipsychotic therapy, the use of antipsychotics in depressive disorders, and antipsychotic treatment issues in the elderly. It is important to note that antidepressants, as their name implies, represent the primary pharmacological option for the treatment of depressive disorders. On the other hand, the use of antipsychotics for certain mood disorders, while common, is currently off-label treatment.

## PRINCIPLES OF ANTIPSYCHOTIC USE

### Conventional Antipsychotic Pharmacology

The modern era of antipsychotic pharmacotherapy began with the discovery of the antipsychotic properties of chlorpromazine in the 1950s. This finding became the foundation for hypotheses of altered dopaminergic transmission in schizophrenia. All of the currently marketed antipsychotics have significant activity at the dopamine$_2$ (D$_2$) receptor, as demonstrated by in vivo D$_2$ receptor studies. The level of occupancy at the D$_2$ receptor suggests that such blockade is necessary for the therapeutic effects of antipsychotics (Schmidt, 2001). Conventional antipsychotics differ from one another mainly in the potency of D$_2$ receptor blockade and their activity at other receptors, most notably histamine, alpha$_1$, and muscarinic/cholinergic (Stahl, 1999).

Blockade of the postsynaptic dopamine receptors in the mesolimbic pathway is thought to mediate antipsychotic efficacy primarily by reducing positive symptoms (Stahl, 1999). Dopamine receptor blockade in the nigrostriatal pathway produces extrapyramidal symptoms. When dopamine receptors are blocked in this region, acetylcholine becomes overly active, leading to a relative dopamine deficiency and an acetylcholine excess. Antimuscarinic activity can cause such side effects as constipation, blurred vision, dry mouth, and drowsiness; histaminic effects lead to weight gain and drowsiness (Stahl, 1999).

While conventional antipsychotics are effective for decreasing the positive symptoms experienced by many psychotic patients, and while numerous clinical trials have shown that conventional agents are effective for both acute exacerbations and long-term maintenance, five decades of experience with these medications have highlighted important drawbacks (Arana and Rosenbaum, 2000). Such disadvantages include the high incidence of acute and chronic motor side effects (i.e., extrapyramidal symptoms, tardive dyskinesia), frequent partial or poor response of positive and negative symptoms in schizophrenia, high rates of nonadherence, and uncertainty about conventional antipsychotic effects on the long-term course of psychotic disorders (Kane, 1999). In addition, negative symptoms tend to be relatively refractory to typical compared with atypical antipsychotic treatment (Arana and Rosenbaum, 2000), a finding with potential treatment implications with regard to the use of conventional antipsychotics in patients with depressive symptoms. Medications targeting primarily positive symptoms leave many patients with schizophrenia substantially undertreated from a functional point of view (Meltzer, 1997).

### Atypical Antipsychotic Pharmacology

The goals in developing new antipsychotics should be to widen the therapeutic ratio between efficacy and adverse effects and to increase the therapeutic range of efficacy, such as increased activity against negative and refractory symptoms (Lieberman, 1996). Atypical antipsychotic agents were first developed in an attempt to achieve these goals (Miyamoto et al., 2001). With the introduction of clozapine, an interest in the development of antipsychotics with dopamine and serotonin (5-HT) activity emerged. Attention to the role of 5-HT in the pharmacological mechanism of action of antipsychotic medications is a result of the gains in efficacy and improvements in some side effects seen with the currently marketed atypical or second-generation antipsychotics. These agents, which are more potent antagonists at the 5-HT$_{2a}$ compared to the D$_2$ receptor, are reported to have greater efficacy than conventional antipsychotics in treating both positive and negative symptoms (anhedonia, anergia, avolition, and withdrawal) of patients with schizophrenia (Arvanitis et al., 1997; Kane et al., 1988; Marder and Meibach, 1994; Meltzer, 2001; Tandon et al., 1997). Not all investigators have reached such positive conclusions when comparing atypical antipsychotics to conventional agents. In a recent review and meta-analysis of randomized, controlled trials comparing atypical with conventional antipsychotics, investigators suggested that atypical agents were more beneficial than conventional antipsychotics only in reducing extrapyramidal side effects (Geddes et al. 2000).

In terms of side effects, 5HT$_{2a}$ antagonism of the nigrostriatal pathway by atypical antipsychotics may lead to reduced extrapyramidal symptoms and tardive dyskinesia (Stahl, 1999). For example, large, randomized, controlled trials have demonstrated reductions in parkinsonian symptoms (Arvanitis et al., 1997; Beasley et al., 1997; Chouinard et al., 1993; Kane et al., 1988; Simpson and Lindenmayer, 1997) and a reduced risk of tardive dyskinesia (Chouinard et al., 1993; Jeste et al., 1999a, 1999b; Kane et al., 1993; Tollefson et al., 1997) in patients treated with atypical antipsychotics. Further study is needed regarding other promising therapeutic aspects of atypical antipsychotics, including the effect of these agents on negative symptoms, cognitive function (Kane, 1999), and depressive signs and symptoms in schizophrenia (Tollefson, 2001).

No uniform definition of an atypical antipsychotic has been widely accepted. The high ratio of 5-HT$_2$ to D$_2$ occupancy seen with clozapine (Goyer et al., 1996) led to the common belief that such activity created an atypical profile. However, it has been suggested that affinity for both 5-HT$_{2a}$ and D$_2$ receptors does not in itself confirm an atypical antipsychotic profile (Schmidt, 2001). Three features that differentiate atypical antipsychotics from conventional agents have been proposed: (1) atypical antipsychotics have less ability to cause extrapyramidal symptoms or tardive dyskinesia; (2) some atypical antipsychotics do not cause hyperprolactinemia; and (3) most atypical agents reduce negative symptoms to a greater extent than the conventional agents (Stahl, 1999). The ability to improve negative symptoms and findings, suggesting greater improvement in depressive signs and symptoms in schizophrenia patients treated with atypical antipsychotics

compared to conventional agents (Tollefson, 2001), has produced excitement regarding atypical antipsychotics' potential efficacy in depressive disorders. It remains to be seen whether atypical antipsychotics are better antidepressants or are less depressogenic than conventional agents. In addition, more research is needed to determine whether antidepressant activity among atypical antipsychotics is a class effect.

## ANTIPSYCHOTICS IN DEPRESSIVE DISORDERS

In addition to having become the treatment of choice in schizophrenia, atypical antipsychotics are widely used for other conditions. A study of atypical antipsychotic use (not restricted to older adults) reported that over 70% of prescriptions were for disorders other than schizophrenia (Buckley, 1999). Unfortunately, the widespread use of atypical antipsychotics for conditions other than schizophrenia is troublesome in that, with a few exceptions, controlled studies are lacking (Glick et al., 2001; Jeste and Dolder, 2002). One such use for antipsychotics is treating psychotic depression.

Addressing psychotic symptoms in depression is an important treatment consideration, as patients with psychotic features commonly have more severe depressive symptoms (Coryell and Tsuang, 1992; Coryell et al., 1984; Lykouras et al., 1986) and may have worse treatment outcomes (Kocsis et al., 1990; Nelson and Bowers, 1978). In general, antipsychotics combined with antidepressants are the pharmacological treatment of choice in psychotic depression (Vega et al., 2000). Meta-analyses comparing tricyclic antidepressant (TCA) monotherapies, conventional antipsychotics, and TCA plus antipsychotic treatment found increased effectiveness with TCA plus antipsychotic therapy (Kroessler, 1985; Parker et al., 1992; Spiker et al., 1985). The efficacy of electroconvulsive therapy (ECT) was examined in the previously mentioned meta-analyses and ECT was generally found to have greater efficacy than pharmacological treatment. Electroconvulsive therapy is indicated in psychotic depression, and its use has been examined in the elderly; however, there are mixed findings regarding the efficacy and tolerability of ECT in elderly patients with psychotic depression compared to younger individuals (Burke et al., 1987; Cattan et al., 1990; Gormley and Rizwan, 1998; Karlinsky and Shulman, 1984; Tomac et al., 1997), although several prospective trials have found at least similar response rates between age groups (O'Connor et al., 2001; Tew et al., 1999; Wilkinson et al., 1993).

In recently published expert consensus guidelines for the treatment of depressive disorders in older patients, experts have recommended the use of antipsychotics only in psychotic depression. In unipolar psychotic depression, the experts preferred the atypical antipsy-

TABLE 20.1. *Dosing of Antipsychotics in Older Patients with Depressive Disorders*

| Antipsychotic | Average Starting Dose (mg/day) | Average Target Dose Range (mg/day) |
|---|---|---|
| Haloperidol | 0.5 | 0.5–5.0 |
| Perphenazine | 2–4 | 4–20 |
| Risperidone | 0.25–0.5 | 0.5–4.0 (authors recommend 0.5–3.0) |
| Olanzapine | 2.5 | 2.5–10.0 |
| Quetiapine | 25–50 | 50–300 (authors recommend 50–250) |

*Source:* Derived from Alexopoulos et al. (2001).

chotics risperidone, olanzapine, or quetiapine and did not recommend clozapine or low-potency conventional antipsychotics. For those patients with unipolar psychotic major depression currently in remission, most experts believe that antipsychotic medication should be continued for 6 months (Alexopoulos et al., 2001). Recommended daily dosages for antipsychotics in older adults with depressive disorders are presented in Table 20.1.

## Conventional Antipsychotics in Psychotic Depression

To date, there is limited literature on the use of conventional antipsychotics in older adults with depression. Investigations of older adults with psychotic depression suggest that the use of antidepressants and antipsychotics must be carefully considered, as improved efficacy with combination treatment is questionable and older persons are more likely to experience medication side effects (Flint and Rifat, 1998; Meyers et al., 1985, 2001; Mulsant et al., 2001; Nelson et al., 1986). Two randomized, double-blind, controlled trials conducted in middle-age patients with psychotic depression who received amitriptyline plus high-dose perphenazine found a high response rate (78%–81%) with combination therapy (Anton and Burch, 1990; Spiker et al., 1985). While a high response rate was found in these two studies, high doses of perphenazine were used (the mean dose ranged from 33 to 54 mg/day) in this group of patients with a mean age of 45 years. It is unlikely that a majority of older patients could tolerate the high doses of conventional antipsychotics that were used in these two trials. Mulsant and colleagues (2001) conducted a double-blind, randomized comparison of nortriptyline plus perphenazine versus nortriptyline alone in middle-age and older adults (i.e., at least 50 years of age) with psychotic depression. Thirty-six patients with a mean age of 72 years were started on nortriptyline in an open-label fashion, and the dose was titrated to a therapeutic level. Participants were then randomized to the ad-

dition of perphenazine (mean dose of 19 mg/day) or placebo and followed for up to 16 weeks. Both treatments were well tolerated, with only two patients dropping out due to treatment-related side effects and no differences between the two groups in side effect rating scales. Rates of response in the two groups were not significantly different (50% in the perphenazine group and 44% in the placebo group). Thus, two of the more important findings from this investigation are that the addition of perphenazine to a TCA did not significantly improve the response rate and the overall rate of response was much lower than that in other published trials in younger patients.

Despite the potential benefits of adding antipsychotics to treatment regimens in patients with psychotic depression (especially young adults), a previous evaluation of the adequacy of pharmacological treatment received by patients with psychotic major depression found that many of these patients referred for ECT had received no or inadequate antipsychotic medication (Mulsant et al., 1997). This finding, suggesting a need for more treatment with antipsychotics, at least in young adults, should be considered in the context of the previously described finding of reduced additive benefit with the use of antipsychotics in older adults with psychotic major depression.

## Atypical Antipsychotics in Psychotic Depression

The use of atypical antipsychotics in psychotic depression in older adults can only be inferred from a small literature on younger samples, comprised mainly of case reports and open-label trials. Nonetheless, the reduced risk of extrapyramidal side effects and the lower incidence of tardive dyskinesia seen in schizophrenia trials (Arvanitis et al., 1997; Beasley et al., 1999; Tran et al., 1997) make atypical antipsychotics an attractive choice for therapy in this patient population.

The place of clozapine in the treatment of psychotic depression is unclear, as there are only a few reports of clozapine's effectiveness in psychotic depression and no double-blind, controlled trials. Generally, authors concluded that clozapine had some efficacy in treatment-resistant mood disorders. Determining clozapine's usefulness in psychotic depression was complicated, as many of the studies examined samples with a variety of diagnoses including schizophrenia, schizoaffective disorder, bipolar disorder, and psychotic depression (Banov et al., 1994; McElroy et al., 1991; Zarate et al., 1995). Ranjan and Meltzer (1996) reported the successful use of clozapine monotherapy in three patients with resistant psychotic depression.

A few small, uncontrolled, open-label studies and case reports have examined the use of risperidone in psychotic depression (Hillert et al., 1992; Jacobsen,

1995; Lane and Chang, 1998). Investigators reported improvements in psychotic (Hillert et al., 1992; Jacobsen, 1995) and depressive symptoms (Hillert et al., 1992). Some evidence also exists for the use of olanzapine in psychotic depression; olanzapine alone and in combination with an antidepressant has been reported to be effective in case reports (Adli et al., 1999; Debattista et al., 1997; Malhi and Checkley, 1999) and in a retrospective, blinded chart review (Rothschild, 1999).

An important consideration in the maintenance treatment of psychotic depression is pharmacological prophylaxis, as the intervals between depressive episodes appear to be shorter in patients with psychotic depression compared to depression without psychotic features and the likelihood of psychotic features redeveloping increases with subsequent episodes (Coryell et al., 1996; Leyton et al., 1995). For those patients receiving antidepressants and antipsychotics, the question of whether antipsychotics should be discontinued is a treatment decision with possible long-term consequences. While the risk of antipsychotic-induced tardive dyskinesia increases over time and the long-term outcomes of other side effects such as diabetes and weight gain should not be ignored, the risk of relapse may increase after discontinuing antipsychotic therapy despite the continuation of antidepressants (Aronson et al., 1987). One suggested therapeutic strategy (Coryell, 1998) is to gradually taper the antipsychotic during full-dose antidepressant maintenance therapy. Family members and the patient should monitor the possible reemergence of depressive or psychotic symptoms in order to adjust or restart antipsychotic therapy.

## Antipsychotics for Depressive Symptoms in Schizophrenia

The use of antipsychotics for depressive symptoms in schizophrenia is another interesting therapeutic area. Depressive signs and symptoms are relatively common among patients with schizophrenia (Siris, 1994; Tollefson, 2001) and are associated with substantial morbidity or mortality over the course of the disease (Roy, 1989; Tollefson, 2001). Reported prevalence rates of depressive signs and symptoms in schizophrenia (25%–64%) suggest that a large proportion of schizophrenia patients will experience at least one depressive episode during their lifetime (Jin et al., 2001; Martin et al., 1985; Tollefson, 2001; Zisook et al., 1999).

The choice of antipsychotic is an important treatment consideration in older schizophrenia patients with depressive symptoms, although data on this topic must be gleaned from younger patients due to a lack of studies in older adults. In a review of the antidepressant effects of conventional antipsychotics, Robertson and

Trimble (1982) cited 34 double-blind trials and suggested little evidence for antidepressant activity with conventional antipsychotics. Furthermore, in a study of depressed and nondepressed patients with acute exacerbations of schizophrenia treated with haloperidol, the authors suggested that while conventional agents may improve the depressive symptoms present in acute psychotic episodes, these agents may also contribute to depression (Krakowski et al., 1997).

There may be biological support for such a conclusion. Conventional antipsychotics, due to their dopamine-blocking activity in frontal regions of the brain, may be associated with the appearance or intensification of depressive signs and symptoms, sometimes referred to as *neuroleptic-induced dysphoria* (Siris, 1994; Tollefson, 2001). While such dysphoria may not encompass all of the criteria for a depressive disorder, it does adversely affect functional well-being (De Arlacon and Carney, 1969; Tollefson, 2001). In a blinded, controlled study of treatment-emergent mood worsening between patients treated with haloperidol or olanzapine for 6 weeks, the incidence of worsened mood (at least 50% worsening on the Montgomery-Asberg Depression rating scale [MADRS] from baseline) was significantly higher in the haloperidol group than in the olanzapine group (Tollefson et al., 1998).

Possible mood effects with risperidone and ziprasidone have also been suggested (Dwight et al., 1994; Hillert et al., 1992; Keck et al., 2001; Marder and Davis, 1997; Muller-Siecheneder et al., 2000). Overall, it would appear that the atypical antipsychotics may be more beneficial in patients with depressive signs and symptoms than conventional antipsychotic agents; however, additional trials to specifically examine such use are needed. While antipsychotic type may be an important treatment consideration, the use of antidepressants in schizophrenia patients with depressive symptoms is also significant. In a 10-week single-blind trial of citalopram versus no citalopram in 19 middle-aged and elderly patients with schizophrenia and depressive symptoms, the addition of citalopram led to significant improvements in depression and clinical impression ratings (Kasckow et al., 2001).

## ANTIPSYCHOTIC TREATMENT ISSUES IN THE ELDERLY

### Pharmacokinetic and Pharmacodynamic Considerations

The use of antipsychotics in older adults is not without risks. Due to physiological changes in older adults and their greater likelihood of taking medications for concomitant illness, practitioners must consider the medication side effects and drug interactions associated with antipsychotics. All of the most common pharmacokinetic parameters (i.e., absorption, distribution, metabolism, and excretion) and pharmacodynamic factors can be affected by age. With respect to antipsychotic therapy in the elderly, changes in body composition, hepatic function, and increased variability among individuals may lead to substantial changes in medication action. Lipid-soluble medications, such as antipsychotics, distribute more widely and may take longer to be eliminated due to a general increase in body fat relative to total body weight with increasing age. Hepatic function may decline with age as a result of decreased hepatic perfusion, reducing metabolic enzyme activity. As a result of the pharmacokinetic and pharmacodynamic changes in the elderly, even wider variations in antipsychotic plasma concentrations can be seen among persons given identical doses of an antipsychotic medication (Maixner et al., 1999; Sweet and Pollock, 1998).

## Antipsychotic Side Effects

Antipsychotic medications carry a risk of side effects such as sedation, hypotension, dry mouth, blurred vision, tachycardia, cardiac effects, amenorrhea, galactorrhea, hyperpyrexia, pigmentary retinopathy, weight gain and associated metabolic changes, allergic reactions, and seizures (Arana and Rosenbaum, 2000). The propensity to cause certain side effects varies among individual medications and with the type of antipsychotic (conventional vs. atypical). Older adults treated with antipsychotics may also be at increased risk for certain medication-induced side effects, such as orthostasis, falls, tardive dyskinesia, and anticholinergic effects.

Orthostatic hypotension is a common side effect of antipsychotics and can be a major contributor to the occurrence of falls, especially in the elderly. The importance of not increasing elderly patients' risk of falling is well known in view of the morbidity and mortality associated with falls. Those antipsychotics most likely to cause orthostasis are low-potency conventional antipsychotics and clozapine; risperidone and quetiapine may also cause orthostatic hypotension (Tandon, 1998). In general, thoughtful titration should be used when initiating therapy with agents that can cause orthostasis in the elderly.

Anticholinergic side effects such as constipation, urinary retention, dry mouth, blurry vision, and cognitive deficits are all adverse effects to which the elderly population is susceptible. Antipsychotics have varying levels of anticholinergic activity; low-potency conventional agents and clozapine have the most anticholinergic effects. Medications with an increased propensity to cause anticholinergic side effects should generally be avoided in elderly individuals. They may also lead to adjuvant medication and polypharmacy in an attempt to treat adverse side effects. Choosing an agent with fewer anticholinergic properties is important in elderly patients (Maixner et al., 1999).

Reduced bone mineral density and osteoporosis are major health concerns in the elderly, especially in postmenopausal women. Elevated prolactin secretion, which can lead to a decrease in bone mineral density, has been noted with conventional antipsychotics and with higher doses of risperidone (Halbreich and Palter, 1996; Halbreich et al. 1995; Klibanski et al., 1980; Maixner et al., 1999). While large, prospective studies of the effects of antipsychotics on bone mineral density in the elderly have not been published, the possibility of reduced bone mineral density combined with the potential for orthostasis and falls in the elderly make the risk of fractures a potential concern.

The possible cardiac effects of antipsychotics are another important consideration in choosing antipsychotic therapy for the elderly. A number of antipsychotics, most notably thioridazine and ziprasidone, have been shown to prolong ventricular repolarization, which appears on the electrocardiogram (ECG) as a prolonged QT interval (although no published data exist in elderly patients treated with ziprasidone) (Fayek et al., 2001; Thomas, 1994; Warner et al., 1996). Some patients can develop the life-threatening cardiac arrhythmia torsades de pointes, with symptoms ranging from asymptomatic palpitations to sudden cardiac death (Fayek et al., 2001; Ray et al., 2001). In the elderly, the combination of such variables as multiple medications, concomitant medications that may increase plasma concentrations of agents that prolong the QT interval, the possibility of cardiac arrhythmias being dose-related, and the elderly's sensitivity to cardiac effects of medications makes it advisable to avoid antipsychotics that produce additional cardiac changes, such as thioridazine (Branchey et al., 1978; Fayek et al., 2001). Baseline ECGs should be performed prior to initiating therapy with an antipsychotic, and regular ECG monitoring may be advisable in some patients.

## Long-Term Side Effects of Antipsychotics

In general, antipsychotics are prescribed for prolonged periods of time, exposing patients to such long-term side effects as tardive dyskinesia, weight gain, diabetes, and cardiac effects. Concern regarding side effects such as weight gain, diabetes, and hyperlipidemia with atypical antipsychotics has increased due to studies conducted primarily in younger adults with schizophrenia. Substantial weight gain may negatively affect long-term patient health by contributing to co-morbid conditions such as diabetes, coronary artery disease, and hypertension (Must et al., 1999). While weight gain has been reported with conventional antipsychotics, more weight gain has been seen with such atypical agents as clozapine, olanzapine, and, to a lesser extent, quetiapine (Meyer, 2001). Unfortunately, increases in weight do not occur without potentially affecting other aspects of health. For example, weight gain leads to an increase in triglyceride levels, which in turn leads to an increased risk of serious events such as coronary artery disease and cerebrovascular accidents (Wirshing, 2001). Additionally, even relatively small increases in visceral adipose tissue can cause insulin resistance (Lebovitz, 2001), worsening existing diabetes or potentially leading to its development in susceptible individuals. While the mechanism is uncertain, hyperglycemia, new-onset diabetes, and worsening of existing diabetes have been associated with the use of atypical antipsychotics, most frequently clozapine and olanzapine (Haupt and Newcomer, 2001; Jin et al., 2002; Wirshing, 2001; Wirshing et al., 1998). The long-term consequences of weight gain, diabetes, and hyperlipidemia should prompt providers to regularly monitor the weight and glucose of patients who are prescribed antipsychotics. Older adults should not be exempt from such monitoring, as old age is not an excuse to ignore such potential long-term side effects of atypical antipsychotics.

An especially bothersome long-term side effect of antipsychotic treatment, especially with conventional agents, is tardive dyskinesia (TD). The TD syndrome consists of abnormal, involuntary movements, usually choreoathetoid in nature (American Psychiatric Association 2000). Typically, orofacial and upper extremity musculature is involved, with orofacial dyskinesias occurring in about 80% of patients who develop TD. In some patients the trunk, lower extremities, pharynx, and diaphragm are also affected. Usually TD appears after at least 3 months of antipsychotic treatment; however, only 1 month of treatment with an antipsychotic is necessary to diagnosis TD in older adults. Unfortunately, other than discontinuation of antipsychotics, there are no consistently reliable treatments for TD. A number of trials have examined the effects of vitamin E, with mixed results, and other small experimental trials have been conducted, but further study is needed (Gupta et al., 1999).

In a review of 76 studies reporting the prevalence of TD published from 1960 to 1990, Yassa and Jeste (1992) reported an overall prevalence of TD of 24.2% in a total population of approximately 40,000 patients. Kane and coworkers (1992) prospectively studied over 850 patients (mean age, 29 years) and determined the incidence of TD after cumulative exposure to conventional antipsychotics to be 5% after 1 year, 18.5% after 4 years, and 40% after 8 years. The incidence in older populations has been found to be much higher. Saltz and colleagues (1991) reported an incidence of 31% after 43 weeks of conventional antipsychotic treatment in a population of elderly patients. Jeste and colleagues (1995, 1999b, 1999c) evaluated 439 psychiatric patients with a mean age of 65 years and found that 28.8% of them met criteria for TD during the first 12 months of study treatment; 50.1% had TD by the end of 24 months and 63.1% by the end of 36 months. Furthermore, aging consistently appears to be the most important risk factor for the development of TD, as the prevalence, severity of dyskinetic symptoms, and intractability of the course of the disease increase with advancing age.

The most important development regarding TD has been the increasing evidence supporting a reduced risk of TD with atypical antipsychotics. The lower risk of extrapyramidal symptoms with atypical agents has led to the belief that these agents would also have a reduced TD risk, a conclusion supported by the low risk of TD seen in clozapine-treated individuals (Kane et al., 1993). A lower incidence of TD has been reported with risperidone. A study of elderly institutionalized dementia patients treated with risperidone found a 1-year cumulative incidence rate of persistent TD of 2.6%. An investigation of the 9-month cumulative incidence of TD in older patients treated with risperidone or haloperidol found that risperidone-treated patients were significantly less likely to develop TD than patients treated with haloperidol (Jeste et al., 1999a, 2000). Furthermore, studies have shown a reduction in TD symptoms in patients with existing TD after they switch from a conventional to an atypical antipsychotic (Jeste et al., 1997; Kane et al., 1993; Littrell et al., 1998; Simpson et al., 1978; Street et al., 2000). While most of the studies involved younger patients, the reduced risk of developing or worsening TD with atypical antipsychotics appears generalizable across age groups. The reduced risk of TD with atypical antipsychotics, when used at appropriate doses, supports their use as therapeutic options and preventive measures for TD.

## SUMMARY

Clearly, due to their improved side effect profile, atypical antipsychotics are preferred over conventional agents in older adults with psychotic disorders. Nevertheless, atypical antipsychotics are not without side effects, an issue that is magnified during prolonged treatment and in disorders for which the efficacy of atypical antipsychotics has not been clearly established, such as psychotic depression in elderly individuals. Based on limited data, the use of atypical antipsychotics is preferred in patients with schizophrenia experiencing depressive signs and symptoms. In addition, the use of an atypical antipsychotic in older adults with psychotic depression is possible, although there are no published data in this area and a recent trial raised questions regarding the efficacy of an antidepressant and conventional antipsychotic combination in older adults with psychotic depression. Due to the pharmacokinetic and pharmacodynamic changes in the elderly and their increased likelihood of experiencing certain medication side effects, the use of atypical antipsychotics in this population must be carefully considered. Controlled studies examining the efficacy and safety of antipsychotics in older adults with depressive and other mood disorders are needed.

ACKNOWLEDGMENTS
This work was supported, in part, by the National Institute of Mental Health Grants MH19934 and MH49671 and by the Department of Veterans Affairs Healthcare System.

REFERENCES

Adli, M., Rossius, W., and Bauer, M. (1999) Olanzapine in the treatment of depressive disorders with psychotic symptoms. *Nervenarzt* 70:68–71.

Alexopoulos, G.S., Katz, I.R., Reynolds, C.F., et al. (2001, October) The expert consensus guideline series: Pharmacotherapy of depressive disorders in older patients. *Postgrad Med* (special report).

American Psychiatric Association. (2000) *Diagnostic and Statistical Manual of Mental Disorders*, 4th ed., text revision. Washington, DC: American Psychiatric Association.

Anton, R.F. and Burch, E.A. (1990) Amoxapine versus amitriptyline combined with perphenazine in the treatment of psychotic depression. *Am J Psychiatry* 147:1203–1208.

Arana, G.W. and Rosenbaum, J.F. (2000) *Handbook of Psychiatric Drug Therapy*, 4th ed. Philadelphia: Lippincott Williams & Wilkins.

Aronson, T., Shukla, S., and Hoff, A. (1987) Continuation therapy after ECT for delusional depression: A naturalistic study of prophylactic treatments and relapse. *Convul Ther* 3:251–259.

Arvanitis, L.A., Miller, B.G., and the Seroquel Trial 13 Study Group. (1997) Multiple fixed doses of "seroquel" (quetiapine) in patients with acute exacerbation of schizophrenia: A comparison with haloperidol and placebo. *Biol Psychiatry* 42:233–246.

Banov, M.D., Zarate, C.A., and Tohen, M. (1994) Clozapine therapy in refractory affective disorders: Polarity predicts response in long-term follow-up. *J Clin Psychiatry* 55:295–300.

Beasley, C.M., et al. (1997) Olanzapine versus haloperidol: Acute phase results of the international double-blind olanzapine trial. *Eur J Neuropsychopharmacol* 7:125–137.

Beasley, C.M., et al. (1999) Randomized double-blind comparison of the incidence of tardive dyskinesia in patients with schizophrenia during long-term treatment with olanzapine or haloperidol. *Br J Psychiatry* 174:23–30.

Branchey, M.H., Lee, J.H., and Ramesh, A. (1978) High- and low-potency neuroleptics in elderly psychiatric patients. *JAMA* 239:1860–1862.

Buckley, P.F. (1999) New antipsychotic agents: Emerging clinical profiles. *J Clin Psychiatry* 60:12–17.

Burke, W.J., et al. (1987) The safety of ECT in geriatric psychiatry. *J Am Geriatr Soc* 35:516–521.

Cattan, R.A., et al. (1990) Electroconvulsive therapy in octogenarians. *J Am Geriatr Soc* 38:753–758.

Chouinard, G., et al. (1993) A Canadian multicenter placebo-controlled study of fixed doses of risperidone and haloperidol in the treatment of chronic schizophrenic patients. *J Clin Psychopharmacol* 13:25–40.

Coryell, W. (1998) The treatment of psychotic depression. *J Clin Psychiatry* 59:22–27.

Coryell, W. (1996) Importance of psychotic features to long-term course in major depressive disorder. *Am J Psychiatry* 153:483–489.

Coryell, W., Pfohl, B., and Zimmerman, M. (1984) The clinical and neuroendocrine features of psychotic depression. *J Ment Disorder* 172:521–528.

Coryell, W., and Tsuang, D. (1992) Hypothalamic-pituitary-adrenal axis hyperactivity and psychosis: Recovery during an 8-year follow-up. *Am J Psychiatry* 149:1033–1039.

De Arlacon, R., and Carney, M.P. (1969) Severe depressive mood changes following slow release intramuscular fluphenazine injections. *Br Med J* 3:564–567.

Debattista, C. et al. (1997) Treatment of psychotic depression. *Am J Psychiatry* 154:1625–1626.

Dwight, M.M., et al. (1994) Antidepressant activity and mania associated with risperidone treatment of schizoaffective disorder. *Lancet* 344:1029–1030.

Fayek, M., et al. (2001) Cardiac effects of antipsychotic medications. *Psychiatr Serv* 52:607–609.

Flint, A.J., and Rifat, S.L. (1998) The treatment of psychotic depression in later life: A comparison of pharmacotherapy and ECT. *Int J Geriatr Psychiatry* 13:23–28.

Geddes, J., et al. (2000) Atypical antipsychotics in the treatment of schizophrenia: Systematic overview and meta-regression analysis. *Br Med J* 321:1371–1376.

Glick, I.D., et al. (2001) Treatment with atypical antipsychotics: New indications and new populations. *J Psychiatr Res* 35:187–191.

Gormley, N., and Rizwan, M.R. (1998) Prevalance and clinical correlates of psychotic symptoms in Alzheimer's disease. *Int J Geriatr Psychiatry* 13:410–414.

Goyer, P.F., et al. (1996) PET measurements of neuroreceptor occupancy by typical and atypical neuroleptics. *J Nucl Med* 37:1122–1127.

Gupta, S., et al. (1999) Tardive dyskinesia: Review of treatments past, present, and future. *Ann Clin Psychiatry* 11:257–266.

Halbreich, U., and Palter, S. (1996) Accelerated osteoporosis in psychiatric patients: Possible pathophysiological processes. *Schizophr Bull* 22:447–454.

Halbreich, U., et al. (1995) Decreased bone mineral density in medicated psychiatric patients. *Psychosom Med* 57:485–491.

Haupt, D.W., and Newcomer, J.W. (2001) Hyperglycemia and antipsychotic medications. *J Clin Psychiatry* 62:15–26.

Hillert, A., et al. (1992) Risperidone in the treatment of disorders with a combined psychotic and depressive syndrome—a functional approach. *Pharmacopsychiatry* 25:213–217.

Jacobsen, F.M. (1995) Risperidone in the treatment of affective illness and obsessive-compulsive disorder. *J Clin Psychiatry* 56:423–429.

Jeste, D.V., and Dolder, C. (2002) Treatment of non-schizophrenic disorder: Focus on atypical antipsychotics. *J Psychiatr Res* (in press).

Jeste, D.V., et al. (1995) Risk of tardive dyskinesia in older patients: A prospective longitudinal study of 266 patients. *Arch Gen Psychiatry* 52:756–765.

Jeste, D.V., et al. (1997) A clinical evaluation of risperidone in the treatment of schizophrenia: A 10-week, open-label, multicenter trial involving 945 patients. *Psychopharmacology* 131:239–247.

Jeste, D.V., et al. (1999a) Lower incidence of tardive dyskinesia with risperidone compared with haloperidol in older patients. *J Am Geriatr Soc* 47:716–719.

Jeste, D.V., et al. (1999b) Incidence of tardive dyskinesia in early stages of low-dose treatment with typical neuroleptics in older patients. *Am J Psychiatry* 156:309–311.

Jeste, D.V., et al. (2000) Low incidence of persistent tardive dyskinesia in elderly patients with dementia treated with risperidone. *Am J Psychiatry* 157:1150–1155.

Jeste, D.V., et al. (1999c) Conventional vs. newer antipsychotics in elderly patients. *Am J Geriatr Psychiatry* 7:70–76.

Jin, H., et al. (2001) Association of depressive symptoms and functioning in schizophrenia: A study in older outpatients. *J Clin Psychiatry* 62:797–803.

Jin, H., Meyer, J.M., and Jeste, D.V. (2002) Phenomenology of and risk factors for new-onset diabetes mellitus and diabetic ketoacidosis associated with atypical antipsychotics: An analysis of 45 published cases. *Ann Clin Psychiatry* 14:59–64.

Kane, J.M. (1999) Pharmacologic treatment of schizophrenia. *Biol Psychiatry* 46:1396–1408.

Kane, J.M., et al. (1988) Clozapine for the treatment resistant schizophrenic: A double-blind comparison with chlorpromazine. *Arch Gen Psychiatry* 45:789–796.

Kane, J.M., et al. (1992) *Tardive Dyskinesia: A Task Force Report of the American Psychiatric Association.* Washington, DC: American Psychiatric Association.

Kane, J.M., et al. (1993) Does clozapine cause tardive dyskinesia? *J Clin Psychiatry* 54:327–330.

Karlinsky, H., and Shulman, K.I. (1984) The clinical use of electroconvulsive therapy in old age. *J Am Geriatr Soc* 32(3):183–186.

Kasckow, J.W., et al. (2001) Citalopram augmentation of antipsychotic treatment in older schizophrenia patients. *Int J Geriatr Psychiatry* 16:1163–1167.

Keck, P.E., Reeves, K.R., and Harrigan, E.P. (2001) Ziprasidone in the short-term treatment of patients with schizoaffective disorder: Results from two double-blind, placebo-controlled, multicenter trials. *J Clin Psychopharmacol* 21:27–35.

Klibanski, A., et al. (1980) Decreased bone density in hyperprolactinemic women. *N Engl J Med* 303:1511–1514.

Kocsis, J.H., et al. (1990) Response to treatment with antidepressants of patients with severe or moderate nonpsychotic depression and of patients with psychotic depression. *Am J Psychiatry* 147:621–624.

Krakowski, M., Czobor, P., and Volavka, J. (1997) Effect of neuroleptic treatment on depressive symptoms in acute schizophrenic episodes. *Psychiatry Res* 71:19–26.

Kroessler, D. (1985) Relative efficacy rates for therapies of delusional depression. *Convuls Ther* 1:173–182.

Lane, H.Y., and Chang, W.H. (1998) Risperidone monotherapy for psychotic depression unresponsive to other treatments. *J Clin Psychiatry* 59:624.

Lebovitz, H.E. (2001) Diagnosis, classification, and pathogenesis of diabetes mellitus. *J Clin Psychiatry* 62:5–9.

Leyton, M., et al. (1995) Psychotic symptoms and vulnerability to recurrent major depression. *J Affect Disord* 33:107–115.

Lieberman, J.A. (1996) Atypical antipsychotic drugs as a first-line treatment of schizophrenia: A rationale and hypothesis. *J Clin Psychiatry* 57:68–71.

Littrell, K.H., et al. (1998) Marked reduction of tardive dyskinesia with olanzapine. *Arch Gen Psychiatry* 55:279–280.

Lykouras, E., et al. (1986) Delusional depression: Phenomenology and response to treatment. A prospective study. *Acta Psychiatr Scand* 73:324–329.

Maixner, S.M., Mellow, A.M., and Tandon, R. (1999) The efficacy, safety, and tolerability of antipsychotics in the elderly. *J Clin Psychiatry* 60:29–41.

Malhi, G.S., and Checkley, S.A. (1999) Olanzapine in the treatment of psychotic depression. *Br J Psychiatry* 174:460–463.

Marder, S.R., and Davis, J.M. (1997) The effects of risperidone on the five dimensions of schizophrenia derived by factor analysis: Combined results of the North American trials. *J Clin Psychiatry* 58:538–546.

Marder, S.R., and Meibach, R.C. (1994) Risperidone in the treatment of schizophrenia. *Am J Psychiatry* 151:825–835.

Martin, R.L., et al. (1985) Frequency and differential diagnosis of depressive syndromes in schizophrenia. *J Clin Psychiatry* 46:6–13.

McElroy, S.L., Dessain, E.C., and Pope, H.G. (1991) Clozapine in the treatment of psychotic mood disorders, schizoaffective disorder, and schizophrenia. *J Clin Psychiatry* 52:411–414.

Meltzer, H.Y. (1997) Treatment-resistant schizophrenia-the role of clozapine. *Curr Med Res Opin* 14:1–20.

Meltzer, H.Y. (2001) Serotonin as a target for antipsychotic drug action. In: Breier, A., Tran, P.V., Herrea, J.M., Tollefson, G.D., and Bymas-

ter, F.P., eds. *Current Issues in the Psychopharmacology of Schizophrenia.* Philadelphia: Lippincott Williams & Wilkins, pp. 289–303.

Meyer, J.M. (2001) Effects of atypical antipsychotics on weight and serum lipid levels. *J Clin Psychiatry* 62:27–34.

Meyers, B.S., et al. (2001) Continuation treatment of delusional depression in older adults. *Am J Geriatr Psychiatry* 9:415–422.

Meyers, B.S., Greenberg, R., and Mei-Tal, V. (1985) Delusional depression in the elderly. In: Shamoian, C., ed. *Treatment of Affective Disorders in the Elderly* Washington, DC: American Psychiatric Press, pp. 19–28.

Miyamoto, S., Duncan, G.E., and Lieberman, J.A. (2001) Olanzapine. In: Breier, A., Tran, P.V., Herrea, J.M., Tollefson, G.D., and Bymaster, F.P., eds. *Current Issues in the Psychopharmacology of Schizophrenia.* Philadelphia: Lippincott Williams & Wilkins, pp. 224–242.

Muller-Siecheneder, F., et al. (2000) Risperidone versus haloperidol and amitriptyline in the treatment of patients with a combined psychotic and depressive syndrome. *J Clin Psychopharmacol* 18:111–120.

Mulsant, B.H., et al. (1997) Low use of neuroleptic drugs in the treatment of psychotic major depression. *Am J Psychiatry* 154:559–561.

Mulsant, B.H., et al. (2001) A double-blind randomized comparison of nortriptyline plus perphenazine versus nortriptyline plus placebo in the treatment of psychotic depression in late life. *J Clin Psychiatry* 62:597–604.

Must, A., et al. (1999) The disease burden associated with overweight and obesity. *JAMA* 282:1523–1529.

Nelson, J.C., and Bowers, M.B., Jr. (1978) Delusional unipolar depression: Description and drug response. *Arch Gen Psychiatry* 35:1321–1328.

Nelson, J.C., Price, L.H., and Jatlow, P.I. (1986) Neuroleptic dose and desipramine concentrations during combined treatment of unipolar delusional depression. *Am J Psychiatry* 143:1151–1154.

O'Connor, M.K., Knapp, R., and Husain, M. (2001) The influence of age on the response of major depression to electroconvulsive therapy. *Am J Geriatr Psychiatry* 9:382–390.

Parker, G., Roy, K., and Hadzi-Pavlovic, D. (1992) Psychotic (delusional) depression: A meta-analysis of physical treatment. *J Affect Disord* 24:17–24.

Ranjan, R., and Meltzer, H.Y. (1996) Acute and long-term effectiveness of clozapine in treatment-resistant psychotic depression. *Biol Psychiatry* 40:253–258.

Ray, W.A., et al. (2001) Antipsychotics and the risk of sudden cardiac death. *Arch Gen Psychiatry* 59:1161–1167.

Robertson, M.M., and Trimble, M.R. (1982) Major tranquillizers used as antidepressants. *J Affect Disord* 4:173–193.

Rothschild, A.J. (1999) Olanzapine response in psychotic depression. *Clin Psychiatry* 60:116–118.

Roy, A. (1989) Suicidal behavior in schizophrenics. In: Williams, R., and Dalby, J.T., eds. *Depression in Schizophrenics.* New York: Plenum, pp. 137–152.

Saltz, B.L., et al. (1991) Prospective study of tardive dyskinesia incidence in the elderly. *JAMA* 266:2402–2406.

Schmidt, M.E. (2001) Neuroimaging and the pharmacological treatment of schizophrenia. In: Breier, A., Tran, P.V., Herrea, J.M., Tollefson, G.D., and Bymaster, F.P., eds. *Current Issues in the Psychopharmacology of Schizophrenia.* Philadelphia: Lippincott Williams & Wilkins, pp. 131–147.

Simpson, G.M., Lee, J.M., and Shrivastava, R.K. (1978) Clozapine in tardive dyskinesia. *Psychopharmacology* 56:75–80.

Simpson, G.M., and Lindenmayer, J.P. (1997) Extrapyramidal symptoms in patients treated with risperidone. *J Clin Psychopharmacol* 17:194–201.

Siris, S.G. (1994) Depression and schizophrenia. In: Hirsch, S.R., and Weinberger, D.R., eds. *Schizophrenia.* Oxford: Blackwell Science, pp. 128–145.

Spiker, D.G., et al. (1985) The pharmacological treatment of delusional depression. *Am J Psychiatry* 142:430–436.

Stahl, S.M. (1999) *Psychopharmacology of Antipsychotics*. London: Martin Dunitz.

Street, J.S., et al. (2000) Olanzapine for psychotic conditions in the elderly. *Psychiatr Ann* 30:191–196.

Sweet, R.A., and Pollock, B.G. (1998) New atypical antipsychotics. Experience and utility in the elderly. *Drugs Aging* 12:115–127.

Tandon, R. (1998) Antipsychotic agents. In: Quitkin, F.M., Adams, D.C., and Bowden, C.L., eds. *Current Psychotherapeutic Drugs*. Philadelphia: Current Medicine, pp. 120–154.

Tandon, R., Harrigan, E., and Zorn, S.H. (1997) Ziprasidone: A novel antipsychotic with unique pharmacology and therapeutic potential. *J Serotonin Res* 4:159–177.

Tew, J.D., et al. (1999) Acute efficacy of ECT in the treatment of major depression in the old-old. *Am J Psychiatry* 156:1865–1870.

Thomas, S.H.L. (1994) Drugs, QT interval prolongation abnormalities, and ventricular arrhythmias. *Adverse Drug Reactions Toxicol Rev* 13:77–102.

Tollefson, G.D. (2001) Role of novel antipsychotics in the treatment of co-morbid mood disorders in schizophrenia. In: Breier, A., Tran, P.V., Herrea, J.M., Tollefson, G.D., and Bymaster, F.P., eds. *Current Issues in the Psychopharmacology of Schizophrenia*. Philadelphia: Lippincott Williams & Wilkins, pp. 497–512.

Tollefson, G.D., et al. (1997) Olanzapine versus haloperidol in the treatment of schizophrenia and schizoaffective and schizophreniform disorders: Results of an international collaborative trial. *Am J Psychiatry* 154:457–465.

Tollefson, G.D., et al. (1998) Depressive signs and symptoms in schizophrenia. A prospective blinded trial of olanzapine and haloperidol. *Arch Gen Psychiatry* 55:250–258.

Tomac, T.A., Rummans, T.A., and Pileggi, T.S. (1997) Safety and efficacy of electroconvulsive therapy in patients over age 85. *Am J Geriatr Psychiatry* 5:126–130.

Tran, P.V., et al. (1997) Extrapyramidal symptoms and tolerability of olanzapine versus haloperidol in the acute treatment of schizophrenia. *J Clin Psychiatry* 58:205–211.

Vega, J.A.W., Mortimer, A.M., and Tyson, P.J. (2000) Somatic treatment of psychotic depression: Review and recommendations for practice. *J Clin Psychopharmacol* 20:504–517.

Warner, J.P., Barnes, T.R.E., and Henry, J.A. (1996) Electrocardiographic changes in patients receiving neuroleptic medication. *Acta Psychiatr Scand* 93:311–313.

Wilkinson, A.M., Anderson, D.N., and Peters, S. (1993) Age and the effects of ECT. *Int J Geriatr Psychiatry* 8:401–406.

Wirshing, D.A. (2001) Adverse effects of atypical antipsychotics. *J Clin Psychiatry* 62:7–10.

Wirshing, D.A., et al. (1998) Novel antipsychotics and new onset diabetes. *Biol Psychiatry* 44:778–783.

Yassa, R., and Jeste, D.V. (1992) Gender differences in tardive dyskinesia: A critical review of the literature. *Schizophr Bull* 18(4): 701–715.

Zarate, C.A., Tohen, M., and Baldessarini, R.J. (1995) Clozapine in severe mood disorders. *J Clin Psychiatry* 56:411–417.

Zisook, S., et al. (1999) Depressive symptoms in schizophrenia. *Am J Psychiatry* 156:1736–1743.

# 21 | Electroconvulsive therapy in late-life depression

HAROLD A. SACKEIM

## USE AND INDICATIONS

Electroconvulsive therapy (ECT) has a special role in the treatment of late-life depression and other psychiatric conditions in the elderly. Compared to those receiving pharmacological treatments, the elderly constitute an especially high proportion of those who receive ECT. For example, a survey of practice in California between 1977 and 1983 indicated that the probability of receiving ECT increased markedly with patient age. While 1.12 persons per 10,000 in the general adult population were treated with ECT, this rate was 3.86 persons per 10,000 people aged 65 years and above (Kramer, 1985). Across diagnoses, Figure 21.1 presents the number of patients treated with ECT in California between 1989 and 1994 as a function of age. (Data for 1993 were not available.) The use of ECT was constant over this period, and the high representation of elderly patients is noteworthy. Similarly, a national survey of inpatient psychiatric facilities conducted by the National Institute of Mental Health (NIMH) indicated that patients aged 61 and older comprised the largest age group receiving ECT (Thompson and Blaine, 1987). In this survey, overall use of ECT had declined substantially in a comparison between the years 1975 and 1980. However, there was no change in the rate of use for inpatients aged 61 years and above. In a follow-up NIMH national survey, Thompson et al. (1994) reported that the use of ECT increased somewhat between 1980 and 1986. Hospital type and age were particularly strong predictors of the use of this modality. Electroconvulsive therapy was far more commonly administered in private general and psychiatric hospitals than in hospitals in the public sector. Individuals aged 65 and older received ECT at a higher rate than persons in any other age group. Indeed, as Figure 21.2 shows, the overall increase in the use of ECT between 1980 and 1986 was fully attributable to its greater use in elderly patients. The national estimate in 1986 was that 15.6% of inpatients with mood disorders received ECT if they were 65 years of age or older, while the rate was only 3.4% among younger inpatients with mood disorder.

Olfson et al. (1998) reported the most comprehensive national study of the factors impacting the use of ECT, using data from the Health Care Cost and Utilization Project (Agency for Health Care Policy and Research, 1993). A representative sample of nearly 25,000 adult inpatients was identified with a discharge diagnosis of recurrent major depression and treated in general hospitals. Overall, it was estimated that nearly 10% of this sample received ECT during their inpatient stay. The factors that most strongly predicted use of ECT were age, race, insurance status, and median income of the patient's home zip code. Older patients, whites, and those who had private insurance and who lived in more affluent areas were most likely to be treated with this modality. Figure 21.3 illustrates the association with age. Before the age of 50, less than 5% of the sample received ECT, while after 65 years of age the rate was 21.2%.

This study also confirmed the fact that, contrary to the popular impression that ECT is most frequently used among the poor and destitute, this modality is administered far more frequently to the economically advantaged. As the median annual income in the patient's zip code rose from less than $15,000 to between $40,001 and $45,000, there was a linear increase in the rate of ECT use from 4.1% to 12.5%. Among African-Americans the rate of ECT use was 2.9%, compared to 8.4% among whites. The effects of these demographic variables were extraordinarily large, and it is unlikely that any psychopharmacological treatment would have comparable disparities in use as a function of income or race. In the case of ECT, the source of these patterns is thought to reflect the skew in treatment availability. It has long been known that ECT is far more readily available in private hospitals, particularly academic institutions, than in public municipal, county, state, or federal institutions (Thompson and Blaine, 1987; Thompson et al., 1994). However, there is considerable geographic heterogeneity across the United States in the availability of ECT (Hermann et al., 1995; Rosenbach et al., 1997), and even among general hospitals that contributed to the Health Care

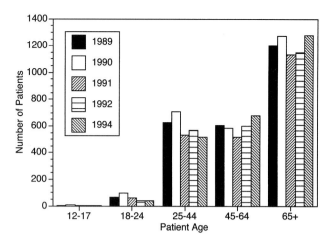

FIGURE 21.1  Patients treated with electroconvulsive therapy in California as a function of age group and year. (Data for 1993 were not available)

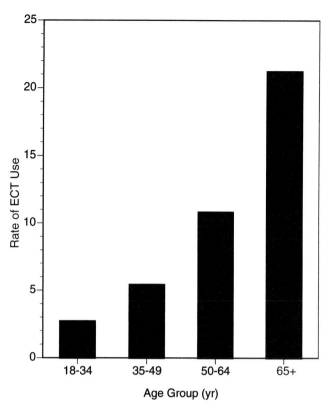

FIGURE 21.3  Rate of electroconvulsive therapy use in a sample of representative inpatients in the United States in 1993 with a diagnosis of recurrent major depression. (After Olfson et al., 1998)

Cost and Utilization Project, it is likely that ECT was more available in academic teaching hospitals than in general community facilities. It should be noted that the elderly are overrepresented among those with low annual incomes and may be underrepresented as patients in academic facilities. In other words, it can be speculated that the sharp increase in ECT among those 65 years and older would represent an underestimate were there greater equivalence in the types of facilities caring for younger and older patients with severe mood disorders.

Despite its frequent use among the elderly, age per se is not a primary indication for the use of ECT in major depression or other diagnostic classifications. Rather, elderly patients are particularly likely to be characterized by the diagnostic and other factors that

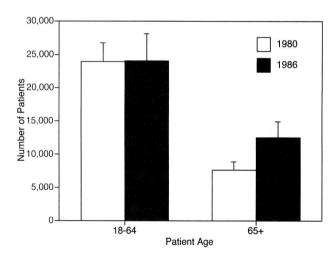

FIGURE 21.2  Patients treated with electroconvulsive therapy in U.S. inpatient facilities in 1980 and 1986 as a function of age. (After Thompson et al., 1994)

impact on the recommendation to proceed with ECT. The vast majority of patients treated with ECT in the United States are experiencing an episode of major depression (unipolar or bipolar). In the NIMH national survey conducted in 1986, 84% of patients who received ECT had a diagnosis of a major mood disorder (Thompson et al., 1994). The next most common diagnostic indications for ECT are schizophrenia (Sackeim, 2003) and mania (Mukherjee et al., 1994). Within the diagnosis of major depression, the primary factors that lead to consideration of ECT are a history of inadequate response to antidepressant medication, intolerance of antidepressant medication, a history of a good ECT response in previous episodes, situations in which the risks of other antidepressant treatments outweigh those of ECT, situations in which there is a particular need for a rapid and definitive clinical response due to the patient's medical or psychiatric status, and patient preference (American Psychiatric Association, 1990, 1993, 2001).

Intolerance of antidepressant medications and the presence of medical conditions, particularly some forms of cardiovascular disease, that preclude or limit pharmacological options are known to be age-related. At least in terms of the morbidity and mortality associated with traditional heterocyclic antidepressants, ECT is believed to present less medical risk, making its use particularly likely in elderly and medically compromised patients (O'Connor et al., 2001; Sackeim et al., 1995; Tew et al., 1999; Zielinski et al., 1993). It is also suspected by some, but not well documented, that resistance to the therapeutic effects of antidepressant medication is age-related, with depression in late life more likely to be medication resistant (Gerson et al., 1988; Himmelhoch et al., 1980; Prudic et al., 1990, 1996). There is also some evidence that resistance to standard pharmacological treatments may be especially likely in late-onset major depression (Alexopoulos et al., 1996; Hickie et al., 1995, 1997; Krishnan et al., 1997).

The issue of the relations between medication resistance and aging requires careful consideration. While there has been controversy about whether the selective serotonin reuptake inhibitors (SSRIs) are less effective than the heterocyclics in severe or melancholic depression (Danish, 1986, 1990; Hirschfeld, 1999; Nelson, 1999; Roose et al., 1994), it may be that aging plays a more important role than symptom severity or diagnostic subtype in mediating responsiveness to SSRIs. Indeed, there are prominent effects of age on serotonergic transmission that may leave insufficient substrate for antidepressant action (Nobler et al., 1999). In general, the rates of response and remission in placebo-controlled studies of SSRIs are not impressive and appear to be smaller than those obtained in the similar, but earlier, study of heterocyclics (Roose and Sackeim, 2002). While the same has not been done as a function of aging, patients with melancholia have been found to rate ECT as the most helpful treatment they have received, with tricyclic antidepressants (TCAs) rated more highly than SSRIs (Parker et al., 2001). The upshot is that SSRIs, the medications that may present the fewest problems in terms of tolerability, may be ineffective in a sizable subgroup of the elderly. It is not uncommon to see elderly patients referred for ECT because of presumed medication resistance who were serially tried on a variety of SSRIs without problems of tolerance and without exposure to newer dual-action antidepressants or TCAs.

In the general population, the likelihood and speed of clinical remission are superior with ECT than with any antidepressant medication regimen (Folkerts et al., 1997; Janicak et al., 1985; Nobler et al., 1997; Rifkin, 1988; Sackeim et al., 1995; Segman et al., 1995). Thus, ECT is also considered when patients present with medical and psychiatric conditions of heightened urgency. Severe inanition, refusal to eat, psychosis, and suicidality are features of depression that may be more common in the elderly. In short, ECT is most frequently considered when alternative biological treatments are too risky or have proven ineffective, or when it is particularly important to ensure a rapid or full clinical response.

## WHEN TO CONSIDER ELECTROCONVULSIVE THERAPY

Given ECT's low rates of morbidity and mortality, and its likely superior short-term efficacy and rapidity of action compared to pharmacological alternatives, the question arises as to why ECT is often used only as a second, third, or last-resort treatment. Put another way, since ECT is frequently recommended when it is particularly important for patients to have a rapid or full response, one can ask: When isn't it important to achieve these goals? What patient doesn't need to get better quickly and fully? Unfortunately, little research has been conducted on the issue of when during the course of antidepressant treatment the use of ECT should be entertained. Like its overall rate of use, the extent to which ECT is used early or late in the course of antidepressant treatment varies markedly from country to country and, within the United States, varies considerably among localities and practitioners (Hermann et al., 1995, 1999).

Often prompting consideration of an earlier use of ECT are the clinical features predictive of the clinical outcome with ECT in major depression. As with pharmacological treatment, the duration of the index depressive episode has been consistently related to ECT response rates, with patients with longer duration showing less benefit, including the elderly (Black et al., 1989; Coryell and Zimmerman, 1984; Fraser and Glass, 1980; Hobson, 1953; Kindler et al., 1991; Prudic et al., 1996, in press). It is not known whether this association reflects an intrinsic aspect of the patient or a consequence of disease chronicity. Some patients may present with a pathophysiology that is not responsive to conventional treatments and, thus, are especially likely to have episodes of long duration. This is the traditional view in which medication resistance is a static property of the patient. On the other hand, the neurobiological effects of increasingly long episode duration may engender treatment resistance. In this view, the use of a weak or ineffective treatment at the beginning of an episode could carry the additional cost of promoting treatment resistance. In other words, the clinician might consider the theoretical possibility that the duration of the episode (and the underlying biology) makes an active contribution to treatment resistance, suggesting earlier use of ECT. Indeed, recent research has raised the possibility that the number of lifetime days in a depressed state is associated with the extent of hippocampal atrophy, with the presumed mechanisms being the atrophic effects of excessive glucocorticoid stimulation. Since the hippocampus has an established role in regulating the hypothalamic-pituitary-adrenal (HPA) axis, the atrophic effects linked to episode duration may lead to increased vulnerability to stress and prolongation of the episode.

Recent research has indicated that resistance to antidepressant medications, particularly heterocyclics, is predictive of an inferior short-term ECT response (Prudic et al., 1990, 1996; Sackeim et al., 2000b, 2001b). This relationship holds for other somatic treatments as well (Sackeim, 2001a, 2001c). As patients do not benefit from increasing numbers of robust medication trials, the percentage that benefit from ECT is reduced. This, in turn, suggests that ECT is likely to be of greater value when it is not restricted to last-resort use.

However, there are other considerations that support less aggressive use of ECT. The three key factors are the cognitive side effect profile of ECT, the need for pharmacological treatment to prevent relapse and recurrence following successful ECT therapy, and patient preference.

Electroconvulsive therapy has more profound short-term and long-term cognitive side effects than any pharmacological alternative (American Psychiatric Association, 2001; Sackeim, 1992, 2000). This is the single most important factor limiting or delaying the use of ECT.

Second, continuation ECT, with treatments spaced over weekly to monthly intervals, is an increasingly used method for relapse prevention (Clarke et al., 1989; Decina et al., 1987; Sackeim, 1994). Nonetheless, the vast majority of patients who respond to ECT are subsequently treated with antidepressant medications (Prudic et al., 2001, in press; Sackeim et al., 2001b), and continuation or maintenance ECT is most commonly recommended only after pharmacological methods of relapse prevention have failed following successful ECT. Since the majority of ECT responders goes on to receive pharmacological treatment, they are exposed to the side effects of both modalities. More critically, for many patients, the decision to treat with ECT only postpones the often trial-and-error identification of an effective long-term pharmacological strategy. Ordinarily, when a patient responds to a medication regimen, that same regimen is used for continuation and maintenance therapy to prevent relapse and recurrence (Frank et al., 1990, 1993; Prien and Kupfer, 1986). There is now evidence that medication regimens that failed during treatment of the acute depressive episode are also ineffective in preventing relapse following ECT (Sackeim, 1994; Sackeim et al., 1990b, 2001b). Therefore, since a large number of patients receive ECT because of medication resistance, the clinician is faced with considerable uncertainty about optimal pharmacological treatment in these patients following successful ECT.

Finally, while there are indications that the public image of ECT has improved in recent years, many patients are reluctant to receive this modality. The personal suffering and costs of chronic depression and the disappointment in not benefiting sufficiently from serial pharmacological trials often provide the motivation to reconsider this decision. In short, the decision to recommend ECT and, if so, when during the course of treatment, is complex. Overall, the clinician and patient must weigh the greater certainty of a short-term response or remission with ECT and its strong medical safety profile against the likelihood of troublesome and often permanent cognitive side effects and uncertainty about the optimal methods of relapse prevention.

The special role of ECT in the treatment of the elderly raises several critical questions. Is the efficacy of ECT different in late-life depression compared to that observed in younger populations or to other treatment alternatives? Are the medical and cognitive risks of ECT different in patients with late-life depression than in younger patients? How should the administration of ECT be modified to augment its efficacy and minimize its side effects when treating the elderly depressed patient? What are the optimal approaches to relapse prevention?

## EFFICACY

### General Considerations

The efficacy of ECT in the treatment of major depression is established. A set of double-blind, random assignment trials conducted in England during the late 1970s and 1980s contrasted real ECT with that of the repeated administration of anesthesia alone—*sham* ECT (Brandon et al., 1984; Gregory et al., 1985; Johnstone et al., 1980; Lambourn and Gill, 1978; West, 1981). With one exception (Lambourn and Gill, 1978), real ECT was found consistently to be more efficacious than sham treatment (see Crow, 1979; Crow and Johnstone, 1986; United Kingdom ECT Review Group, "Efficacy and safety," 2003; Sackeim, 1989, for reviews. The exceptional Lambourn and Gill (1978) study used a form of real ECT now known to have limited efficacy (McCall et al., 2000; Sackeim et al., 1987a, 1993, 2000b). Overall, these studies demonstrated that the passage of an electrical stimulus and/or the elicitation of a generalized seizure was necessary for ECT to exert antidepressant effects. Furthermore, the use of repeated administration of anesthesia as a sham or active placebo condition may have underestimated its true therapeutic effects. There is some concern that repeated administration of anesthesia, by itself, may have mild antidepressant effects (O'Brien, 1989; Sackeim, 1986b, 1989).

Taking this body of findings one step further, it has been demonstrated more recently that particular forms of ECT reliably lack therapeutic properties, despite the use of general anesthesia, the application of an electrical stimulus, and the production of "adequate" generalized seizures. In independent, random-assignment, double-blind studies, the Columbia University group found that right unilateral (RUL) ECT administered at very low stimulus intensity (just above the seizure threshold) was decidedly ineffective, producing a response rate of approximately 20% (Sackeim et al., 1987a, 1993, 2000b). In contrast, in the same studies, other forms of ECT, involving different electrode placements or stimulus intensity, had short-term response rates of approximately 70%. This work was critical in demonstrating the intrinsic efficacy of ECT. Since patients in all the treatment conditions not only received repeated general anesthesia but also had adequate generalized seizures, the marked differences in remission rates were attributable to the specific manipulations of electrode placement and stimulus dosing. These findings also suggested that with careful patient selection, placebo and other nonspecific effects make small contributions to response rates in ECT samples (Sobin et al., 1996).

Subsequent research at Columbia and elsewhere has shown that the efficacy of RUL ECT is highly dependent on the dosage relative to the seizure threshold and that at high stimulus intensity (e.g., six times the seizure threshold), the efficacy of RUL ECT is comparable to that of a robust form of bilateral (BL) ECT (McCall et al., 2000; Sackeim et al., 2000b). These research efforts establishing dose-response relationships in ECT also go beyond sham-controlled trials as demonstrations of the intrinsic efficacy of ECT. The fact that efficacy is dependent on the technical parameters of stimulation necessitates the conclusion that the intervention has antidepressant properties that are mediated by the biological consequences of the dosage manipulations.

In recent years, there have been limited and primarily retrospective comparisons of ECT to other forms of biological treatment (Dinan and Barry, 1989; Folkerts et al., 1997; Philibert et al., 1995). Indeed, since ECT is now most commonly used when patients have already failed adequate pharmacological treatments or when the risks of such treatment are too high, it is unlikely that controlled, random assignment trials contrasting the efficacy of ECT and antidepressant medications in the treatment of acute episodes of depression would be feasible. This is especially true in elderly patients, in whom compromised medical status and the high representation of psychotic depression often compel the use of ECT. However, soon after the introduction of TCAs and monoamine oxidase inhibitors (MAOIs), such comparisons were conducted, with ECT used as the gold standard by which to evaluate the efficacy of the newer treatments (Bruce et al., 1960; Fay et al., 1963; Gangadhar et al., 1982; Greenblat et al., 1964; Harris and Robins, 1960; Kiloh et al., 1960; Robin and Harris, 1962; Shephard, 1965; Wilson et al., 1963). Janicak et al. (1985), in a meta-analysis of these studies, reported that the average response rate

to ECT was 20% higher when compared to TCAs and 45% higher when compared to MAOIs. No study has ever found a pharmacological regimen to have superior antidepressant effects to ECT. Rather, ECT has consistently been found to have either equal or superior efficacy. At the same time, it should be recognized that this literature is characterized by methodological limitations. Most critically, the era in which these trials were conducted had different standards regarding the dose and duration of adequate pharmacological treatment. By modern standards (Keller et al., 1986; Prudic et al., 1996; Quitkin, 1985; Sackeim et al., 1990b), the pharmacological treatments used were often suboptimal. In addition, given that patients must recognize whether they are receiving a medication or ECT, such comparisons could not be double-blind.

In a more recent study, Folkerts et al. (1997) randomized 39 patients to treatment with paroxetine or ECT. Entry criteria required that, at minimum, patients had inadequate improvement in at least two antidepressant trials in the current episode. Antidepressant effects were markedly superior with ECT. Of course, the choice of an SSRI as the comparator for medication-resistant patients can be questioned. The majority of these patients had not responded to treatment with an SSRI, and it is doubtful whether the use of another SSRI would be the optimal therapeutic strategy. Indeed, Dinan and Barry (1989) conducted the only study to suggest an advantage for a pharmacological regimen relative to ECT. Thirty patients resistant to treatment with a TCA were randomized to continuing on the TCA with the addition of lithium or switching to ECT. Overall, 21 of the 30 patients were rated as much improved at the end of 3 weeks, with no difference between the two groups in extent of benefit. However, onset of improvement was quicker with the combination treatment, with a significant difference observed after 7 days. Lithium augmentation of an antidepressant medication, especially a TCA, is one of the best-documented treatments in terms of efficacy in patients with medication-resistant depression (Nemeroff, 1996–97; Rouillon and Gorwood, 1998). Of note, the combination of nortriptyline and lithium appears to be especially useful in relapse prevention following ECT (Sackeim et al., 2001b). It is conceivable that this combination pharmacological strategy overlaps more in its spectrum of action with ECT than do SSRIs.

Another issue intrinsic to the comparison of ECT and other biological interventions concerns the quality of the clinical response. In pharmacological trials, patients are usually categorized as clinical responders based on the extent of their reduction in symptom scores on instruments such as the Hamilton Rating Scale for Depression (HRSD) (Hamilton, 1967). Various criteria have been used, with a 50% reduction in symptoms after treatment relative to the pretreatment baseline being the most common. Since ECT is frequently administered to patients with severe and often psychotic depressive illness, such a criterion is inappropriate. Regardless of their baseline level of symptomatology, patients who have HRSD scores of 20 or greater following somatic treatment are still seriously depressed, require additional treatment, and in the clinical community would not ordinarily be considered remitted. Consequently, in ECT trials it is common to use more stringent outcome criteria (Andrade and Gangadhar, 1989; Petrides et al., 2001). This approach with ECT is now becoming more generalized, as it is widely acknowledged that the goal of treatment should be remission recovery, and not just response (Paykel, 1998; Thase and Ninan, 2002)

Surprisingly, the extent of residual symptomatology following pharmacological treatment and ECT has rarely been compared. Hamilton (1982), in a naturalistic open study, reported that a considerably higher percentage of depressed patients became asymptomatic after receiving ECT compared to a similar group treated with a TCA. This finding, which is in line with our experience, is of considerable clinical importance. Residual symptomatology in the context of an incomplete response to antidepressant medications often has a significant impact on the quality of life, particularly since the residual symptoms may become chronic (Paykel, 2002). Further, the extent of such symptoms has been one of the few consistent predictors of the likelihood of relapse following pharmacological treatment (Prien and Kupfer, 1986).

Another critical issue in considering the relative efficacy of ECT and pharmacological treatments is the speed of symptom reduction. There have been no trials contrasting speed of response with these modalities in mixed-age or elderly samples. Nonetheless, it is highly doubtful that any pharmacological strategy produces as rapid symptomatic improvement as ECT (Nobler et al., 1997; Sackeim et al., 1995; Segman et al., 1995). In the United States, a schedule of three treatments per week is standard, and the typical ECT course requires eight or nine treatments to achieve a full response. Consequently, approximately 3 weeks are needed to produce maximal gains, and significant clinical improvement is usually seen with the first few treatments. This speed of improvement is less common with antidepressant medications. Many believe that the elderly are especially likely to have delayed improvement (Georgotas et al., 1989), although this has never been adequately demonstrated.

## Aging and the Efficacy of Electroconvulsive Therapy

The short-term efficacy of ECT in the general depressed population is impressive. Since there is usually a high representation of the elderly in such samples, the implication is that ECT is an effective treatment in late-life depression. However, the impact of aging on the short-term efficacy of ECT has been examined more directly. Table 21.1 provides a selective summary of studies addressing the relations between patient age and ECT outcome. The findings in this area have been somewhat inconsistent. A number of authorities have suggested that the response rate to ECT is higher in older relative to younger patients (Abrams, 2002a; Fraser, 1981; Sackeim, 1993; Weiner, 1982). Indeed, an impressive number of both early and recent investigations found positive associations between patient age and the degree of clinical improvement following ECT. In contrast, a variety of studies have not found aging effects, and there are some data suggesting that older individuals may have a diminished response to unilateral but not bilateral ECT (Heshe et al., 1978; Pettinati et al., 1986) or that older patients may require longer courses of treatment to achieve the same level of remission as younger patients (Ottosson, 1960; Rich et al., 1984).

In general, the findings in this area suggest that older depressed patients have a superior outcome with ECT than younger patients. This pattern is unusual in the somatic treatment of major depression, and is of particular note since most of the work in this area preceded the discovery that the extent to which the intensity of the electrical stimulus in ECT exceeds the individual patient's seizure threshold determines the efficacy of right unilateral ECT and the speed of response, regardless of electrode placement (Sackeim et al., 1987a–1987c, 1991, 1993). These discoveries are of special relevance since age is one of the more reliable predictors of seizure threshold (Sackeim et al., 1987c; Watterson, 1945; Weiner, 1980), with the oldest patients generally having the highest thresholds. Since, in the vast majority of ECT studies, all patients in a given study received the same fixed electrical dosage, elderly patients were treated in a fashion that would delay or diminish the therapeutic response. Given that, in the past, older patients were particularly likely to receive suboptimal forms of ECT, the findings of a positive association between patient age and short-term ECT outcome are all the more impressive.

The positive association between patient age and ECT outcome may reflect on some of the clinical factors that determine when ECT is used and that are related to efficacy. Due to the high representation of medication intolerance, medical complications, and psychotic depression in elderly compared to younger patients, the elderly treated with ECT often have a shorter episode duration and a lower representation of medication resistance. As indicated, a short duration of index episode (Black et al., 1989; Coryell and Zim-

TABLE 21.1. *Studies Examining the Efficacy of Electroconvulsive Therapy (ECT) as a Function of Age*

| Study* | Patients | Study Design | ECT Treatment | Results/Comments |
|---|---|---|---|---|
| Prudic et al. (2004) | 347 patients with major depression treated at seven hospitals in the New York metropolitan area | Prospective, naturalistic study of ECT practices and outcomes in community settings; evaluations before, immediately after, and monthly for 6 months following ECT | Modified ECT given three times/week; diverse electrode placement and dosing practices | Age, treated as a continuous variable, was not related to symptom improvement or categorical clinical outcomes |
| O'Connor et al. (2001) | 253 patients with major depression treated openly with titrated (50% above seizure threshold) bilateral ECT | Prospective naturalistic acute phase study followed by double-blind continuation trial comparing nortriptyline and lithium with continuation ECT; acute response to ECT contrasted in three patient groups: young adults (<45 years), older adults (46 to 64 years), and elderly patients (65 years and older) | Modified ECT given three times/week; patients titrated at first session and treated afterward with a suprathreshold intensity 50% above threshold | The youngest age group had a lower remission rate (70%) than either the older adults (89.8%) or the elderly (90%). When these dimensions were treated as continuous variables, age was also related to outcome. |
| Sackeim et al. (2000) | 80 inpatients with major depression randomized to four groups (right unilateral at 1.5, 2.5, or 6 times seizure threshold or bilateral ECT at 2.5 times seizure threshold); free of all medications except lorazepam (up to 3 mg/day PRN) | Double-blind, prospective study of effects of electrical dosage and electrode placement; patients evaluated before ECT and regularly during and after treatment course | Modified ECT given three times/week; patients randomized to three forms of right unilateral ECT (1.5, 2.5, or 6 times seizure threshold) or bilateral ECT (2.5 times seizure threshold) | High-dosage right unilateral ECT (6 times threshold) and bilateral ECT (2.5 times threshold) equal in efficacy and superior to lower-dosage right unilateral ECT; no age-related effects seen |
| Tew et al. (1999) | 268 patients with major depression treated openly with suprathreshold unilateral or bilateral ECT; free of all medications except lorazepam (up to 3 mg/day PRN) | Prospective, naturalistic acute phase study followed by a double-blind continuation pharmacotherapy trial; acute response to ECT contrasted in three patient groups: adults (59 years and younger), the young-old (60 to 74 years), and the old-old (75 years and older) | Modified ECT given three times/week; patients titrated at first session and treated with a suprathreshold intensity selected by the treating psychiatrist | Both older age groups had a greater physical illness burden and greater cognitive impairment than the adult group. Both older groups had shorter depressive episodes and were less likely to be medication resistant. The adult patients had a lower rate of ECT response (54%) than the young-old patients (73%), while the old-old patients had an intermediate response (67%). |
| Sackeim et al. (1993) | 96 inpatients with major depression randomized to four groups (unilateral or bilateral ECT at low or high stimulus intensity); free of all medications except lorazepam (up to 3 mg/day PRN); age range, 22–80; mean, 56.4 | Double-blind, prospective study of effects of electrical dosage and electrode placement; patients evaluated before ECT and regularly during and after treatment course | Modified ECT given three times/week; patients titrated at first session and treated either at just above threshold or at 2.5 times initial seizure threshold | Electrical dosage determined unilateral ECT efficacy and speed of response for unilateral and bilateral ECT; no age-related effects seen |

*(continued)*

| Study* | Patients | Study Design | ECT Treatment | Results/Comments |
|---|---|---|---|---|
| Black et al. (1993) | 423 depressed inpatients between 1970 and 1981 | Retrospective chart review using multiple logistic regression to identify response predictors | Modified ECT given three times/week; bilateral, unilateral, and mixed courses included | Patients rated as recovered ($n = 295$) were older than those rated as unrecovered ($n = 128$) |
| Sackeim et al. (1987a) | 52 inpatients with major depression randomized to unilateral or bilateral ECT; patients free of all medications except lorazepam (up to 3 mg/day PRN); age range, 25–83; mean, 61.3 | Double-blind, prospective study comparing low-dose, titrated bilateral and unilateral ECT; patients evaluated before ECT and following treatments 1, 3, 5, 6, and every treatment thereafter | Bilateral or right unilateral modified ECT given three times/week; patients titrated and treated at just above threshold | Low-dosage right unilateral ECT ineffective; regardless of ECT modality, age unrelated to clinical outcome |
| Coryell and Zimmerman (1984) | 31 patients with unipolar depression selected prospectively | Prospective study of ECT response predictors; ratings made on HRSD at weekly intervals by blind raters | Most treatments unilateral; most patients had at least six treatments; patients with fewer than four treatments excluded | Age independently associated with outcome on more than one of three outcome measures; superior outcome found in older patients |
| Rich et al. (1984) | Data from two groups of patients pooled: 66 with major depressive episode or organic affective syndrome; antidepressant medications either stopped prior to ECT or held constant | Prospective study of response rate to conventional ECT by identifying point of maximal improvement; patients rated on HRSD before first ECT and at 36–48 hours after each treatment | Modified ECT given three times/week; right unilateral ECT used with >80% of patients; mean no. of treatments for each of two groups was 8.6 and 8.3 | Age associated with longer time to achieve a response; study flawed by use of different rating scales and different ECT devices for the two groups |
| Fraser and Glass (1980) | 29 depressed (Feigner criteria) elderly (64–86 years) randomized to unilateral or bilateral ECT | Prospective, double-blind, randomized study; postictal recovery times, memory changes, and clinical improvement assessed by HRSD | Modified ECT with twice-weekly treatment until patient recovered or ECT had to be stopped | No age difference between good- and moderate-outcome groups |
| Heshe et al. (1978) | 51 patients with endogenous depression randomized to unilateral or bilateral ECT | Prospective, blind evaluations before ECT, at end of ECT, and 3 months after final treatment | Patients received either modified unilateral (average, 9.2 treatments) or bilateral ECT (average, 8.5 treatments) two treatments per week; number of treatments decided by treating clinician | In patients over 60, bilateral ECT produced a significantly better therapeutic effect than unilateral treatment, regardless of ECT modality; satisfactory results in 75% of patients >60 years and in 96% of patients <60 years—a significant difference |
| Herrington et al. (1974) | 43 consecutive severely depressed patients (aged 25–69) randomized to ECT or L-tryptophan (up to 8 g/day); 40 patients included in efficacy analysis | Patients rated on day before treatment and weekly thereafter for 4 weeks | ECT given twice weekly for total of six to eight treatments | Age unrelated to outcome |
| Strömgren (1973) | 100 patients with endogenous unipolar or bipolar depression; aged 19–65; patients drug-free except for hypnotics and mild sedatives | Prospective, double-blind study contrasting unilateral and bilateral ECT | Minimum of six treatments given; duration of current individualized; average of 9 treatments given to younger patients, 8.7 to older patients | Of 53 patients aged 19–44, 17 were resistant; 7 of 47 aged 45–65 showed overt resistance—a significant difference; efficacy of both bilateral and unilateral ECT superior in older patients *(continued)* |

TABLE 21.1. *Studies Examining the Efficacy of Electroconvulsive Therapy (ECT) as a Function of Age*

| Study[*] | Patients | Study Design | ECT Treatment | Results/Comments |
|---|---|---|---|---|
| Folstein et al. (1973) | 118 consecutive patients who received ECT; diagnoses of schizophrenia, neurotic reactions, and affective disorders | Retrospective chart review: progress notes at time of discharge stated whether or not patient had improved | Nature and duration of ECT not described | Improvement related to older age and shorter hospital stay; no significance tests provided; mean age of patients rated improved ($n = 86$) 50, compared with 31 inpatients rated not improved ($n = 32$) |
| Mendels (1965a, 1965b) | 53 consecutive inpatients evaluated before ECT and 1 and 3 months after ECT; ages 21–76, mean, 48.8 | Prospective study: patients rated with HRSD; evaluators not blind to treatment history | 4–11 treatments (mean, 6.4) with modified ECT | Superior outcome in patients over 50 at 3-month follow-up but not at 1-month follow-up |
| Carney et al. (1965) | 129 depressed inpatients | Prospective study to establish predictive factors; patients scored for presence or absence of 35 features and followed up at 3 and 6 months post-ECT; outcome criteria defined | Patients received three or more treatments | Better response in endogenous depressives at 3 and 6 months (per factor analysis); in patients over age 40, type of depression not associated with outcome |
| Nystrom (1964) | Two series of patients: 254 in Gothenburg series, 188 in Lund series; most cases depressed but other diagnoses included | Prospective, blind evaluation; outcome criteria specified | Modified bilateral ECT, 2 treatments per week initially; average number in Lund series 6.9, 4.4 in Gothenberg series | Lund series: positive association between age and degree of improvement in females; Gothenberg series age <25 years negatively related to outcome |
| Greenblatt et al. (1962) | 128 patients randomized to four treatment groups; diagnosis of schizophrenia, psychoneurotic and psychotic depressive reactions, and involutional psychosis; 28 received ECT; age range, 16–70; mean, 46 | Prospective study compared ECT and antidepressant medications; explicit outcome criteria used | ECT modified by succinylcholine given three times weekly for at least 3 weeks, more at discretion of psychiatrist | Medications and ECT equally effective in youngest age group; ECT significantly more effective than medications in oldest age group |
| Ottoson (1960) | 44 patients (18 males, 26 females) with endogenous depression; age range, 36–70; mean, 55.8 | Prospective study with blind raters; efficacy evaluated by outcome 1 week after fourth treatment, 1 week after end of ECT course, and by total number of treatments required | Modified bilateral ECT with intervals between first three treatments of 2–4 days and between following treatments of 3–7 days; dose adjusted upward for age; patients divided into two groups: one received stimulus grossly above threshold, one moderately above threshold | Age not significantly related to efficacy; therapeutic response tended to appear later in older patients |
| Hamilton and White (1960) | 49 hospitalized male patients with severe depression; age range, 21–69; mean, 51.7 | Patients assessed prospectively and 1 month after end of ECT | Usual course 6 treatments, maximum 10; 14 patients had second course | Age unrelated to outcome |

(*continued*)

249

TABLE 21.1. *Studies Examining the Efficacy of Electroconvulsive Therapy (ECT) as a Function of Age (Continued)*

| Study* | Patients | Study Design | ECT Treatment | Results/Comments |
|---|---|---|---|---|
| Roberts (1959a, 1959b) | 50 female patients 41–60 years of age | Prospective study of predictors of ECT response; patients scored on clinical features prior to ECT and on presence or absence of symptoms at 1 and 3 months post-ECT | Patients received twice-weekly modified ECT until maximum benefit achieved; averaged between seven and eight treatments | Symptom scores at 1 month had significant inverse correlation with age (older women more improved); no correlation at 3 months |
| Herzberg (1954) | 227 cases selected from all patients who had received ECT; diagnoses of schizophrenia, manic-depressive psychoses, involutional melancholia | Retrospective chart review of patients rated along several criteria: initial response to ECT, continued response, and no relapse after discharge | Nature and duration of ECT not described | Patients in fourth decade showed superior outcome on sustained improvement compared with patients in other age groups |
| Hobson (1953) | 150 patients at Maudsley Hospital; no diagnostic criteria used, but almost all patients were depressed; 127 included in analyses | Prospective study to identify predictors of ECT response; patients categorized as either free of symptoms or still having marked symptoms after ECT | Nature and number of of ECT treatments not described | Age unrelated to outcome; several other predictors identified |
| Rickles and Polan (1948) | 200 private patients treated with ECT; diverse diagnostic categories included schizophrenia | Retrospective study of why patients failed ECT; treatment considered failed when improvement not maintained for at least 1 year | Usual course 10–12 treatments; patients with schizophrenia also received 24–40 subcoma insulin shocks | Authors believed that ECT failed if patient was menopausal or postmenopausal; statistics not presented |
| Gold and Chiarello (1944) | 121 consecutive male patients; 103 diagnosed as schizophrenic; age range, 15–60 | Prospective study of outcome predictors and outcome; patients placed in one of four categories from *much improved* to *no change* | Type and number of treatments not described | Superior clinical outcome in older age groups |

merman, 1984; Fraser and Glass, 1980; Hobson, 1953; Kindler et al., 1991) and the absence of medication resistance (Flint and Rifat, 1996; Prudic and Sackeim, 1990; Prudic et al., 1990, 1996; Sackeim et al., 2000b) are consistent predictors of a positive ECT outcome. There is also evidence that, unlike the case with pharmacotherapy, patients with delusional or psychotic depression may preferentially respond to ECT (Buchan et al., 1992; Nobler and Sackeim, 1996; Petrides et al., 2001; Sobin et al., 1996). However, it is especially likely that elderly patients with psychotic depression do not receive an adequate medication trial (Wolfersdorf et al., 1995) prior to receiving ECT (Mulsant et al., 1997). Consequently, the low representation of medication resistance among patients with psychotic depression may account for their superior rate of response to ECT (Prudic et al., 1990; Sackeim, 1994). Although not established, it is also likely that, among patients who receive ECT, the elderly have a lower rate of comorbid Axis II

pathology, and this factor may also contribute to a superior ECT response rate (Black et al., 1993; Prudic et al., in press).

In previous work, only the linear relation between patient age and clinical outcome has been examined, with age treated as a continuous variable. In particular, while a variety of case reports and retrospective studies document the efficacy of ECT in the very old (Alexopoulos et al., 1984; Cattan et al., 1990b; Karlinsky and Shulman, 1984; Kramer, 1987), only in the past few years has there been prospective documentation of ECT efficacy in the oldest age groups and comparison to younger patients.

O'Connor et al. (2001) conducted a similar study of 253 patients treated with ECT at four hospitals. However, in this study the age groupings were defined differently. The elderly comprised those 65 years of age and above, while the younger patients were divided into a group at least 56 years of age but less than 65 and a group 45 years of age and below. All patients were treated with dose-titrated bilateral ECT (50% above the seizure threshold). A weakness in this study was that the outcome was assessed immediately following the ECT course, usually within a day. This practice may produce unreliable estimates of benefit due to the confounding effects of confusion and acute memory loss on symptom assessment. In any case, the oldest age group (≥65 years) had a remission rate of 90%, and the next oldest group had a rate of 89.8%, while the youngest patients had a rate of 70%. Here again, age was a positive predictor of ECT outcome.

Overall, across these studies, the efficacy of ECT tends to have a positive relation with patient age. However, the magnitude of this effect is relatively small, and age alone does not constitute an indication for the use of ECT. Given that the efficacy of ECT is strong in the general mixed-age population, the fact that this effect may be enhanced with aging indicates that ECT is particularly useful in the treatment of late-life depression. Indeed, one is hard pressed to identify other treatments whose efficacy is greater in older than younger patients.

Post (1972) suggested that prior to the introduction of ECT, the elderly depressed often manifested a chronic course or died of intercurrent medical illnesses in psychiatric institutions. A number of studies have contrasted the clinical outcome of depressed patients who received inadequate or no biological treatment to that of patients who received ECT. While none of this work involved prospective, random assignment designs, the findings have been largely uniform. In the elderly, ECT results in decreased chronicity, decreased morbidity, and possibly decreased mortality (Avery and Winokur, 1976; Babigian and Guttmacher, 1984; Philibert et al., 1995; Wesner and Winokur, 1989). Indeed, in much of this work, the advantages of ECT were particularly pronounced in elderly compared to younger populations. For example, in a retrospective comparison of elderly depressed patients treated with ECT or pharmacotherapy, Philibert et al. (1995) found that at long-term follow-up, rates of mortality and significant depressive symptomatology were higher in the pharmacotherapy group. There have been no prospective, random assignment trials contrasting ECT with adequate pharmacotherapy with a focus on elderly depressives. However, as indicated, because ECT is so often used in the elderly due to medication resistance, medication intolerance, or safety factors, at this time the practicality and clinical significance of such a comparison would be dubious.

## Psychotic Depression

Electroconvulsive therapy has a special role in the treatment of elderly patients with psychotic or delusional depression. Due to the gravity of the condition, its high rate of response to ECT, and the relatively poor rate of response to monotherapy with antidepressants, many consider ECT as a primary treatment for patients with psychotic depression (American Psychiatric Association, 1990, 2001; Royal College of Psychiatrists, 1995). In mixed age samples, approximately 30%–40% of depressed patients who receive ECT present with psychotic depression (Sackeim et al., 2000b; Sobin et al., 1996). This rate is likely higher among the elderly, who are more likely to present with psychotic depression than younger age groups (Parker et al., 1991).

### Phenomenology and diagnosis

Identification of psychotic features in the elderly depressed patient is critical. Such patients have special needs with regard to treatment (Dubovsky, 1994) and have a considerably increased risk of suicide (Coryell and Zimmerman, 1984; Roose et al., 1983; Spiker et al., 1985a). Psychotic depression is often underrecognized, particularly in the elderly, because a subgroup of these patients deny having delusions or hallucinations. Indeed, a telltale sign of psychotic depression is found in the elderly patient who, despite having psychomotor retardation, anorexia, markedly diminished social interactions, or other symptoms of depression, denies being depressed. Further complicating identification of psychotic depression is the distinction between over-valued ideas or "near-delusional status" and delusions (Nelson et al., 1994). In the elderly patient, diagnostic uncertainty may arise particularly in distinguishing between hypochondriasis and somatic delusions.

Between 20% and 45% of hospitalized elderly depressed patients present with psychotic depression (Avery and Lubrano, 1979; Nelson and Bowers, 1978; Schatzberg and Rothschild, 1992). Typically, the elderly patient with psychotic features has severe depressive illness, although the overall severity of depression may be comparable in some patients with melancholic, nonpsychotic depression, indicating that psychosis does not result invariably from severe illness. Among the elderly, the psychotic features far more commonly involve delusions than hallucinations.

There is evidence that the manifestations of psychotic depression tend to be consistent from episode to episode, suggesting a trait-like quality (Aronson et al., 1988; Coryell et al., 1984, 1994). Furthermore, psychotic depression appears to be familial, and relatives may share the same psychotic content (Aronson et al., 1988; Kendler et al., 1986). Mood-incongruent features, delusions, or hallucinations whose content is inconsistent with depressive themes are compatible with a diagnosis of psychotic depression by DSM-IV. However, mood-incongruent features may be more common among the younger depressed groups and/or those with bipolar depression. Indeed, the presence of mood-incongruent psychotic features in an elderly patient should trigger consideration of possible bipolarity or an organic affective disorder. Psychotic depression is overrepresented in bipolar relative to unipolar depression (Dubovsky, 1994), and the elderly bipolar patient with psychotic depression may be particularly likely to present with psychomotor retardation and sleep disturbance. In contrast, psychotic depression that appears as a first episode after 50 years of age is frequently unipolar in course. Late-onset psychotic depression may be particularly difficult to treat, subject to a relapsing course, and possible later development of dementia (Alexopoulos et al., 1992; Aronson et al., 1988). In contrast to the delusions in persons with psychotic depression, the patient with a psychotic organic affective disorder usually has delusions that are less systematized and less congruent with depressive themes. The delusions in the elderly patient with psychotic depression usually are highly organized and reflect unrealistic or bizarre ideas about somatic illness, nihilism, persecution, guilt, or jealousy. The elderly patient with psychotic depression may also be particularly likely to manifest gross global cognitive deterioration (*pseudodementia*), which reverses with successful treatment of the mood disorder (Caine, 1986). There is evidence that such patients later develop a dementing illness (Mitchell and Dening, 1962).

### Pharmacological treatment

Controlled and uncontrolled investigations have established that patients with psychotic depression have a remarkably poor rate of response to monotherapy with heterocyclic antidepressants, MAOIs, or neuroleptics, regardless of dosage (Avery and Lubrano, 1979; Glassman and Roose, 1981; Janicak et al., 1988; Khan et al., 1987; Parker et al., 1992; Spiker et al., 1985b). Rates of spontaneous recovery and placebo response rates are also remarkably low among patients with psychotic depression (Aronson et al., 1988; Glassman and Roose, 1981).

Combination treatment with antidepressant medications and neuroleptics is effective in psychotic depression (Parker et al., 1992). Controlled and uncontrolled studies indicate that the combination of heterocyclic antidepressants (amitriptyline, desipramine, nortriptyline) and neuroleptics (chlorpromazine, haloperidol, perphenazine) results in marked improvement in approximately 70% of patients with psychotic depression (Aronson et al., 1988; Nelson and Bowers, 1978; Spiker et al., 1985b). There is some evidence that the combination of an SSRI and a neuroleptic may also be effective (Rothschild et al., 1993; Wolfersdorf et al., 1995).

While the evidence regarding the efficacy of combination antidepressant-neuroleptic treatment is compelling, practicality is often a problem when treating the elderly, psychotically depressed patient. The dosage of a traditional neuroleptic needed to achieve remission is often higher than elderly patients can tolerate. In a dose-finding study, Nelson et al. (1986) found a remarkably poor response rate to the combination of desipramine (150 mg/day) and perphenazine when the perphenazine dose was 32 mg/day or less. The response rate was excellent when the perphenazine dose was 45 mg/day or greater. Spiker et al. (1985b), in a double-blind controlled study, titrated the perphenazine dose to achieve a response. Three-fourths of the patients treated with combination amitriptyline and perphenazine required a perphenazine dose of 64 mg/day.

Traditional neuroleptics and heterocyclic antidepressants have additive anticholinergic and cardiac effects. Neuroleptics can also substantially raise heterocyclic plasma concentrations. The available evidence suggests that the dose of traditional antipsychotic medication needs to be comparable to at least 400 mg/day chlorpromazine equivalents to be effective in combination treatment of psychotic depression (Mulsant et al., 1997). It has not been determined whether this value also approximates the threshold for benefit when translated into comparable units for the newer atypical antipsychotic medications. Independent of the additive and synergistic effects with the antidepressant, many elderly patients cannot tolerate the extrapyramidal and anticholinergic side effects of this level of neuroleptic treatment, whether treated with a traditional or an atypical antipsychotic.

In a largely elderly sample, Mulsant et al. (1997) reviewed the medication trials of 52 patients with psychotic depression who ultimately received ECT. Of note, only 2 of the 52 patients (4%) had received an adequate combination antidepressant-neuroleptic trial prior to ECT. Nearly half of the patients had been treated with a neuroleptic sometime during the index episode, often in combination with an antidepressant. However, virtually none of the patients achieved a dose of at least 400 mg/day chlorpromazine equivalents, and very few achieved even half of this dose.

Recently, evidence has been presented from open case series that monotherapy with other classes of antidepressants (fluvoxamine, venlafaxine) is effective in mixed-age patients with psychotic depression (Gatti et al., 1996). Until such reports are confirmed in controlled trials, there is reason for skepticism. Indeed, in a recent open trial, Simpson and colleagues (2003) treated patients in a major depressive episode with and without psychotic features with sertraline, up to 200 mg/day for an 8-week period. Unlike the enthusiastic reports of SSRI effectiveness in psychotic depression, in this study sertraline was much more effective in the nonpsychotic patients. There is also considerable controversy about whether the newer antidepressants, particularly the SSRIs, are as effective as the traditional heterocyclics in the treatment of severe or melancholic, nonpsychotic major depression (Danish, 1986, 1990; Roose et al., 1994). That monotherapy with the newer agents would show greater efficacy in psychotic depression seems unlikely.

## Electroconvulsive therapy

In contrast to the controversy surrounding pharmacological treatment, the debate in the field of ECT is whether or not the patient with psychotic depression has a higher rate of response to ECT than the nonpsychotic patient (Petrides et al., 2001; Sobin et al., 1996), and, if so, why. In essence, there is the possibility of a double dissociation: the elderly with psychotic depression respond at a lower rate to pharmacological treatment (particularly monotherapy) than the nonpsychotic patient but at a higher rate to ECT.

Early investigations of the symptomatic features associated with the ECT outcome reported that specific delusions, and more generally vegetative or melancholic symptoms, predicted a favorable response (Hamilton and White, 1960; Hobson, 1953; Mendels, 1965a–1965c). In more recent research, the majority of studies that have compared the response of psychotic and nonpsychotic to ECT have found a higher rate of response among the psychotic subgroup (see Nobler and Sackeim, 1996, for a review). There was also evidence from the British trials comparing real and sham ECT that the relative advantage of real treatment was most marked among patients with psychotic features and/or motor retardation (Buchan et al., 1992). Both psychotic depression and motor retardation are more commonly expressed in older than younger depressed patients, and there continues to be evidence that psychomotor disturbance may be a favorable prognostic indicator of an ECT response (Hickie et al., 1990; Sobin et al., 1996). A meta-analysis comparing response rates to ECT and combined antidepressant-neuroleptic treatment in psychotic depression suggests that ECT has superior efficacy (Parker et al., 1992).

There is no doubt that ECT is a highly effective treatment for psychotic depression (Petrides et al., 2001). At issue may be the reason for the possibly superior rate of response in this subgroup. Psychotically depressed patients are often treated with ECT without having failed an adequate combination antidepressant-neuroleptic medication trial (Mulsant et al., 1997; Prudic et al., 1990). This low rate of medication resistance is found particularly in the elderly with psychotic depression, while medication resistance is considerably more frequent among nonpsychotic patients. The higher rate of medication resistance in nonpsychotic patients is due in part to the different standards for adequate pharmacotherapy in nonpsychotic depression, the lesser gravity of the nonpsychotic state—allowing for extended and multiple medication trials—and the younger age of nonpsychotic patients and consequently their greater tolerance of higher dosages. When ECT response or remission rates were compared in psychotic and nonpsychotic depressed patients as a function of medication resistance, it was found that medication resistance, and not psychosis, was predictive of the outcome. Patients who have not failed an adequate medication trial respond to ECT at extraordinarily high rates (i.e., >85%), while response rates are lower (i.e., 50%) in patients with established medication resistance. The psychotically depressed are particularly likely not to have failed an adequate medication trial.

Some consideration should be given to whether methods of ECT administration should be altered in the patient with psychotic depression. The key issues are the choice of electrode placement and the concomitant pharmacotherapy. It has been suggested that BL ECT may be more effective in psychotic depression than RUL ECT (Parker et al., 1992). However, this issue has never been prospectively studied in a controlled fashion, and the evidence preceded much of the newer information regarding the optimization of unilateral ECT (Sackeim et al., 1993, 2000b). For many practitioners, particularly in an elderly psychotic patient with debilitating medical illness or significant suicidality, bilateral ECT remains the gold standard. Just a few years ago, it was said with assurance that no elderly patient should be considered resistant unless he or she had failed a full course (e.g., at least 10 treatments) of suprathreshold bilateral treatment. However, recent evidence indicates that high-dosage RUL ECT is at least equal to BL ECT in efficacy and that long-term amnesia is accentuated especially by the use of BL electrode placement. Therefore, a more reasonable conclusion at this time is that no patient should be considered ECT resistant unless he or she has not benefited from a course of either high-dosage RUL or BL ECT. In the case of RUL ECT, this is defined as treatment at least six times the seizure threshold. In the case of BL ECT, it is defined as treatment that is administered at 2.5 times the seizure threshold.

In the treatment of schizophrenia, there is consistent evidence that the combination of ECT and neuroleptics produces more powerful antipsychotic effects than either treatment alone (Sackeim, 2003). While there are no comparable data on the combination in psychotic depression, similar benefit would not be unexpected. Particularly since the benzodiazepines used to limit anxiety and agitation are frequently problematic in the elderly and may interfere with the therapeutic properties of ECT (Pettinati et al., 1990), use of small or moderate doses of a neuroleptic in combination with ECT is common and does not usually raise issues of safety. Especially in the elderly patient with psychotic depression who shows a slow or insufficient response to ECT, the addition of a neuroleptic may be considered. There has been a series of reports on the combination of ECT with newer antipsychotic medications, specifically clozapine (Benatov et al., 1996; Bhatia et al., 1998; Cardwell and Nakai, 1995; James and Gray, 1999; Meltzer, 1992) and rispiradone (Farah et al., 1995; Tang and Ungvari, 2002). In younger and elderly patients, untoward effects have not been reported. However, since ECT has prominent antiparkinsonism properties, the extrapyramidal side effects usually encountered with traditional neuroleptics are often reduced or eliminated when these agents are combined with ECT (Ananth et al., 1979; Andersen et al., 1987; Balldin et al., 1980; Fall and Granerus, 1999; Goswami et al., 1989).

The goal of ECT is complete resolution of the episode of psychotic depression, including both psychotic and nonpsychotic features. It is sometimes thought that vegetative or melancholic depressive features are particularly responsive to ECT and should resolve prior to nonvegetative symptoms. However, the empirical evidence does not indicate that any group of depressive symptoms is more likely to respond or respond more quickly. In elderly patients with psychotic depression, it is common to observe early resolution of the appetite and sleep disturbances and of the delusionality, with later improvement in subjective mood and feelings of self-worth. It is also common to observe that elements of the delusionality may be late in demonstrating improvement. Indeed, it is probably more common than not that aspects of delusionality gradually recede over the course of ECT. Progressive changes are seen in the bizarreness of delusions, the extent to which they impact on the patient's behavior, the conviction with which they are held, awareness of the delusionality, and so on. The progression in the resolution of delusions can be a guide later in treating an incipient relapse. The patient who progressed with ECT from somatic delusion to somatic concern to full insight without somatic preoccupation may express a somatic concern as a prodrome to full relapse. Issues in relapse prevention in psychotic depression are discussed below.

The psychotically depressed patient who fails ECT is a source of concern. In this circumstance, the first consideration should be whether the course of ECT was adequate. In an earlier era, the average number of ECT treatments given in the United States for major depression was approximately six; at present, the average is approximately eight or nine, likely reflecting the increasing treatment resistance of the patients receiving ECT and the use of lower-intensity stimulation. Some depressed patients begin to show clinical benefit only after extended courses of ECT, that is, after 10 to 12 treatments. There is documentation of elderly, psychotically depressed patients not improving after a

course of standard BL ECT and then showing rapid improvement when BL ECT is continued, but at a much higher stimulus intensity relative to threshold (Sackeim, 1991b). The utility of combining ECT with a neuroleptic has been emphasized. Nonetheless, if clinical progress is insufficient with ECT or if the patient cannot tolerate the treatment, purely pharmacological strategies will be tried. Highly diverse pharmacological approaches have been used successfully in patients who have benefited insufficiently from an adequate course of ECT (Rothschild, 1996; Sackeim et al., 1990a). In the elderly psychotic patient, these include lithium supplementation of antidepressant-neuroleptic combinations, markedly increasing the neuroleptic dosage or switching to a newer class of neuroleptics, and, paradoxically, use of psychostimulants.

## MEDICAL COMPLICATIONS AND RELATIVE CONTRAINDICATIONS

Electroconvulsive therapy is often described as safer than the older heterocyclic antidepressant medications, particularly among the frail elderly (American Psychiatric Association, 2001; Benbow, 1989; Weiner, 1982). Direct controlled comparisons are not available to support this claim. However, the rate of ECT-associated mortality is very low, estimated to be about 1 per 10,000 mixed-aged patients treated and comparable to that observed with general anesthesia in minor surgery (Abrams, 1997, 2002a; American Psychiatric Association, 2001). With ECT, cardiovascular complications are the leading cause of mortality and significant morbidity (Welch and Lambertus, 1989) and, surprising to some, cerebrovascular complications are rare. In part, the relatively strong safety profile of ECT is related to the fact that the generalized seizure is a short-lived event, usually on the order of 40–60 seconds. Consequently, the peripheral hemodynamic and cerebrovascular changes during and following the ictus are transient events that are typically well tolerated, even in the frail elderly, despite their intensity. Further, when cardiovascular and other medical complications arise, they usually occur in the immediate postictal period. During this period, patients' physiological functions are monitored and patients are attended to by trained medical staff, usually including a psychiatrist, an anesthesiologist, and nursing personnel. In contrast, the physiological alterations associated with pharmacological treatment are ever present and, in the absence of defined periods of increased risk, cannot be subject to enhanced monitoring.

It should be noted that the prevailing belief that ECT is less dangerous than pharmacological treatment in many of the elderly and those with preexisting medical conditions biases the assessment of the base rates of

ECT-related medical complications and comparison to pharmacological alternatives. At many centers, those most likely to experience medical complications with any somatic intervention—the medically compromised elderly—are preferentially referred for ECT (Rice et al., 1994; Zielinski et al., 1993).

The strong safety profile of ECT and the recognition that the evaluation of treatment options must always include not only assessment of the likely risks and benefits of specific interventions, but also the risks of no treatment, resulted in the 1990 APA Task Force Report on ECT (American Psychiatric Association, 1990) stating that there are no absolute contraindications for ECT, a position restated in the 2001 report (American Psychiatric Association, 2001). In some cases, the risks of performing ECT will be decidedly increased, but the risks of alternative treatments or of no biological intervention may be greater. Patients at substantially increased risk are those with space-occupying cerebral lesions or other conditions that increase intracranial pressure, recent myocardial infarction associated with unstable cardiac function, recent intracerebral hemorrhage, unstable vascular aneurysm or malformation, pheochromocytoma, or any patient rated at American Society of Anesthesiologists level 4 or 5. In the main, the clinician should be concerned about the use of ECT in any patient in whom a substantial, transient increase in heart rate, blood pressure, intracranial pressure, or intraocular pressure is likely to lead to medical complications. The prevalence of these conditions clearly increases with aging. As noted below, a variety of steps may be taken during the administration of ECT to lessen the probability of medical complications.

Retrospective studies have observed widely varying rates of medical complications during the course of ECT in the elderly, with the range being 0% to 77% of patients developing one or more complications (Alexopoulos et al., 1984; Braddock et al., 1986; Burd and Kettl, 1998; Burke et al., 1985, 1987; Cattan et al., 1990a; de and Kohn, 2000; Fraser, 1981; Fraser and Glass, 1978, 1980; Gaspar and Samarasinghe, 1982; Gerring and Shields, 1982; Huuhka et al., 2003; Kramer, 1987; Rice et al., 1994; Tomac et al., 1997; Zielinski et al., 1993; Zorumski et al., 1988; Zwil and Pelchat, 1994). This variability reflects differences among investigators in their thresholds for what was considered a complication, as well as differences in the medical status of the patient samples. Nonetheless, there is strong consistency in this literature in documenting that ECT-related medical complications are considerably more likely in the elderly (particularly the oldest age groups), in those with preexisting medical conditions (particularly cardiac illness), and in those receiving concurrent medication for medical conditions. Cardiovascular complications and falls are the most common medical problems encountered in the elderly,

and patients older than 75 with preexisting cardiac illness require especially careful monitoring. It is particularly useful to note that the nature of the preexisting heart disease, whether ischemic or ventricular in origin, strongly predicts the nature of the cardiac complications encountered during the course of ECT (Zielinski et al., 1993).

Since cardiovascular complications are the most common cause of medical morbidity and mortality with ECT, especially in the elderly (American Psychiatric Association, 2001), it is surprising that there has been little prospective, controlled work evaluating the possible protection afforded by medication strategies that modify the acute hemodynamic effects of the treatment. Over the past 15 years, prophylactic use of beta-adrenergic blocking agents, such as labetalol or esmolol, has become common, with the aim of lessening the hypertensive and tachycardic effects of seizure induction (Avramov et al., 1998; Blanch et al., 2001; Castelli et al., 1995; Dannon et al., 1998; Drop et al., 1998; Figiel et al., 1993, 1994; Howie et al., 1990; Kovac et al., 1991; McCall et al., 1991; O'Connor et al., 1996; Stoudemire et al., 1990; Zvara et al., 1997). Other agents that are similarly used include nitrates (Ciraulo et al., 1978), hydralazine (Foster and Ries, 1988; Gaines and Rees, 1992), calcium channel blockers (Antkiewicz-Michaluk et al., 1993; Avramov et al., 1998; Ding and White, 2002; Wajima et al., 2002; Wells et al., 1989), diazoxide (Kraus and Remick, 1982), and ganglionic blockers such as trimethaphan (Petrides and Fink, 1996a). Likewise, in recent years, a growing number of centers have routinely used propofol as the anesthesia-induction agent, instead of methohexital or thiopental, partly because propofol results in a smaller magnitude of hemodynamic changes (Avramov et al., 1995; Boey and Lai, 1990; Bone et al., 1988; Dwyer et al., 1988; Fredman et al., 1994; Geretsegger et al., 1998; Hasan and Woolley, 1994; Kirkby et al., 1995; Lim et al., 1996; Martensson et al., 1994; Nguyen et al., 1997; Saito et al., 2000; Zaidi and Khan, 2000). The belief driving this practice is that the frequency and/or severity of postictal arrhythmias, cardiac ischemia, and other cardiovascular adverse events are reduced by the use of prophylactic strategies that result in a lower magnitude of heart rate and blood pressure increases (Figiel et al., 1994; Maneksha, 1991; O'Connor et al., 1996). However, whether any of these approaches are effective in limiting cardiovascular morbidity has not been well documented, as there has been little comparative study of the rates of cardiac complications with or without such an intervention in the relevant population—patients with preexisting cardiac illness (Castelli et al., 1995; Stoudemire et al., 1990). Indeed, when Castelli et al. (1995) compared esmolol (1.3 or 4.4 mg/kg) and labetalol (0.13 or 0.44 mg/kg) with placebo in patients at elevated cardiac risk, the beta blockers were found to have successfully reduced ECT-induced hemodynamic elevations, but there was no evidence of benefit with respect to cardiac complications. This was because there were no adverse events, including significant ST-segment changes, in any treatment group, including the group treated with placebo.

Judgment is needed about when to use such a strategy. Three major considerations suggest judicious use. First, an unintended side effect of administering agents that decrease the heart rate, particularly beta blockers, is the occurrence of asystole during ECT (Decina et al., 1984; Kaufman, 1994; McCall, 1996). Application of the electrical stimulus results in vagal stimulation, regardless of whether a seizure is induced. This parasympathetic discharge almost invariably results in a decreased heart rate unless patients are premedicated with an anticholinergic agent, either atropine or glycopperrolate (McCall et al., 1994). The induction of the seizure produces a sympathetic discharge, an outpouring of catecholamine, and a conversion from bradycardia to tachycardia (Mann et al., 1990). Following the end of the seizure, there may be reflex bradycardia. For a variety of reasons, subconvulsive stimulation (the administration of an electrical stimulus below the seizure threshold) can occur at any time during ECT. In this case, the parasympathetic discharge is unopposed, and in the presence of a beta blocker, asystole may result (Decina et al., 1984; McCall, 1996). Similarly, postseizure reflex bradycardia can be exaggerated by medications that limit heart rate increases.

Second, one of the most common circumstances for considering the use of an agent to limit hemodynamic changes is tachycardia or hypertension prior to treatment. The concern here is that such patients will not tolerate further increases in heart rate or blood pressure. The two studies that examined predictors of the magnitude of the peak hemodynamic changes during ECT concurred in indicating that patients with baseline tachycardia or hypertension (or elevated rate pressure product) showed the smallest absolute increases following seizure induction (Prudic et al., 1987; Webb et al., 1990). In other words, the patients often of most concern typically show the least dramatic increases in hemodynamic variables without any alteration of the procedure. In part, this may be due to the fact that pre-ECT anxiety may be associated with sympathetic discharge, and further increases with seizure induction are limited by ceiling effects.

Finally, there is a theoretical concern that pretreating to limit hemodynamic changes may be counterproductive with respect to other side effects of ECT. During electrically induced seizures, cerebral blood flow increases markedly, on the order of 300%. Oxygen use and glucose metabolism also increase, with estimates in the order of 200% (Ackermann et al., 1986;

Siesjö et al., 1986). The increased cardiac output and peripheral hypertension associated with the seizure may be necessary to sustain the profound ictal increase in cerebral blood flow, as autoregulation is not maintained given the magnitude of the hemodynamic changes associated with ECT. In turn, the enhanced cerebral blood flow provides the transport of the oxygen and carbohydrate supplies that are necessary to sustain the large ictal increase in cerebral metabolic rate. It has been speculated that by limiting the peripheral hemodynamic surge, the oxygen and carbohydrate supplies to the brain may be reduced. This could account for the reduced seizure duration associated with a variety of these agents, including beta blockers and propofol, and could contribute to cognitive side effects.

In this light, we are conservative in the use of pharmacological modifications of standard ECT, with the rationale echoed in the 2001 APA Task Force Report on ECT. In patients who are unequivocally at increased risk for vascular complications, such as those with unstable aneurysms and those in whom ECT is conducted as a high-risk or lifesaving intervention, we may attempt to fully block the hemodynamic changes that accompany seizure induction, and do so prophylactically at all treatments (Devanand et al., 1990). In patients with unstable hypertension or other cardiac conditions and in whom ECT is not conducted on an emergency basis, we typically attempt to stabilize the medical condition before introducing ECT. In most patients, with or without preexisting cardiac illness, we forgo prophylactics and closely monitor cardiovascular changes at the initial treatments. The occasional sustained hypertension and/or significant arrhythmia following seizure induction are treated emergently, and prophylaxis is considered for subsequent treatments. Following these procedures, we have documented that 38 of 40 patients with prospectively determined serious cardiac illness successfully completed an ECT course (Zielinski et al., 1993). Naturally, a strong working relationship with the anesthesiologist, and informed consultation with the cardiologist, are helpful in optimizing management of the elderly patient with significant cardiac illness. It is a mistake, however, to place either the authority or the burden of deciding whether to proceed with ECT on the views of a cardiologist or other consultant. At many centers, internists routinely clear patients for ECT. This judgment assumes that the internist (or other specialist) can uniquely weigh the relative risks and likely benefits of receiving or not receiving this treatment, including those of the viable alternatives. Rather, especially because thoughtful evaluation of the likely benefits is even more critical in high-risk situations, the final recommendations regarding treatment modality (ECT, pharmacology, etc.) must reside with the treating psychiatrist.

## COGNITIVE SIDE EFFECTS

Adverse cognitive effects are the primary factor limiting the use of ECT. In conceptualizing these adverse effects, four key points should be considered. First, the cognitive effects of ECT are highly stereotyped. Knowledge of the short- and long-term deficits that are expected with ECT is essential for adequate informed consent and clinical care (Lisanby et al., 2000; McElhiney et al., 1995; Sackeim, 1992; Squire, 1986). Second, the methods used to administer ECT can impact profoundly the magnitude and persistence of cognitive side effects. The clinician has a number of ways to limit these cognitive changes (Krueger et al., 1992; Sackeim, 1992; Sackeim et al., 1986, 1993, 2000b; Weiner et al., 1986). Third, there are individual differences in the magnitude and persistence of cognitive side effects. An appreciation of which patients are at greater risk for more persistent cognitive deficits can assist the clinician in matching aspects of treatment technique to patient needs (Sobin et al., 1995; Zervas et al., 1993). Finally, independent of objective changes in neuropsychological function, patients' perceptions of their capacity to learn and remember are often altered (Prudic et al., 2000). While many patients report subjective improvement in cognitive function within a few days of ECT (Coleman et al., 1996; Pettinati et al., 1994; Sackeim et al., 2000b), a small minority state that ECT has had a devastating impact on their cognitive abilities (Donahue, 2000; Sackeim, 2000). Understanding the factors leading to these heterogeneous changes in subjective report is important.

### The Nature of Cognitive Side Effects

Similar to the consequences of generalized seizures in epilepsy, in the immediate postictal period following ECT, patients may manifest transient neurological abnormalities, alterations of consciousness (disorientation, attentional dysfunction), sensorimotor abnormalities, and disturbance in higher cognitive functions, particularly learning and memory (Sackeim, 1992). The severity and persistence of these acute effects are exquisitely sensitive to technical factors in ECT administration. These factors determine, for instance, whether patients on average require a few minutes to achieve full reorientation following seizure elicitation or several hours (Daniel and Crovitz, 1983a, 1983b, 1986; Sackeim, 1992; Sackeim et al., 1993, 2000b; Weiner et al., 1986).

Recovery of cognitive function following a single treatment is rapid. However, with forms of ECT that produce more severe acute cognitive effects, recovery often is incomplete by the time of the next treatment. In such cases, repeated acute assessment at the same time points relative to seizure induction demonstrates deterioration over the treatment course (Calev et al., 1991c; Daniel and Crovitz, 1983a, 1986; Fraser and Glass, 1978, 1980; Summers et al., 1979). In practical terms, this progressive deterioration causes some patients to develop an organic mental syndrome with marked disorientation during the ECT course (Daniel and Crovitz, 1986; Figiel et al., 1990). This persistent confusional state presents management problems for the clinical staff, as patients may have difficulty carrying out routine activities of daily life and the mental confusion can be frightening to family members. Furthermore, the development of an organic mental syndrome may result in interruption or premature termination of ECT, thereby reducing its efficacy, and commonly results in extended hospitalization (Miller et al., 1986). Following termination of ECT, organic mental syndromes typically resolve within 2–10 days (Summers et al., 1979). It is noteworthy that with milder forms of ECT, cumulative deterioration in cognitive functions rarely occurs. Indeed, with specific alterations of ECT technique (see below), cumulative improvement in some acute cognitive measures has been demonstrated (Calev et al., 1995; Sackeim, 1986a; Sackeim et al., 2000b).

Associations between the magnitude of most cognitive effects and ECT treatment parameters diminish rapidly as the time from ECT increases. More than a week or two following the end of the ECT course, differences in the cognitive effects of BL and RUL electrode placement are difficult to discern in domains other than retrograde amnesia (memory for events prior to receiving ECT) (Lisanby et al., 2000; Sackeim, 1992; Sackeim et al., 1993, 2000b; Weiner et al., 1986). Furthermore, within days of the end of the ECT course, depressed patients manifest superior performance in most cognitive domains relative to their pretreatment baseline. Indeed, scores on tests of intelligence, including those of the elderly, are higher shortly following ECT relative to the untreated depressed state (Malloy et al., 1982; Sackeim, 1992). Similarly, prior to treatment, depressed patients often manifest deficits in the acquisition of information, as revealed by tests of immediate recall or recognition of item lists (Sackeim and Steif, 1988; Steif et al., 1986; Sternberg and Jarvik, 1976; Zakzanis et al., 1998). Within several days following the ECT course, patients are typically unchanged or improved in immediate memory scores, with the change in clinical state being the critical predictor of the magnitude of improvement (Cronholm and Ottosson, 1963a; Sackeim et al., 1993, 2000b; Steif et al., 1986). In contrast, patients often manifest a marked disturbance in their ability to retain information over a delay. This reflects a double dissociation between the effects of depression and ECT on anterograde learning and memory (Sackeim, 1992). Depression is associated with an acquisition deficit, most likely related to disturbances in attention and concentration, that frequently recedes following treatment with ECT. In contrast, ECT introduces a new deficit in consolidation or retention, so that information that is newly learned is rapidly forgotten (Cronholm and Ottosson, 1963a).

Clinically, this pattern is expressed by pronounced problems with attention and concentration prior to the start of ECT. Patients may be unable to follow the plot of a TV program or take in information about ward rules, the side effects of medications, and so on. Often some of the first evidence of improvement with ECT is manifested in patients' activities. After a few treatments with ECT, they begin to read books, attend group meetings, and are capable of following more complex instructions. However, despite this improvement in attention and concentration, patients may not retain information over a delay. Thus, the fact that a book was read or a conversation was held in the morning will be forgotten by the afternoon. Given this, it is important that ward staff and family members be sensitive to the possibility of anterograde amnesia. Not infrequently, patients will repeatedly request information about a pass for the weekend or an expected visit from a relative. These repeated requests are sometimes interpreted as reflecting ambivalence about participating in the activity or a need for reassurance. In fact, these requests are repeated because the information is quickly forgotten. Determining that the anterograde amnesia has receded is key in determining the duration of the post-ECT convalescence period. It makes no sense for a surgeon to operate in the afternoon after having learned and forgotten the details of the case presented in the morning.

During and following a course of ECT, patients also display retrograde amnesia. Deficits in the recall or recognition of both personal and public information are usually evident, and these deficits are usually greatest for events that occurred temporally closest to the treatment (Lisanby et al., 2000; McElhiney et al., 1995; Squire, 1986; Weiner et al., 1986). Therefore, while memory for more remote events is intact, patients may have difficulty recalling events that transpired during and several months to years prior to the ECT course (Squire, 1975). The retrograde amnesia is rarely dense; patients typically show a spotty memory for recent events. This is important to convey to patients prior to the start of ECT, since it is frequently feared that whole segments of life will be lost. Furthermore, as the time from treatment increases, retrograde memory typically improves, with a return of more distant memories (McElhiney et al., 1995; Squire and Chace, 1975; Weeks et al., 1980; Weiner et al., 1986). This tempo-

rally graded pattern indicating greatest vulnerability for more recent events is compatible with similar findings of the effects of repeated electroconvulsive shock (ECS) in animals (Andrade et al., 2002; Fochtmann, 1994; Krueger et al., 1992; Zornetzer, 1974). Both anterograde and retrograde amnesia are most marked for explicit or declarative memory, while no effect is expected on implicit or procedural memory (Sackeim et al., 1992; Squire et al., 1984, 1985).

Until recently, objective evidence of a persistent cognitive deficit was difficult to document a few weeks following the end of ECT (Sackeim et al., 1993; Squire and Chace, 1975). The anterograde amnesia typically resolves within a few weeks of ECT termination (Sackeim, 1992; Sackeim et al., 1993). It is questionable that ECT alone ever results in a persistent deficit in forming new memories, that is, permanent anterograde amnesia. This fact is often critical in communications with prospective patients. Adequate new learning and memory are essential to job performance.

Retrograde amnesia will often show a more gradual reduction, and over time there will be substantial return of memory for events that were seemingly forgotten immediately following the treatment course. Many, but not all, patients report that they could not spontaneously remember an autobiographical event, such as a family trip, but that after being reminded of the event, they experienced full recall and subsequent retention. This phenomenon implies that much of the retrograde amnesia associated with ECT reflects disruption in the retrieval of memories, as opposed to permanent loss of memory contents. However, persistent effects of ECT have been identified (McElhiney et al., 1995; Sackeim et al., 2000b; Weiner et al., 1986). Most likely due to a combination of retrograde and anterograde effects, even when tested at substantial time periods after treatment, patients may manifest persistent amnesia for some events that transpired in the several months prior to and following the ECT course (McElhiney et al., 1995; Weiner, 1984; Weiner et al., 1986). In rare instances, the retrograde amnesia may extend back several years prior to ECT.

In short, all patients should be informed that ECT exerts characteristic effects on learning and memory. While most cognitive functions improve shortly following ECT, there will be a period in which newly learned information is rapidly forgotten. This anterograde amnesia may last for only a few days or, at most, a few weeks. However, given this rapid forgetting, it is important that the recovery period following ECT be supervised. The rapidity of resolution of this amnesia should shape recommendations for when patients may drive on their own, make important personal and financial decisions, and so on. Patients should also be informed that ECT produces a loss of memory for events that occur prior to the treatment, during the treatment course, and in the weeks following the course. This spotty memory loss will concern events in the life of the patient (autobiographical memory), as well as information learned about the world (public events). While there will also be recovery in this domain, some degree of permanent temporally graded retrograde amnesia will likely occur in all patients who receive ECT. The vast majority of patients consider this a small price for the symptomatic relief obtained (Pettinati et al., 1994). However, as with any other medical intervention, there are individual differences in the magnitude and persistence of side effects (see below). A rare, but possible, profound complication of ECT is a persistent and dense retrograde amnesia that extends back in time for a period of several years. In my experience, such complications are associated with extended courses of especially intense forms of ECT (e.g., sine wave stimulation, BL electrode placement), often where patients continue to receive ECT despite manifesting an organic mental syndrome.

## Treatment Technique

A variety of technical factors determine the magnitude and persistence of the cognitive side effects of ECT. These include the nature of the electrical waveform, anatomical positioning of the stimulating electrodes (electrode placement), electrical stimulus intensity, the spacing or frequency of treatments, the total number of treatments, the duration of seizures, the type and dosage of anesthetic agent, the adequacy of oxygenation, and the use of concomitant medications (American Psychiatric Association, 2001; Sackeim, 1992). Table 21.2 summarizes the steps that can be taken to minimize cognitive side effects by altering the ECT technique.

### Electrical waveform

Up to the past several years, many patients were treated with ECT devices that used constant-voltage, sine wave stimulation. While this form of stimulation has not been eliminated (Prudic et al., in press), its rate of use

TABLE 21.2. *Treatment Technique Factors and the Severity of Cognitive Side Effects of Electroconvulsive Therapy (ECT)*

| Treatment Factor | Effects on Cognitive Parameters | Methods to Reduce Cognitive Side Effects | References* |
|---|---|---|---|
| Stimulus waveform | Sine wave stimulation grossly increases cognitive side effects | Use square wave, brief pulse stimulation | Daniel and Crovitz (1983a) Valentine et al. (1968) Weinter et al. (1986) |
| Electrode placement | Standard bilateral (bifrontotemporal) ECT results in more widespread, severe, and persistent cognitive side effects | Switch to right unilateral ECT | Daniel and Crovitz (1983b) McElhiney et al. (1995) Sackeim et al. (1986, 1993, 2000b) Weiner et al. (1986) |
| Stimulus dosage | Grossly suprathreshold stimulus intensity increases acute and short-term cognitive side effects | Adjust stimulus intensity to needs of individual patients by dosage titration | Sackeim et al. (1993) Sackeim et al. (1986) Sobin et al. (1995) Squire and Zouzounis (1986) |
| Number of treatments | Progressive cognitive decline occurs with high-intensity treatments (sine wave, bilateral, or grossly suprathreshold) | Limit treatments to the number necessary to achieve maximal clinical gains | Calev et al. (1991) Daniel and Crovitz (1983a) Fraser and Glass (1978, 1980) Sackeim et al. (1986a) |
| Frequency of treatments | More frequent treatments (three to five per week) result in greater cognitive deficits | Decrease frequency of ECT | Lerer et al. (1995) McAllister et al. (1987) |
| Oxygenation | Poor oxygenation can result in hypoxia and increased cognitive deficits | Use pulse oximetry to monitor oxygen saturation and administer 100% oxygen prior to seizure induction | APA (1990, 2001) |
| Concomitant medications | High anesthetic dose may increase cognitive effects; some psychotropics can augment cognitive effects | Reduce anesthetic dose to produce light level of anesthesia; decrease or discontinue psychotropic dosage; discontinue lithium prior to ECT | APA (1990, 2001) Miller et al. (1985) Mukherjee (1993) Small and Milstein (1990) |

*Complete reference citations occur at the end of the chapter.
*Source:* Adapted from American Psychiatric Association (2001) with permission.

is very low. Relative to constant-current, brief pulse stimulation, sine wave stimululation is intrinsically inefficient in its capacity to produce seizures. In essence, considerable excess current must be passed with a sine wave device to produce a seizure compared to that produced by a brief pulse device (Weiner, 1980). Not surprisingly, there is a profound difference between sine wave and brief pulse stimulation in cognitive side effects (Valentine et al., 1968; Weiner et al., 1986). No difference has ever been observed with respect to efficacy (Carney and Sheffield, 1974; Valentine et al., 1968; Weiner et al., 1986). As noted in the APA Task Force Report (American Psychiatric Association, 2001), there is no justification for the continued use of sine wave stimulation. Indeed, the report indicates substantially increased liability if sine wave stimulation is used.

There are two main reasons why sine wave stimulation is inefficient in producing neuronal depolarization and seizure induction. The stimulus is slow to reach its peak and substantial stimulation is given after neuronal polarization, during the refractory and relatively refractory phases. It has long been recognized that stimuli that reach peak current density instantaneously, such as with brief or ultrabrief pulses (Fig. 21.4), are more efficient than stimuli that are slow-rising. The sine wave stimulus, given at 60 Hz in the United States, delivers 60 positive-going and 60 negative-going waves per second. Each wave lasts 8.33 ms. Thus, the sine wave stimulus takes 4.17 ms to reach peak, while this is virtually instantaneous with a brief pulse or ultrabrief pulse stimulus. Not only is excessive stimulation given with a sine wave because much of the stimulus is delivered below the threshold for neuronal depolarization, but this very inefficiency actively raises the threshold. Through the principle of accommodation, a slow-rising stimulus will require a greater peak current density than a brief or ultrabrief pulse (Sackeim et al., 1994).

After reaching its peak, the sine wave stimulus requires 4.17 ms to complete the phase. The width of a standard brief rectangular pulse is 0.5–2.0 ms, and ultrabrief stimuli are defined as having a pulse width of less than 0.5 ms. A large literature has indicated that the chronaxie for the optimal pulse width to produce neuronal depolarization is on the order of 0.1–0.2 ms. Thus, the 4.17 ms-period from peak to offset of the sine wave stimulus indicates that a considerable amount of stimulation is given during the neuronal refractory and relatively refractory periods.

Abandonment of sine wave stimulation dramatically reduced the acute cognitive side effects of ECT. Recent research indicates that the standard brief pulse stimulus uses an excessively wide pulse width and results in substantial stimulation after neuronal depolarization. In a study contrasting a traditional pulse width (1.5 ms) with ultrabrief pulse stimulation (0.3 ms), the Columbia University group found that the initial seizure threshold is approximately three to four times less with ultrabrief stimulation. In this study, patients were also randomized to treatment with RUL stimulation (6× [ST]) or BL (2.5× ST) ECT. The magnitude of the advantage of ultrabrief stimulation over standard brief pulse stimulation on effects on cognition was as large as or larger than the difference between RUL and BL ECT on adverse cognitive effects.

The finding that ultrabrief pulse stimulation profoundly reduced adverse cognitive effects had been anticipated, given the findings of earlier studies (Cronholm and Ottoson, 1963a; 1963b; Robin and De Tissera, 1982; Valentine et al., 1968). However, the efficacy findings of the recent Columbia University trial were surprising. Ultrabrief pulse (0.3 ms) RUL ECT administered at six times the initial seizure threshold was comparable in efficacy to standard pulse width (1.5 ms) BL (2.5× ST) or RUL (6× ST) ECT. In contrast, ultrabrief pulse (2.5× ST) BL ECT lacked efficacy. This study provided the first demonstration of an instance where BL ECT had markedly inferior therapeutic effects compared to RUL ECT. The explanation offered for this surprising finding was that the dosage relative to the seizure threshold in the ultrabrief BL ECT condition was insufficient. With a 0.3-ms pulse width, an electrical intensity that is 2.5 times the initial seizure threshold is insufficient to maximize the efficacy of BL

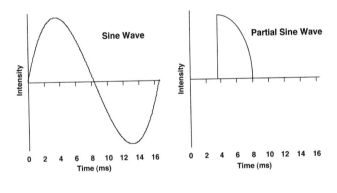

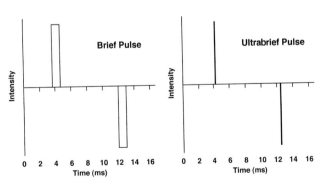

FIGURE 21.4 Examples of some of the waveforms used in ECT. Top left: sine wave; top right: chopped, rectified sine wave; bottom left: brief pulse, square wave; bottom right: ultrabrief pulse, square wave. (After Sackeim et al., 1994)

ECT. This is because the size of the population of neurons participating in seizure onset with this form of ECT is too small to provoke an adequate inhibitory response following the seizure, leading to diminished efficacy. While this explanation predicts that more intense stimulation would convert the ultrabrief BL treatment into an effective form of ECT, this possibility is only of academic interest. This study also produced the first instance in which a treatment with a superior cognitive side effect profile was also superior in efficacy (ultrabrief RUL ECT vs. ultrabrief BL ECT). Since ultrabrief RUL ECT (0.3 ms and 6× ST) is highly effective and has a profoundly reduced side effect profile, in the future it is likely to be widely adopted as the standard form of ECT.

### Electrode placement

For the past 30 years, one of the most contentious areas in ECT has been the anatomical positioning of stimulating electrodes, and specifically the use of BL versus RUL ECT. This debate has centered on efficacy and on the issue of whether BL ECT accentuates long-term amnesia (Abrams, 2002a; Kellner, 2001; Sackeim, 2000; Sackeim et al., 2001a). It is widely recognized that BL ECT results in more profound acute and short-term cognitive side effects than RUL ECT (Sackeim, 1992). In the immediate postictal period, the duration of disorientation is considerably greater with BL relative to RUL ECT (Daniel and Crovitz, 1986; Sackeim et al., 1986, 1993; Sobin et al., 1995). During the administration of ECT and in the days following the termination of ECT, BL ECT results in greater retrograde amnesia for personal and public information (Lisanby et al., 2000; McElhiney et al., 1995; Sackeim et al., 1993; Weiner et al., 1986). Anterograde amnesia, particularly for verbal material, is also greater following BL ECT (Daniel and Crovitz, 1983b; Sackeim et al., 1993; Steif et al., 1986; Weiner et al., 1986).

Weiner et al. (1986) provided some of the first objective evidence of long-term cognitive sequelae following ECT. Compared to depressed patients treated with medications, those who received RUL ECT did not show greater retrograde amnesia for autobiographical information 6 months after the ECT course. However, there was impairment at this time point in patients treated with BL ECT. The difference between RUL and BL ECT in long-term amnesia was greater in magnitude than the difference between brief pulse and sine wave stimulation. However, the small sample size studied at 6 months left considerable doubt about the consistency and clinical relevance of this effect. This issue was especially controversial since a difference between the ECT modalities in long-term amnesia means that at least some form of ECT can produce long-term or permanent amnesia, a possibility that until recently was denied by most authorities.

Broad and intensive neuropsychological evaluation was incorporated in the randomized, double-blind efficacy trials conducted at Columbia University (Sackeim et al., 1987a, 1993, 2000b). In the most recent studies, 2 months following the completion of ECT, patients treated with the BL electrode placement had greater retrograde amnesia for both personal and public information than patients treated with RUL ECT. The dosage of electricity used for treatment had no effect at this long-term time point. However, these findings also derived from relatively small samples, and unlike the 6 month time point, follow-up at 2 months may be too soon to quantify permanent amnestic effects. Of note, significant between-group differences in small samples may arise either because the effect size is large and there is a genuine difference or because the results are unreliable and heavily influenced by outliers or measurement errors.

There was also a neuropsychological component in the recent naturalistic, prospective study of ECT practices and outcomes for patients treated in community settings (Prudic et al., in press). In the first phase of this study, nearly 400 patients, treated at seven hospitals were enrolled. The neuropsychological battery was administered just prior to the start of ECT, during the week following ECT, and 6 months after completion of the acute ECT course. Time constraints for patient involvement dictated the use of a streamlined and, in some respects, superficial neuropsychological battery. For example, the Columbia University Autobiographical Memory Interview: Short Form was used instead of the long form, the former taking about 20 minutes to administer and the latter about 1.5–2.5 hours. Nonetheless, on this primary measure of retrograde amnesia, the memory loss was greater at 6 months in patients treated with BL ECT than in those who received RUL ECT. At this time point, and unlike the assessments immediately following ECT, there were no effects of stimulus waveform. However, the number of treatments received during the ECT course, and specifically the number of BL ECT treatments, had a significant linear relationship with the extent of memory loss.

In short, there is now compelling evidence from a community-based trial that is fully consonant with the results of recent controlled trials. The traditional BL electrode placement substantially increases the severity of memory loss following ECT, both short- and long-term. It is generally agreed that material subject to amnesia 6 months following ECT is unlikely to be recovered spontaneously; that is, the amnesia is permanent. There is also reason to suspect that elderly patients are particularly sensitive to the adverse cognitive effects of BL ECT (Fraser and Glass, 1980; Sackeim, 1992; Zervas et al., 1993). When effects of aging on amnesia are seen, they indicate greater vulnerability in the elderly.

The choice of electrode placement has also been a contentious issue because of claims about efficacy

(Ottosson, 1991; Sackeim, 1991b). Particularly in the United States and England, there has been concern that RUL ECT has inherently inferior therapeutic properties relative to BL ECT (American Psychiatric Association, 1990; Royal College of Psychiatrists, 1995). Indeed, the recent National Institute for Clinical Excellence report concluded from its meta-analysis that bilateral ECT is more effective than unilateral ECT in the treatment of major depression ("Efficacy and safety," 2003). However, after approximately 40 comparative studies, this issue has been resolved in a manner that would not be reflected in a meta-analysis. It is now evident that the efficacy of both RUL and BL ECT can be undone, depending on the parameters of stimulation (Sackeim et al., 1987a, 1993, 2000b). Thus, it is not appropriate to ask whether either electrode placement is intrinsically superior or inferior. One must ask whether there is a difference in efficacy when both are administered in an optimal fashion. The efficacy of RUL ECT is especially sensitive to electrical dosage. When stimulus intensity is near the seizure threshold, RUL ECT lacks therapeutic properties. This lack of efficacy is not relative. Even patients who ordinarily respond to ECT at extraordinarily rapid rates—that is, the elderly without established medication resistance, with short episode duration, and/or with psychotic depression—fail to respond to low-dosage RUL ECT (Sackeim et al., 1987a, 1993). This issue is particularly germane to the treatment of the elderly. In the recent past, most practitioners administered a fixed electrical dosage to all patients. Since age is a reliable predictor of seizure threshold, because of the use of a fixed electrical dose, older patients were treated closer to their thresholds (Coffey et al., 1995a, 1995b; Enns and Karvelas, 1995; Sackeim et al., 1987c, 1991). When RUL ECT was used, older patients were particularly likely to receive ineffective treatment. Since the electrical dosage determines the speed of response regardless of electrode placement (Sackeim et al., 1991, 1993), with a fixed electrical dose older patients often received too many treatments, even with BL ECT.

The efficacy of RUL ECT improves as the dosage relative to the seizure threshold is escalated (Sackeim et al., 1993, 2000b). As we and others have shown, at markedly suprathreshold dosing (e.g., 6 times the initial seizure threshold), RUL ECT achieves an efficacy equivalent to that of robust forms of BL ECT (e.g., 2.5 times the initial seizure threshold)(McCall et al., 2000; Sackeim et al., 2000b). However, if one has to increase the electrical dose of RUL ECT to such high levels, the key clinical question is whether advantages are retained with respect to cognitive side effects. The available data suggest that even at grossly suprathreshold stimulus intensities, RUL ECT retains significant advantages with respect to cognitive parameters (Sackeim et al., 2000b). Indeed, while clear-cut adverse effects of electrical dos-

age can be seen in measures taken acutely during the ECT course, the effects of electrode placement are more extensive and persistent. Long after the completion of ECT, effects on cognition will be linked to the electrode placement used and not to the dosing range. Particularly since the elderly are highly sensitive to the cognitive side effects of BL ECT, in my view, use of suprathreshold forms of RUL ECT should be routine in this population. Indeed, given the marked cognitive benefits of ultrabrief stimulation, optimal treatment might involve dose-titrated, ultrabrief stimulation, using markedly suprathreshold RUL ECT.

From a practical point of view, at many centers BL ECT is reserved for patients in whom ECT is conducted in the context of a psychiatric or medical emergency or in medically high-risk patients in whom the number of treatments must be minimized. When patients are started on BL ECT, and show substantial clinical progress but unacceptable cognitive side effects, a switch to RUL ECT should be considered. Patients who show inadequate progress when treated with RUL ECT may be given an increased stimulus dosage before a switch to BL ECT is considered.

Brain imaging and other findings have led to the hypothesis that modulation of functional activity in frontal cortex (e.g., medial-orbital cortex) is key to efficacy, while the persistent amnesia is due to deregulation in medial temporal lobe structures (Nobler et al., 1994, 2001; Sackeim, 1999, 2001b; Sackeim et al., 1983, 1996, 2000a). Thus, forms of ECT that avoid primary stimulation in or secondary generalization to the hippocampus and other medial temporal lobe structures might be preferred. With this theory in mind, a group at Queens University in Kingston, Ontario, Canada developed the bifrontal electrode placement (Delva et al., 2000; Lawson et al., 1990; Letemendia et al., 1993). The hope was that this placement would mimic the action of BL ECT in frontal lobe structures but have diminished short- and long-term amnestic effects. Due to the inhomogeneity of the skull in impedance, it is doubtful that the current paths in the brain differ for BL and bifrontal placements, as suggested by initial studies of voltage gradients produced by both types of ECT as measured in multicontact, indwelling electrodes in the brains of nonhuman primates (Lisanby, 2003; Lisanby et al., 2003). In this work, BL and bifrontal ECT did not differ in voltage gradients in contacts in the medial temporal lobe. Furthermore, while immediately following the treatment course a slight cognitive advantage was seen with bifrontal relative to BL ECT in one study (Bailine et al., 2000), other studies found that high-dose RUL ECT had both superior cognitive and superior efficacy profiles compared to bifrontal ECT (Heikman et al., 2002). The theory guiding the development of bifrontal ECT may be correct, but its current instantiation may hardly differ from traditional BL ECT in neurophysiological and behavioral effects. Indeed, in our study of ECT in community settings, the profile of cognitive effects immediately after this treatment and 6 months later in patients treated with the bifrontal placement was indistinguishable from that of patients treated only with bilateral ECT.

### Stimulus dosing

In general clinical practice, using brief pulse, constant current stimulation, patients vary at least 50-fold in their initial seizure threshold (the minimum electrical intensity necessary to produce an adequate generalized seizure) (Boylan et al., 2000; Lisanby et al., 1996; Sackeim, 1991a). Indeed, when one factors in the greater efficiency in seizure elicitation with an ultrabrief stimulus and RUL placement, thresholds with this combination are often below 10 mC, while patients with exceptionally high thresholds using a conventional stimulus configuration may have thresholds greater than 1000 mC (Lisanby et al., 1996; Sackeim, 1991a).

The three factors that reliably predict seizure threshold are electrode placement, gender, and age (Coffey et al., 1995b; Colenda and McCall, 1996; Enns and Karvelas, 1995; Sackeim et al., 1987b, 1987c, 1991). Seizure threshold is higher with BL than with RUL electrode placement, in males relative to females, and in older patients. However, the combined predictive power of these features is insufficient to base the choice of electrical dosage on a formula (American Psychiatric Association, 2001; Colenda and McCall, 1996; Sackeim, 1997). Regardless, the patients with the highest thresholds are elderly males treated with BL ECT (Lisanby et al., 1996; Sackeim, 1991a). In some cases, the current generation of ECT devices available in the United States will be insufficient to ensure optimal treatment of such patients even with maximal stimulus output. There is reason to suspect that elderly male patients with cardiac disease may be particularly represented in the subgroup with an extraordinarily high seizure threshold (Lisanby et al., 1996). The use of ultrabrief stimulation may partially solve this problem. Since this form of stimulation is considerably more efficient, seizure thresholds are greatly reduced, allowing a greater effective range for dosing relative to threshold.

With respect to efficacy, speed of response, and cognitive side effects, the degree to which the ECT stimulus exceeds the seizure threshold is critical. Markedly suprathreshold dosing will improve the efficacy of RUL ECT, enhance the speed of clinical improvement with RUL and BL ECT, and result in more severe acute and short-term cognitive side effects (Sackeim et al., 1986, 1993; Sobin et al., 1995; Squire and Zouzounis, 1986). These effects are not attributable to the absolute electrical dosage administered—that is, where the practi-

tioner sets the ECT device parameters—but rather are due to the extent to which the absolute dose exceeds the threshold for the individual patient (McCall et al., 2000; Sackeim et al., 1987a, 1987b, 1991, 1993, 1994, 2000b). Consequently, when a fixed or formula-based approach is used to determine electrical dosing, some patients may be treated with electrical stimuli that are far in excess of threshold, thereby contributing to cognitive side effects, while other patients may be treated with barely suprathreshold stimuli, thereby comprising efficacy.

Duration of the seizure is not a guide to the adequacy of stimulus dosing. Brief and inadequate seizures are observed when the electrical dose is right at the seizure threshold and when the electrical dose is markedly suprathreshold (Sackeim et al., 1991). This counterintuitive fact has important implications for selection of the electrical dose. The longest seizures, often weak in electroencephalographic (EEG) amplitude, are obtained when the patient is treated just above the seizure threshold. As the electrical dosage is increased, the seizures become more robust in EEG amplitude (Krystal et al., 1995) but shorter in duration. Independent of electrical dosage, older patients have seizures of shorter duration (Krystal et al., 1993; Nobler et al., 1993; Perera et al., in press; Sackeim et al., 1987; Sackeim et al., 1991). Some practitioners have held the mistaken view that short but robust seizures lack therapeutic properties (Maletzky, 1978) and that increasing the stimulus intensity invariably results in longer seizure duration. In elderly patients already being treated at suprathreshold stimulus intensity, further increments in stimulus dosage only result in a further decrease in seizure duration and more severe cognitive side effects.

These considerations suggest that knowledge of the patient's seizure threshold, particularly at the outset of ECT, is key to guiding selection of the stimulus dosage. The danger of underdosage is ineffective or inefficient treatment, despite an apparently adequate seizure duration. The danger of overdosage is excessive side effects. In particular, clinicians should consider a decrease in stimulus dosage in patients who have received significantly suprathreshold stimulation with unacceptable cognitive side effects.

Some investigators have recommended that the choice of stimulus dosing be based solely on age, setting the percentage of maximal device output to match the age of the patient (Abrams, 2002b; Petrides and Fink, 1996b, 1996c). Age-based dosing cannot be recommended, as it provides a poor approximation of the seizure threshold and the greatest errors, resulting in overdosing of the oldest patients. Figure 21.5 presents the threshold data for 245 patients treated primarily with RUL ECT in a multicenter study (Boylan et al., 2001). As in all previous studies reporting associations between age and seizure threshold (Coffey et al., 1995b;

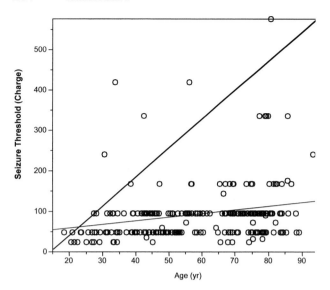

FIGURE 21.5 Initial seizure threshold as a function of age for 245 patients treated with right unilateral electroconvulsive therapy (Boylan et al., 2000). The diagonal line represents the dosage patients would receive based on age-based dosing—for example, 50% of device output for a 50-year-old patient. The lower line is the fit of the regression of age on seizure threshold. While there is a significant relationship ($r = 0.19$ for raw values), there is marked variability. Dosing based solely on age provides a poor approximation of dosing needs and results in the greatest overdosing in the oldest patients.

Colenda and McCall, 1996; Enns and Karvelas, 1995; Krueger et al., 1993; Sackeim et al., 1987c), while a significant association was obtained, the magnitude of the effect was modest.

### Number and schedule of treatments

The cognitive side effects of ECT are sensitive to the frequency with which the treatment is administered and the total number of treatments given (Lerer et al., 1995; McAllister et al., 1987; Sackeim et al., in prep.). This is particularly the case when the most intense forms of ECT are used, that is, markedly suprathreshold, bilateral treatment. The most common schedule in the United States is three treatments per week. In England, it is two treatments per week. It appears that the former schedule results in more rapid improvement, but with greater short-term cognitive side effects (Lerer and Shapira, 1986; Lerer et al., 1995; Shapira et al., 1991). Again, sensitivity to treatment frequency and number is likely increased in the elderly (Calev et al., 1991b; Daniel and Crovitz, 1983a; Fraser and Glass, 1978, 1980; Sackeim et al., 1986). In our practice, it is common to reduce the frequency of treatment to twice a week in elderly patients who show progressive clinical improvement but excessive cognitive side effects. Our study of ECT outcomes in the community found that the overall number of ECT treatments during the acute phase predicted the extent of neuropsychological deficits

at 6-month follow-up. The number of BL treatments but not the number of RUL treatments administered was associated with a poorer cognitive long-term outcome (Sackeim et al., unpublished). Therefore, if BL ECT is used, minimizing exposure to that required for maximal improvement will minimize untoward cognitive effects.

### Concomitant medications

There is some evidence that the dose of anesthetic agent may contribute to the severity of cognitive side effects in the postictal recovery period (Miller et al., 1985). Not surprisingly, an excessive anesthetic dose may result in prolonged postictal disorientation. The purpose of the anesthetic agent in ECT is to render the patient unconscious during the period of muscle paralysis produced by the succinylcholine. The ECT electrical stimulus itself produces immediate loss of consciousness, so the lack of awareness of paralysis before and after the seizure is the primary role of the anesthetic agent. The elderly commonly require lower doses of anesthetic agents than younger patients. This is particularly important since the dose of the anesthetic may impact on seizure expression (Krueger et al., 1993; Sackeim et al., 1991). Also, independent of the anesthetic dose, the elderly manifest seizures with the shortest duration and the lowest EEG amplitude (Krystal et al., 1995; Nobler et al., 1993; Sackeim et al., 1991).

The use of agents with significant central anticholinergic activity is usually avoided in elderly patients due to their propensity to worsen cognitive deficits and produce delirium. However, a small dose of a muscarinic anticholinergic agent (0.4–0.8 mg atropine or 0.2–0.4 mg glycopyrrolate) is commonly administered intravenously in ECT, just prior to the anesthetic agent. The anticholinergic serves to block vagal outflow and limit the bradycardia produced by the ECT stimulus. An anticholinergic is strongly recommended whenever there is the possibility of subconvulsive stimulation or when patients are administered a beta blocker (Zielinski et al., 1993). Theoretically, glycopyrrolate might be preferred, since under normal circumstances it does not cross the blood–brain barrier. However, ECT results in transient disruption of the blood–brain barrier, likely as a function of the central hypertension (Bolwig, 1988; Bolwig et al., 1977a–1977c), and the cognitive effects of anesthesia, electrical stimulation of the brain, and seizure induction are likely to outweigh by far the effects of a small dose of the anticholinergic agent. Indeed, randomized comparisons with atropine have not shown any advantage for glycopyrrolate with respect to cognitive effects during ECT (Greenan et al., 1983; Kellway et al., 1986; Kramer, 1993; Kramer et al., 1986; Simpson et al., 1987; Sommer et al., 1989; Swartz and Saheba, 1989). We prefer atropine, since protection against bradycardia is less certain with glycopyrrolate and the incidence of postictal nausea is higher (Kramer et al., 1986; Swartz and Saheba, 1989).

In sensitive patients, a variety of psychotropic agents may intensify the adverse cognitive effects of ECT. Lithium carbonate has been of greatest concern, since approximately 1 in 15 patients develop an acute confusional state when lithium is continued during ECT and, more rarely, status epilepticus (Milstein and Small, 1988; Mukherjee, 1993; Small and Milstein, 1990; Small et al., 1980; Weiner et al., 1980). Discontinuation of lithium just prior to the start of ECT avoids these complications. When lithium is an integral part of continuation or maintenance pharmacotherapy and ECT is also used to prevent relapse or recurrence, lithium can be withheld both the night and the morning before ECT. In the elderly, concurrent use of benzodiazepines, neuroleptics, or other psychotropic agents, in principle, can be responsible for augmented cognitive side effects. In such cases, dose reduction or discontinuation may be needed. In practice, benzodiazepines and anticonvulsant medications are of significant concern due to their possible interference with ECT efficacy (Greenberg and Pettinati, 1993; Pettinati et al., 1990).

The equivalent of ECT in animals, ECS, is the most common paradigm used to produce amnesia and screen pharmacological agents for protective effects on memory. Approximately 50–100 compounds have shown beneficial effects in animal work, but there have been few attempts to test the potential of pharmacological protection in human ECT (Andrade et al., 2000; Fochtmann, 1994; Krueger et al., 1992). Although some initial findings have been encouraging (Khan et al., 1994; Levin et al., 1987; Prudic et al., 1999; Stern et al., 1991), the work in this area has been preliminary and no pharmacological intervention is established as effective in reducing the amnestic effects of ECT.

## Individual Differences

Regardless of how ECT is performed, patients vary considerably in the magnitude of cognitive side effects. There are two key clinical questions: (1) Are there signs available during the ECT course that predict which patients will develop more severe and/or persistent short- and long-term cognitive deficits? (2) Can we identify the patients most at risk for severe and/or persistent amnesia prior to the start of ECT? Over the 70-year history of convulsive therapy, there have been numerous investigations of the technical factors that influence the magnitude of cognitive side effects. Surprisingly, only in the past few years has there been investigation of the patient factors that predict variability in these deficits.

As indicated, the most intense cognitive deficits are seen in the acute postictal period. Patients vary considerably both in the severity of postictal cognitive changes and in their speed of recovery. Furthermore, on theoretical grounds, there is reason to suspect that specific postictal deficits reflect a more intense form of the amnesia that is observed following the ECT course. For example, the disorientation for name, place, and date seen in the postictal state has been viewed as a form of rapidly shrinking retrograde amnesia (Daniel and Crovitz, 1986; Sobin et al., 1995). It is not uncommon to observe elderly patients "age" with progressive recovery from disorientation. When first asked, 80-year-old patients frequently report that they are 20 years old. With repeated questioning, their reports of their age gradually approach their current status, likely reflecting a remarkably rapid resolution of retrograde amnesia. Similarly, bilingual patients often awaken speaking their first language and only with time respond in English. Consequently, it is important to determine whether the severity of postictal disorientation predicts the magnitude of amnesia following termination of ECT.

The one study on this issue examined the time needed to recover orientation in the postictal period in relation to the magnitude of amnesia for autobiographical events in the 1 week and 2 months following the end of ECT (Sobin et al., 1995). Patients who had more prolonged postictal disorientation had more severe retrograde amnesia at both post-ECT time points (Fig. 21.5). This effect was independent of the method of ECT administration (electrical placement or electrical dosage). While clearly in need of replication and extension to measures of anterograde amnesia, these findings are of clinical importance. They provide the clinician with a behavioral guide as to which patients may be most at risk for severe or prolonged retrograde amnesia. When methods of ECT administration are standardized (electrode placement, stimulus dosing, anesthetic dosing, etc.), some patients take twice or three times as long to reorient and be capable of leaving the recovery room. Indeed, as noted, some patients develop an organic mental syndrome, that is, a continuous confusional state (Daniel and Crovitz, 1986; Summers et al., 1979). While there is rapid improvement in global cognitive status immediately following termination of ECT, patients with prolonged postictal disorientation are likely to develop the most severe and persistent retrograde amnesia. These findings support the utility of monitoring the time to the recovery of orientation in the postictal state, at least at a gross level, and suggest that the treatment technique should be modified to reduce the intensity of postictal and long-term deficits in patients who initially present with prolonged disorientation (see Table 21.2).

A variety of retrospective studies have indicated that patient age and medical status are predictors of the development of persistent confusion during the ECT course (Alexopoulous et al., 1989; Burke et al., 1985,

1987; Fraser and Glass, 1978, 1980; Gaspar and Sama-rasinghe, 1982; Kramer, 1987; Miller et al., 1986). Older patients and those with a compromised medical status are most at risk for prolonged confusion during the course of ECT. Zervas et al. (1993) found that older depressed patients had more severe anterograde and retrograde amnesia immediately following the end of ECT relative to younger patients, with some of the differences persisting at 1-month follow-up. Unfortunately, in this work, a cutoff of 65 years was used for the oldest patients in the sample.

Sobin et al. (1995) examined the relations of preexisting cognitive impairment to the magnitude of retrograde amnesia for autobiographical information immediately and 2 months following the end of ECT. In a sample restricted to patients with major depression without known neurological disease or insult (e.g., stroke, parkinsonism, epilepsy, etc.), pre-ECT baseline scores on the modified Mini-Mental State Examination (MMSE) predicted the magnitude of retrograde amnesia at both time points. Patients with impaired global cognitive status at the pre-ECT baseline manifested the greatest retrograde amnesia following ECT. In this work, both the duration of postictal disorientation and the baseline MMMS score uniquely predicted long-term retrograde amnesia. Of particular note, patients with impaired global cognitive status at baseline showed the greatest improvement in MMMS scores at long-term follow-up, indicating the dissociation between improvement in global cognitive status following ECT and the severity of amnesia (Fig. 21.6). Consequently, these findings indicate that monitoring changes in patients' global cognitive status with instruments like the MMMS is insufficient to gauge the depth of amnesia. Furthermore, the findings support the notion that patients with preexisting cognitive impairment, even outside the context of frank neurological disease, are at risk for more prolonged retrograde amnesia and require appropriate modification of the ECT technique to reduce the cognitive side effects (see Table 21.2). Finally, the findings suggest that the global cognitive impairment seen in the depressed state is a vulnerability factor for the amnestic effects of seizure induction. While *pseudodemented* patients (Caine, 1986) often show dramatic improvement in global cognitive status during and following ECT, they are at heightened risk for more prolonged and deeper amnesia. Consequently, baseline cognitive impairment in the elderly depressed patient may not simply be another depressive feature that fully reverses with symptomatic response, but may denote a subgroup whose memory function is more fragile. It is important to determine whether such patients are more likely to manifest dementia at long-term follow-up.

Increasingly, ECT is being used to treat psychiatric manifestations in a variety of patient populations with frank neurological illness, including Parkinson's disease

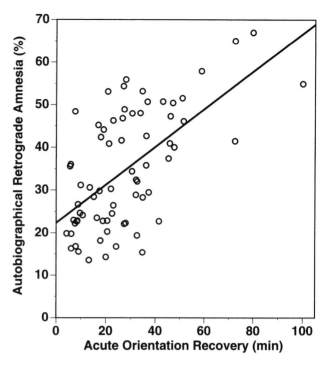

FIGURE 21.6  Relationship between the duration of acute postictal disorientation and retrograde amnesia for autobiographical information during the week following the electroconvulsive therapy course. (After Sobin et al., 1995)

(Andersen et al., 1987; Asnis, 1977; Balldin et al., 1980; Douyon et al., 1989; Fromm, 1959; see Faber and Trimble, 1991, and Kellner et al., 1994, for reviews), poststroke depression (Gustafson et al., 1995; Hsiao et al., 1987; Murray et al., 1986), and, to a lesser extent, dementing disorders (Nelson and Rosenberg, 1991; Price and McAllister, 1989). Across a variety of neurological disorders, there is evidence that ECT is effective in the treatment of primary or secondary mood disorders. In the case of Parkinson's disease, ECT frequently produces beneficial effects on aspects of the movement disorder, and it has been used as a primary treatment for the neurological condition. The limitation here is that the longevity of the antiparkinsonian effects is unpredictable, with some patients losing benefit within days and others maintaining the improvement in the movement disorder for months or longer (Pridmore and Pollard, 1996). The role of continuation or maintenance ECT in sustaining the improvement in the movement disorder is largely undocumented, although clinical experience indicates that such long-term treatment can be highly effective. Of note, however, is the fact that patients with Parkinson's disease who receive ECT may be at increased risk for prolonged confusion or delirium (Figiel et al., 1991, 1992). Similarly in poststroke depression and major depression in the context of dementing illness, the efficacy of ECT is apparent, as well as a propensity for more severe cognitive side effects.

A recent retrospective study of 21 patients with depression and dementia reported a generally favorable clinical outcome, with an increased tendency toward transient postictal confusion compared to similarly aged nondemented, depressed patients (Nelson and Rosenberg, 1991). Similar findings were reported in a retrospective study of 135 ECT patients with concomitant dementia-like syndromes (Price and McAllister, 1989). While there has been little prospective study in this area, it is clear that ECT is an effective treatment for psychiatric manifestations in a variety of neurological conditions, and such patients are likely to experience greater adverse cognitive side effects. It is routine in our practice to inform patients of this heightened risk when they present with preexisting cognitive impairment and/or neurological illness, regardless of their age.

## Patient Attitudes

Both prior to and following ECT, patients' subjective evaluations of their memory function often are discrepant with the findings with objective neuropsychological tests (Prudic et al., 2000). Using a variety of instruments to elicit self-reports and to assess memory, with one possible exception (Coleman et al., 1996), no investigator has observed a significant relation between changes in subjective and objective measures of memory functioning at short- or long-term testing intervals following ECT (Calev et al., 1991a; Cronholm and Ottosson, 1963a; Frith et al., 1983; Sackeim et al., 1993, 2000b; Shellenberger et al., 1982; Squire and Slater, 1983; Squire and Zouzounis, 1988; Weiner et al., 1986). This lack of association is not unique to psychiatric samples, as the relations between objective impairment and subjective reports are generally weak or nonexistent in healthy and neurological samples (Bennett-Levy and Powell, 1980; Broadbent et al., 1982; Hinkin et al., 1996; Larrabee and Levin, 1986; Rabbitt, 1982). Age per se has little impact on the relations between subjective and objective measures of memory function.

Early studies by Squire and colleagues (Squire and Chace, 1975; Squire and Cohen, 1979; Squire and Slater, 1983) suggested that shortly after RUL ECT there was no change in the level of patients' memory complaints, but that with BL ECT there was an increase in memory complaints and a redistribution in the nature of perceived deficits. On being tested several months after ECT, patients who had received BL ECT showed a reduction of memory complaints, reaching the global level that was observed in RUL ECT patients, but nonetheless showing a persistent redistribution in the nature of complaints. However, as with objective cognitive side effects, technical factors in the way ECT is performed may impact on alterations in subjective complaints. The work by Squire and colleagues typically involved high-intensity (sine wave) electrical stimulation in patients who were not randomly assigned to RUL or BL electrode placements.

Since then, a large set of studies has demonstrated marked improvement in patients' subjective reports of memory function within days of the end of ECT principally using the Squire Memory Complaint Questionnaire (SMCQ) (Calev et al., 1991a; Coleman et al., 1996; Mattes et al., 1990; Pettinati and Rosenberg, 1984; Sackeim et al., 1993; Weiner et al., 1986). Pettinati and Rosenberg (1984) found that shortly following ECT, patients randomly assigned to brief pulse RUL or BL ECT showed pronounced improvement in self-evaluations of memory functioning. There was no evidence that the treatment groups differed in the global level or distribution of perceived memory difficulties. Likewise, Weiner et al. (1986) observed that within 2 to 3 days following ECT termination, there was a marked improvement in global self-ratings of memory function compared to pre-ECT baseline, with no differences between ECT patients and non-ECT matched controls. Similarly, in several studies, the Columbia University group repeatedly observed that the great majority of patients reported fewer memory difficulties within a week of the ECT course than they had prior to the course (Sackeim et al., 1993, 2000b). In one study by this group, the memory self-ratings of patients at 2-month follow-up were generally indistinguishable from those of healthy controls (Coleman et al., 1996). No evidence has been obtained in any of the recent work that ECT results in a redistribution of the nature of perceived memory problems.

Therefore, with group data from mixed-age samples it appears that ECT has little, if any, persistent effect on self-evaluation of memory functioning. It may be surprising that most current research indicates that memory complaints decrease during the course of ECT. However, three issues are relevant here. First, across psychiatric, neurological, and healthy samples, the most powerful predictor of memory self-evaluation is the current mood state (Coleman et al., 1996; Frith et al., 1983; Hinkin et al., 1996; Larrabee and Levin, 1986; Weiner et al., 1986). Subjective memory complaints increase when people are depressed, regardless of the population. This is illustrated in Figure 21.7, where the improvement in memory self-evaluation following ECT was most marked in patients who manifested the greatest clinical improvement. Second, it should be recalled that a large group of cognitive functions show improvement shortly following the ECT course, particularly in domains sensitive to the adequacy of attention and concentration. It is unlikely that, within their own subjective experience, patients can readily tease out deficits related to the retention of information over delays or the recall of recent events from improvements

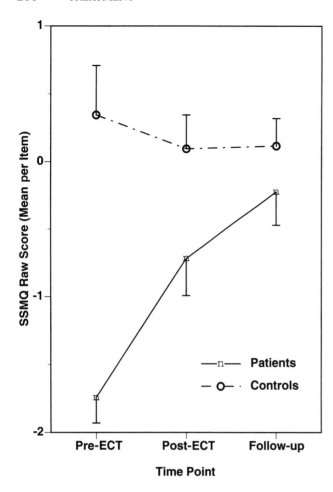

FIGURE 21.7 Score on the Squire Subjective Memory Questionnaire before and after the treatment course in electroconvulsive therapy responders and nonresponders. A score of 0 indicates no change in memory relative to before the episode of depression. (After Coleman et al., 1996)

in the capacity to acquire new information or to attend to their surroundings. Consequently, with the marked change in clinical state that typically occurs with ECT, there is often improvement in self-evaluations of cognitive capacities. Finally, the SMCQ is an awkward instrument, requiring patients to rate their current cognitive functioning to the period before they first became ill. This is a difficult cognitive leap for many patients, especially when expressing a major depressive disorder. The seeming improvement may in fact be a result of confounded assessment. Indeed, in our ongoing study at Columbia, the SMCQ shows consistent improvement following ECT, while the Cognitive Failures Questionnaire (Broadbent et al., 1982), which only requires a judgment about the work in the here and now, shows substantial deterioration.

A small minority of patients report that ECT has had a devastating and persistent impact on their cognitive function. Indeed, ECT is one of the few areas in psychiatry that has attracted vocal opponents, who have frequently called for its ban. The reasons why a small minority of the patients who receive ECT subsequently report profound impairment have been poorly studied. This is understandable, since the prevalence of the phenomenon is low and no single center treats a sufficient number of patients with ECT to recruit a meaningful sample. Nonetheless, the following factors should be kept in mind.

First, global or discrete neuropsychological deterioration is part of the natural history of some of the conditions treated with ECT. In younger populations, it is well established that global cognitive deterioration may occur prior to or following the first psychotic episode (Wyatt, 1991), particularly in the context of schizophrenia or schizoaffective disorder.

Among the elderly, a subset of patients who receive ECT present with or develop a dementia. Due to the public and scientific attention that has been given to the cognitive side effects of ECT and the often exhaustive nature of the informed consent process, patients who receive this modality are often primed to attribute perceived changes in cognitive functioning to ECT relative to other treatments or to the aging process (Squire, 1986). It is useful to recognize that ECT results in stereotyped cognitive side effects. When there are profound adverse effects of ECT on cognitive function, they should be expressed as a dense, persistent retrograde amnesia for autobiographical and public events that occurred months to years prior to the treatment. Complaints about attentional dysfunction, impaired creativity, global intellectual decline, global amnesia, and/or persistent anterograde amnesia are highly unlikely to be consequences of ECT. When patients have such complaints without complicating psychiatric presentations, a neurological work-up is particularly recommended, as is examination of the patient's opportunities for secondary gain.

Second, as noted, the patient's current mood state or, more generally, psychiatric status heavily determines the subjective evaluation of cognitive function. Freeman et al. (1980) conducted the only study that systematically evaluated a sample of former patients who believed that ECT had resulted in long-term negative consequences. In comparison to controls, evidence for objective cognitive deficits was not impressive in the patients with persistent complaints. However, major differences were identified in the frequency of concurrent psychiatric illness and the ongoing use of psychotropic medications. In order not to appear to be blaming the victim, it is understandable that this type of evidence has been downplayed within the psychiatric profession. Nonetheless, it is likely that lack of clinical benefit from ECT and ongoing psychiatric disturbance contribute to some of the reports of persistent adverse cognitive effects. Here also identification of the nature of the complaints is critical, as cognitive complaints in the context of ongoing psychopathology rarely have a profile compatible with a negative ECT outcome.

Finally, in the past, the field of ECT was reluctant to acknowledge that persistent and profound retrograde amnesia could result from the treatment. Indeed, the field has more readily acknowledged death and significant medical morbidity as rare ECT outcomes than persistent cognitive deficits (American Psychiatric Association, 1990; American Psychiatric Association Task Force on ECT, 1978). This is surprising, since the side effects that limit the more general use of ECT are cognitive in nature and are experienced by virtually all patients. The fact that there are individual differences in the magnitude and persistence of such side effects is established, and the recent APA Task Force Report on ECT now states that the treatment will result in retrograde amnesia in all patients. While for the great majority this will be trivial since the amnesia is time-limited, for rare patients a dense amnesia will be produced that is distressing to the patient (American Psychiatric Association, 1990). In my experience, profound cognitive deficits that appear to be a result of ECT are extremely rare. When they occur, they are usually marked by a dense retrograde amnesia and associated with large numbers of high-intensity treatments (e.g., sine wave, markedly suprathreshold BL ECT), often in patients with preexisting cognitive impairment. Attention to the quality of ECT and ongoing monitoring of the tolerability of the treatment for the individual patient may prevent these rare and unfortunate outcomes.

ACKOWLEDGMENTS
A version of this chapter also appears in C. Salzman, ed., *Geriatric Psychopharmacology*, 4th ed. (Baltimore: Williams & Wilkins, 2004). Preparation of this chapter was supported in part by Grants MH35636, MH59069, MH60884, and MH61609.

REFERENCES

Abrams, R. (1997) The mortality rate with ECT. *Convuls Ther* 13:125–127.

Abrams, R. (2002a) *Electroconvulsive Therapy*, 4th ed. New York: Oxford University Press.

Abrams, R. (2002b) Stimulus titration and ECT dosing. *J ECT* 18:3–9.

Ackermann, R., Engel, J.J., and Baxter, L. (1986) Positron emission tomography and autoradiographic studies of glucose utilization following electroconvulsive seizures in humans and rats. *Ann NY Acad Sci* 462:263–269.

Agency for Health Care Policy and Research. (1993) *General Information for the HCUP-3 Nationwide Inpatient Sample, Release 2.* Springfield, VA: National Technical Information Service.

Alexopoulos, G., Meyers, B., Young, R., Kakuma, T., Feder, M., Einhorn, A., et al. (1996) Recovery in geriatric depression. *Arch Gen Psychiatry* 53:305–312.

Alexopoulos, G., Shamoian, C., Lucas, J., Weiser, N., and Berger, H. (1984) Medical problems of geriatric psychiatric patients and younger controls during electroconvulsive therapy. *J Am Geriatr Soc* 32:651–654.

Alexopoulous, G.S., Young, R.C., and Abrams, R.C. (1989) ECT in the high-risk geriatric patient. *Convuls Ther* 5:75–87.

Alexopoulos, G.S., Young, R.C., and Shindledecker, R.D. (1992) Brain computed tomography findings in geriatric depression and primary degenerative dementia. *Biol Psychiatry* 31:591–599.

American Psychiatric Association. (1990) *The Practice of ECT: Recommendations for Treatment, Training and Privileging.* Washington, DC: American Psychiatric Press.

American Psychiatric Association. (1993) Practice guideline for major depressive disorder in adults. *Am J Psychiatry* 150:1–26.

American Psychiatric Association. (2001) *The Practice of ECT: Recommendations for Treatment, Training and Privileging,* 2nd ed. Washington, DC: American Psychiatric Press.

American Psychiatric Association Task Force on ECT. (1978) *Electroconvulsive Therapy, Task Force Report #14.* Washington, DC: American Psychiatric Association.

Ananth, J., Samra, D., and Kolivakis, T. (1979) Amelioration of drug-induced parkinsonism by ECT. *Am J Psychiatry* 136:1094.

Andersen, K., Balldin, J., Gottfries, C., Granérus, A., Modigh, K., Svennerholm, L., et al. (1987) A double-blind evaluation of electroconvulsive therapy in Parkinson's disease with on-off: phenomena. *Acta Neurol Scand* 76:191–199.

Andrade, C., and Gangadhar, B.N. (1989) When is an ECT responder, an ECT responder? *Convuls Ther* 5:190–191.

Andrade, C., Sudha, S., and Venkataraman, B.V. (2000) Herbal treatments for ECS-induced memory deficits: A review of research and a discussion on animal models. *J ECT* 16:144–156.

Andrade, C., Suresh, S., Krishnan, J., and Venkataraman, B.V. (2002) Effects of stimulus parameters on seizure duration and ECS-induced retrograde amnesia. *J ECT* 18:31–37.

Antkiewicz-Michaluk, L., Michaluk, J., Romanska, I., and Vetulani, J. (1993) The effect of calcium channel blockade during electroconvulsive treatment on cerebral cortical adrenoceptor subpopulations in the rat. *Pol J Pharmacol* 45:197–200.

Aronson, T., Shukla, S., Hoff, A., and Cook, B. (1988) Proposed delusional depression subtypes: Preliminary evidence from a retrospective study of phenomenology and treatment course. *J Affect Disord* 14:69–74.

Asnis, G. (1977) Parkinson's disease, depression, and ECT: A review and case study. *Am J Psychiatry* 134:191–195.

Avery, D., and Lubrano, A. (1979) Depression treated with imipramine and ECT: The DeCarolis study reconsidered. *Am J Psychiatry* 136:559–562.

Avery, D., and Winokur, G. (1976) Mortality in depressed patients treated with electroconvulsive therapy and antidepressants. *Arch Gen Psychiatry* 33:1029–1037.

Avramov, M.N., Husain, M.M., and White, P.F. (1995) The comparative effects of methohexital, propofol, and etomidate for electroconvulsive therapy. *Anesth Analg* 81:596–602.

Avramov, M.N., Stool, L.A., White, P.F., and Husain, M.M. (1998) Effects of nicardipine and labetalol on the acute hemodynamic response to electroconvulsive therapy. *J Clin Anesth* 10:394–400.

Babigian, H., and Guttmacher, L. (1984) Epidemiologic considerations in electroconvulsive therapy. *Arch Gen Psychiatry* 41:246–253.

Bailine, S.H., Rifkin, A., Kayne, E., Selzer, J.A., Vital-Herne, J., Blieka, M., et al. (2000) Comparison of bifrontal and bitemporal ECT for major depression. *Am J Psychiatry* 157:121–123.

Balldin, J., Edén, S., Granérus, A., Modigh, K., Svanborg, A., Walinder, J., et al. (1980) Electroconvulsive therapy in Parkinson's syndrome with on-off: phenomenon. *J Neural Transm* 47:11–21.

Benatov, R., Sirota, P., and Megged, S. (1996) Neuroleptic-resistant schizophrenia treated with clozapine and ECT. *Convuls Ther* 12:117–121.

Benbow, S.M. (1989) The role of electroconvulsive therapy in the treatment of depressive illness in old age. *Br J Psychiatry* 155:147–152.

Bennett-Levy, J., and Powell, G.E. (1980) The subjective memory questionnaire (SMQ). An investigation into the self-reporting of "real-life" memory skills. *Br J Soc Clin Psychol* 19:177–188.

Bhatia, S.C., Bhatia, S.K., and Gupta, S. (1998) Concurrent administration of clozapine and ECT: A successful therapeutic strategy for a patient with treatment-resistant schizophrenia. *J ECT* 14:280–283.

Black, D.W., Hulbert, J., and Nasrallah, A. (1989) The effect of somatic treatment and comorbidity on immediate outcome in manic patients. *Compr Psychiatry* 30:74–79.

Black, D.W., Winokur, G., and Nasrallah, A. (1989) Illness duration and acute response in major depression. *Convuls Ther* 5:338–343.

Black, D.W., Winokur, G., and Nasrallah, A. (1993) A multivariate analysis of the experience of 423 depressed inpatients treated with electroconvulsive therapy. *Convul Ther* 9:112–120.

Blanch, J., Martinez-Palli, G., Navines, R., Arcega, J.M., Imaz, M.L., Santos, P., et al. (2001) Comparative hemodynamic effects of urapidil and labetalol after electroconvulsive therapy. *J ECT* 17:275–279.

Boey, W.K., and Lai, F.O. (1990) Comparison of propofol and thiopentone as anaesthetic agents for electroconvulsive therapy. *Anaesthesia* 45:623–628.

Bolwig, T.G. (1988) Blood–brain barrier studies with special reference to epileptic seizures. *Acta Psychiatr Scand* (Suppl) 345:15–20.

Bolwig, T.G., Hertz, M., and Holm-Jensen, J. (1977a) Blood–brain barrier during electroshock seizures in the rat. *Eur J Clin Invest* 7:95–100.

Bolwig, T.G., Hertz, M., Paulson, O., Spotoft, H., and Rafaelsen, O. (1977b) The permeability of the blood–brain barrier during electrically induced seizures in man. *Eur J Clin Invest* 7:87–93.

Bolwig, T.G., Hertz, M.M., and Westergaard, E. (1977c) Acute hypertension causing blood–brain barrier breakdown during epileptic seizures. *Acta Neurol Scand* 56:335–342.

Bone, M.E., Wilkins, C.J., and Lew, J.K. (1988) A comparison of propofol and methohexitone as anaesthetic agents for electroconvulsive therapy. *Eur J Anaesthesiol* 5:279–286.

Boylan, L.S., Devanand, D.P., Lisanby, S.H., Nobler, M.S., Prudic, J., and Sackeim, H.A. (2001) Focal prefrontal seizures induced by bilateral ECT. *J ECT* 17:175–179.

Boylan, L.S., Haskett, R.F., Mulsant, B.H., Greenberg, R.M., Prudic, J., Spicknall, K., et al. (2000) Determinants of seizure threshold in ECT: Benzodiazepine use, anesthetic dosage, and other factors. *J ECT* 16:3–18.

Braddock, L., Cowen, P., Elliott, J., Fraser, S., and Stump, K. (1986) Binding of yohimbine and imipramine to platelets in depressive illness. *Psychol Med* 16:765–773.

Brandon, S., Cowley, P., McDonald, C., Neville, P., Palmer, R., and Wellstood-Eason, S. (1984) Electroconvulsive therapy: Results in depressive illness from the Leicestershire trial. *Br Med J (Clin Res)* 288:22–25.

Broadbent, D.E., Cooper, P.F., Fitzgerald, P., and Parkes, K.R. (1982) The cognitive failures questionnaire (CFQ) and its correlates. *Br J Clin Psychol* 21:1–16.

Bruce, E.M., Crone, N., Fitzpatrick, G., Frewin, S.J., Gillis, A., Lascelles, C.F., et al. (1960) A comparative trial of ECT and Tofranil. *Am J Psychiatry* 117:76–80.

Buchan, H., Johnstone, E., McPherson, K., Palmer, R.L., Crow, T.J., and Brandon, S. (1992) Who benefits from electroconvulsive therapy? Combined results of the Leicester and Northwick Park trials. *Br J Psychiatry* 160:355–359.

Burd, J., and Kettl, P. (1998) Incidence of asystole in electroconvulsive therapy in elderly patients. *Am J Geriatr Psychiatry* 6:203–211.

Burke, W., Rubin, E., Zorumski, C., and Wetzel, R. (1987) The safety of ECT in geriatric psychiatry. *J Am Geriatr Soc* 35:516–521.

Burke, W., Rutherford, J., Zorumski, C., and Reich, T. (1985) Elec-

troconvulsive therapy and the elderly. *Compr Psychiatry* 26:480–486.

Caine, E. (1986) The neuropsychology of depression: The pseudodementia syndrome. In: Grant, I., and Adams, K.M., eds. *Neuropsychological Assessment of Neuropsychiatric Disorders*. New York: Oxford University Press, pp. 221–243.

Calev, A., Gaudino, E.A., Squires, N.K., Zervas, I.M., and Fink, M. (1995) ECT and non-memory cognition: A review. *Br J Clin Psychol* 34(Pt 4):505–515.

Calev, A., Kochav-lev, E., Tubi, N., Nigal, D., Chazan, S., Shapira, B., et al. (1991a) Change in attitude toward electroconvulsive therapy: Effects of treatment, time since treatment, and severity of depression. *Convuls Ther* 7:184–189.

Calev, A., Nigal, D., Shapira, B., Tubi, N., Chazan, S., and Ben-Yehuda, Y. (1991b) Early and long-term effects of electroconvulsive therapy and depression on memory and other cognitive functions. *J Nerv Ment Dis* 179:526–533.

Calev, A., Phil, D., Cohen, R., Tubi, N., Nigal, D., Shapira, B., et al. (1991c) Disorientation and bilateral moderately suprathreshold titrated ECT. *Convuls Ther* 7:99–110.

Cardwell, B.A., and Nakai, B. (1995) Seizure activity in combined clozapine and ECT: A retrospective view. *Convuls Ther* 11:110–113.

Carney, M.W.P., Roth, M., and Garside, R.F. (1965) The diagnosis of depressive syndromes and the prediction of ECT response. *Br J Psychiatry* 111:659–674.

Carney, M.W.P., and Sheffield, B. (1974) The effects of pulse ECT in neurotic and endogenous depression. *Br J Psychiatry* 125:91–94.

Castelli, I., Steiner, L.A., Kaufmann, M.A., Alfille, P.H., Schouten, R., Welch, C.A., et al. (1995) Comparative effects of esmolol and labetalol to attenuate hyperdynamic states after electroconvulsive therapy. *Anesth Analg* 80:557–561.

Cattan, R.A., Barry, P.P., Mead, G., Reefe, W.E., Gay, A., and Silverman, M. (1990a) Electroconvulsive therapy in octogenarians. *J Am Geriatr Soc* 38:753–758.

Cattan, R.A., Barry, P.P., Mead, G., Reefe, W.E., Gay, A., and Silverman, M. (1990b) Electroconvulsive therapy in octogenarians. *J Am Geriatr Soc* 38:753–758.

Ciraulo, D., Lind, L., Salzman, C., Pilon, R., and Elkins, R. (1978) Sodium nitroprusside treatment of ECT-induced blood pressure elevations. *Am J Psychiatry* 135:1105–1106.

Clarke, T.B., Coffey, C.E., Hoffman, G.W., and Weiner, R.D. (1989) Continuation therapy for depression using outpatient electroconvulsive therapy. *Convuls Ther* 5:330–337.

Coffey, C.E., Lucke, J., Weiner, R.D., Krystal, A.D., and Aque, M. (1995a) Seizure threshold in electroconvulsive therapy (ECT) II. The anticonvulsant effect of ECT. *Biol Psychiatry* 37:777–788.

Coffey, C.E., Lucke, J., Weiner, R.D., Krystal, A.D., and Aque, M. (1995b) Seizure threshold in electroconvulsive therapy: I. Initial seizure threshold. *Biol Psychiatry* 37:713–720.

Coleman, E.A., Sackeim, H.A., Prudic, J., Devanand, D.P., McElhiney, M.C., and Moody, B.J. (1996) Subjective memory complaints before and after electroconvulsive therapy. *Biol Psychiatry* 39:346–356.

Colenda, C.C., and McCall, W.V. (1996) A statistical model predicting the seizure threshold for right unilateral ECT in 106 patients. *Convuls Ther* 12:3–12.

Coryell, W., Pfohl, B., and Zimmerman, M. (1984) The clinical and neuroendocrine features of psychotic depression. *J Nerv Ment Dis* 172:521–528.

Coryell, W., Winokur, G., Shea, T., Maser, J.D., Endicott, J., and Akiskal, H.S. (1994) The long-term stability of depressive subtypes. *Am J Psychiatry* 151:199–204.

Coryell, W., and Zimmerman, M. (1984) Outcome following ECT for primary unipolar depression: A test of newly proposed response predictors. *Am J Psychiatry* 141:862–867.

Cronholm, B., and Ottosson, J.-O. (1963a) The experience of memory function after electroconvulsive therapy. *Br J Psychiatry* 109:251–258.

Cronholm, B., and Ottosson, J.-O. (1963b) Ultrabrief stimulus technique in electroconvulsive therapy. I. Influence on retrograde amnesia of treatments with the Elther ES electroshock apparatus, Siemens Konvulsator III and of lidocane-modified treatment. *J Nerv Ment Dis* 137:117–123.

Cronholm, B., and Ottoson, J.-O. (1963c) Ultrabrief stimulus technique in electroconvulsive therapy. II. Comparative studies of therapeutic effects and memory disturbances in treatment of endogenous depression with the Elther ES electroshock apparatus and Siemens Konvulsator III. *J Nerv Ment Dis* 137:268–276.

Crow, T.J. (1979) The scientific status of electro-convulsive therapy. *Psychol Med* 9:401–408.

Crow, T.J., and Johnstone, E.C. (1986) Controlled trials of electroconvulsive therapy. *Ann NY Acd Sci* 462:12–29.

Daniel, W., and Crovitz, H. (1983a) Acute memory impairment following electroconvulsive therapy. 1. Effects of electrical stimulus waveform and number of treatments. *Acta Psychiatr Scand* 67:1–7.

Daniel, W., and Crovitz, H. (1983b) Acute memory impairment following electroconvulsive therapy. 2. Effects of electrode placement. *Acta Psychiatr Scand* 67:57–68.

Daniel, W., and Crovitz, H. (1986) Disorientation during electroconvulsive therapy. Technical, theoretical, and neuropsychological issues. *Ann NY Acad Sci* 462:293–306.

Danish, U., Antidepressant, Group (DUAG). (1986) Citalopram: Clinical effect profile in comparison with clomipramine. A controlled multicenter study. *Psychopharmacology* 90:131–138.

Danish, U., Antidepressant, Group (DUAG). (1990) Paroxetine: A selective serotonin reuptake inhibitor showing better tolerance, but weaker antidepressant effect than clomipramine in a controlled multicenter study. *J Affect Disord* 18:289–299.

Dannon, P.N., Iancu, I., Hirschmann, S., Ross, P., Dolberg, O.T., and Grunhaus, L. (1998) Labetalol does not lengthen asystole during electroconvulsive therapy. *J ECT* 14:245–250.

de Carle, A.J., and Kohn, R. (2000) Electroconvulsive therapy and falls in the elderly. *J ECT* 16:252–257.

Decina, P., Guthrie, E.B., Sackeim, H.A., Kahn, D., and Malitz, S. (1987) Continuation ECT in the management of relapses of major affective episodes. *Acta Psychiatr Scand* 75:559–562.

Decina, P., Malitz, S., Sackeim, H., Holzer, J., and Yudofsky, S. (1984) Cardiac arrest during ECT modified by beta-adrenergic blockade. *Am J Psychiatry* 141:298–300.

Delva, N.J., Brunet, D., Hawken, E.R., Kesteven, R.M., Lawson, J.S., Lywood, D.W., et al. (2000) Electrical dose and seizure threshold: Relations to clinical outcome and cognitive effects in bifrontal, bitemporal, and right unilateral ECT. *J ECT* 16:361–369.

Devanand, D.P., Malitz, S., and Sackeim, H.A. (1990) ECT in a patient with aortic aneurysm. *J Clin Psychiatry* 51:255–256.

Dinan, T.G., and Barry, S. (1989) A comparison of electroconvulsive therapy with a combined lithium and tricyclic combination among depressed tricyclic nonresponders. *Acta Psychiatr Scand* 80:97–100.

Ding, Z., and White, P.F. (2002) Anesthesia for electroconvulsive therapy. *Anesth Analg* 94:1351–1364.

Donahue, A.B. (2000) Electroconvulsive therapy and memory loss: A personal journey. *J ECT* 16:133–143.

Douyon, R., Serby, M., Klutchko, B., and Rotrosen, J. (1989) ECT and Parkinson's disease revisited: A naturalistic study. *Am J Psychiatry* 146:1451–1455.

Drop, L., Castelli, I., and Kaufmann, M. (1998) Comparative doses and cost: Esmolol versus labetalol during electroconvulsive therapy. *Anesth Analg* 86:916–917.

Dubovsky, S.L. (1994) Challenges in conceptualizing psychotic mood disorders. *Bull Menninger Clin* 58:197–214.

Dwyer, R., McCaughey, W., Lavery, J., McCarthy, G., and Dundee, J.W. (1988) Comparison of propofol and methohexitone as anaesthetic agents for electroconvulsive therapy. *Anaesthesia* 43:459–462.

United Kingdom ECT Review Group, Efficacy and safety of electroconvulsive therapy in depressive disorders: a systematic review and meta-analysis. (2003) *Lancet* 361:799–808.

Enns, M., and Karvelas, L. (1995) Electrical dose titration for electroconvulsive therapy: A comparison with dose prediction methods. *Convuls Ther* 11:86–93.

Faber, R., and Trimble, M.R. (1991) Electroconvulsive therapy in Parkinson's disease and other movement disorders. *Mov Disord* 6:293–303.

Fall, P.A., and Granerus, A.K. (1999) Maintenance ECT in Parkinson's disease. *J Neural Transm* 106:737–741.

Farah, A., Beale, M.D., and Kellner, C.H. (1995) Risperidone and ECT combination therapy: A case series. *Convuls Ther* 11:280–282.

Figiel, G.S., Coffey, C.E., Djang, W.T., Hoffman, G.J., and Doraiswamy, P.M. (1990) Brain magnetic resonance imaging findings in ECT-induced delirium. *J Neuropsychiatry Clin Neurosci* 2:53–58.

Figiel, G.S., DeLeo, B., Zorumski, C.F., Baker, K., Goewert, A., and Jarvis, M. (1993) Combined use of labetalol and nifedipine in controlling the cardiovascular response from ECT. *J Geriatr Psychiatry Neurol* 6:20–24.

Figiel, G.S., Hassen, M.A., Zorumski, C., Krishnan, K.R., and Doraiswamy, P.M. (1991) ECT-induced delirium in depressed patients with Parkinson's disease. *J Neuropsychiatry Clin Neurosci* 3:405–411.

Figiel, G.S., McDonald, L., and LaPlante, R. (1994) Cardiovascular complications of ECT [letter; comment]. *Am J Psychiatry* 151:790–791.

Figiel, G.S., Zorumski, C.F., Doraiswamy, P.M., Mattingly, G.W., and Jarvis, M.R. (1992) Simultaneous major depression and panic disorder: treatment with electroconvulsive therapy. *J Clin Psychiatry* 53:12–15.

Flint, A.J., and Rifat, S.L. (1996) The effect of sequential antidepressant treatment on geriatric depression. *J Affect Disord* 36:95–105.

Fochtmann, L.J. (1994) Animal studies of electroconvulsive therapy: Foundations for future research. *Psychopharmacol Bull* 30:321–444.

Folkerts, H.W., Michael, N., Tolle, R., Schonauer, K., Mucke, S., and Schulze-Monking, H. (1997) Electroconvulsive therapy vs. paroxetine in treatment-resistant depression—a randomized study. *Acta Psychiatr Scand* 96:334–342.

Folstein, M., Folstein, S., and McHugh, P. (1973) Clinical predictors of improvement after electroconvulsive therapy of patients with schizophrenia, neurotic reactions, and affective disorders. *Biol Psychiatry* 7:147–152.

Foster, S., and Ries, R. (1988) Delayed hypertension with electroconvulsive therapy. *J Nerv Ment Dis* 176:374–376.

Frank, E., Kupfer, D.J., Perel, J.M., Cornes, C., Jarrett, D.B., Mallinger, A.G., et al. (1990) Three-year outcomes for maintenance therapies in recurrent depression. *Arch Gen Psychiatry* 47:1093–1099.

Frank, E., Kupfer, D.J., Perel, J.M., Cornes, C., Mallinger, A.G., Thase, M.E., et al. (1993) Comparison of full-dose versus half-dose pharmacotherapy in the maintenance treatment of recurrent depression. *J Affect Disord* 27:139–145.

Fraser, R.M., and Glass, I. (1978) Recovery from ECT in elderly patients. *Br J Psychiatry* 133:524–528.

Fraser, R., and Glass, I. (1980) Unilateral and bilateral ECT in elderly patients. A comparative study. *Acta Psychiatr Scand* 62:13–31.

Fraser-R.M. (1981) ECT and the elderly. In: Palmer, R.L., ed. Electroconvulsive Therapy: An Appraisal. New York: Oxford University Press, pp. 55–60.

Fredman, B., Husain, M.M., and White, P.F. (1994) Anaesthesia for electroconvulsive therapy: Use of propofol revisited. *Eur J Anesthesiol* 11:423–425.

Freeman, C., Weeks, D., and Kendell, R. (1980) ECT: II: Patients who complain. *Br J Psychiatry* 137:17–25.

Frith, C., Stevens, M., Johnstone, E., Deakin, J., Lawler, P., and Crow, T.J. (1983) Effects of ECT and depression on various aspects of memory. *Br J Psychiatry* 142:610–617.

Fromm, G. (1959) Observations on the effect of electroshock treatment on patients with parkinsonism. *Bull Tulane Med Faculty* 18:71–73.

Gaines, G.Y.D., and Rees, D.I. (1992) Anesthetic considerations for electroconvulsive therapy. *South Med J* 85:469–482.

Gangadhar, B., Kapur, R., and Kalyanasundaram, S. (1982) Comparison of electroconvulsive therapy with imipramine in endogenous depression: a double blind study. *Br J Psychiatry* 141:367–371.

Gaspar, D., and Samarasinghe, L. (1982) ECT in psychogeriatric practice—a study of risk factors, indications and outcome. *Compr Psychiatry* 23:170–175.

Gatti, F., Bellini, L., Gasperini, M., Perez, J., Zanardi, R., and Smeraldi, E. (1996) Fluvoxamine alone in the treatment of delusional depression. *Am J Psychiatry* 153:414–416.

Georgotas, A., McCue, R.E., Cooper, T.B., Nagachandran, N., and Friedhoff, A. (1989) Factors affecting the delay of antidepressant effect in responders to nortriptyline and phenelzine. *Psychiatry Res* 28:1–9.

Geretsegger, C., Rochowanski, E., Kartnig, C., and Unterrainer, A.F. (1998) Propofol and methohexital as anesthetic agents for electroconvulsive therapy (ECT): A comparison of seizure-quality measures and vital signs. *J ECT* 14:28–35.

Gerring, J., and Shields, H. (1982) The identification and management of patients with a high risk for cardiac arrhythmias during modified ECT. *J Clin Psychiatry* 43:140–143.

Gerson, S.C., Plotkin, D.A., and Jarvik, L.F. (1988) Antidepressant drug studies, 1964–1985: Empirical evidence for aging patients. *J Clin Pharmacol* 8:311–322.

Glassman, A.H., and Roose, S.P. (1981) Delusional depression. A distinct clinical entity? *Arch Gen Psychiatry* 38:424–427.

Gold, L., and Chiarello, C.J. (1944) Prognostic value of clinical findings in cases treated with electroshock. *J Nerv Ment Dis* 100:577–583.

Goswami, U., Dutta, S., Kuruvilla, K., Papp, E., and Perenyi, A. (1989) Electroconvulsive therapy in neuroleptic-induced parkinsonism. *Biol Psychiatry* 26:234–238.

Greenan, J., Dewar, M., and Jones, C. (1983) Intravenous glycopyrrolate and atropine at induction of anaesthesia: A comparison. *J R Soc Med* 76:369–371.

Greenberg, R.M., and Pettinati, H.M. (1993) Benzodiazepines and electroconvulsive therapy. *Convuls Ther* 9:262–273.

Greenblatt, M., Grooser, G.H., and Wechsler, H.A. (1964) Differential response of hospitalized depressed patients in somatic therapy. *Am J Psychiatry* 120:935–943.

Greenblatt, M., Grosser, G.H., and Wechsler, H.A. (1962) A comparative study of selected antidepressant medications and EST. *Am J Psychiatry* 119:144–153.

Gregory, S., Shawcross, C., and Gill, D. (1985) The Nottingham ECT Study. A double-blind comparison of bilateral, unilateral and simulated ECT in depressive illness. *Br J Psychiatry* 146:520–524.

Gustafson, Y., Nilsson, I., Mattsson, M., Astrom, M., and Bucht, G. (1995) Epidemiology and treatment of post-stroke depression. *Drugs Aging* 7:298–309.

Hamilton, M. (1967) Development of a rating scale for primary depressive illness. *Br J Soc Clin Psychol* 6:278–296.

Hamilton, M. (1982) The effect of treatment on the melancholias (depressions). *Br J Psychiatry* 140:223–230.

Hamilton, M., and White, J. (1960) Factors related to the outcome of depression treated with ECT. *J Ment Sci* 106:1031–1041.

Harris, J.A., and Robin, A.A. (1960) A controlled trial of phenelzine in depressive reactions. *J Ment Sci* 106:1432–1437.

Hasan, Z.A., and Woolley, D.E. (1994) Comparison of the effects of propofol and thiopental on the pattern of maximal electroshock seizures in the rat. *Pharmacol Toxicol* 74:50–53.

Heikman, P., Kalska, H., Katila, H., Sarna, S., Tuunainen, A., and Kuoppasalmi, K. (2002) Right unilateral and bifrontal electroconvulsive therapy in the treatment of depression: A preliminary study. *J ECT* 18:26–30.

Hermann, R.C., Dorwart, R.A., Hoover, C.W., and Brody, J. (1995) Variation in ECT use in the United States. *Am J Psychiatry* 152:869–875.

Hermann, R.C., Ettner, S.L., Dorwart, R.A., Langman-Dorwart, N., and Kleinman, S. (1999) Diagnoses of patients treated with ECT: A comparison of evidence-based standards with reported use. *Psychiatr Serv* 50:1059–1065.

Herrington, R., Bruce, A., and Johnstone, E. (1974) Comparative trial of L-tryptophan and E.C.T. in severe depressive illness. *Lancet* 2:731–734.

Herzberg, F. (1954) Prognostic variables for electro-shock therapy. *J Gen Psychol* 50:79–86.

Heshe, J., Röder, E., and Theilgaard, A. (1978) Unilateral and bilateral ECT. A psychiatric and psychological study of therapeutic effect and side effects. *Acta Psychiatr Scand Suppl* 275:1–180.

Hickie, I., Parsonage, B., and Parker, G. (1990) Prediction of response to electroconvulsive therapy. Preliminary validation of a sign-based typology of depression. *Br J Psychiatry* 157:65–71.

Hickie, I., Scott, E., Mitchell, P., Wilhelm, K., Austin, M.P., and Bennett, B. (1995) Subcortical hyperintensities on magnetic resonance imaging: Clinical correlates and prognostic significance in patients with severe depression. *Biol Psychiatry* 37:151–160.

Hickie, I., Scott, E., Wilhelm, K., and Brodaty, H. (1997) Subcortical hyperintensities on magnetic resonance imaging in patients with severe depression—a longitudinal evaluation. *Biol Psychiatry* 42:367–374.

Himmelhoch, J.M., Neil, J.F., May, S.J., Fuchs, C.Z., and Licata, S.M. (1980) Age, dementia, dyskinesia, and lithium response. *Am J Psychiatry* 137:941–945.

Hinkin, C., Van Gorp, W.G., and Satz, P. (1996) Actual versus self-reported cognitive dysfunction in HIV-1 infection: Memory–metamemory dissociations. *J Clin Exp Neuropsychol* 18:431–443.

Hirschfeld, R.M. (1999) Efficacy of SSRIs and newer antidepressants in severe depression: Comparison with TCAs. *J Clin Psychiatry* 60:326–335.

Hobson, R.F. (1953) Prognostic factors in ECT. *J Neurol Neurosurg Psychiatry* 16:275–281.

Howie, M.B., Black, H.A., Zvara, D., McSweeney, T.D., Martin, D.J., and Coffman, J.A. (1990) Esmolol reduces autonomic hypersensitivity and length of seizures induced by electroconvulsive therapy. *Anesth Analg* 71:384–388.

Hsiao, J.K., Messenheimer, J.A., and Evans, D.L. (1987) ECT and neurological disorders. *Convuls Ther* 3:121–136.

Huuhka, M.J., Seinela, L., Reinikainen, P., and Leinonen, E.V. (2003) Cardiac arrhythmias induced by ECT in elderly psychiatric patients: Experience with 48-hour olter monitoring. *J ECT* 19:22–25.

James, D.V., and Gray, N.S. (1999) Elective combined electroconvulsive and clozapine therapy. *Int Clin Psychopharmacol* 14:69–72.

Janicak, P.G., Davis, J.M., Gibbons, R., Ericksen, S., Chang, S., and Gallagher, P. (1985) Efficacy of ECT: A meta-analysis. *Am J Psychiatry* 142:297–302.

Janicak, P.G., Pandey, G.N., Davis, J.M., Boshes, R., Bresnahan, D., and Sharma, R. (1988) Response of psychotic and nonpsychotic depression to phenelzine. *Am J Psychiatry* 145:93–95.

Johnstone, E.C., Deakin, J.F.W., Lawler, P., Frith, C.D., Stevens, M., McPherson, K., et al. (1980) The Northwick Park electroconvulsive therapy trial. *Lancet* 2:1317–1320.

Karlinsky, H., and Shulman, K. (1984) The clinical use of electroconvulsive therapy in old age. *J Am Geriatr Soc* 32:183–186.

Kaufman, K.R. (1994) Asystole with electroconvulsive therapy. *J Intern Med* 235:275–277.

Keller, M., Lavori, P., Klerman, G., Andreasen, N., Endicott, J., Coryell, W., et al. (1986) Low levels and lack of predictors of somatotherapy and psychotherapy received by depressed patients. *Arch Gen Psychiatry* 43:458–466.

Kellner, C.H. (2001) Towards the modal ECT treatment. *J ECT* 17:1–2.

Kellner, C.H., Beale, M.D., Pritchett, J.T., Bernstein, H.J., and Burns, C.M. (1994) Electroconvulsive therapy and Parkinson's disease: the case for further study. *Psychopharmacol Bull* 30:495–500.

Kellway, B., Simpson, K., Smith, R., and Halsall, P. (1986) Effects of atropine and glycopyrrolate on cognitive function following anaesthesia and electroconvulsive therapy. *Int Clin Psychopharm* 1:296–302.

Kendler, K.S., Gruenberg, A.M., and Tsuang, M.T. (1986) A DSM-III family study of the nonschizophrenic psychotic disorders. *Am J Psychiatry* 143:1098–1105.

Khan, A., Cohen, S., Stowell, M., Capwell, R., Avery, D., and Dunner, D.L. (1987) Treatment options in severe psychotic depression. *Convuls Ther* 3:93–99.

Khan, A., Mirolo, M.H., Claypoole, K., Bhang, J., Cox, G., Horita, A., et al. (1994) Effects of low-dose TRH on cognitive deficits in the ECT postictal state. *Am J Psychiatry* 151:1694–1696.

Kiloh, L.G., Child, J.P., and Latner, G. (1960) A controlled trial of iproniazid in the treatment of endogenous depression. *J Ment Sci* 106:1139–1144.

Kindler, S., Shapira, B., Hadjez, J., Abramowitz, M., Brom, D., and Lerer, B. (1991) Factors influencing response to bilateral electroconvulsive therapy in major depression. *Convuls Ther* 7:245–254.

Kirkby, K.C., Beckett, W.G., Matters, R.M., and King, T.E. (1995) Comparison of propofol and methohexitone in anaesthesia for ECT: Effect on seizure duration and outcome. *Aust NZ J Psychiatry* 29:299–303.

Kovac, A.L., Goto, H., Pardo, M.P., and Arakawa, K. (1991) Comparison of two esmolol bolus doses on the haemodynamic response and seizure duration during electroconvulsive therapy. *Can J Anaesth* 38:204–209.

Kramer, B.A. (1985) Use of ECT in California, 1977–1983. *Am J Psychiatry* 142:1190–1192.

Kramer, B. (1987) Electroconvulsive therapy use in geriatric depression. *J Nerv Ment Dis* 175:233–235.

Kramer, B.A., Allen, R., and Friedman, B. (1986) Atropine and glycopyrrolate as ECT preanesthesia. *J Clin Psychiatry* 47:199–200.

Kramer, B.A. (1993) Anticholinergics and ECT. *Convuls Ther* 9:293–300.

Kraus, R., and Remick, R. (1982) Diazoxide in the management of severe hypertension after electroconvulsive therapy. *Am J Psychiatry* 139:504–505.

Krishnan, K.R., Hays, J.C., and Blazer, D.G. (1997) MRI-defined vascular depression. *Am J Psychiatry* 154:497–501.

Krueger, R.B., Fama, J.M., Devanand, D.P., Prudic, J., and Sackeim, H.A. (1993) Does ECT permanently alter seizure threshold? *Biol Psychiatry* 33:272–276.

Krueger, R.B., Sackeim, H.A., and Gamzu, E.R. (1992) Pharmacological treatment of the cognitive side effects of ECT: A review. *Psychopharmacol Bull* 28:409–424.

Krystal, A.D., Weiner, R.D., and Coffey, C.E. (1995) The ictal EEG as a marker of adequate stimulus intensity with unilateral ECT. *J Neuropsychiatry Clin Neurosci* 7:295–303.

Krystal, A.D., Weiner, R.D., McCall, W.V., Shelp, F.E., Arias, R., and Smith, P. (1993) The effect of ECT stimulus dose and electrode

placement on the ictal electroencephalogram: An intraindividual crossover study. *Biol Psychiatry* 34:759–767.

Lambourn, J., and Gill, D. (1978) A controlled comparison of simulated and real ECT. *Br J Psychiatry* 133:514–519.

Larrabee, G.J., and Levin, H.S. (1986) Memory self-ratings and objective test performance in a normal elderly sample. *J Clin Exp Neuropsychol* 8:275–284.

Lawson, J.S., Inglis, J., Delva, N.J., Rodenburg, M., Waldron, J.J., and Letemendia, F.J. (1990) Electrode placement in ECT: Cognitive effects. *Psychol Med* 20:335–344.

Lerer, B., and Shapira, B. (1986) Optimum frequency of electroconvulsive therapy: Implications for practice and research. *Convuls Ther* 2:141–144.

Lerer, B., Shapira, B., Calev, A., Tubi, N., Drexler, H., Kindler, S., et al. (1995) Antidepressant and cognitive effects of twice- versus three-times-weekly ECT. *Am J Psychiatry* 152:564–570.

Letemendia, F.J., Delva, N.J., Rodenburg, M., Lawson, J.S., Inglis, J., Waldron, J.J., et al. (1993) Therapeutic advantage of bifrontal electrode placement in ECT. *Psychol Med* 23:349–360.

Levin, Y., Elizur, A., and Korczyn, A. (1987) Physostigmine improves ECT-induced memory disturbances. *Neurology* 37:871–875.

Lim, S.K., Lim, W.L., and Elegbe, E.O. (1996) Comparison of propofol and methohexitone as an induction agent in anaesthesia for electroconvulsive therapy. *West Afr J Med* 15:186–189.

Lisanby, S.H. (2003) Focal brain stimulation with repetitive transcranial magnetic stimulation (rTMS): Implications for the neural circuitry of depression. *Psychol Med* 33:7–13.

Lisanby, S.H., Devanand, D.P., Nobler, M.S., Prudic, J., Mullen, L., and Sackeim, H.A. (1996) Exceptionally high seizure threshold: ECT device limitations. *Convuls Ther* 12:156–164.

Lisanby, S.H., Maddox, J.H., Prudic, J., Devanand, D.P., and Sackeim, H.A. (2000) The effects of electroconvulsive therapy on memory of autobiographical and public events. *Arch Gen Psychiatry* 57:581–590.

Lisanby, S.H., Morales, O., Payne, N., Kwon, E., Fitzsimons, L., Luber, B., et al. (2003) New developments in electroconvulsive therapy and magnetic seizure therapy. *CNS Spectr* 8:529–536.

Maletzky, B. (1978) Seizure duration and clinical effect in electroconvulsive therapy. *Compr Psychiatry* 19:541–550.

Malloy, F., Small, I., Miller, M., Milstein, V., and Stout, J.R. (1982) Changes in neuropsychological test performance after electroconvulsive therapy. *Biol Psychiatry* 17:61–67.

Maneksha, F.R. (1991) Hypertension and tachycardia during electroconvulsive therapy: To treat or not to treat? [clinical note]. *Convuls Ther* 7:28–35.

Mann, J.J., Manevitz, A.Z., Chen, J.S., Johnson, K.S., Adelsheimer, E.F., Azima-Heller, R., et al. (1990) Acute effects of single and repeated electroconvulsive therapy on plasma catecholamines and blood pressure in major depressive disorder. *Psychiatry Res* 34:127–137.

Martensson, B., Bartfai, A., Hallen, B., Hellstrom, C., Junthe, T., and Olander, M. (1994) A comparison of propofol and methohexital as anesthetic agents for ECT: Effects on seizure duration, therapeutic outcome, and memory. *Biol Psychiatry* 35:179–189.

Mattes, J.A., Pettinati, H.M., Stephens, S., Robin, S.E., and Willis, K.W. (1990) A placebo-controlled evaluation of vasopressin for ECT-induced memory impairment. *Biol Psychiatry* 27:289–303.

McCall, W.V. (1996) Asystole in electroconvulsive therapy: Report of four cases. *J Clin Psychiatry* 57:199–203.

McCall, W.V., Reboussin, D.M., Weiner, R.D., and Sackeim, H.A. (2000) Titrated moderately suprathreshold vs. fixed high-dose right unilateral electroconvulsive therapy: Acute antidepressant and cognitive effects. *Arch Gen Psychiatry* 57:438–444.

McCall, W.V., Reid, S., and Ford, M. (1994) Electrocardiographic and cardiovascular effects of subconvulsive stimulation during titrated right unilateral ECT. *Convuls Ther* 10:25–33.

McCall, W.V., Shelp, F.E., Weiner, R.D., Austin, S., and Harrill, A.

(1991) Effects of labetalol on hemodynamics and seizure duration during ECT. *Convuls Ther* 7:5–14.

McAllister, D., Perri, M., Jordan, R., Rauscher, F., and Sattin, A. (1987) Effects of ECT given two vs. three times weekly. *Psychiatry Res* 21:63–69.

McElhiney, M.C., Moody, B.J., Steif, B.L., Prudic, J., Devanand, D.P., Nobler, M.S., et al. (1995) Autobiographical memory and mood: Effects of electroconvulsive therapy. *Neuropsychology* 9:501–517.

Meltzer, H.Y. (1992) Treatment of the neuroleptic-nonresponsive schizophrenic patient. *Schizophr Bull* 18:515–542.

Mendels, J. (1965a) Electroconvulsive therapy and depression. I. The prognostic significance of clinical factors. *Br J Psychiatry* 111:675–681.

Mendels, J. (1965b) Electroconvulsive therapy and depression. II. Significance of endogenous and reactive syndromes. *Br J Psychiatry* 111:682–686.

Mendels, J. (1965c) Electroconvulsive therapy and depression. III. A method for prognosis. *Br J Psychiatry* 111:687–690.

Miller, A., Faber, R., Hatch, J., and Alexander, H. (1985) Factors affecting amnesia, seizure duration, and efficacy in ECT. *Am J Psychiatry* 142:692–696.

Miller, M., Siris, S., and Gabriel, A. (1986) Treatment delays in the course of electroconvulsive therapy. *Hosp Commun Psychiatry* 37:825–827.

Milstein, V., and Small, J.G. (1988) Problems with lithium combined with ECT. *Am J Psychiatry* 145:1178.

Mitchell, A.J., and Dening, T.R. (1962) Depression-related cognitive impairment: Possibilities for its pharmacological treatment. *J Affect Disord* 36:79–87.

Mukherjee, S. (1993) Combined ECT and lithium therapy. *Convuls Ther* 9:274–284.

Mukherjee, S., Sackeim, H.A., and Schnur, D.B. (1994) Electroconvulsive therapy of acute manic episodes: A review of 50 years' experience. *Am J Psychiatry* 151:169–176.

Mulsant, B.H., Haskett, R.F., Prudic, J., Thase, M.E., Malone, K.M., Mann, J.J., et al. (1997) Low use of neuroleptic drugs in the treatment of psychotic major depression. *Am J Psychiatry* 154:559–561.

Murray, G., Shea, V., and Conn, D. (1986) Electroconvulsive therapy for poststroke depression. *J Clin Psychiatry* 47:258–260.

Nelson, J.C. (1999) A review of the efficacy of serotonergic and noradrenergic reuptake inhibitors for treatment of major depression. *Biol Psychiatry* 46:1301–1308.

Nelson, J.C., and Bowers, M.B.J. (1978) Delusional unipolar depression: Description and drug response. *Arch Gen Psychiatry* 35:1321–1328.

Nelson, J.C., Mazure, C.M., and Jatlow, P.I. (1994) Characteristics of desipramine-refractory depression. *J Clin Psychiatry* 55:12–19.

Nelson, J.C., Price, L.H., and Jatlow, P.I. (1986) Neuroleptic dose and desipramine concentrations during combined treatment of unipolar delusional depression. *Am J Psychiatry* 143:1151–1154.

Nelson, J.P., and Rosenberg, D.R. (1991) ECT treatment of demented elderly patients with major depression: A retrospective study of efficacy and safety. *Convuls Ther* 7:157–165.

Nemeroff, C.B. (1996–97) Augmentation strategies in patients with refractory depression. *Depress Anxiety* 4:169–181.

Nguyen, T.T., Chhibber, A.K., Lustik, S.J., Kolano, J.W., Dillon, P.J., and Guttmacher, L.B. (1997) Effect of methohexitone and propofol with or without alfentanil on seizure duration and recovery in electroconvulsive therapy. *Br J Anaesth* 79:801–803.

Nobler, M.S., Mann, J.J., and Sackeim, H.A. (1999) Serotonin, cerebral blood flow, and cerebral metabolic rate in geriatric major depression and normal aging. *Brain Res Rev* 30:250–263.

Nobler, M.S., Oquendo, M.A., Kegeles, L.S., Malone, K.M., Campbell, C.C., Sackeim, H.A., et al. (2001) Decreased regional brain metabolism after ECT. *Am J Psychiatry* 158:305–308.

Nobler, M.S., and Sackeim, H.A. (1996) Electroconvulsive therapy: Clinical and biological aspects. In: Goodnick, P.J., ed. *Predictors of Response in Mood Disorders*. Washington, DC: American Psychiatric Press, pp. 177–198.

Nobler, M.S., Sackeim, H.A., Moeller, J.R., Prudic, J., Petkova, E., and Waternaux, C. (1997) Quantifying the speed of symptomatic improvement with electroconvulsive therapy: Comparison of alternative statistical methods. *Convuls Ther* 13:208–221.

Nobler, M.S., Sackeim, H.A., Prohovnik, I., Moeller, J.R., Mukherjee, S., Schnur, D.B., et al. (1994) Regional cerebral blood flow in mood disorders, III. Treatment and clinical response. *Arch Gen Psychiatry* 51:884–897.

Nobler, M.S., Sackeim, H.A., Solomou, M., Luber, B., Devanand, D.P., and Prudic, J. (1993) EEG manifestations during ECT: Effects of electrode placement and stimulus intensity. *Biol Psychiatry* 34:321–330.

Nystrom, S. (1964) On relation between clinical factors and efficacy of ECT in depression. *Acta Psychiatr Neurol Scand (Suppl)*, 181:11–135.

O'Brien, D.R. (1989) The effective agent in electroconvulsive therapy: Convulsion or coma? *Med Hypotheses* 28:277–280.

O'Connor, C., Rothenberg, D., Soble, J., Macioch, J., McCarthy, R., Neumann, A., et al. (1996) The effect of esmolol pretreatment on the incidence of regional wall motion abnormalities during electroconvulsive therapy. *Anesth Analg* 82:143–147.

O'Connor, M.K., Knapp, R., Husain, M., Rummans, T.A., Petrides, G., Smith, G., et al. (2001) The influence of age on the response of major depression to electroconvulsive therapy: A C.O.R.E. Report. *Am J Geriatr Psychiatry* 9:382–390.

Oh, J.J., Rummans, T.A., O'Connor, M.K., and Ahlskog, J.E. (1992) Cognitive impairment after ECT in patients with Parkinson's disease and psychiatric illness [letter]. *Am J Psychiatry* 149:271.

Olfson, M., Marcus, S., Sackeim, H.A., Thompson, J., and Pincus, H.A. (1998) Use of ECT for the inpatient treatment of recurrent major depression. *Am J Psychiatry* 155:22–29.

Ottosson, J.-O. (1960) Experimental studies of the mode of action of electroconvulsive therapy. *Acta Psychiatr Scand* (Suppl) 145:1–141.

Ottosson, J.-O. (1991) Is unilateral nondominant ECT as efficient as bilateral ECT? A new look at the evidence. *Convuls Ther* 7:190–200.

Parker, G., Hadzi-Pavlovic, D., Hickie, I., Mitchell, P., Wilhelm, K., Brodaty, H., et al. (1991) Psychotic depression: A review and clinical experience. *Aust NZ J Psychiatry* 25:169–180.

Parker, G., Roy, K., Hadzi-Pavlovic, D., and Pedic, F. (1992) Psychotic (delusional) depression: A meta-analysis of physical treatments. *J Affect Disord* 24:17–24.

Parker, G., Roy, K., Wilhelm, K., and Mitchell, P. (2001) Assessing the comparative effectiveness of antidepressant therapies: A prospective clinical practice study. *J Clin Psychiatry* 62:117–125.

Paykel, E.S. (1998) Remission and residual symptomatology in major depression. *Psychopathology* 31:5–14.

Paykel, E.S. (2002) Achieving gains beyond response. *Acta Psychiatr Scand (Suppl)* 41:12–17.

Perera, T.D., Luber, B., Nobler, M.S., Prudic, J., Anderson, C., and Sackeim, H.A. (in press) Seizure expression during electroconvulsive therapy: Relationships with clinical outcome and cognitive side effects. *Neuropsychopharmacology*.

Petrides, G., and Fink, M. (1996a) Atrial fibrillation, anticoagulation, and electroconvulsive therapy. *Convuls Ther* 12:91–98.

Petrides, G., and Fink, M. (1996b) Choosing a dosing strategy for electrical stimulation in ECT [letter; comment]. *J Clin Psychiatry* 57:487–488.

Petrides, G., and Fink, M. (1996c) The "half-age" stimulation strategy for ECT dosing. *Convuls Ther* 12:138–146.

Petrides, G., Fink, M., Husain, M.M., Knapp, R.G., Rush, A.J., Mueller, M., et al. (2001) ECT remission rates in psychotic versus nonpsychotic depressed patients: A report from CORE. *J ECT* 17:244–253.

Pettinati, H.M., Mathisen, K.S., Rosenberg, J., and Lynch, J.F. (1986) Meta-analytical approach to reconciling discrepancies in efficacy between bilateral and unilateral electroconvulsive therapy. *Convuls Ther* 2:7–17.

Pettinati, H.M., and Rosenberg, J. (1984) Memory self-ratings before and after electroconvulsive therapy: Depression versus ECT induced. *Biol Psychiatry* 19:539–548.

Pettinati, H.M., Stephens, S.M., Willis, K.M., and Robin, S.E. (1990) Evidence for less improvement in depression in patients taking benzodiazepines during unilateral ECT. *Am J Psychiatry* 147: 1029–1035.

Pettinati, H.M., Tamburello, T.A., Ruetsch, C.R., and Kaplan, F.N. (1994) Patient attitudes toward electroconvulsive therapy. *Psychopharmacol Bull* 30:471–475.

Philibert, R.A., Richards, L., Lynch, C.F., and Winokur, G. (1995) Effect of ECT on mortality and clinical outcome in geriatric unipolar depression. *J Clin Psychiatry* 56:390–394.

Post, F. (1972) The management and nature of depressive illnesses in late life: A follow-through study. *Br J Psychiatry* 121:393–404.

Price, T.R., and McAllister, T.W. (1989) Safety and efficacy of ECT in depressed patients with dementia: A review of clinical experience. *Convuls Ther* 5:61–74.

Pridmore, S., and Pollard, C. (1996) Electroconvulsive therapy in Parkinson's disease: 30 month follow-up. *J Neurol Neurosurg Psychiatry* 60:693.

Prien, R., and Kupfer, D. (1986) Continuation drug therapy for major depressive episodes: How long should it be maintained? *Am J Psychiatry* 143:18–23.

Prudic, J., Fitzsimons, L., Nobler, M.S., and Sackeim, H.A. (1999) Naloxone in the prevention of the adverse cognitive effects of ECT: A within-subject, placebo controlled study. *Neuropsychopharmacology* 21:285–293.

Prudic, J., Haskett, R.F., Mulsant, B., Malone, K.M., Pettinati, H.M., Stephens, S., et al. (1996) Resistance to antidepressant medications and short-term clinical response to ECT. *Am J Psychiatry* 153:985–992.

Prudic, J., Olfson, M., Marcus, S.C., Fuller, R.B., and Sackeim, H.A. (2004) The effectiveness of electroconvulsive therapy in community settings. *Biol Psychiatry* 55:301–312.

Prudic, J., Olfson, M., and Sackeim, H.A. (2001) Electro-convulsive therapy practices in the community. *Psychol Med* 31:929–934.

Prudic, J., Peyser, S., and Sackeim, H.A. (2000) Subjective memory complaints: A review of patient self-assessment of memory after electroconvulsive therapy. *J ECT* 16:121–132.

Prudic, J., and Sackeim, H. (1990) Refractory depression and electroconvulsive therapy. In: Roose, S.P., and Glassman, A.H., eds. *Treatment of Refractory Depression*. Washington, DC: American Psychiatric Press, pp. 109–128.

Prudic, J., Sackeim, H., Decina, P., Hopkins, N., Ross, F., and Malitz, S. (1987) Acute effects of ECT on cardiovascular functioning: Relations to patient and treatment variables. *Acta Psychiatr Scand* 75:344–351.

Prudic, J., Sackeim, H.A., and Devanand, D.P. (1990) Medication resistance and clinical response to electroconvulsive therapy. *Psychiatry Res* 31:287–296.

Quitkin, F. (1985) The importance of dosage in prescribing antidepressants. *Br J Psychiatry* 147:593–597.

Rabbitt, P. (1982) Development of methods to measure changes in activities of daily living in the elderly. In: Corkin, S., Davis, K.L., Growdon, J.H., Usdin, E., and Wurtman, R., eds. *Alzheimer's Disease: A Report of Progress in Research*. New York: Raven Press, pp. 127–131.

Rice, E.H., Sombrotto, L.B., Markowitz, J.C., and Leon, A.C. (1994) Cardiovascular morbidity in high-risk patients during ECT. *Am J Psychiatry* 151:1637–1641.

Rich, C., Spiker, D., Jewell, S., Neil, J., and Black, N. (1984) The efficiency of ECT: I. Response rate in depressive episodes. *Psychiatry Res* 11:167–176.

Rickles, N.K., and Polan, C.G. (1948) Causes of failure in treatment with electric shock: Analysis of thirty-eight cases. *Arch Neurol Psychiatry* 59:337–346.

Rifkin, A. (1988) ECT versus tricyclic antidepressants in depression: A review of the evidence. *J Clin Psychiatry* 49:3–7.

Roberts, J.M. (1959a) Prognostic factors in the electroshock treatment of depressive states. II. The application of specific tests. *J Ment Sci* 105:703–713.

Roberts, J.M. (1959b) Prognostic factors in the electroshock treatment of depressive states: (1) clinical features from testing and examination. *J Ment Sci* 105:693–702.

Robin, A., and De Tissera, S. (1982) A double-blind controlled comparison of the therapeutic effects of low and high energy electroconvulsive therapies. *Br J Psychiatry* 141:357–366.

Robin, A.A., and Harris, J.A. (1962) A controlled comparison of imipramine and electroplexy. *J Ment Sci* 108:217–219.

Roose, S.P., Glassman, A.H., Attia, E., and Woodring, S. (1994) Comparative efficacy of selective serotonin reuptake inhibitors and tricyclics in the treatment of melancholia. *Am J Psychiatry* 151:1735–1739.

Roose, S.P., Glassman, A.H., Walsh, B.T., Woodring, S., and Vital-Herne, J. (1983) Depression, delusions, and suicide. *Am J Psychiatry* 140:1159–1162.

Roose, S.P., and Sackeim, H.A. (2002) Clinical trials in late-life depression: Revisited. *Am J Geriatr Psychiatry* 10:503–505.

Rosenbach, M.L., Hermann, R.C., and Dorwart, R.A. (1997) Use of electroconvulsive therapy in the Medicare population between 1987 and 1992. *Psychiatr Serv* 48:1537–1542.

Rothschild, A.J. (1996) Management of psychotic, treatment-resistant depression. *Psychiatr Clin North Am* 19:237–252.

Rothschild, A.J., Samson, J.A., Bessette, M.P., and Carter-Campbell, J.T. (1993) Efficacy of the combination of fluoxetine and perphenazine in the treatment of psychotic depression. *J Clin Psychiatry* 54:338–342.

Rouillon, F., and Gorwood, P. (1998) The use of lithium to augment antidepressant medication. *J Clin Psychiatry* 59(Suppl 5):32–39; discussion 32–39, 40–41.

Royal College of Psychiatrists (1995) *The ECT Handbook: The Second Report of the Royal College of Psychiatrists' Special Committee on ECT*. London: Royal College of Psychiatrists.

Sackeim, H.A. (1986a) Acute cognitive side effects of ECT. *Psychopharm Bull* 22:482–484.

Sackeim, H.A. (1986b) The efficacy of electroconvulsive therapy: Discussion of Part I. *Ann NY Acad Sci* 462:70–75.

Sackeim, H.A. (1989) The efficacy of electroconvulsive therapy in treatment of major depressive disorder. In: Fisher, S., and Greenberg, R.P., eds. *The Limits of Biological Treatments for Psychological Distress: Comparisons with Psychotherapy and Placebo*. Hillsdale, NJ: Erlbaum, pp. 275–307.

Sackeim, H.A. (1991a) Are ECT devices underpowered? *Convuls Ther* 7:233–236.

Sackeim, H.A. (1991b) Optimizing unilateral electroconvulsive therapy. *Convuls Ther* 7:201–212.

Sackeim, H.A. (1992) The cognitive effects of electroconvulsive therapy. In: Moos, W.H., Gamzu, E.R., and Thal, L.J., eds. *Cognitive Disorders: Pathophysiology and Treatment*. New York: Marcel Dekker, pp. 183–228.

Sackeim, H.A. (1993) The use of electroconvulsive therapy in late life depression. In: Schneider, L.S., Reynolds, C.F., III, Liebowitz, B.D., and Friedhoff, A.J., eds. *Diagnosis and Treatment of Depression in Late Life*. Washington, DC: American Psychiatric Press, pp. 259–277.

Sackeim, H.A. (1994) Continuation therapy following ECT: Directions for future research. *Psychopharmacol Bull* 30:501–521.

Sackeim, H.A. (1997) Comments on the "half-age" method of stimulus dosing. *Convuls Ther* 13:37–43.

Sackeim, H.A. (1999) The anticonvulsant hypothesis of the mechanisms of action of ECT: Current status. *J ECT* 15:5–26.

Sackeim, H.A. (2000) Memory and ECT: From polarization to reconciliation. *J ECT* 16:87–96.

Sackeim, H.A. (2001a) The definition and meaning of treatment-resistant depression. *J Clin Psychiatry* 62(Suppl 16):10–17.

Sackeim, H.A. (2001b) Functional brain circuits in major depression and remission. *Arch Gen Psychiatry* 58:649–650.

Sackeim, H.A. (2003) Electroconvulsive therapy and schizophrenia. In: Hirsch, S.R., and Weinberger, D., eds. *Schizophrenia*, 2nd ed. Oxford: Blackwell, pp. 517–551.

Sackeim, H.A., Decina, P., Kanzler, M., Kerr, B., and Malitz, S. (1987a) Effects of electrode placement on the efficacy of titrated, low-dose ECT. *Am J Psychiatry* 144:1449–1455.

Sackeim, H.A., Decina, P., Portnoy, S., Neeley, P., and Malitz, S. (1987b) Studies of dosage, seizure threshold, and seizure duration in ECT. *Biol Psychiatry* 22:249–268.

Sackeim, H.A., Decina, P., Prohovnik, I., and Malitz, S. (1987c) Seizure threshold in electroconvulsive therapy. Effects of sex, age, electrode placement, and number of treatments. *Arch Gen Psychiatry* 44:355–360.

Sackeim, H.A., Decina, P., Prohovnik, I., Malitz, S., and Resor, S.R. (1983) Anticonvulsant and antidepressant properties of electroconvulsive therapy: A proposed mechanism of action. *Biol Psychiatry* 18:1301–1310.

Sackeim, H.A., Devanand, D.P., Lisanby, S.H., Nobler, M.S., Prudic, J., Heyer, E.J., et al. (2001a) Treatment of the modal patient: Does one size fit nearly all? *J ECT* 17:219–222.

Sackeim, H.A., Devanand, D.P., and Nobler, M.S. (1995) Electroconvulsive therapy. In: Bloom, F., and Kupfer, D., eds. *Psychopharmacology: The Fourth Generation of Progress*. New York: Raven Press, pp. 1123–1142.

Sackeim, H.A., Devanand, D.P., and Prudic, J. (1991) Stimulus intensity, seizure threshold, and seizure duration: Impact on the efficacy and safety of electroconvulsive therapy. *Psychiatr Clin North Am* 14:803–843.

Sackeim, H.A., Haskett, R.F., Mulsant, B.H., Thase, M.E., Mann, J.J., Pettinati, H.M., et al. (2001b) Continuation pharmacotherapy in the prevention of relapse following electroconvulsive therapy: a randomized controlled trial. *JAMA* 285:1299–1307.

Sackeim, H.A., Long, J., Luber, B., Moeller, J.R., Prohovnik, I., Devanand, D.P., et al. (1994) Physical properties and quantification of the ECT stimulus: I. Basic principles. *Convuls Ther* 10:93–123.

Sackeim, H.A., Luber, B., Katzman, G.P., Moeller, J.R., Prudic, J., Devanand, D.P., et al. (1996) The effects of electroconvulsive therapy on quantitative electroencephalograms. Relationship to clinical outcome. *Arch Gen Psychiatry* 53:814–824.

Sackeim, H.A., Luber, B., Moeller, J.R., Prudic, J., Devanand, D.P., and Nobler, M.S. (2000a) Electrophysiological correlates of the adverse cognitive effects of electroconvulsive therapy. *J ECT* 16:110–120.

Sackeim, H.A., Nobler, M.S., Prudic, J., Devanand, D.P., McElhinney, M., Coleman, E., et al. (1992) Acute effects of electroconvulsive therapy on hemispatial neglect. *Neuropsychiatry Neuropsychol Behav Neurol* 5:151–160.

Sackeim, H.A., Portnoy, S., Neeley, P., Steif, B.L., Decina, P., and Malitz, S. (1986) Cognitive consequences of low-dosage electroconvulsive therapy. *Ann NY Acad Sci* 462:326–340.

Sackeim, H.A., Prudic, J., and Devanand, D.P. (1990a) Treatment of medication-resistant depression with electroconvulsive therapy. In: Tasman, A., Goldfinger, S.M., and Kaufmann, C.A., eds. *Annual Review of Psychiatry*, Vol. 9. Washington, DC: American Psychiatric Press, pp. 91–115.

Sackeim, H.A., Prudic, J., Devanand, D.P., Decina, P., Kerr, B., and Malitz, S. (1990b) The impact of medication resistance and continuation pharmacotherapy on relapse following response to electroconvulsive therapy in major depression. *J Clin Psychopharmacol* 10:96–104.

Sackeim, H.A., Prudic, J., Devanand, D.P., Kiersky, J.E., Fitzsimons, L., Moody, B.J., et al. (1993) Effects of stimulus intensity and electrode placement on the efficacy and cognitive effects of electroconvulsive therapy. *N Engl J Med* 328:839–846.

Sackeim, H.A., Prudic, J., Devanand, D.P., Nobler, M.S., Lisanby, S.H., Peyser, S., et al. (2000b) A prospective, randomized, double-blind comparison of bilateral and right unilateral electroconvulsive therapy at different stimulus intensities. *Arch Gen Psychiatry* 57:425–434.

Sackeim, H.A., Prudic, J., Olfson, M., and Fuller, R.B. (unpublished). Short- and long-term cognitive effects of electroconvulsive therapy in community settings.

Sackeim, H.A., Rush, A.J., George, M.S., Marangell, L.B., Husain, M.M., Nahas, Z., et al. (2001c) Vagus nerve stimulation (VNS) for treatment-resistant depression: Efficacy, side effects, and predictors of outcome. *Neuropsychopharmacology* 25:713–728.

Sackeim, H.A., and Steif, B.L. (1988) The neuropsychology of depression and mania. In: Georgotas, A., and Cancro, R., eds. *Depression and Mania*. New York: Elsevier, pp. 265–289.

Saito, S., Kadoi, Y., Nara, T., Sudo, M., Obata, H., Morita, T., et al. (2000) The comparative effects of propofol versus thiopental on middle cerebral artery blood flow velocity during electroconvulsive therapy. *Anesth Analg* 91:1531–1536.

Schatzberg, A.F., and Rothschild, A.J. (1992) Psychotic (delusional) major depression: Should it be included as a distinct syndrome in DSM-IV? *Am J Psychiatry* 149:733–745.

Segman, R.H., Shapira, B., Gorfine, M., and Lerer, B. (1995) Onset and time course of antidepressant action: Psychopharmacological implications of a controlled trial of electroconvulsive therapy. *Psychopharmacology (Berl)* 119:440–448.

Shapira, B., Calev, A., and Lerer, B. (1991) Optimal use of electroconvulsive therapy: Choosing a treatment schedule. *Psychiatr Clin North Am* 14:935–946.

Shellenberger, W., Miller, M., Small, I., Milstein, V., and Stout, J.R. (1982) Follow-up study of memory deficits after ECT. *Can J Psychiatry* 27:325–329.

Shepherd, M. (1965) Clinical trial of the treatment of depressive illness. *Br Med J* 1:881–886.

Siesjö, B.K., Ingvar, M., and Wieloch, T. (1986) Cellular and molecular events underlying epileptic brain damage. *Ann NY Acad Sci* 462:207–223.

Simpson, G.M., El Sheshai, A., Rady, A., Kingsbury, S.J., and Fayek, M. (2003) Sertraline as monotherapy in the treatment of psychotic and nonpsychotic depression. *J Clin Psychiatry* 64:959–965.

Simpson, K.H., Smith, R.J., and Davies, L.F. (1987) Comparison of the effects of atropine and glycopyrrolate on cognitive function following general anaesthesia. *Br J Anaesth* 59:966–969.

Small, J.G., Kellams, J.J., Milstein, V., and Small, I.F. (1980) Complications with electroconvulsive treatment combined with lithium. *Biol Psychiatry* 15:103–112.

Small, J.G., and Milstein, V. (1990) Lithium interactions: Lithium and electroconvulsive therapy. *J Clin Psychopharmacol* 10:346–350.

Sobin, C., Prudic, J., Devanand, D.P., Nobler, M.S., and Sackeim, H.A. (1996) Who responds to electroconvulsive therapy? A comparison of effective and ineffective forms of treatment. *Br J Psychiatry* 169:322–328.

Sobin, C., Sackeim, H.A., Prudic, J., Devanand, D.P., Moody, B.J., and McElhiney, M.C. (1995) Predictors of retrograde amnesia following ECT. *Am J Psychiatry* 152:995–1001.

Sommer, B.R., Satlin, A., Friedman, L., and Cole, J.O. (1989) Glycopyrrolate versus atropine in post-ECT amnesia in the elderly. *J Geriatr Psychiatry Neurol* 2:18–21.

Spiker, D.G., Stein, J., and Rich, C.L. (1985a) Delusional depression and electroconvulsive therapy: One year later. *Convuls Ther* 1:167–172.

Spiker, D.G., Weiss, J.C., Dealy, R.S., Griffin, S.J., Hanin, I., Neil, J.F., et al. (1985b) The pharmacological treatment of delusional depression. *Am J Psychiatry* 142:430–436.

Strömgren, L. (1973) Unilateral versus bilateral electroconvulsive therapy. Investigations into the therapeutic effect in endogenous depression. *Acta Psychiatr Scand [Suppl]* 240:8–65.

Squire, L. (1975) A stable impairment in remote memory following electroconvulsive therapy. *Neuropsychologia* 13:51–58.

Squire, L. (1986) Memory functions as affected by electroconvulsive therapy. *Ann NY Acad Sci* 462:307–314.

Squire, L.R., and Chace, P. (1975) Memory functions six to nine months after electroconvulsive therapy. *Arch Gen Psychiatry* 32:1557–1564.

Squire, L.R., and Cohen, N. (1979) Memory and amnesia: Resistance to disruption develops for years after learning. *Behav Neural Biol* 25:115–125.

Squire, L.R., Cohen, N., and Zouzounis, J. (1984) Preserved memory in retrograde amnesia: Sparing of a recently acquired skill. *Neuropsychologia* 22:145–152.

Squire, L.R., Shimamura, A., and Graf, P. (1985) Independence of recognition memory and priming effects: A neuropsychological analysis. *J Exp Psychol (Learn Mem Cogn)* 11:37–44.

Squire, L.R., and Slater, P. (1983) Electroconvulsive therapy and complaints of memory dysfunction: A prospective three-year follow-up study. *Br J Psychiatry* 142:1–8.

Squire, L.R., and Zouzounis, J.A. (1986) ECT and memory: Brief pulse versus sine wave. *Am J Psychiatry* 143:596–601.

Squire, L.R., and Zouzounis, J.A. (1988) Self-ratings of memory dysfunction: Different findings in depression and amnesia. *J Clin Exp Neuropsychol* 10:727–738.

Steif, B., Sackeim, H., Portnoy, S., Decina, P., and Malitz, S. (1986) Effects of depression and ECT on anterograde memory. *Biol Psychiatry* 21:921–930.

Stern, R.A., Nevels, C.T., Shelhorse, M.E., Prohaska, M.L., Mason, G.A., and Prange, A.J.J. (1991) Antidepressant and memory effects of combined thyroid hormone treatment and electroconvulsive therapy: Preliminary findings. *Biol Psychiatry* 30:623–627.

Sternberg, D.E., and Jarvik, M.E. (1976) Memory function in depression: Improvement with antidepressant medication. *Arch Gen Psychiatry* 33:219–224.

Stoudemire, A., Knos, G., Gladson, M., Markwalter, H., Sung, Y.F., Morris, R., et al. (1990) Labetalol in the control of cardiovascular responses to electroconvulsive therapy in high-risk depressed medical patients. *J Clin Psychiatry* 51:508–512.

Summers, W., Robins, E., and Reich, T. (1979) The natural history of acute organic mental syndrome after bilateral electroconvulsive therapy. *Biol Psychiatry* 14:905–912.

Swartz, C.M., and Saheba, N.C. (1989) Comparison of atropine with glycopyrrolate for use in ECT. *Convuls Ther* 5:56–60.

Tang, W.K., and Ungvari, G.S. (2002) Efficacy of electroconvulsive therapy combined with antipsychotic medication in treatment-resistant schizophrenia: A prospective, open trial. *J ECT* 18:90–94.

Tew, J.D.J., Mulsant, B.H., Haskett, R.F., Prudic, J., Thase, M.E., Crowe, R.R., et al. (1999) Acute efficacy of ECT in the treatment of major depression in the old-old. *Am J Psychiatry* 156:1865–1870.

Thase, M.E., and Ninan, P.T. (2002) New goals in the treatment of depression: Moving toward recovery. *Psychopharmacol Bull* 36(Suppl 2):24–35.

Thompson, J.W., and Blaine, J.D. (1987) Use of ECT in the United States in 1975 and 1980. *Am J Psychiatry* 144:557–562.

Thompson, J.W., Weiner, R.D., and Myers, C.P. (1994) Use of ECT in the United States in 1975, 1980, and 1986. *Am J Psychiatry* 151:1657–1661.

Tomac, T.A., Rummans, T.A., Pileggi, T.S., and Li, H. (1997) Safety and efficacy of electroconvulsive therapy in patients over age 85. *Am J Geriatr Psychiatry* 5:126–130.

Valentine, M., Keddie, K., and Dunne, D. (1968) A comparison of techniques in electro-convulsive therapy. *Br J Psychiatry* 114:989–996.

Wajima, Z., Yoshikawa, T., Ogura, A., Imanaga, K., Shiga, T., Inoue, T., et al. (2002) Intravenous verapamil blunts hyperdynamic responses during electroconvulsive therapy without altering seizure activity. *Anesth Analg* 95:400–402.

Watterson, D. (1945) The effect of age, head resistance and other physical factors of the stimulus threshold of electrically induced convulsions. *J Neurol Neurosurg Psychiatry* 8:121–125.

Webb, M.C., Coffey, C.E., Saunders, W.R., Cress, M.M., Weiner, R.D., and Sibert, TR. (1990) Cardiovascular response to unilateral electroconvulsive therapy. *Biol Psychiatry* 28:758–766.

Weeks, D., Freeman, C., and Kendell, R. (1980) ECT: III: Enduring cognitive deficits? *Br J Psychiatry* 137:26–37.

Weiner, R.D. (1980) ECT and seizure threshold: Effects of stimulus wave form and electrode placement. *Biol Psychiatry* 15:225–241.

Weiner, R.D. (1982) The role of electroconvulsive therapy in the treatment of depression in the elderly. *J Am Geriatr Soc* 30:710–712.

Weiner, R.D. (1984) Does ECT cause brain damage? *Behav Brain Sci* 7:1–53.

Weiner, R.D., Rogers, H.J., Davidson, J.R., and Squire, L.R. (1986) Effects of stimulus parameters on cognitive side effects. *Ann NY Acad Sci* 462:315–325.

Weiner, R.D., Volow, M.R., Gianturco, D.T., and Cavenar, J.O.J. (1980) Seizures terminable and interminable with ECT. *Am J Psychiatry* 137:1416–1418.

Welch, C.A., and Lambertus, L.J. (1989) Cardiovascular effects of ECT. *Convuls Ther* 5:35–43.

Wells, D.G., Davies, G.G., and Rosewarne, F. (1989) Attenuation of electroconvulsive therapy induced hypertension with sublingual nifedipine. *Anaesth Intens Care* 17:31–33.

Wesner, R.B., and Winokur, G. (1989) The influence of age on the natural history of unipolar depression when treated with electroconvulsive therapy. *Eur Arch Psychiatry Neurol Sci* 238:149–154.

West, E. (1981) Electric convulsion therapy in depression: A double-blind controlled trial. *Br Med J (Clin Res)* 282:355–357.

Wilson, I.C., Vernon, J.T., Guin, T., and Sandifer, M.G.J. (1963) A controlled study of treatments of depression. *J Neuropsychiatry* 4:331–337.

Wolfersdorf, M., Barg, T., Konig, F., Leibfarth, M., and Grunewald, I. (1995) Paroxetine as antidepressant in combined antidepressant-neuroleptic therapy in delusional depression: Observation of clinical use. *Pharmacopsychiatry* 28:56–60.

Wyatt, R.J. (1991) Neuroleptics and the natural course of schizophrenia. *Schizophr Bull* 17:325–351.

Zaidi, N.A., and Khan, F.A. (2000) Comparison of thiopentone sodium and propofol for electro convulsive therapy (ECT). *J Pak Med Assoc* 50:60–63.

Zakzanis, K.K., Leach, L., and Kaplan, E. (1998) On the nature and pattern of neurocognitive function in major depressive disorder. *Neuropsychiatry Neuropsychol Behav Neurol* 11:111–119.

Zervas, I.M., Calev, A., Jandorf, L., Schwartz, J., Gaudino, E., Tubi, N., et al. (1993) Age-dependent effects of electroconvulsive therapy on memory. *Convuls Ther* 9:39–42.

Zielinski, R.J., Roose, S.P., Devanand, D.P., Woodring, S., and Sackeim, H.A. (1993) Cardiovascular complications of ECT in depressed patients with cardiac disease. *Am J Psychiatry* 150:904–909.

Zornetzer, S. (1974) Retrograde amnesia and brain seizures in rodents: Electrophysiological and neuroanatomical analyses. In: Fink, M., Kety, S., McGaugh, J., and Williams, T.A., eds. *Psychobiology of Convulsive Therapy*. Washington, DC: V.H. Winston, pp. 99–128.

Zorumski, C.F., Rubin, E.H., and Burke, W.J. (1988) Electroconvulsive therapy for the elderly: A review. *Hosp Commun Psychiatry* 39:643–647.

Zvara, D.A., Brooker, R.F., McCall, W.V., Foreman, A.S., Hewitt, C., Murphy, B.A., et al. (1997) The effect of esmolol on ST-segment depression and arrhythmias after electroconvulsive therapy. *Convuls Ther* 13:165–174.

Zwil, A.S., and Pelchat, R.J. (1994) ECT in the treatment of patients with neurological and somatic disease. *Int J Psychiatry Med* 24:1–29.

# 22 | Pharmacological treatment of depression in Alzheimer's disease

JOHN L. BEYER AND P. MURALI DORAISWAMY

The incidence of depression in patients with Alzheimer's disease (AD) varies widely across studies, from 0% (Knesevich et al., 1983) to 86% (Merriam et al., 1988), depending on the type of measurement and the definition of depression used. After reviewing the wide range of estimates and considering the factors that caused the variations, Greenwald (1995) estimated that up to 15% of patients with AD have a major depressive episode, while 25% have a minor depression. Fifty percent of all AD patients exhibit depressive features. Lykestsos et al. (1997), reviewing their population sample, similarly found that 20%–25% of patients with AD had a major depressive episode. Depression occurs at all stages and severities of the dementia (Payne et al., 1998) and causes greater functional impairment (Alexopoulos and Abrams, 1991; Lykestos et al., 1997).

Pharmacological treatment has been demonstrated to be effective across phenomenological subgroups of AD, but the greatest improvement occurs in patients who meet criteria for a co-morbid major depression (Greenwald et al., 1989; Zubenko et al., 1992). However, although depression is a significant problem in AD and is responsive to treatment, there are remarkably few systematic studies of the treatment response in these patients.

A review of the literature (MEDLINE 1966–2002) found only 11 published controlled clinical trials of depression in AD (or probable AD) (Tables 22.1 and 22.2). Interestingly, only three of the eight placebo-controlled clinical trials demonstrated a significant improvement with the study medication compared to placebo. Possible explanations include the poor efficacy of antidepressants in this population, inadequate dosing, inadequate length of treatment, or underpowered studies. These trials varied significantly in the intensity of depressive symptoms, with many focusing on AD patients with minor depression. They also varied significantly in the patient's level of cognitive functioning.

Medications studied have included three selective serotonin reuptake inhibitors (SSRIs) (fluoxetine, paroxetine, citalopram), three tricyclics (imipramine, clomipramine, amytriptyline), and a reversible monoamine oxidase inhibitor (MAOI) (moclobimide). Even when case reports are considered (Table 22.3), the published literature on the pharmacological treatment of depression in AD remains limited, but it does include a tetracyclic (mianserine), a monoamine oxidase inhibitor (tranylcypromine), and electroconvulsive therapy (ECT).

In making treatment decisions for depression in AD, the physician must consider not only the diagnosis, but also the potential side effects of the medications. As with the general considerations for the treatment of depression, the goals of treatment in AD should be to achieve remission of symptoms, prevent relapse and recurrence, and improve the patient's quality of life and functional capacity (Lebowitz et al., 1997).

## TRICYCLIC ANTIDEPRESSANTS

Tricyclics were among the first of the antidepressants to be systematically reviewed for efficacy. Reifler et al. (1986) conducted a retrospective chart review of depressed outpatients with AD and found an 85% treatment response rate to standard tricyclics. He and his colleagues (1989) followed up these findings by conducting a placebo-controlled, randomized trial of imipramine in 61 AD subjects, 33 of whom had depression. They found no clinically significant difference between active treatment and placebo, though both groups had marked improvement in their depressive symptoms. This study was criticized because it used a fixed dose schedule and a relatively high dose of imipramine in an elderly population (average daily dose, 82 mg; average plasma level, 119 ng/ml). Imipramine was associated with significant improvements in Mini-Mental State Examination (MMSE) scores and none of the subjects developed anticholinergic delirium, but imipramine was also associated with significant worsening on the Mattis Dementia Rating Scale, a more sensitive assessment of cognitive functioning.

Katona et al. (1997) also conducted a trial of imipramine, comparing it to paroxetine. A total of 198 AD patients with major depression were studied for 8

279

TABLE 22.1. Placebo-Controlled Clinical Trials for Treatment of Depression in Alzheimer's Disease

| Study | Medication | Dose | Sample Size | Study Design | Length of Study | Diagnosis of Depression | Diagnosis of Alzheimer's Disease | Findings |
|---|---|---|---|---|---|---|---|---|
| Reifler et al. (1989) | Imipramine | Mean dose = 83 mg (average plasma level = 119 ng/ml) | 61: 28 AD with depression 33 AD without depression | Double-blind, PBO (outpatients) | 8 weeks | Mean HAM-D = 18.9 | Mean MMSE = 17.5 | Depressive symptoms improved in both imipramine and placebo groups without significant difference. |
| Nyth and Gottfries (1990) | Citalopram | 10–30 mg | 98: 65 AD/SDAT 24 VD | 4-week double-blind PBO phase, with 8-week open trial, followed by 4-week double-blind rerandomization | 16 weeks | Mean MADRS = 8.1 (only 2 patients identified as MDE with MADRS >26) | GBS | AD subjects had reduced emotional blunting, confusion, irritability, anxiety, fear, depressed mood, and restlessness. No improvement in depressive symptoms for VD subjects. |
| Nyth et al. (1992) | Citalopram | 10–40 mg | 149: 29 AD with depression 120 depression without cognitive impairment | Double-blind, PBO (inpatients and outpatients) | 6 weeks | Mean HAM-D = 21.7 | GBS | Citalopram demonstrated significant improvement over placebo in treatment of depression in full sample. Improvement in anxiety and depressed mood in AD subjects measured on GBS. |
| Fuchs et al. (1993) | Maprotiline | 25 mg | 127 (minor depression) | Double-blind, PBO | 8 weeks | Mean GDS = 8 | Mean MMSE = 20 | Maprotiline was significantly better than placebo for depressive symptoms, but no difference was noted on CGI. |
| Petracca et al. (1996) | Clomipramine | 100 mg | 21 NINCDS/ ADRDA 8 MDE 13 Dysthymia | Double-blind Crossover, PBO, (outpatients) | 14 weeks (6 weeks on each cross-over arm, with 2 weeks washout) | Mean HAM-D = 17.5 | Mean MMSE = 21.5 | Clomipramine was significantly more effective than placebo during the first 6-week treatment period, but no difference occurred after crossover. MMSE score declined on clomipramine. |

| Study | Drug | Dose | Sample | Design | Duration | Baseline (depression) | Baseline (cognition) | Outcome |
|---|---|---|---|---|---|---|---|---|
| Roth et al. (1996) | Meclobemide | 400 mg | 694 511 MDE with dementia 183 MDE with cognitive impairment | Double-blind, PBO, 4-day minimum placebo lead-in, multicenter | 6 weeks | Mean HAM-D = 24.5 | Mean MMSE = 20.2 | Improvement in depression and cognition in both depressed groups compared with placebo. |
| Lyketsos et al. (2000) | Sertraline | 25–125 mg (mean, 81 mg) | 22 | Double-blind PBO with 1-week placebo lead-in (outpatient) | 12 weeks | Mean Cornell Scale = 12.4 HAM-D = 23.2 | Mean MMSE = 15.8 | Sertraline was superior to placebo on Cornell Scale. No difference on HAM-D. |
| Magai et al. (2000) | Sertraline | 100 mg | 31 NINCDS/ADRDA 6 MDE 25 Dysthymic | Double-blind, PBO multicenter (nursing homes) | 8 weeks | Cornell Scale ≥3, Gestalt Scale ≥1 | Late-stage dementia (GDS Stages 6 and 7) | No significant difference between groups |
| Petracca et al. (2001) | Fluoxetine | 40 mg | 41 NINCDS-ADRDA 31 MDE 10 dysthymic | Double-blind, PBO, parallel | 6 weeks | Mean HAM-D = 16.6 | Mean MMSE = 23.2 | Fluoxetine did not differ signficantly from placebo for the treatment of depression in AD |
| Lyketsos et al. (2003) | Sertraline | 50–150 mg (mean 95 mg) | 44 NINCDS-ADRDA | Double-blind, PBO, parallel (outpatient) | 12 weeks | Mean HAM-D = 22.8 | Mean MMSE = 16.6 | Sertraline was superior to placebo on Cornell Scale and HAM-D. |

GDS, Global Deterioration Scale; AD, Alzheimer's disease; CGI, Clinical Global Impression scale; GBS, Gottries-Brane-Steen geriatric rating scale; HAM-D, Hamilton Depression Rating Scale; MADRS, Montgomery-Asberg Depression Rating Scale; MDE, major depressive episode; MMSE, Mini-Mental State Examination; NINCDS/ADRDA, National Institute of Neurological Diseases and Stroke/Alzheimer's Disease and Related Disorders Association; VD, vascular dementia; PBO, placebo; SDAT, senile dementia of Alzheimer type.

TABLE 22.2. *Antidepressant Comparator Clinical Trials for the Treatment of Depression in Alzheimer's Disease*

| Study | Medication | Dose | Sample Size | Study Design | Length of Study | Diagnosis of Depression | Diagnosis of Alzheimer's Disease | Findings |
|---|---|---|---|---|---|---|---|---|
| Taragano et al. (1997) | Fluoxetine vs. amitriptyline | 10 mg vs. 25 mg | 37 | Double-blind, fixed dose | 6 weeks | Mean HAM-D = 25.8 | Mean MMSE = 19.4 | Fluoxetine and amitriptyline are equally efficacious for the treatment of depressive symptoms, but amitriptyline is less well tolerated even at a low dose. |
| Katona et al. (1998) | Paroxetine vs. imipramine | 20–40 mg (mean 25mg) vs. 50–100 mg (mean 60 mg) | 198 | Double-blind, parallel with 3- to 7-day placebo lead-in, multicenter | 8 weeks | Mean MADRS = 28.2 | Mean MMSE = 19.9 | No significant difference in depressive response between groups |

HAM-D, Hamilton Depression Rating Scale; MADRS, Montgomery-Asberg Depression Rating Scale; MMSE, Mini-Mental State Examination.

weeks using an average daily dose of 50–100 mg imipramine or 20–40 mg paroxetine. The researchers found that both medications were effective, but paroxetine appeared to be better tolerated. Cognitive scores were not assessed at the end of the study, but 10% of the patients treated with imipramine, compared with 3% of the paroxetine group, experienced confusion.

Petracca et al. (1996) conducted a trial of clomipramine in 21 depressed patients with AD using a double-blind, crossover study. Eight of the subjects met the criteria for a major depressive episode, while 13 had dysthymia. The researchers found that mood improved significantly on both clomipramine (100 mg dose) and placebo, but clomipramine was significantly more effective during the first 6-week treatment period. Patients who started on clomipramine maintained their improvement during the 2-week washout period of the crossover, but those who started on the placebo worsened. However, like Reifler's findings with imipramine, the use of clomipramine was associated with lower MMSE scores.

Tarango et al. (1997) conducted a similar study comparing amitriptyline (25 mg) and fluoxetine (10 mg) in 37 depressed AD patients. They also found that the medications were equally effective for treatment of the depressive symptoms, but fluoxetine was much better tolerated than amitriptyline, even at this low dose. Given the fact that no separation between imipramine and placebo was found in Reifler's study (1989), the lack of a placebo arm in these two comparator studies prevents a clear separation between active treatment and placebo response.

The increasing cognitive impairment with tricyclic antidepressant treatment in this population remains an issue. Preserving cognitive functioning at the beginning of treatment is important to the successful treatment of depression in AD (Tune, 1998) and may affect treatment compliance (Amado-Boccaro et al., 1995). Elderly patients, especially those with dementia, are particularly sensitive to the anticholinergic effects of all med-ications. Impairments in memory and attention induced by tricyclic antidepressants may replicate what is seen in the early cases of dementia. The secondary amine tricyclics, nortriptyline and desipramine, have less anticholinergic activity than the tertiary amine tricyclics (such as amitriptyline, imipramine, and clomipramine). However, even the secondary amine tricyclics have been noted to impair the performance on cognitive tests of older adults. When severe, the effects of memory impairment and confusion may offset the gains in depressive symptoms (Oxman, 1996).

## SELECTIVE SEROTONIN REUPTAKE INHIBITORS

Due to the unwanted side effects of the tricyclic antidepressants, SSRIs have been increasingly used for the treatment of depression. Five placebo-controlled studies and two comparator studies have been conducted with this group.

Nyth and Gottfries (1990) conducted the first study of SSRIs in depressed patients with mixed etiology of dementia using citalopram. No improvement in depressive symptoms was noted in subjects with vascular dementia, but AD subjects showed improvement in emotional blunting, confusion, irritability, anxiety, fear, depressed mood, and restlessness. The lack of efficacy in the vascular dementia group may have been due to their relatively minimal depressive symptoms. Only 2 of the 98 patients studied actually met the criteria for a major depressive episode on the Montgomery-Asberg Depression Rating Scale (MADRS >26), while the mean baseline MADRS score was just over 8.

Nyth et al. (1992) conducted a second study of citalopram in 149 depressed patients with probable AD. In this study, the patients met the criteria for a major depressive disorder (the mean Hamilton Depression Scale score was 21.7). Citalopram demonstrated significant improvement over placebo. In their discussion, the au-

TABLE 22.3. *Case Reports of Antidepressant Treatment of Depression in Alzheimer's Disease*

| Study | Medication | Dose | Sample Size | Study Design | Length of Study | Diagnosis of Depression | Diagnosis of Alzheimer's Disease | Findings |
|---|---|---|---|---|---|---|---|---|
| Jenike (1985) | Tranylcypromine | 20 mg bid | 2 | Case report | 6–8 months | Clinical impression | MDRS = 125, 135 | Clinical observation of improved functioning without significant orthostasis. |
| Haupt (1991) | Mianserine | 20 mg/day | 1 | Case report | 6 weeks | Clinical impression and DMAS = 40 | Clinical impression NINCDS-ADRDA, CCE = 6 | Clinical observation of improvement in depressive symptoms without significant side effects. |

DMAS, Dementia Mood Assessment Scale; MDRS, Mattis Dementia Rating Scale; NINCDS/ADRDA, National Institute of Neurological Diseases and Stroke/Alzheimer's Disease and Related Disorder Association.

thors noted that a dose of 20–30 mg was the most effective, since patients with a higher plasma level showed the greatest improvement.

As noted in the previous section, two SSRIs have been studied in comparator trials with tricyclics. Fluoxetine (10 mg) (Tarango et al., 1997) and paroxetine (20–40 mg) (Katona et al., 1998) were found to be effective (and well tolerated) in depressed AD patients.

More recently, sertraline has been investigated for the treatment of depression in AD, but with differing results. Lyketsos et al. (2000) randomized 22 AD patients with depression to either clomipramine or placebo for 12 weeks. Sertraline was titrated to the highest tolerated dose (mean dose, 81 mg). After 12 weeks, 9 of the 11 patients treated with sertraline and 2 of the 10 patients given placebo showed at least a partial response. In a second study, Lyketsos et al. (2003) randomized 44 AD patients with depression to either sertraline (n = 24) or placebo (n = 20) for 12 weeks. Sertraline was titrated to the highest tolerated dose (mean dose = 95 mg). In the sertraline-treated group, 38% of the patients were full reponders and 46% were partial responders, compared with the placebo group in which only 20% were full responders and 15% partial responders. Magai et al. (2000) randomized 31 nursing home AD patients with depressive symptoms to either placebo or sertraline. Although similar doses of sertraline were used, no signficant differences were noted. However, several differences between these two studies should be noted. Lyketsos' study sample was composed of more highly functioning outpatients, while Magai's subject sample consisted of nursing home patients with late-stage AD in whom assessment for depressive symptoms and response had to be conducted using nonverbal responses.

In contrast to the tricyclics, some of the SSRIs have been noted to have positive effects on cognitive measures. Fluoxetine, sertraline, and low-dose paroxetine have all been found to have some cognition-enhancing effects (Amado-Baccaro et al., 1995; Hindmarch and Bhatti, 1988; Knegtering et al., 1994; Oxman, 1996). In the clinical trials with SSRIs mentioned above, Taragano et al. (1997) found fluoxetine improved the MMSE, but Lyketsos et al. (2000) did not find similar improvements with sertraline.

## MONOAMINE OXIDASE INHIBITORS

Monoamine oxidase inhibitors have been used to treat depression in dementia due to two observations: several case studies show that depressive symptoms are responsive to MAOIs (Jenicke, 1985), and behavioral symptoms in AD that are possibly related to depression have been noted to improve (Tariot et al., 1987). Jenike (1985) reported two patients successfully treated with tranylcypromine after previous trials of tricyclic antidepressants failed. He noted that the central cholinergic deficit in AD patients makes them particularly prone to develop memory impairment and other anticholinergic side effects of standard tricyclics. Since MAOIs do not produce clinically significant anticholinergic effects, he reasoned that they should be considered in depressed AD patients. However, MAOIs are often associated with other side effects, primarily orthostatic hypotension and insomnia. They also require patients to be on a specialized diet and avoid taking other medications such as SSRIs, narcotic analgesics, or sympathomimetic agents. For these reasons, MAOIs have been used only in treatment-refractory patients or those who have been unable to tolerate other antidepressant treatment.

A second MAOI that has been used frequently for dementia is donepezil. In an open-label study of emotional and behavioral symptoms in AD patients, Weiner et al. (2000) noted that donepezil had a mildly positive effect on mood over a 12-month period. However, none of these patients was formally diagnosed with depression.

## NEWER ANTIDEPRESSANT AGENTS

Research has shown that the newer antidepressant agents such as venlafaxine, bupropion, nefazodone, and mirtazepine may be effective in the treatment of depression in the elderly. However, these agents have not been studied in depressed AD patients. Their efficacy

TABLE 22.4. *Electroconvulsive Therapy for the Treatment of Depression in Alzheimer's Disease*

| Study | Therapy | Sample Size | Study Design | Length of Study | Diagnosis of Depression | Diagnosis of Alzheimer's Disease | Findings |
|---|---|---|---|---|---|---|---|
| Rao and Lyketsos (2000) | ECT: 22 unilateral 9 bilateral Number of treatments = 1–23 | 31: 17 VD, 4 AD, 10 unknown etiology | Chart review | NA | Mean MADRS = 27.5 | Mean MMSE = 18.8 | Improvement in depressive symptoms and cognition; 49% became delirious. |

MADRS, Montgomery-Asberg Depression Rating Scale; MMSE, Mini-Mental State Examination.

profile in other elderly depressed groups and their limited side effect profile do make them attractive for use in the AD population.

## ELECTROCONVULSIVE THERAPY

The efficacy and safety of ECT for the treatment of depression in the elderly are well established (Weiner, 1982), though the efficacy and safety in patients with AD have been very poorly studied (American Psychiatric Association 1997). Rao and Lyketsos (2000) conducted a chart review of 31 depressed patients with dementia who received ECT (Table 22.4). Seventeen of the patients had vascular dementia, 4 had AD, and 10 had a dementia of unknown etiology. The patients received between 1 and 27 ECT treatments (mean, 9). Twenty-two received unilateral ECT and nine received bilateral treatment. At discharge, these patients had significant improvement in depressive symptoms as measured by the MADRS, as well as a significant mean increase in MMSE. However, 49% of the patients developed a delirium during the ECT course.

## GUIDELINES FOR TREATMENT

The 1997 Practice Guideline for the Treatment of Patients with Alzheimer's Disease and Other Dementias of Late Life published by the American Psychiatric Association (1997) reviewed the current literature and presented recommendations regarding the treatment of depressive symptoms. Three major recommendations (Katz, 1998) were:

1. Patients with depression should be carefully monitored for their suicidal potential.
2. Depressed mood may respond to improvements in the living situation, but patients with severe or persistent depressed mood should be treated with antidepressant medications.
3. The choice among antidepressant agents is based on the side effect profile and the characteristics of a given patient.

In general, SSRIs are believed to be the first-line treatment, although one of the newer agents may be more appropriate for some patients (Katz, 1998). Tricyclics should be considered if the other agents are not effective, but agents with significant anticholinergic effects should be avoided. Electroconvulsive therapy is effective in the treatment of depressed AD patients who do not respond to other agents, though delirium and memory loss may occur during the course of therapy. The use of unilateral treatment and the decreased frequency of therapy (twice weekly) may decrease the risk of delirium. As with all pharmacological agents in elderly patients, the maxim "start low and go slow" also applies to the treatment of depressed AD patients with antidepressants.

## REFERENCES

Alexopoulos, G.S., and Abrams, R.C. (1991) Depression in Alzheimer's disease. *Psychiatr Clin North Am* 14:327–340.

Amado-Bocarra, I., Gougoulis, N., Poirer Littre, M.F., Galinowski, A., and Loo, A. (1995) Effects of antidepressants on cognitive functions: A review. *Neurosci Biobehav Rev* 19:479–493.

American Psychiatric Association. (1997) Practice Guidelines for the Treatment of Patients with Alzheimer's Disease and Other Dementias of Late Life. *Am J Psychiatry* 154(5):1–39.

Fuchs, A., Hehnke, U., Erhart, C., Schell, C., Pramshohler, B., Danninger, B., and Schautzer, F. (1993) Video rating analysis of effect of maprotiline in patients with dementia and depression. *Pharmacopsychiatry* 26(2):37–41.

Greenwald, B. (1995) Depression in Alzheimer's disease and related dementias. In: Lawlor, B., ed. *Behavioral Complications in Alzheimer's Disease*. Washington, DC: American Psychiatric Press, pp. 19–53.

Greenwald, B.S., Kramer-Ginsberg, E., Marin, D.B., Laitman, L.B., Hermann, C.K., Mohs, R.C., and Davis, K.L. (1989) Dementia with coexistent major depression. *Am. J. Psychiatry* 146(11): 1472–1478.

Haupt, M. (1991) Depression in Alzheimer's disease significantly improved under treatment with mianserine. *J Am Geriatr Soc* 39: 1141–1144.

Hindmarch, I., and Bhatti, J.Z. (1988) The effects of paroxetine and other antidepressants in combination with alcohol in psychomotor activity related to car driving. *Hum Psychopharmacol* 3:13–20.

Jenike, M. (1985) Monoamine oxidase inhibitors as treatment for depressed patients with primary degenerative dementia (Alzheimer's disease). *Am J Psychiatry* 142(6):763–764.

Katona, C.L., Hunter, B.N., and Bray, J. (1998) A double-blind comparison of the efficacy and safety of paroxetine and imipramine in the treatment of depression with dementia. *Int J Geriatr Psychiatry* 2:100–108.

Katona, C.L.E., Hunter, B.N., and Bray, J. (1997) A double-blind comparison of the efficacy and safety of paroxetine and imipramine in the treatment of depression with dementia. *Int J Geriatr Psychiatry* 13:100–108.

Katz, I.R. (1998) Diagnosis and treatment of depression in patients with Alzheimer's disease and other dementias. *J Clin Psychiatry* 59(suppl 9):38–44.

Knegtering, H., Eijck, M., and Huijsman, A. (1994) Effects of antidepressants on cognitive functioning of elderly patients: A review. *Drugs Aging* 5:192–199.

Knesevich, J.W., Martin, R.L., and Berg, L. (1983) Preliminary report on affective symptoms in the early stages of senile dementia of the Alzheimer's type. *Am J Psychiatry* 140:233–235.

Lebowitz, B.D., Pearson, J.L., Sccneider, L.S., Reynolds, C.F., Alexopoulos G.S., Bruce, M.L., Conwell Y., Katz, I.R., Meyers, B.S., Morrison, M.F., Mossey, J., Niederehe, G., and Parmelee, P. (1997) Diagnosis and treatment of depression in late life: Consensus statement update. *JAMA* 278(14):1186–1190.

Lyketsos, C.G., Baker, L., Warren, A., Steele, C., Brandt, J., Steinberg, M., Kopunek, S., and Baker, A. (1997) Major and minor depression in Alzheimer's disease: Prevalence and impact. *J Neuropsychiatry Neurosci* 9:556–561.

Lyketsos, C.G., DelCampo, L., Steinberg, M., Miles, Q., Steele, C.D., Munro, C., Baker, A.S., Sheppard, J.M., Frangakis, C., Brandt, J., and Rabins, P.V. (2003) Treating depression in Alzheimer disease: efficacy and safety of sertraline therapy, and the benefits of depression reduction: the DIADS. *Arch Gen Psychiatry* 60(7): 737–746.

Lyketsos, C.G., Sheppard, J-M.E., Steele, C.D., Kopunek, S., Steinberg, M., Baker, A.S., Brandt, J., and Rabins, P.V. (2000) Randomized, placebo-controlled, double-blind clinical trial of sertraline in the treatment of depression complicating Alzheimer's disease: Initial results from the depression in Alzheimer's disease study. *Am J Psychiatry* 157:1686–1689.

Magai, C., Kennedy, G., Cohen, C.I., and Gomberg, D. (2000) A controlled clinical trial of sertraline in the treatment of depression in nursing home patients with late-stage Alzheimer's disease. *Am J Geriatr Psychiatry* 8:66–74.

Merriam, A.E., Aronson, M.K., Gaston, P., Wey, S.L., and Katz, I. (1988) The psychiatric symptoms of Alzheimer's disease. *J Am Geriatr Soc* 36:7–12.

Nyth, A.L., and Gottfries, C.G. (1990) The clinical efficacy of citalopram in treatment of emotional disturbances in dementia disorders: A Nordic multicenter study. *Br J Psychiatry* 157:894–901.

Nyth, A.L., Gottfries, C.G., Lyby, K., Smedegaard-Andersen, L., Gylding-Sabroe, J., Kristensen, M., Refsum, H-E., Ofsti, E., Eriksson, S., and Syversen, S. (1992) A controlled multicenter clinical study of citalopram and placebo in elderly depressed patients with and without concomitant dementia. *Acta Psychiatr Scand* 86: 138–145.

Oxman, T. (1996) Antidepressants and cognitive impairment in the elderly. *J Clin Psychiatry* 57(suppl 5):38–44.

Payne, J.L., Lyketsos, C.G., Baker, L., Warren, A., Steele, C., Brandt, J., Steinberg, M., Kopunek, S., and Baker, A. (1998) The relationship of cognitive and functional impairment to depressive features in Alzheimer's disease and other dementias. *J Neuropsychiatry Clin Neurosci* 10:440–447.

Petracca, G.M., Chemerinski, E., and Starkstein, S.E. (2001) A double-blind, placebo-controlled study of fluoxetine in depressed patients with Alzheimer's disease. *Intl Psychogeriatr* 13(2):233–240.

Petrecca, G.M., Teson, A., Chemerinski, E., Leiguarda, R., and Starkstein, S.E. (1996) A double-blind placebo-controlled study of clomipramine in depressed patients with Alzheimer's disease. *J Neuropsychiatry Clin Neurosci* 8:270–275.

Rao, V., and Lyketsos, C.G. (2000) The benefits and risks of ECT for patients with primary dementia who also suffer from depression. *Int J Geriatr Psychiatry* 15:729–735.

Reifler, B.V., Teri, L., Rasking, M., Veith, R., Barnes, R., White, E., and McLean, P. (1989) Double-blind trial of imipramine in Alzheimer's disease patients with and without depression. *Am J Psychiatry* 146(1):45–49.

Reifler, B.V., Larson, E., Teri, L., and Poulsen, M. (1986) Dementia of the Alzheimer's type and depression. *J Am Geriatr Soc* 34(12): 855–859.

Roth, M., Mountjoy, C.Q., Amrein, R., and the International Collaborative Study Group (1996) Moclobemide in elderly patients with cognitive decline and depression. *Br J Psychiatry* 168: 149–157.

Taragano, F.E., Lyketsos, C.G., Mangone, C.A., Allegri, R.F., and Comesana-Diaz, E. (1997) A double-blind, randomized, fixed-dose trial of fluoxetine vs. amitriptyline in the treatment of major depression complicating Alzheimer's disease. *Psychosomatics* 38(3):246–252.

Tariot, P.N., Cohen, R.M., Sunderland, T., Newhouse, P.A., Yount, D., Mellow, A.M., Weingartner, H., Mueller, E.A., and Murphy, D.L. (1987) L-deprenyl in Alzheimer's disease. Preliminary evidence for behavioral change with monoamine oxidase B inhibition. *Arch Gen Psychiatry* 44(5):427–433.

Tune, L. (1998) Depression and Alzheimer's disease. *Depress Anxiety* 8(suppl 1):91–95.

Weiner, M.F., Martin-Cook, M.S., Foster, B.M., Saine, K., Fontaine, C.S., and Svetlik, D.A. (2000) Effects of donepezil on emotional/behavioral symptoms in Alzheimer's disease patients. *J Clin Psychiatry* 61(7):487–492.

Weiner, R.D. (1982) The role of electroconvulsive therapy in the treatment of depression in the elderly. *J Am Soc Geriatr* 30:710–712.

Zubenko, G.S., Rosen, J., Sweet, R.A., Mulsant, B.H., and Rifai, A.H. (1992) Impact of psychiatric hospitalization on behavioral complications of Alzheimer's disease. *Am J Psychiatry* 149(11): 1484–1491.

# 23 | Psychotherapy in old-age depression: Progress and challenges

CHARLES F. REYNOLDS III, PATRICIA A. AREAN, THOMAS R. LYNCH, AND ELLEN FRANK

## RATIONALE FOR PSYCHOSOCIAL INTERVENTIONS AND FOR PSYCHOTHERAPY IN THE TREATMENT OF DEPRESSION IN LATER LIFE

Both biological and psychosocial risk factors operate in old-age depression. Nonmodifiable risk factors (such as gender and race) may be critical in understanding causal pathways, as well as identifying groups at high risk for depression or suicide. The targets of intervention are *modifiable* risk factors, and many of them are psychosocial in nature, thus providing a rationale for psychosocial interventions (Bruce, 2002). To understand how psychosocial interventions might work, it is important to distinguish which factors mediate, and which moderate, risk in the chain of events. Mediators are in the chain of events (e.g., social isolation could mediate the effect of disability on depression), while moderators influence the impact of one variable upon another (e.g., social support or ways of coping moderate the impact of loss of a spouse on depression). Even, or perhaps especially, when considering co-morbid medical or neurological illness (such as cardiovascular disease or neurodegenerative disorders such as Alzheimer's dementia or Parkinson's disease) as a risk for depression, it is important clinically to consider *both* biological *and* psychosocial consequences of the disease. Many dementing disorders (Alzheimer's disease, Parkinson's disease) are associated with depression in the elderly, and psychosocial variables act as mediators and moderators of depression associated with neurodegenerative illnesses. Depression in old age occurs in an interpersonal and psychosocial as well as a biological context. Interpersonal and psychosocial factors are both antecedent and consequent to old-age depression.

Psychosocial risk factors for major depression in later life, either new onset or recurrent, frequently involve negative life events such as bereavement and other events characterized by loss and/or disability. It is useful clinically and scientifically to consider key dimensions of these events, such as undesirability, uncontrollability, magnitude and duration, changes in lifestyle, loss of independence, and self-perception. Psychosocial risk factors are nodes in a web of causation with many potential interconnections; they may be both additive and interactive. The most important and best-studied risk factors for new-onset and recurrent depression in late life are bereavement, caregiver strain, interpersonal conflict, role transitions, social isolation, disability from medical illness, and need for rehabilitation (Bruce, 2002).

Psychosocial factors also represent important mediators and moderators of the risk of suicide in the elderly. Risk factors for suicide in the elderly include mood disorder (especially major depression), previous attempts, physical illness (increased risk mediated by psychological factors such as hopelessness and certain personality traits such as avoidance of new stimuli), stressful events, and strength of social ties. In late life, the suicide risk is higher in men compared to women and in whites compared to nonwhites (Conwell et al., 2002).

Depression is also a risk factor in *nonsuicide* mortality in the elderly. Depression is linked to mortality in diverse elderly populations, with a crude relative risk of approximately 2.00 (Schulz et al., 2001). While there are multiple candidate mediator variables, it is plausible to hypothesize that certain aspects of depression account for increased risk (e.g., hopelessness, motivational depletion). Psychotherapeutic and psychosocial treatments may be especially helpful in ameliorating these dimensions of depression in later life, whether related to suicide or nonsuicide mortality.

Psychosocial treatments endorsed by North American academic geriatric psychiatrists in the recent development of consensus-based treatment guidelines (Alexopoulos et al., 2001) include both psychotherapy (especially cognitive-behavioral therapy [CBT] problem solving therapy, interpersonal psychotherapy [IPT], and supportive psychotherapy) and psychosocial interventions (such as psychoeducation, family counseling, visiting nurse services, bereavement groups, and senior citizen center programs).

The latter group of interventions are considered by the majority of respondents in the survey (Alexopoules et al., 2001) to be adjunctive to primary treatment with pharmacotherapy, psychotherapy, or both.

A majority of the psychotherapy studies in late-life depression have involved CBT and IPT, with or without combined pharmacotherapy. Dialectical behavior therapy (DBT) is being adapted to the treatment of older depressed patients with personality disorders and shows promise in these patients. In a recent review of psychotherapy and combined psychotherapy/pharmacotherpy for late-life depression, Arean and Cook (2002) suggested that the evidence base be evaluated with respect to quality of data, generalizability, and long-term effects of treatment. We take this approach here. In addition, we review the role of psychotherapy in the management of suicidal elderly depressed patients, and we propose an agenda for future research.

## COGNITIVE-BEHAVIORAL THERAPY

As recently reviewed by Arean and Cook (2002), the effectiveness of CBT as an intervention for the treatment of late-life depression has been studied more extensively than any other type of psychotherapeutic intervention. Actually, CBT is not one type of therapy, but rather a group of therapies that are all based in learning theory: psychopathology is thought to be largely attributable to the way people learn to manage their psychosocial environment, modulate their mood, and interpret the events that happen around them. While cognitive-behavioral theorists all agree that genetics and biology play a role in how people respond to psychosocial stress, they believe that biological vulnerability to depression can be mediated by skill acquisition and lifetime learning. Cognitive-behavioral interventions that have been evaluated for late-life depression include cognitive therapy (Beck, 1976), social problem solving therapy (SPST) (Nezu and Perri, 1989), problem solving therapy for primary care (PST-PC) (Mynors-Wallis, 1996), and self-management therapy (Rokke et al., 2000). These interventions have been evaluated in different settings and with different populations, including the medically ill elderly, the rural and homebound elderly, and cognitively impaired subjects. Most of the trials have focused on major depression; there are limited data on dysthymia and minor depression. Though CBT is short-term (often 6–20 weeks in length), its purpose is to train patients in mood management and coping skills so that they can better negotiate their psychosocial environment.

Randomized trials enrolling elderly depressed outpatients have found CBT superior to usual care (Campbell, 1992), to wait-list controls (Arean et al., 1993), to pill-placebo (Jarvik et al., 1982), and to no treatment (Viney et al., 1989). There is also evidence for persistence of treatment-attributable gains over time in a 1-year follow-up study (Rokke et al., 2000). In this study, a large percentage of subjects in the self-management therapy and educational group therapy groups (71% and 61%, respectively) made clinically significant improvements in their depressive symptoms even over the follow-up period, indicating substantial and persistent improvements as a result of treatment. As demonstrated in Figures 23.1 and 23.2, a substantial decrease in depression scores on both the Hamilton Depression Rating Scale and the Beck Depression Inventory are seen following CBT interventions as baseline scores drop significantly from baseline assessment to assessment after treatment. Although only one study (Arean et al., 1993) contained raw scores 3 months post treatment, the persistent decrease in depression ratings from baseline scores suggests promising long-term results for CBT with the elderly. Further studies are necessary to offer additional support for the long-term effectiveness and maintenance of CBT.

Cognitive-behavioral therapy has been compared to several other psychotherapies in the elderly (see Figs. 23.1 and 23.2). Thompson et al. (1987) compared CBT,

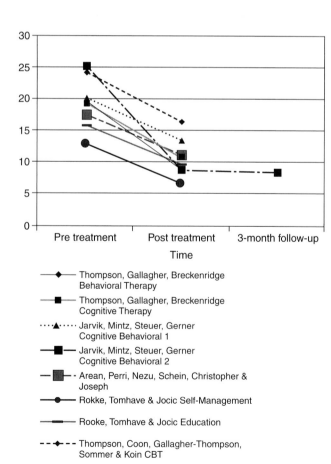

FIGURE 23.1 Mean Hamilton Depression Rating Scale scores across cognitive-behavioral therapy studies.

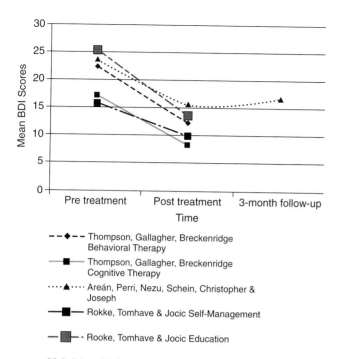

Legend:

- - ◆ - -  Thompson, Gallagher, Breckenridge
         Behavioral Therapy

———■———  Thompson, Gallagher, Breckenridge
         Cognitive Therapy

····▲····  Areán, Perri, Nezu, Schein, Christopher &
         Joseph

———■———  Rokke, Tomhave & Jocic Self-Management

—·■·—  Rooke, Tomhave & Jocic Education

FIGURE 23.2 Mean Beck Depression Inventory scores across studies.

behavioral therapy (BT), and brief dynamic therapy (BDT) in 91 older adults with current major depression. All active treatments were superior to wait-list controls and showed maintenance of positive outcomes over 1 year (70% showed significant improvement or remission of depression). Areán et al. (1993) reported that PST was superior to both a waiting-list control and to reminiscence therapy (RT) (64% showed significant improvement or remission post treatment). Further supporting cognitive behavioral strategies for treating depression, only 11% of the subjects in PST continued to display depressive symptomology post treatment, while 60% of subjects in RT continued to show symptoms. As RT is more insight-oriented, while PST is more skills oriented, this study suggests that a skills-based approach might be a more effective approach with older populations. These results further imply that improvement in coping skills is linked to amelioration of depression in adults, also suggested in previous studies looking at depression and coping skills (Nezu, 1986; Nezu and Perri, 1989). The improvements seen following PST indicated a permanent change, even at the 3-month follow-up. Areán and Cook (2002) suggest that the *flexibility* of PST makes it especially amenable to the needs of older depressed patients. For example, Gallagher-Thompson and Steffen (1994) found that CBT's problem-solving approach was especially helpful to elderly depressed caregivers in coping with the challenge of cognitive decline in a family member. The ability of CBT to be more or less structured strengthens CBT's potential effectiveness and, more specifically, its potential effectiveness in populations with specific needs.

Two studies have compared CBT to psychotropic medication in elderly subjects with major depressive episodes. Beutler and colleagues (1987) tested the relative and combined effectiveness of alprazolam and group cognitive therapy. Subjects randomized to cognitive therapy had greater and more persistent treatment outcomes and were also less apt to end their treatment prematurely compared to the participants in other study conditions. In addition, alprazolam (a type of benzodiazepine) is not a recommended medication for depression.

Thompson et al. (2001) found that CBT and combined CBT and desipramine (DMI) were superior to DMI alone. A total of 102 depressed elderly patients were randomly assigned to groups of CBT alone, DMI alone, or combined CBT and DMI. Results demonstrated that there was little difference between CBT alone and CBT combined with DMI, but that both were significantly more effective than DMI alone. This evidence shows that the efficacy of CBT may surpass that of DMI, although combining the two interventions also results in significant alleviation of depression. No research has been published comparing CBT to selective serotonin reuptake inhibitor (SSRI) antidepressants. Although data are limited, it appears that elderly subjects who respond to CBT maintain those treatment gains for up to 1 year without relapsing (Arean and Cook, 2002).

Data on CBT's efficacy in late-life dysthymia and minor depression are limited. In a small study, Leung and Orrell (1993) reported a 50% remission rate for elderly subjects with minor depression or dysthymia. A large primary care study in both elderly and younger adult patients compared paroxetine, PST, and pill-placebo (Williams et al., 2000). The authors observed that PST was not as effective as paroxetine in decreasing depressive symptoms and improving functioning. The study has been criticized, however, for using a version of PST that had not been adapted for older adults. In this study, PST was much shorter in length and duration than usual. Typical sessions lasted 30 minutes, and patients had only four to six meetings. Moreover, the model was discussed only once, in the initial meeting, and was merely reviewed in follow-up sessions. The brevity and condensation of PST-PC may be detrimental in helping older depressed patients learn this complex set of skills. PST (and other psychosocial interventions) may need to be modified by slowing the pace, emphasizing repeated review, and relying on multiple modes of tracking adherence and practice of problem-solving shifts.

In summary, the published data support the efficacy of CBT for older outpatients with current major depressive episodes, but more data are needed with respect to CBT's efficacy in minor depression and dysthymia. The limitations of the literature include relatively small sample sizes and inadequate evaluation of CBT in the minority elderly, the frail elderly, and those with mild cognitive impairment (Arean and Cook, 2002).

## INTERPERSONAL PSYCHOTHERAPY

Like CBT, IPT was originally designed as a short-term psychotherapy (Weissman, 1999). The therapeutic focus in IPT is on four broad problems that are prevalent in the lives of older depressed patients: abnormal grief, role transitions, role or interpersonal disputes, and interpersonal deficits (often resulting in social isolation). Generally, IPT employs techniques of exploration, clarification, encouragement of affect, communication analysis, and encouragement to attempt alternative coping strategies. Interpersonal therapy is based in part on empirical data focusing on intimacy and social support (Brown et al., 1977), stressors inducing depression (Pearlin and Lieberman, 1979), and the role of marital disputes in depression (Weissman et al., 1974).

In bereavement-related major depression in late life, *acute treatment* over 16 weeks with a combination of nortriptyline and IPT was associated with the highest rate of remission (69%), followed by nortriptyline plus supportive medication clinic (56%), placebo plus supportive medication clinic (45%), or placebo with IPT (29%) (Reynolds et al., 1999b). Another recent study focusing on *maintenance treatment* addressed the longer-term outcome of recurrent major depression in later life (MTLD) (Reynolds et al., 1999a). This study of maintenance therapies in late-life depression built on the earlier work of Frank et al. (1991) in maintenance treatment of nongeriatric adults with recurrent major

depression. In the MTLD study, 180 elderly subjects with recurrent unipolar depression were treated with combined weekly IPT and a nortriptyline plasma concentration of 80–120 ng/ml. A remission rate of 78% (140/180) was attained. Of the 140 subjects who remitted, 124 maintained remission for 4 months and were eligible for random assignment to one of four maintenance treatments. Recurrence rates of major depressive episodes over 3 years were lowest in patients who received nortriptyline (80–120 ng/ml) plus monthly maintenance IPT (20%). Maintenance treatment with nortriptyline plus medication clinic (without IPT) was associated with a recurrence rate of 43%; monthly maintenance IPT plus placebo, 64%; and placebo plus medication clinic, 90%. Combined treatment with nortriptyline and IPT was superior to the other three maintenance treatments. Subjects aged 70 years and older had higher and more rapid rates of recurrence than those aged 60–69. Among subjects aged 70 and older, only the group that received combination therapy sustained recovery over 3 years (Reynolds et al., 1999a). These outcomes are shown in Figure 23.3.

The question of which patients can remain well on which treatments has considerable clinical importance. We observed that patients whose pretreatment scores on the 17-item Hamilton Depression Rating Scale were below 20 were able to remain well on monthly maintenance IPT (Taylor et al., 1999). Patients with pretreatment Hamilton scores of 20 or higher required the addition of nortriptyline (steady-state plasma levels of 80–120 ng/ml) to remain well. In further analyses, we learned that subjects whose depression remitted within 4–5 weeks were able to survive depression-free on monotherapy (IPT alone or nortriptyline alone), while those who took longer to remit required combination treatment (nortriptyline plus IPT) during maintenance

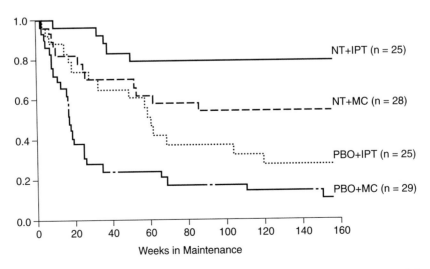

FIGURE 23.3 Survival analysis: recurrence rates of major depressive episodes. IPT, interpersonal therapy; MC, medication clinic; NT, nortriptyline; PBO, placebo. (From Reynolds et al., 1999a)

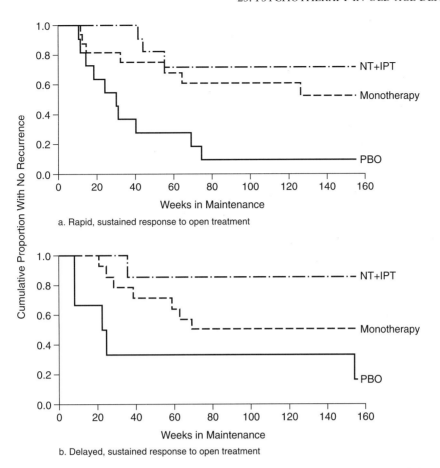

FIGURE 23.4 Early response trajectory correlate with maintenance response. IPT, interpersonal therapy; MC, medication clinic; NT, nortriptyline; PBO, placebo. (From Dew et al., 2001)

to remain depression-free for 3 years (Dew et al., 2001). These relationships are depicted in Figure 23.4.

The advantage of continuing combined treatment during maintenance was not only in the greater prolongation of recovery (relative to either monotherapy), but also in the better maintenance of treatment-attributable gains in social adjustment. Subjects receiving combined treatment with nortriptyline and IPT continued to demonstrate better scores on the Social Adjustment Scale than those on maintenance drug alone or IPT alone (Lenze et al., 2002), especially in the continuing reduction of interpersonal or role conflict. Our previous report had shown the advantages of combining nortriptyline and IPT in prolonging recovery in depressed elderly patients (Reynolds et al., 1999a, 1999b). Our subsequent study of social adjustment during maintenance treatment (Lenze et al., 2002) demonstrated that combination treatment enhanced not only the length but also the quality, of the recovery. This finding was comparable to that of a previous study in younger adults in maintenance treatment for depression (Weissman et al., 1974), which reported significant improvement in social adjustment attributable to combined IPT and maintenance medication. In the

elderly, combined treatment provided better *retention* of the gains that had already been made during acute and continuation treatment, especially in the domain of interpersonal conflict.

As noted earlier, the four most common foci of IPT in acute treatment were role transitions, interpersonal disputes, interpersonal deficits, and abnormal grief. Indeed, the majority of subjects (57%) had more than one IPT focus (Wolfson et al., 1997). Types of role transitions included changes such as retirement, relocating from one's home, and having the last adult child leave home. Role disputes, generally involving a spouse or another family member, often emerged as a secondary focus after role transitions were resolved.

These observations suggest the pathways, such as reduction in interpersonal conflict, whereby IPT may work with medication to bring about and to maintain better social functioning in older persons with depression. Further, in our studies of bereavement-related major depression in later life (Reynolds et al., 1999c), we concluded that while nortriptyline was superior to placebo in achieving remission of depressive episodes, it was the *combination* of medication and IPT that was associated with the highest rate of treatment comple-

- Further reduce clinical distance between the clinician and patient.

- Allow more reminiscence.

- In the face of long-standing marital disputes, emphasize reevaluation of expectations rather than changes in the relationship.

FIGURE 23.5 Modifications of interpersonal therapy treatment of the elderly.

tion. This result supports the use of pharmacological treatment of major depressive episodes in the wake of a serious life stressor such as bereavement, but also suggests that treatment is more likely to succeed when combined with a psychosocial component such as IPT. Case vignettes of IPT interventions are illustrated in Figures 23.5 to 23.11.

As we noted above, patients with milder major depression who remitted within 6 weeks were protected against a recurrence of major depression with monthly maintenance IPT. Self-reported normalization of sleep quality also correlated with maintenance of recovery with monthly maintenance IPT (Reynolds et al., 1997), as did lower levels of residual anxiety symptoms following acute phase treatment (Lenze et al., 2003).

We also observed that the use of IPT supported good compliance with antidepressant pharmacotherapy, and that encouragement and extensive education (directed at both patients and family members) were essential to subject retention and treatment adherence (Miller et al., 1999; Sherrill et al., 1997).

We are currently pursuing new research using IPT and paroxetine for elderly depressed patients with cognitive impairment (Miller et al., 2001). We have observed that IPT therapists' ratings of subjects' ability to engage, focus, and recall declined progressively with increasing cognitive impairment. Nonetheless, subjects with cognitive impairment remitted no less frequently with combined treatment involving paroxetine (mean dose, 22.4 mg/day) and weekly IPT. We have found the use of informants to be critical in permittng accurate

**Interventions**

- Point out the couple's indirect style of communication.

- Help the patient to see her husband's peace offerings as a form of apology.

- Reinforce the patient's recognition of the limited options available to her.

- Point out the advantage of reducing her threats of divorce.

FIGURE 23.7 Example of role disputes: "What am I going to do? Go cry on my mother's grave?"

assessment of status and change, especially for patients with a score of 120 or lower on the Mattis Dementia Rating Scale. We have also regularly included input from accompanying family members or caregivers in order to carry out IPT with cognitively impaired subjects. Thus IPT therapists use caregiver reports to review events between sessions and to reinforce strategies for interpersonal changes aimed at reducing depressive symptoms.

## DIALECTICAL BEHAVIOR THERAPY

### Psychotherapeutic Management of Depression in Personality Disordered Older Adult Patients

Although some researchers have suggested a lower prevalence of personality disorders in the elderly compared to younger adults (Kroessler, 1990), others argue that that rate of personality disorder among the elderly is essentially equivalent to that in younger age groups (Abrams and Horowitz, 1999; Fogel and Westlake, 1990; Morse and Lynch, 2000). In addition, DSM-IV states that some types of personality disorders (notably, antisocial and borderline personality disorders) tend to become less evident or to remit with age, whereas this appears to be less true for some other types (e.g., obsessive-compulsive and schizotypal personality disorders) (American Psychiatric Association, 1994). Lynch and Aspnes (2001) have argued that this discrepancy may be due to age-related improvements in emotion/impulse regulation skills and/or to the degree

**Description**

Sixty-two-year-old woman married to a rigid, authoritarian, egotistical man incapable of admitting his mistakes or of apologizing following their frequent and violent arguments, after which the patient frequently threatened divorce.

Within a day of these arguments, the husband invariably came home with a bag of cookies or box of candy.

FIGURE 23.6 Example of role disputes: "What am I going to do? Go cry on my mother's grave?"

**Description**

Seventy-two-year-old man, widowed for 3 years, incapable of using or discarding anything that had belonged to his wife or of cultivating any interpersonal relationships despite intense loneliness.

FIGURE 23.8 Example of unresolved grief: "No one can ever replace my angel, Rosa:"

======= Interventions =======

• Help the patient to achieve a more realistic view of his wife and their relationship.

• Help the patient to see that his wife would not have wanted him to remain alone and unhappy.

• Underscore the naturalness of his interpersonal and sexual needs.

FIGURE 23.9 Example of unresolved grief: "No one can ever replace my angel, Rosa:"

======= Interventions =======

• Encourage the patient to dedicate part of each day to activities pleasing just to her.

• Help the patient to accept and make use of other family members' interest in caring for her mother.

• Point out that the quality of her interactions with her mother improved when she was *less* available.

FIGURE 23.11 Example of a role transition: "It's all right to do something just for myself?"

to which an individual encounters corrective interpersonal feedback. Thus, Cluster B, which is characterized by emotional displays, benefits from both improved regulation and feedback from the community that maladaptive behavior (e.g., suicidal, histrionic, antisocial) is inappropriate. In contrast, higher rates for Cluster A (e.g., paranoid, schizoid) and Cluster C (e.g., avoidant, obsessive-compulsive) may reflect chronic attempts to avoid discrepant feedback from others. For example, dependent individuals may seek out the company of those who perceive them as they see themselves: as fragile and in need of guidance. Paranoid individuals may severely limit social contact, effectively reducing opportunities to receive feedback that their pervasive distrust and suspiciousness of others is unwarranted. Thus, rigid maladaptive coping patterns are maintained and/or worsen over time.

With regard to treatment, there is growing empirical evidence to suggest that elderly depressed patients with a co-morbid personality disorder are generally less responsive to treatment, including antidepressant medications and psychotherapy (Abrams and Horowitz, 1996; Pilkonis and Frank, 1988; Vine and Steingart, 1994; also see Gradman et al., 1999, for a review). However, with the exception of case studies, no published outcome study has specifically focused on treating late-life personality disorders. Gradman et al. (1999) reviewed seven older adult treatment studies in which personality disorder was examined. However, only one study included a randomized control (Thompson et al., 1988). Methodological differences across studies also limited the ability to reach definitive con-

clusions. Treatments were often not clearly defined, standardized instruments varied across studies or were not used at all, and measures of treatment adherence were not obtained.

Interventions that specifically target vulnerability factors, functional status, cognitive dysregulation, and noncompliance may have greater utility for addressing late-life personality disorders (Morse and Lynch, 2000). De Leo et al. (1999), in their review of the literature on personality disorders in late life, suggested that a more suitable therapy for personality disorders in the elderly may be DBT. This form of therapy has the advantage of proven efficacy for treatment of personality disorders in nongeriatric adults (Linehan, 1993; Linehan and Kehrer, 1993; Linehan et al., 1991, 1993, 1994).

One of the authors (Lynch) has modified standard DBT for use with depressed elderly individuals with co-morbid personality disorder. The goal of treatment is to teach patients to relax extreme stances in favor of more flexible and adaptive responses. We have published a pilot randomized clinical trial in which 34 depressed individuals aged 60 and older were randomly assigned to antidepressant medication (MED) plus clinical management, either alone or with the addition of a DBT skills training group plus weekly half-hour scheduled telephone coaching sessions (Lynch et al., 2003). At the 6-month follow-up, 73% of MED+DBT patients and 38% of MED patients were asymptomatic, a significant difference. The MED + DBT patients also improved significantly more than the MED patients due to excessive concern to please others. Only patients receiving DBT showed significant changes from pre- to post-treatment on hopelessness and on several variables proposed to create vulnerability to depression. A second randomized trial using DBT and MED, but now focused on treatment-resistant elderly depressed personality disordered patients, is currently being conducted by Lynch and colleagues at Duke University.

For depressed older adults with co-morbid personality disorders, Lynch (2000) articulated four dialectical tensions, adapted in part from dilemmas defined by Linehan (1993). When rigidly adhered to, these dialectical tensions (polarized positions) are hypothesized

======= Description =======

Sixty-seven-year-old woman who became depressed after placing her mother in a nursing home (something she had vowed she would never do). Prior to the mother's placement, the patient cared for her mother day and night and dedicated her life to trying to meet her mother's endless demands.

FIGURE 23.10 Example of a role transition: "It's all right to do something just for myself?"

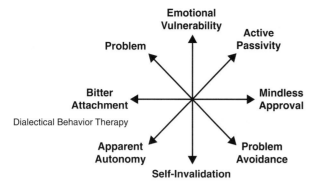

FIGURE 23.12 Dialectical dilemmas for the elderly: dialectical behavior therapy.

to maintain depression and/or enhance the likelihood of depressive relapse (Fig. 23.12).

The first dilemma relates to *acceptance of reality* and whether fighting reality or nonresistance has a history of reinforcement during times of stress. In this dilemma, depression and/or relapse may be more likely when an older adult refuses to accept loss despite evidence that a desired outcome may be unlikely to be achieved through effort (*bitter attachment*). By contrast, consistently acquiescing, not resisting, and giving up despite evidence that a desired outcome may be obtainable (*Mindless Approval*), represents the other pole of the dilemma.

The second dilemma relates to styles of *changing reality or solving problems*. Over time, individuals are hypothesized to develop a characteristic style of either attending to or avoiding problems. Rigid attempts to solve all problems despite evidence that there may not be a solution (*problem brooding*) may increase vulnerability to unwanted emotions and depression. The opposite stance, pervasive experiential avoidance and/or unwillingness to problem solve (*problem avoidant*), may paradoxically exacerbate distress, reduce the chance that effective change may take place, and increase the likelihood that inhibited or traumatic grief will occur. As with the first dilemma, each style can prove adaptive when less rigidly followed. For example, worry can help orient a person to solving important problems and activate resources, while avoidance can help a person attend to other tasks that require more immediate attention.

The third dilemma involves managing *interpersonal relationships* during times of stress. Some persons may withdraw from potential sources of social support when negative life events occur and may say that they are not depressed even though they are (*apparent autonomy*). Others may demand nurturance and care from others when under stress (*active passivity*). Clinically, we have observed *apparently autonomous* older adults become dysregulated when others try to assist them. The *actively passive* older adult may focus on be-

ing cared for, demand support, look to others for solutions, and/or become dysregulated when nurturance is not provided.

The fourth dilemma relates to *self-validation*. One extreme consists of wallowing in self-pity and self-validating that life is sad/distressing (*emotion vulnerability*). Although wallowing in emotion may have a soothing component, it may also result in stimuli associated with loss becoming more salient and consequently exacerbating depression. The other extreme consists of displaying no self-pity, engaging in self-hate, and/or rejecting personal experience (*self-invalidation*). A self-deprecating attributional style has been empirically linked to depressive experience, and self-invalidation may block functional behavior (Linehan, 1993) and/or elicit repeated caregiving responses from social supports who eventually "burn out" (Coyne, 1976).

## PSYCHOTHERAPEUTIC MANAGEMENT OF SUICIDAL OLDER ADULT PATIENTS

In a recent review of the assessment and prevention of suicidal behavior in the elderly (Szanto et al., 2002), we recommended that the following questions always be asked of elderly depressed patients:

1. Have you been feeling so sad lately that you were thinking about death or dying?
2. Have you thought that life is not worth living?
3. Have you been thinking about harming yourself?

In addition, we recommended asking patients whether they have thought about a specific method of suicide and whether they have access to lethal means, including firearms. Although most suicide attempts in the United States involve overdosage of medication, the majority of completed suicides are via firearms, especially in elderly men. The assessment of suicide risk in the elderly should also include the assessment of other risk factors such as previous suicide attempts, any diagnosis involving psychosis or mania, severity of depression and hopelessness, substance abuse, poor impulse control, treatment noncompliance, lack of social support, lack of reasons for living, and recent stressful life events.

With respect to intervention to ensure the patient's safety, we recommend hospitalization if a patient reports suicidal ideation with a plan and lethal means are available. Otherwise, if the patient endorses suicidal ideation but does not have a plan, is not psychotic, has good judgment, and has no history of a high-lethality attempt, then the patient's social support network needs to be activated. Brown et al. (2001) have recently published a comprehensive description of high-risk management strategies for elderly suicidal patients.

The use of *no-suicide* contracts, in which patients

agree that they will inform a relative, friend, or health-care provider of their suicidal intent and not act on it, although widely recommended, is *not* supported by any evidence that these contracts are helpful (Szanto et al., 2002). In fact, they reduce the clinician's vigilance without materially affecting the patient's suicidal intent.

The U.S. National Institutes of Health Consensus Conference on Late Life Depression (1991) and the subsequent Depression and Bipolar Support Alliance's Consensus Conference on Unmet Needs in the Diagnosis and Treatment of Mood Disorders in Later Life (2003) concluded that psychotherapies, including IPT, CBT, and PST, are as effective as antidepressant drugs in the acute treatment of elderly outpatients with mild to moderate nonpsychotic major depression. As noted earlier in this chapter, IPT is a brief, focused psychotherapy that addresses four factors that are often part of the interpersonal context of older suicidal patients: abnormal grief, role transitions, role disputes, and interpersonal deficits leading to social isolation. When combined with nortriptyline, IPT constitutes a highly effective acute, continuation, and maintenance treatment for geriatric major depression (Reynolds et al., 1999a), including patients with suicidal ideation (Szanto et al., 2001).

Cognitive-behavioral therapy combined with DMI was found to be more effective than DMI alone in the acute treatment of geriatric depression (Thompson et al., 1991). In addition, CBT has been used successfully to treat suicidal persons, including the elderly (Beck and Weishaar, 1990; Beck et al., 1979). As we have recently indicated (Szanto et al., 2002), CBT challenges the cognitive constriction that narrows and devalues problem-solving options. It identifies helplessness and hopelessness in depressed suicidal persons and assists them in using problem-solving methods. Lynch and colleagues (2001), using DBT with depressed older adults, reported significant improvements in hopelessness from pre- to posttreatment, and these gains were maintained at follow-up. Finding interventions that impact hopeless thinking will likely prove particularly useful for reducing the risk of suicide among older adults.

Treatments targeting improvements in hopeless thinking may operate by helping the patient form a more precise description of the problem, separate the problem from the depressed mood, and consider alternative solutions. When this happens, suicide no longer represents the only option. For elderly men especially, it may be unacceptable to express dependency needs; moreover, the loss of work, health, and mental capacity may trigger a narcissistic crisis, necessitating the use of both IPT and CBT techniques and the activation and involvement of the patient's support system.

Currently, one suicide prevention study is underway to assess the effectiveness of improved treatment of depression in elderly patients in primary care, including the use of psychosocial interventions (specifically psychoeducation of patients and their families and the use of IPT). The U.S. National Institute of Mental Health–sponsored PROSPECT study (Prevention of Suicide in Primary Care Elderly: Collaborative Trial) specifically targets a geriatric population (Mulsant et al., 2001). The goal of PROSPECT is to determine if placement of a depression care manager in primary care practices will reduce the rates of depression, hopelessness, and suicidal ideation in primary care elderly patients with major depression, treatable minor depression, or dysthymia. The PROSPECT study randomly assigns patients to either the intervention arm or a treatment-as-usual arm. A total of 20 practices and over 600 patients have been recruited. Patients aged 75 and older have been oversampled because the highest suicide rate occurs in older males. Preliminary analysis at the Pittsburgh site of PROSPECT indicated a 75% depression remission rate in the intervention-arm practices versus 25% in the treatment-as-usual control practices (Mulsant, 2001). Remission rates in primary care elderly equal those of elderly treated in the mental health specialty sector but take longer to achieve (Thomas et al., 2002).

## OTHER PSYCHOSOCIAL INTERVENTIONS

A recent survey of academic geriatric psychiatrists in the United States, designed to formulate expert consensus guidelines for the pharmacotherapy of late-life depression (Alexopoulos et al., 2001), reported that more than 75% of the experts surveyed rated CBT, IPT, PST, and supportive psychotherapy as first-line treatment. There was no consensus on the role of psychodynamic psychotherapy in treating depression in the elderly, with only 26% of respondents rating this as first-line treatment. The experts gave strong support to psychosocial interventions such as psychoeducation, family counseling, visiting nurse services, bereavement groups, and programs at senior citizens centers. The choice of such interventions depends upon the patient's needs and the availability of such services in the community. Such psychosocial interventions were not regarded by survey respondents as specific treatments in their own right but as adjuncts to other treatments and components of a humane treatment plan.

We have used a family group workshop for educating our elderly depressed patients and their caregivers and as a measure of improving the process of informal consent. The workshop focuses on the causes and clinical presentation of depression in old age, the nature of treatment, the outcomes of treatment and the importance of treatment adherence, steps caregivers can take to protect their own health and well-being, and recognizing warning signs of suicide. Participation by patients and family members in this workshop has been associated with higher levels of subject retention and treatment compliance than were observed in nonparticipants (Sherrill et al., 1997).

## SUMMARY AND CONCLUSIONS

Severe life events and ongoing difficulties, as well as the depletion of psychosocial resources, form a major part of the substrate of depression in later life, whether first episode or recurrent, and contribute to suicidality in late-life depression. We and other clinician investigators have found that it is clinically important and scientifically well justified to address these issues via the use of psychosocial treatments, such as CBT, IPT, DBT, and PST, as well as adjunctive psychosocial interventions such as educational workshops. These methods, especially in combination with pharmacotherapy, bring about high remission rates and sustain recovery, often in association with better maintenance of social adjustment and improved quality of life.

Future research should address three specific issues: (1) the value of adding psychosocial treatment to first-line pharmacotherapy in patients who do not show evidence of an optimal response and recovery (often 40%–50% of elderly patients in our experience); (2) the value and efficacy of psychotherapeutic approaches to suicidality in late-life depression; and (3) the use of psychosocial interventions as a form of primary or secondary prevention in elderly patients who respond with sadness, loneliness, or insomnia to the vicissitudes of later life and who are therefore at risk for developing clinically significant depression.

ACKNOWLEDGMENTS
This work was supported in part by Grants P30 MH52247, R37 MH43832, R01 MH37869, R01 MH59318, 1 R29 MH51956, 1 U0 AG13289, P30 AG5272, UD2 SM52643, K23 MH01614, and P30 MH30915.

REFERENCES

Abrams, R.C., and Horowitz, S.V. (1996) Personality disorders after age 50: A meta-analysis. *J Person Disord* 10:271–281.

Abrams, R.C., and Horowitz, S.V. (1999). Personality disorders after age 50: A meta-analytic review of the liturature. In: Rosowsky, E., Abrams, R.C., and Zweig, R.A., eds. *Personality Disorders in Older Adults: Emerginng Issues in Diagnosis and Treatment*. Mahwah, NJ: Erlbaum, pp. 55–68.

Alexopoulos, G.S., Katz, I., Reynolds, C.F., Carpenter, D., Docherty, J.P., and Ross, R.W. (2001) Pharmacotherapy of depressive disorders in older patients: A summary of the expert consensus guidelines. *J Psychiatr Pract* 7(6):361–376.

American Psychiatric Association. (1994) *Diagnostic and Statistical Manual of Mental Disorders*, 4th ed. Washington, DC: American Psychiatric Press.

Arean, P.A., and Cook, B.L. (2002). Psychotherapy and combined psychotherapy/pharmacotherapy for late-life depression. *Biol Psychiatry* 52(3):293–303.

Arean, P.A., Perri, M.G., Nezu, A.M., Schein, R.L., Christopher, F., and Joseph, T.X. (1993) Comparative effectiveness of social problem-solving therapy and reminiscence therapy as treatments for depression in older adults. *J Consult Clin Psychol* 61(6):1003–1010.

Beck, A.T. (1976) *Cognitive Therapy and the Emotional Disorders*. New York: International Universities Press.

Beck, A.T., Kovacs, M., and Weissman, A. (1979) Assessment of suicidal intention: The Scale for Suicide Ideation. *J Consult Clin Psychol* 47:343–352.

Beck, A.T., and Weishaar, M.E. (1990) Suicide risk assessment and prediction. *Crisis* 11:22–30.

Beutler, L.E., Scogin, F., Kirkish, P., Schretlen, D., Corbishley, A., Hamblin, D., Meredith, K., Potter, R., Bamford, C.R., and Levenson, A.I. (1987) Group cognitive therapy and alprazolam in the treatment of depression in older adults. *J Consult Clin Psychol* 55(4):550–556.

Brown, G.K., Bruce, M.L., and Pearson, J.L. (2001) High-risk management guidelines for elderly suicidal patients in primary care settings. *Int J Geriatr Psychiatry* 16(6):593–601.

Brown, G.W., Harris, T., and Copeland, J.R. (1977) Depression and loss. *Br J Psychiatry* 130:1–18.

Bruce, M.L. (2002) Psychosocial risk factors for depression in later life. *Biol Psychiatry* 52:175–180.

Campbell, J.M. (1992) Treating depression in well older adults: Use of diaries in cognitive therapy. *Issues Ment Health Nurs* 13(1):19–29.

Conwell, Y., Duberstein, P.R., and Caine, E.D. (2002) Risk factors for suicide in later life. *Biol Psychiatry* 52:193–204.

Coyne, J.C. (1976) Depression and the response of others. *J Abnorm Psychol* 85(2):186–193.

Charney, D., Reynolds, C.F., Lewis, L., Lebowitz, B.D., Sunderland, T., Alexopoulos, G.S., Blazer, D.G., Katz, I.R., Meyers, B.S., Arean, P.A., Borson, S., Brown, C., Bruce, M.L., Callahan, C.M., Charlson, M.E., Conwell, Y., Cuthbert, B.N., Devanand, D.P., Gibson, J.M., Gottlieb, G.L., Krishnan, K.R., Laden, S.K., Lyketsos, C.G., Mulsant, B.H., Niederehe, G., Olin, J.T., Oslin, D.W., Pearson, J., Persky, T., Pollock, B.G., Raetzman, S., Reynolds, M., Salzman, C., Schulz, R., Schwenk, T.L., Scolnick, E., Unüntzer, J., Weissman, M.M., and Young, R.C. (2003) Depression and Bipolar Support Alliance Consensus Conference Report on Unmet Needs in the Diagnosis and Treatment of Mood Disorders in Late Life. *Arch Gen Psychiatry* 60:664–672.

De Leo, D., Scocco, P., and Meneghel, G. (1999) Pharmacological and psychotherapeutic treatment of personality disorders in the elderly. *Int Psychogeriatr* 11(2):191–206.

Dew, M.A., Reynolds, C.F., Mulsant, B.H., Frank, E., Houck, P.R., Mazumdar, S., Begley, A.E., and Kupfer, D.J. (2001) Initial recovery patterns may predict which maintenance therapies for depression will keep older adults well. *J Affect Disord* 65:155–166.

Fogel, B.S., and Westlake, R. (1990) Personality disorder diagnoses and age in inpatients with major depression. *J Clin Psychiatry* 51(6):232–235.

Frank, E., Kupfer, D.J., Wagner, E.F., McEachran, A.B., and Cornes, C. (1991) Efficacy of interpersonal psychotherapy as a maintenance treatment of recurrent depression: Contributing factors. *Arch Gen Psychiatry* 48:1053–1059.

Gallagher-Thompson, D., and Steffen, A.M. (1994) Comparative effects of cognitive-behavioral and brief psychodynamic psychotherapies for depressed family caregivers. *J Consult Clin Psychol* 62(3):543–549.

Gradman, T.J., Thompson, L.W., and Gallagher-Thompson, D. (1999) Personality disorders and treatment outcome. In: Rosowsky, E., Abrams, R.C., and Zweig, R.A., eds. *Personality Disorders in Older Adults: Emerging Issues in Diagnosis and Treatment*. Mahwah, NJ: Erlbaum, pp. 69–94.

Jarvik, L.F., Mintz, J., Steuer, J., and Gerner, R. (1982) Treating geriatric depression: A 26-week interim analysis. *J Am Geriatr Soc*
30(11):713–717.

Kroessler, D. (1990) Personality disorder in the elderly. *Hosp Commun Psychiatry* 41(12):1325–1329.

Lenze, E.J., Dew, M.A., Mazumdar, S., Begley, A.E., Cleon, C., Miller,
M.D., Imber, S.D., Frank, E., Kupfer, D.J., and Reynolds, C.F.
(2002) Combined pharmacotherapy and psychotherapy in maintenance treatment for late-life depression: Effects on social adjustment, quality of life and perception of health. *Am J Psychiatry* 159(3):466–468.

Lenze, E.J., Mulsant, B.H., Dew, M.A., Shear, M.K., Houck, P., Pollock, B.G., and Reynolds, C.F. (2003) Good treatment outcomes
in late-life depression with co-morbid anxiety. *J Affect Disord*
77:247–254.

Leung, S.N., and Orrell, M.W. (1993) A brief cognitive behavioural
therapy group for the elderly: Who benefits? *Int J Geriatr Psychiatry* 8(7):593–598.

Linehan, M.M. (1993) *Cognitive-Behavioral Treatment of Borderlin
Personality Disorder*. New York: Guilford Press.

Linehan, M.M., Armstrong, H.E., Suarez, A., Allmon, D., and Heard,
H.L. (1991) Cognitive-behavioral treatment of chronically para-
suicidal borderline patients [see comments]. *Arch Gen Psychiatry* 48(12):1060–1064.

Linehan, M.M., Heard, H.L., and Armstrong, H.E. (1993) Naturalistic follow-up of a behavioral treatment for chronically parasui-
cidal borderline patients. *Arch Gen Psychiatry* 50(12):971–974.

Linehan, M.M., and Kehrer, C.A. (1993) Borderline personality disorder. In: Barlow, D.H., ed. *Clinical Handbook of Psychological
Disorders*. New York: Guilford Press, pp. 396–441.

Linehan, M.M., Tutek, D.A., Heard, H.L., and Armstrong, H.E.
(1994) Interpersonal outcome of cognitive behavioral treatment
for chronically suicidal borderline patients. *Am J Psychiatry*
151(12):1771–1776.

Lynch, T.R. (2000) Treatment of elderly depression with personality
disorder co-morbidity using dialectical behavior therapy. *Cogn
Behav Pract* 7:468–477.

Lynch, T.R., and Aspnes, A. (2001) Personality disorders in older
adults: Diagnostic and theoretic issues. *Clin Gerontol* 9(11):64–68.

Lynch, T.R., Morse, J.Q., Mendelson, T., and Robins, C.J. (2003)
*Dialectical Behavior Therapy for Depressed Elderly. Am J Geri-
atr Psychiatry* 11:1–13.

Miller, M.D., Cornes, C., Frank, E., Ehrenpreis, L., Silberman, R.,
Schlernitzauer, M.A., Tracey, B., Richards, V., Wolfson, L., Zalt-
man, J., Bensasi, S., and Reynolds, C.F. (2001) Interpersonal psychotherapy for late-life depression: Past, present and future. *J Psychother Pract Res* 10(4):231–238.

Miller, M.D., Frank, E., and Reynolds, C.F. (1999) The art of clinical
management in pharmacologic trials with depressed elderly patients—Lessons from the Pittsburgh study of maintenance therapies in late-life depression. *Am J Geriatr Psychiatry* 7(3):228–234.

Morse, J.Q., and Lynch, T.R. (2000) Personality disorders in late life.
*Curr Psychiatry Rep* 2(1):24–31.

Mulsant, B.H. (2001) Outcomes of depression treatment in the elderly in primary care and in specialty care (ACNP Study Group).
In: Anonymous. Kona, Hawaii: American College of Neuropsychopharmacology.

Mulsant, B.H., Alexopoulos, G.S., Reynolds, C.F., Katz, I., Abrams,
R.C., Oslin, D.W., and Schulberg, H.C. (2001) Pharmacologic
treatment of depression in elderly primary care patients: The
PROSPECT algorithm. *Int J Geriatr Psychiatry* 16(6):585–592.

Mynors-Wallis, L. (1996) Problem-solving treatment: Evidence for
effectiveness and feasibility in primary care. *Int J Psychiatry Med*
26(3):249–262.

Nezu, A.M. (1986) Cognitive appraisal of problem solving effectiveness: Relation to depression and depressive symptoms. *J Clin
Psychol* 42(1):42–48.

Nezu, A.M., and Perri, M.G. (1989) Social problem-solving therapy
for unipolar depression: An initial dismantling investigation. *J
Consult Clin Psychol* 57(3):408–413.

Pearlin, L.I., and Lieberman, M.A. (1979) Social sources of emotional distress. In: Simmons, R., ed. *Research in Community and
Mental Health*. Greenwich, CT: JAI Press, pp. 217–248.

Pilkonis, P.A., and Frank, E. (1988) Personality pathology in recurrent depression: Nature, prevalence, and relationship to treatment
response. *Am J Psychiatry* 145(4):435–441.

Reynolds, C.F., Frank, E., Dew, M.A., Houck, P.R., Miller, M.D.,
Mazumdar, S., Perel, J.M., and Kupfer, D.J. (1999a) Treatment
in 70+ year olds with major depression: Excellent short-term but
brittle long-term response. *Am J Geriatr Psychiatry* 7(1):64–69.

Reynolds, C.F., Frank, E., Houck, P.R., Mazumdar, S., Dew, M.A.,
Cornes, C., Buysse, D.J., and Kupfer, D.J. (1997) Which elderly
patients with remitted depression remain well with continued interpersonal psychotherapy after discontinuation of antidepressant
medication? *Am J Psychiatry* 154(7):958–962.

Reynolds, C.F., Frank, E., Perel, J.M., Imber, S.D., Cornes, C., Miller,
M.D., Mazumdar, S., Houck, P.R., Dew, M.A., Stack, J.A., Pollock, B.G., and Kupfer, D.J. (1999b) Nortriptyline and interpersonal psychotherapy as maintenance therapies for recurrent major depression: A randomized controlled trial in patients older
than 59 years. *JAMA* 281(1):39–45.

Reynolds, C.F., Miller, M.D., Pasternak, R.E., Frank, E., Perel, J.M.,
Cornes, C., Houck, P.R., Mazumdar, S., Dew, M.A., and Kupfer,
D.J. (1999c) Treatment of bereavement-related major depressive
episodes in later life: A controlled study of acute and continuation treatment with nortriptyline and interpersonal psychotherapy. *Am J Psychiatry* 156(2):202–208.

Rokke, P.D., Tomhave, J.A., and Jocic, Z. (2000) Self-management
therapy and educational group therapy for depressed elders. *Cogn
Ther Res* 24(1):99–119.

Schulz, R., Martire, L.M., Beach, S., and Scheier, M.F. (2001) Depression and mortality in the elderly. *Curr Dir Psychol Sci* 9:204–208.

Sherrill, J.T., Frank, E., Geary, M., Stack, J.A., and Reynolds, C.F.
(1997) An extension of psychoeducational family workshops to
elderly patients with recurrent major depression: Description and
evaluation. *Psychiatr Serv* 48(1):76–81.

Szanto, K., Gildengers, A.G., Mulsant, B.H., Brown, G., Alexopoulos,
G., and Reynolds, C.F. (2002) Identification of suicidal ideation and
prevention of suicidal behavior in the elderly. *Drugs Aging* 19:11–24.

Szanto, K., Mulsant, B.H., Houck, P.R., Miller, M.D., Mazum
dar, S., and Reynolds, C.F. (2001) Treatment outcome in suicidal
versus non-suicidal elderly. *Am J Geriatr Psychiatry* 9(3):261–268.

Taylor, M.P., Reynolds, C.F., Frank, E., Cornes, C., Miller, M.D.,
Stack, J.A., Begley, A.E., Mazumdar, S., Dew, M.A., and Kupfer,
D.J. (1999) Which elderly depressed patients remain well on
maintenance interpersonal psychotherapy alone? A report from
the Pittsburgh study of maintenance therapies in late-life depression. *Depress Anxiety* 10(2):55–60.

Thomas, L., Mulsant, B.H., Solano, F.X., Black, A.M., Bensasi, S.,
Flynn, T., Harman, J.S., Rollman, B.L., Post, E.P., Pollock, B.G.,
and Reynolds, C.F. (2002) Speed and rate of late-life depression
remission in primary and specialty care. *Am J Geriatr Psychiatry*
10:583–591.

Thompson, L.W., Coon, D.W., Gallagher-Thompson, D., Sommer, B.R.,
and Koin, D. (2001) Comparison of desipramine and cognitive/
behavioral therapy in the treatment of elderly outpatients with mild-
to-moderate depression. *Am J Geriatr Psychiatry* 9(3):225–240.

Thompson, L.W., Gallagher, D.E., and Breckenridge, J.S. (1987)
Comparative effectiveness of psychotherapies for depressed elders. *J Consult Clin Psychol* 55:385–390.

Thompson, L.W., Gallagher, D., and Czirr, R. (1988) Personality disorder and outcome in the treatment of late-life depression. *J Geriatr Psychiatry* 21:133–153.

Thompson, L.W., Gallagher-Thompson, D., Hanser, S.B., and et al.

(1991) Treatment of late-life depression with cognitive. Presented at the 99th annual convention of the American Psychological Association, San Francisco, August.

Vine, R.G., and Steingart, A.B. (1994) Personality disorder in the elderly depressed. *Can J Psychiatry* 39(7):392–398.

Viney, L.L., Benjamin, Y.N., and Preston, C.A. (1989) An evaluation of personal construct therapy for the elderly. *Br J Med Psychol* 62(pt 1):35–41.

Weissman, M.M. (1999) *Comprehensive Guide to Interpersonal Psychotherapy*. New York: Basic Books.

Weissman, M.M., Klerman, G.L., Paykel, E.S., Prusoff, B., and Hanson, B. (1974) Treatment effects on the social adjustment of depressed patients. *Arch Gen Psychiatry* 30(6):771–778.

Williams, J.W., Barrett, J., Oxman, T., Frank, E., Katon, W., Sullivan, M., Cornell, J., and Sengupta, A. (2000) Treatment of dysthymia and minor depression in primary care: A randomized controlled trial in older adults. *JAMA* 284(12):1519–1526.

Wolfson, L.K., Miller, M., Houck, P.R., Ehrenpreis, L., Stack, J.A., Frank, E., Cornes, C., Mazumdar, S., Kupfer, D.J., and Reynolds, C.F. (1997) Foci of interpersonal psychotherapy (IPT) in depressed elders: Clinical and outcome correlates in a combined IPT/nortriptyline protocol. *Psychother Res* 7(1):45–55.

# 24 | Treatment of depression in residential settings

IRA R. KATZ AND JOEL STREIM

## THE CONTEXT: NURSING HOMES IN AMERICA

Approximately 4% of older Americans, 1.6 million individuals, live in nursing homes. This figure, however, underestimates the number of those who use nursing home services (Katz et al., 2000; Strahan, 1997). In 1995, 1.7 million people were admitted to nursing homes; two-thirds to three-fourths of them were admitted for rehabilitation or convalescent care, and most of them were discharged after a matter of weeks.

It has been estimated that the number of nursing home residents will double by 2020 and triple by 2040, and that more than 40% of the U.S. population will require nursing home care at some point in their lives (Rhoades and Krauss, 1999). With the aging of the population and the increase in the number of elderly patients with chronic diseases and disability, long-term care has become an increasingly important issue in political and economic as well as clinical terms. It is also an area that is in flux. Over the 10 years from 1985 to 1995, the number of nursing home beds increased by 9% (National Center for Health Statistics, 1987). However, the number of homes decreased and their occupancy rate declined. Thus, in spite of an 18% increase in the population over age 65, the number of nursing home residents increased by only 4%. As a result of these changes, the ratio of nursing home residents to the general population over age 65 decreased from approximately 46.2 per 1000 in 1985 to 41.3 in 1995. These changes in the use of nursing homes have been accompanied by changes in the nature of the population served. In recent years, the resident population has become older, sicker, and more disabled.

The decline in the proportion of older people living in nursing homes probably reflects, in part, the significant growth of other forms of long-term care, including home health care, hospice care, and various forms of assisted living. Other recent changes in long-term care have occurred within nursing homes in response to marketplace incentives as well as clinical needs. Nursing homes now provide many of the rehabilitation services historically provided on inpatient units, step-down care units for medical/surgical or poststroke patients, and special care units (SCUs) for patients with Alzheimer's disease.

Nursing home care represents almost 10% of the nation's total health-care costs, but the burden of payment is markedly different from that of other aspects of health care, with approximately 50% of the costs borne directly by residents and their families and most of the remainder shared equally by the federal and state governments through Medicaid programs. Medicare coverage is limited to brief periods of care, usually after acute hospitalization. In spite of recent trends toward a leveling of growth, the number of nursing homes and nursing home beds has increased dramatically since the mid-1960s, when Medicaid programs were first developed. In parallel, there has been increasing recognition of the problems with nursing home care and the need for reform.

As stated in the 1986 Institute of Medicine report *Improving the Quality of Care in Nursing Homes* "many nursing homes provide good care, but in many other government certified nursing homes, individuals who are admitted receive very inadequate—sometimes shockingly deficient—care that is likely to hasten the deterioration of their physical, mental, and emotional health. They also are likely to have their rights violated and may even be subject to physical abuse." Several of the major issues raised about the quality of nursing home care were related to its psychiatric aspects; they included concerns that physical and chemical restraints were being used inappropriately to control residents' behavior, and that psychiatric disorders, primarily depressions, were being undertreated. Estimates of the prevalence of the use of physical restraints, such as wrist or ankle cuffs, belts, vest restraints, or geriatric chairs designed to restrict mobility, ranged from 25% to 85%. Use of these devices was endemic in spite of evidence from observational studies that they do not safely control agitated behavior, as well as suggestions from cross-national studies that it is possible to manage similar patient populations without their use (Evans and Strumpf, 1989).

Surveys of medication use in long-term care facilities found prevalence rates up to 74% for psychotropic medications (Institute of Medicine, 1986). Antipsychotic agents were the most frequently prescribed psychotropic medications, with most reports of prevalence ranging from 20% to 50%. Evidence demonstrating a history of misuse of these drugs came from findings that variables unrelated to patient characteristics, including facility size, ratio of patients to staff, and the size of the physician's nursing home practice, were directly associated with the use of drugs. Substantial numbers of patients received psychotropic drugs without any diagnosis of mental disorder and without any chart note indicating the presence of relevant target symptoms (Ray et al., 1980). The importance of this issue for patients, families, and advocacy groups was poignantly captured by the newspaper headline "America's Other Drug Problem." In addition, advocates for improving the quality of long-term care were concerned about issues such as the lack of mental health services for patients who need long-term care as a result of dementia or psychiatric disorders associated with medical illnesses.

## THE REGULATORY ENVIRONMENT

In 1987 the federal government, as the largest single source of payment for nursing home care, used Medicaid and Medicare legislation to mandate nursing home reform that was enacted in the Omnibus Budget Reconciliation Act (OBRA) of 1987. The OBRA 1987 act (with modification in 1990) required Preadmission Screening and Annual Resident Review (PASARR) to ensure that patients who belonged in psychiatric hospitals were not inappropriately admitted to nursing homes. Other regulations stated that "the resident has a right to be free from any physical and chemical restraints imposed for purposes of discipline or convenience and not required to treat the resident's medical symptoms." The OBRA 1987 act requires that "residents who have not used antipsychotic drugs are not given these drugs unless antipsychotic drug therapy is necessary to treat a specific condition as diagnosed and documented in the clinical record" and that "residents who use antipsychotic drugs receive gradual dose reductions and behavioral interventions, unless clinically contraindicated, in an effort to discontinue these drugs." Regulations also state that each resident must be free from unnecessary drugs, which are defined as any drug used in an excessive dose, for an excessive duration, without adequate monitoring, without indications for use, or in the presence of adverse consequences that indicate that the dose should be reduced or discontinued. Although the definition of unnecessary drugs is rather general, guidelines used by surveyors to monitor facilities' compliance with OBRA regulations focus on antipsychotic, anxiolytic, and sedative hypnotic drugs.

In addition to the PASARR and psychotropic drug regulations, there are requirements related to the treatment of mental health problems. Under the general quality-of-care provision that "each resident must receive and the facility must provide the necessary care and services to attain or maintain the highest practicable physical, mental, and psychosocial well-being," there is a specific provision related to mental health stating that a facility must ensure that "a resident who displays mental or psychosocial adjustment difficulty receives appropriate treatment and services to correct the assessed problem." However, implementation of these OBRA requirements for mental health treatment has lagged behind the other provisions related to psychiatric disorders, despite compelling evidence in the clinical literature that psychiatric treatment is a critical part of nursing home care.

The OBRA regulations state that each facility's staff must conduct regularly scheduled assessments of all residents using a standardized resident assessment instrument, the Minimum Data Set (MDS), that was designed to identify clinical problems, including mental health problems. The MDS includes sections related to mental health/mental illness that evaluate customary routines, cognitive patterns, mood and behavior patterns, psychosocial well-being, and activity pursuit patterns. When certain *trigger* signs are identified, facilities are required to complete resident assessment protocols (RAPs) that provide guidelines for determining whether the resident's treatment plan should be modified. The RAPs address delirium, cognitive loss/dementia, psychosocial well-being, mood state, behavior symptoms, activities, psychotropic drug use, and physical restraints. The MDS is also used as a tool to define Resource Utilization Groups that determine case-based reimbursement rates for Medicare admissions and, in some states, for Medicaid. It is also used to define and measure quality indicators that are used for clinical management.

It is important to note that the federal regulations govern the activities of the nursing homes, not those of the physicians who provide care to patients living in these facilities. Presumably, it is the role of each facility's medical director to work with other providers to ensure that medical care is aligned with regulatory requirements. However, the role of the physician and strategies for ensuring alignment are not explicitly addressed in federal regulations.

## CLINICAL PSYCHIATRY IN THE NURSING HOME

Research conducted in the late 1980s demonstrated that the prevalence of psychiatric disorders in a series of new admissions to nursing homes was approximately

80% (Rovner et al., 1990; Streim and Katz, 1996). Of these, 67.4% had dementia, including 6.3% with dementia complicated by depression, 10.5% with hallucinations or delusions, and 7% with delirium. A total of 10.5% of patients had a depressive disorder, and 2.4% had schizophrenia and other primary psychoses. Other studies, whose estimates included patients with milder depressions, found a prevalence of 90% (Parmelee et al., 1989a). Although the work was completed before implementation of OBRA regulations, only 8.5% of the residents admitted to a nursing facility, or 10.6% of those with a diagnosable psychiatric disorder, had a history of previous psychiatric hospitalization. That statistic demonstrates that the high prevalence of psychiatric disorders among nursing home residents cannot be attributed to transinstitutionalization and the admission of chronic psychiatric patients. Instead, it is explained by conditions such as dementia and depression related to disabling medical and neurological illnesses that make nursing home care necessary.

## Clinical Features of Depression

Depressive disorders are second only to dementia in their prevalence in nursing home residents. Most studies in U.S. nursing homes have demonstrated prevalence rates of 15%–60%, depending on the population studied and the instruments used, whether major depression or depressive symptoms are reported, and whether primary depression and depression occurring secondary to dementia are considered together or separately (Rovner and Katz, 1993). Studies from other countries have shown similar rates. Thus, the high rates of depression cannot be attributed solely to problems in the U.S. approach to long-term care for the elderly. Approximately 6%–10% of all nursing home residents, and 20%–25% of those who are cognitively intact, met criteria for major depression; the latter figures are an order of magnitude greater than the rates reported in the community-dwelling elderly. The prevalence of less severe but clinically significant (e.g., minor or subsyndromal) depression was even higher. Less is known about the incidence of depression. One study reported that the 1-year incidence of major depression was 9.4% and that patients with preexisting minor depression were at increased risk; the incidence of minor depression among those who were euthymic at baseline was 7.4% (Parmelee et al., 1992a). Other, smaller-scale studies have shown comparable rates. Thus, minor depression in nursing home residents appears to be a risk factor for major depression and may represent an opportunity for preventive treatment in this population.

Depression among nursing home residents tends to be persistent. Although there may be moderate decreases in self-rated depression in the initial 2 weeks after nursing home admission, one study found that only 17% of patients with diagnosable depressive disorders had recovered after an average 3.6-year period of follow-up (Ames et al., 1989). Moreover, depression is associated with substantial morbidity. Evidence for morbidity includes increases in complaints of pain among residents with depression (Parmelee et al., 1991a) and an association between depression and biochemical markers of subnutrition (Katz et al., 1993). Other studies have shown that residents with depression deteriorate more rapidly, both in functional capacity (basic physical self-maintenance activities) (Katz and Parmelee, 1997) and in cognitive performance (Parmelee et al., 1991b). In addition to its association with morbidity, depression is associated with an increase in mortality, with effect sizes ranging from 1.6 to 3 (Ashby et al., 1991; Katz et al., 1989; Parmelee et al., 1996; Rovner et al., 1991; Samuels et al., 1996). There is, however, controversy about the mechanism involved. Although some studies reported that the increased mortality associated with depression remained apparent after controlling for the patients' medical diagnoses and level of disability, others suggested that the effect could be attributed to the interrelationships among depression, disability, and physical illness. Resolution of this issue will require further study.

Recurring questions about the validity of applying diagnostic criteria developed for younger and healthier adults to patients with significant psychiatric-medical co-morbidity are a prominent part of the literature on depression in patients with significant medical illness. It might seem logical to expect that the somatic and vegetative symptoms that characterize major depression in other populations lose their diagnostic value among long-term care residents and that long-term care patients who have symptoms consistent with a diagnosis of major depressive disorder may instead be experiencing a combination of medical symptoms and an existential reaction to disability, disease, and residential care placement. However, it has been demonstrated that standard diagnostic criteria remain valid as predictors of specific responses to treatment with the standard antidepressant nortriptyline (Katz et al., 1990; Streim et al., 2000). Therefore, even in nursing homes, the symptoms of major depression characterize a disease similar to that which occurs among younger adult psychiatric patients.

Although limited, there are also data from controlled clinical trials showing that responses to antidepressant treatment have ecological significance specifically in the nursing home environment (Datto et al., 2002). Responses are apparent in surveys conducted by the facilities' staff as well by investigators. Moreover, decreases in standard ratings of depressive symptoms are associated with increases in the positive affect experienced by the residents, and by measures of their initiative and involvement in the life of the nursing home. Thus, treatment of depression can have a substantially positive impact on patients' quality of life, even in nursing homes.

The most important conclusion to be drawn from this body of research is that in spite of the high levels of medical and cognitive co-morbidity in nursing home residents, depression can still be diagnosed using standard criteria, and standard treatments can remain effective. However, superimposed upon this theme are other findings—such as that there are also significant variations, and that specific treatment-relevant subtypes of depression can be found in nursing home populations. In addition to the high level of complexity that characterizes major depression among nursing home residents, there is evidence for heterogeneity in these patients that may reflect the existence of clinically relevant subtypes of depression.

The salience of one subtype of depression was suggested in a study that evaluated predictors of the response to nortriptyline and demonstrated that measures of self-care deficits and serum levels of albumin were highly intercorrelated, and that both predicted a failure to respond to treatment. The co-occurrence of symptoms of major depression with high levels of disability and low levels of albumin has been discussed in terms of the concept of *failure to thrive* in the elderly (Braun et al., 1988; Katz et al., 1993; Mago et al., 2000). Data on treatment responses for this putative syndrome are limited. However, it predicts decreased responses to a range of antidepressant medications, and patients with this cluster of symptoms may benefit from early referral for electroconvulsive therapy.

Findings from another nortriptyline study demonstrated significant differences in plasma level–response relationships between residents who were cognitively intact and those who had moderate degrees of dementia (Streim et al., 2000). Moreover, the contrasts could not be attributed to differences in nortriptyline metabolism or to drug-related cognitive impairment. Together, these findings suggest that the pharmacodynamics of nortriptyline differ between cognitively intact elderly patients and those with significant dementia (Olin et al., 2002a, 2002b). The conclusions to be drawn from these findings extend beyond those related to the utility of nortriptyline. If there is evidence for alterations in the pharmacodynamics of antidepressants in patients with dementia, then it may not be possible to extrapolate from findings on the efficacy of medications in intact patients to draw inferences about treatment in those with dementia. These findings must be viewed as part of a compelling body of evidence demonstrating that depression in Alzheimer's disease and related dementias should be viewed as a distinct disorder for which specific treatment studies will be necessary.

## Clinical Trials and Outcomes Research on Antidepressants in Nursing Homes

At this time, the literature includes reports of seven controlled studies of pharmacological treatment for depression in residents of nursing homes and related settings (Burrows et al., 2002; Kaplitz, 1975; Katz et al., 1990; Magai et al., 2000; Oslin et al., 2000, 2003; Streim et al., 2002). There have been two double-blind, randomized clinical trials evaluating the efficacy and safety of nortriptyline (Katz et al., 1990; Streim et al., 2002). The first was a small-scale, 7-week, placebo-controlled, fixed-plasma-level study of patients with major depression that found significant drug–placebo differences. Of those who completed treatment with nortriptyline, 7 of 12 (57%) were judged to be much or very much improved compared to 1 of 11 (9%) on placebo. However, 6 of 18 (33%) patients on nortriptyline versus 1 of 12 (8.5%) on placebo required early termination for side effects or adverse events. The second study was a 10-week randomized trial of regular (60–75 mg/day) versus low-dose (10–12.5 mg/day) nortriptyline for residents with major and minor depression. Significant, expected dose– and plasma level–response relationships were observed in cognitively intact residents and those with mild cognitive impairment but not in those with more severe dementia. For intact residents, these findings confirmed those from the earlier trial. The response rate was 42% at regular doses of nortriptyline versus 17% at lower doses. Together these studies demonstrate that nortriptyline is efficacious in nursing home residents and that depression is a treatable disorder even in nursing homes. However, in this population, as in others, the frequency of adverse events raises concerns about whether nortriptyline is a useful treatment.

Unfortunately, little information about selective serotonin reuptake inhibitors (SSRIs) is available. Reports of two small-scale, randomized clinical trials of SSRIs have been published. One of them investigated sertraline versus placebo for patients with late-stage dementia and major or minor depression (Magai et al., 2000). The other studied paroxetine versus placebo for residents with nonmajor depression (Burrows et al., 2002). Neither study showed significant drug–placebo differences; however, both were significantly underpowered.

Another approach to evaluating outcomes with reference to a control condition was used in parallel with the second nortriptyline study described above (Oslin et al., 2000). Patients with contraindications to nortriptyine, or with patient or provider preferences against entering the regular versus low-dose study, were treated with sertraline under open-label conditions. The response rate was 18%, significantly less than that of contemporaneous treatment with regular doses of nortriptyline; the rate for early termination was comparable to that for nortriptyline. There have also been three other reports of outcomes from open-label SSRI treatment. One study reported a remission rate of 75% for residents with minor depression (Rosen et al., 2000), but in the absence of any control condition, this observation is difficult to interpret. Two other studies reported lower response rates in patients with dementia or cerebrovascular disease than in cognitively intact patients (Trappler and Cohen, 1996, 1998). Taken together, these findings raise concerns about both the efficacy and the safety of using SSRIs in the older and frail patients who reside in nursing homes.

Prompted by suggestions that the dual serotonin and norepinephrine reuptake inhibitor venlafaxine may be more effective than SSRIs in a number of patient populations, a recent double-blind, randomized clinical trial compared venlafaxine with sertraline (Oslin et al., 2003). The hypothesis was that the rate of response and remission would be higher for venlafaxine than for sertraline, but that tolerability would be comparable. During the course of the 10-week trial, 12 patients (9 on venlafaxine and 3 on sertraline) experienced serious adverse events requiring early termination. (For venlafaxine, they were cerebrovascular accident (two), delirium (two), rapid atrial fibrillation, hypertension, hyponatremia, worsened chronic obstructive pulmonary disease, and congestive heart failure. For sertraline, they were hyponatremia, psychosis, and chest pain/delirium.) One other subject (on sertraline) experienced a severe adverse event (SAE) (worsening of previous heart failure) that interrupted treatment, but was restarted on medication after hospitalization (without breaking the blind). In addition, five other subjects (four on venlafaxine and one on sertraline) withdrew from the study because of side effects not deemed by the investigators to be serious. Two other subjects (both on venlafaxine) withdrew consent because of irritability, but with no other significant side effects. The serious adverse events were, in general, complex; they were judged at the time of their occurrence to be, at most, possibly related to the study medication. Yet, event history analyses showed significantly earlier termination for patients randomized to venlafaxine. (Comparison of medication groups for termination due to SAEs gave log-rank statistic = 5.28, $p$ = .022; for termination or interruption due to SAEs, log-rank statistic = 3.41, $p$ = .065; for termination due to SAEs or withdrawal related to side effects, log-rank statistic = 8.08, $p$ = .005; for termination due to SAEs or withdrawal related to side effects or withdrawn consent, log rank statistic = 10.04, $p$ = .002.) Thus venlafaxine appears to be less well tolerated, and possibly less safe, than sertraline. In applying these findings, it is important to recognize that this study was conducted with immediate-release venlafaxine; it is possible, in principle, that the extended-release preparation would have been better tolerated. Nevertheless, given these findings, there is a clear need for caution in using venlafaxine (and possibly other dual-action serotonin and norepinephrine reuptake inhibitors) in frail elderly patients.

Finally, in considering alternatives for the treatment of depression and related symptoms in nursing home residents, it is important to recall classic findings demonstrating the benefits of methylphenidate versus placebo for "withdrawn apathetic geriatric patients" (Kaplitz, 1975). Further research on the efficacy and safety of stimulants and related medications would be useful.

Clinical trials and outcome studies can be informative about the utility of instruments for evaluating treatment. The two nortriptyline studies that demonstrated specific drug responses both used the Hamilton Depression Rating Scale as a primary measure; therefore, the findings serve to validate it in this context (Katz et al., 1990; Streim et al., 2002). However, use of the Hamilton scale in nursing homes required the development of a manual defining assessment procedures. For the above studies, one key convention was the use of inclusive criteria for ratings, avoiding attempts to factor symptoms into components due to physical illness and those due to depression. Although this strategy was useful in optimizing reliability, it may have led to an overestimation of the magnitude of symptoms, most critically at the conclusion of treatment. Other defined protocols included guidelines for the ascertainment of symptoms through interviews with the resident, direct observations of his or her behavior, and structured inquiries with facility staff. These assessment protocols were similar to those used for the Cornell Scale for Depression in Dementia, an instrument that has been validated for use in older patients, both those who are cognitively intact and those who have dementia (Alexopoulos et al., 1988a, 1988b); the similarities in content and procedures suggest that the Cornell scale should also be of use in nursing home residents. Other promising approaches to assessment include the use of self-rating scales. The Geriatric Depression Scale has been validated as a measure of depression in nursing home residents. Available data demonstrate that it is reliable and valid in both cognitively intact patients and those with mild to moderate dementia, down to Mini-Mental State Examination (MMSE) scores of at least 15 (McGivney et al., 1994; Parmelee et al., 1989). Although it is well evaluated as a state measure of depression in the elderly, the major concerns about its use for monitoring treatment effects must be the limited data evaluating its sensitivity as a measure of change.

The conclusions that can be drawn from the available literature are that nortriptyline is an efficacious antidepressant in nursing home residents, specifically in those who are cognitively intact or mildly demented. However, in nursing homes, as in other geriatric treatment settings, its use may be limited by its well-known side effects and by drug–disease interactions. There has been relatively little controlled research on the SSRIs, but the available data from clinical trials and outcome studies raise questions both about whether these medications are efficacious in frail elderly patients and about whether they are significantly safer than secondary amine tricyclic agents. These concerns have been reinforced by recent epidemiological findings demonstrating that the rate of falls for nursing home residents and other older individuals taking SSRIs is comparable to the rate for those taking tricyclic antidepressants (43%–47%). Although venlafaxine is often considered a second-line agent of choice, to be used in older patients who do not respond to SSRIs, the available data suggest that it may be poorly tolerated, and possibly unsafe, in nursing home residents. Finally, a classic older study suggests that stimulant medications may be efficacious for treating depression and related states such as apathy.

## EVOLUTION IN THE EPIDEMIOLOGY OF DEPRESSION AND ITS TREATMENT

Before the 1986 Institute of Medicine report that called for nursing home reform, only 10% of residents with a known diagnosis of depression were receiving treatment with antidepressants (Heston et al., 1992). However, for 1997, the government estimated that 24.8% of all U.S. nursing home residents were receiving an antidepressant medication (Health Care Financing Administration, 1998).

Extending earlier work (Datto et al., 2002), our research group evaluated the use of antidepressants in residents from 12 nursing homes and found that they were used in almost 45% of residents, with rates for individual facilities ranging from about 20% to 60% (unpublished data). Of those residents who were cognitively intact or mildly to moderately impaired, 34.4% had Geriatric Depression Scale (GDS) scores >10 and thus had clinically significant depressive symptoms. Approximately 8.0% had major depression and 16.3% had minor depression. It is interesting to compare the rates of depression observed now with those reported a decade or more ago. The current rate of major depression, approximately 8.0%, appears substantially below earlier estimates of 20% or even higher. Moreover, this apparent difference has occurred despite trends demonstrating that long-term care patients in nursing homes are becoming older and sicker. Although our comparisons may confound differences across times with differences across facilities, as well as cohort effects and period effects, they suggest that the rate of

depression in nursing home residents is lower now than in the past. This change suggests that there has been a major public health benefit from increased rates of treatment for depression.

Although there has been substantial progress, significant problems remain. Further insight into current issues can be derived from cross-tabulations of rates of depression and of drug treatment. We found that 14.0% of nursing home residents had symptoms of depression (GDS score >10) without treatment; 20.4% had depressive symptoms in spite of taking antidepressant medication; and 26% were receiving antidepressants and did not have significant depression. If we assume that those patients taking antidepressants without significant depressive symptoms had depression in remission, these figures support the suggestion that these medications are having a significant effect. In the sample as a whole, the specific antidepressant classes/agents were SSRIs (27.2% of the population), venlafaxine (2.0%), nefazodone (0.6%), bupropion (0.9%), mirtazepine (8.0%), trazadone (8.7%), tricyclic antidepressants (TCAs) (1.9%), and monoamine oxidase inhibitors (MAOIs) (0.1%). The SSRIs and venlafaxine were more likely to be used in more intact residents, while trazadone was more likely to be used in more demented individuals. Among the more intact, the overall rate of antidepressant use was 46.4%, and the use of classes/agents was: SSRIs (30.8% of the population), venlafaxine (3.3%), nefazodone (0.6%), bupropion (1.0%), mirtazepine (8.6%), trazadone (5.2%), TCAs (4.0%), and MAOIs (0.2%). Among the more intact patients, antidepressant use in general and use of SSRIs, venlafaxine, and TCAs, but not the other agents, was greater among those with current depressive symptoms. The profile for the use of mirtazepine and trazadone is consistent with clinical lore that many providers may use these as hypnotics or for other indications (e.g., to manage agitation [trazadone] or to stimulate appetite and weight gain [mirtazepine]). Other analyses found that 27% of patients receiving an antidepressant were receiving doses less than those recommended by an expert consensus guide to the pharmacotherapy of depressive disorders in older patients (Alexopoulos et al., 2001); 35% were receiving minimal recommended target doses, and 38% were receiving doses above the minimal targets. For SSRIs, the distribution of doses in these three categories was 24%, 42%, and 34%, respectively.

Findings from the cross-tabulation of depressive symptoms and use of antidepressant medications can be used to define areas of clinical concern. The observation that 14% of nursing home residents had significant depressive symptoms without treatment suggests that, in spite of high rates of prescribing, the old problem of undertreatment remains significant. The observation that approximately 20% of residents had significant depressive symptoms even though they were being treated with antidepressants demonstrates that there is a need to conduct research on the efficacy of treatments for those who do not respond to front-line agents. It is also important to develop strategies for service delivery that go beyond emphasizing the importance of diagnosing depression and initiating treatment to include systematic monitoring of treatment outcomes and modification or intensification of treatment when necessary. Finally, the observation that 26% of residents are taking an antidepressant without having current symptoms of depression demonstrates the importance of careful evaluation of such patients to identify those with multiple previous episodes who will require ongoing maintenance treatment and those who may benefit from drug discontinuation with monitoring. Findings suggesting that SSRIs may lead to falls underline the importance of this distinction (Ensrod et al., 2002; Kallin et al., 2002; Liu et al., 1998; Thapa et al., 1998).

## DELIVERY OF CLINICAL CARE

### Nursing Homes as Clinical Settings

The clinical issues that arise in the care of nursing home residents with depression are similar to those that arise with other older patients. However, in nursing homes, psychiatric–medical co-morbidity and/or the co-occurrence of dementia and depression are essentially universal. Although the patient population does not present unique problems, work in the nursing home environment does require specific knowledge. Clinicians providing care in nursing homes must be aware of the unique characteristics of these facilities, both with respect to the specific homes where they see patients and with respect to the state and federal policy and regulatory environments. To evaluate residents thought to have depression, clinicians must be aware of the social environment within each facility, and about recreational activities and the opportunities for pleasurable events. To obtain information about residents' symptoms, they must know who on the nursing staff is able to provide information. Often, developing and maintaining a network of staff members who can report on residents' behaviors will require an ongoing process of formal and informal staff training. Clinicians must also be aware of the federal regulations that govern the nursing homes, and they should be prepared to help facilities establish and maintain compliance.

### Guidelines for Pharmacological Treatment of Depression

In working with depressed nursing home residents, as with other groups of old-old and frail patients, clini-

cians must struggle with an evidence base that demonstrates the value of treatment but provides little guidance about what treatments are most safe and effective. In this context, it is not possible to make specific recommendations about agents or doses. Instead, it is reasonable to shift the focus away from questions about which drug is optimal and to consider what sequences or combinations of drugs and psychosocial or environmental treatments are most appropriate. The key, then, is to think not in terms of individual agents, but in terms of treatment algorithms. At this time, the most relevant set of recommendations may be those of a recent Expert Consensus Guide (Alexopoulos et al., 2001). In these, as in the Agency for Health Care Policy and Research Clinical Practice Guidelines for Depression in Primary Care (Depression Guideline Panel, 1993), priority must be given to monitoring patients' responses to medications, and modifying or intensifying treatment if there is no evidence of a response after approximately 6 weeks and if residual symptoms remain after about 12 weeks. However, based on the findings discussed above, it may be reasonable at this time to modify the Expert Consensus Guide to de-emphasize the potential value of venlafaxine. Taking this into account, the guidelines would recommend the SSRIs, citalopram, sertraline, or paroxetine as first-line agents, and buproprion, and possibly nortriptyline or mirtazapine, as second-line antidepressants for modification or augmentation of treatment, as needed.

There have been major advances over the past decade in the availability of drug treatments for depression in nursing home residents, and there are early suggestions that this has had a public health impact. Nevertheless, significant issues remain. These include the need to develop strategies to ensure that both psychosocial and pharmacological treatment is availabe to all of those who require it. Another issue is to develop strategies to ensure that those who do not respond to first-line treatments receive the downstream components of care that they require. Finally, given the exceptionally high rates of antidepressant use among nursing home residents, it is important to develop an evidence base and clinical strategies to facilitate decision making about when patients should receive long-term maintenance treatment and when these agents should be discontinued. Thus, one can view the past decade from a continuous quality improvement perspective; there have been profound gains with respect to the historic problem of undertreatment of depression, but new problems have emerged.

REFERENCES

Alexopoulos, G.S., Abrams, R.C., Young, R.C., and Shamoian, C.A. (1988a) Cornell Scale for Depression in Dementia. *Biol Psychiatry* 23:271–284.

Alexopoulos, G.S., Abrams, R.C., Young, R.C., and Shamoian, C.A. (1988b) Use of the Cornell scale in nondemented patients. *J Am Geriatr Soc* 36:230–236.

Alexopoulos, G.S., Katz, I.R., Reynolds, C.F., 3rd, Carpenter, D., and Docherty, J.P. (2001) The expert consensus guideline series: Pharmacotherapy of depression in older patients. *Postgrad Med* (special report).

Ames, D., Ashby, D., Mann, A.H., et al. (1989) Psychiatric illness in elderly residents of part III homes in one London borough: Prognosis and review. *Age Aging* 17:249–256.

Arfken, C.L., Wilson, J.G., and Aronson, S.M. (2001) Retrospective review of selective serotonin reuptake inhibitors and falling in older nursing home residents. *Int Psychogeriatr* 13:85–91.

Ashby, D., Ames, D., West, C.R., et al. (1991) Psychiatric morbidity as prediction of mortality for residents of local authority homes for the elderly. *Int J Geriatr Psychiatry* 6:567–575.

Braun, J.V., Wykle, M.H., and Cowling, W.R. (1988) Failure to thrive in older persons: A concept derived. *Gerontologist* 28:809–812.

Burrows, A.B., Salzman, C., Satlin, A., Noble, K., Pollock, B.G. and Gersh, T. (2002) A randomized, placebo-controlled trial of paroxetine in nursing home residents with non-major depression. *Depress Anxiety* 15:102–110.

Datto, C., Oslin, D., Streim, J., Scheinthal, S., DiFilippo, S., and Katz, I. (2002) Pharmacological treatment of depression in nursing home residents: A mental health services perspective. *J Geriatr Psychiatry Neurol* 15:141–146.

Depression Guideline Panel. (1993) *Depression in Primary Care*, vol. 2, *Treatment of Major Depression*. Clinical Practice Guideline, Number 5 (AHCPR Pub. No. 93-0551). Rockville, MD: U.S. Department of Health and Human Services, Public Health Service, Agency for Health Care Policy and Research.

Ensrud, K.E., Blackwell, T.L., Mangione, C.M., et al. (2002) Central nervous system—active medications and risk of falls in older women. *J Am Geriatr Soc* 50:1629–1637.

Evans, L.K., and Strumpf, N.E. (1989) Tying down the elderly. A review of the literature on physical restraint. *J Am Geriatr Soc* 37:65–74.

Health Care Financing Administration. (1998) *A Report to Congress: Study of Private Accreditation (Deeming) of Nursing Homes, Regulatory Incentives and Non-Regulatory Incentives, and Effectiveness of the Survey and Certification System*. Available at www.cms.hhs.gov/medicaid/reports/deemovw.asp checked 1/20/04.

Heston, L.L., Garrard, J., Makris, L., Kane, R.L., Cooper, S., Dunham, T., and Zelterman, D. (1992) Inadequate treatment of depressed nursing home elderly. *J Am Geriatr Soc* 40:1117–1122.

Institute of Medicine, Committee on Nursing Home Regulation. (1986) *Improving the Quality of Care in Nursing Homes*. Washington, DC: National Academy Press.

Kallin, K., Lundin-Olsson, L., Jensen, J., Nyberg, L., and Gustafson, Y. (2002) Predisposing and precipitating factors for falls among older people in residential care. *Public Health* 116:263–271.

Kaplitz, S.E. (1975) Withdrawn, apathetic geriatric patients responsive to methylphenidate. *J Am Geriatr Soc* 23:271–276.

Katz, I.R., Beaston-Wimmer, P., Parmelee, P.A., et al. (1993) Failure to thrive in the elderly: Exploration of the concept and delineation of psychiatric components. *J Geriatr Psychiatry Neurol* 6:161–169.

Katz, I.R., Lesher, E., Kleban, M., et al. (1989) Clinical features of depression in the nursing home. *Int Psychogeriatr* 1:5–15.

Katz, I.R., and Parmelee, P. (1997) Overview. In: Rubinstein, R.L., and Lawton, M.P., eds. *Depression in Long Term and Residential Care*. New York: Springer, pp. 1–25.

Katz, I.R., Simpson, G.M., Curlik, S.M., Parmelee, P.A., and Muhly, C. (1990) Pharmacologic treatment of major depression for elderly patients in residential care settings. *J Clin Psychiatry* 51:41–47.

Katz, I.R., Streim, J.E., and Smith, B.D. (2000) Psychiatric aspects of long-term care. In: Sadock, B.J., and Sadock, V.A., eds. *Kaplan and Sadock's Comprehensive Textbook of Psychiatry*, vol. II, 7th ed. Baltimore: Lippincott, Williams & Wilkins, pp. 3145–3150.

Liu, B., Anderson, G., Mittmann, N., To, T., Axcell, T., and Shear, N. (1998) Use of selective serotonin-reuptake inhibitors or tricyclic antidepressants and risk of hip fractures in elderly people. *Lancet* 351:1303–1307.

Magai, C., Kennedy, G., Cohen, C.I., et al. (2000) A controlled clinical trial of sertraline in the treatment of depression in nursing home patients with late-stage Alzheimer's disease. *Am J Geriatr Psychiatry* 8:66–74.

Mago, R., Warren, B., Ten Have, T., Harralson, T., Streim, J., Parmalee, P., and Katz, I.R. (2000) Clinical laboratory measures in relation to depression, disability, and cognitive impairment in the elderly. *Am J Geriatr Psychiatry* 8:1–6.

McGivney, S.A., Mulvihill, M., and Taylor, B. (1994) Validating the GDS Depression Screen in the Nursing Home. *J A Geriatr Soc* 42:490–492.

National Center for Health Statistics. (1987) Use of nursing homes by the elderly: Preliminary data from the 1985 National Nursing Home Survey (DHHS Publ No PHS 87-1250). Hyattsville, MD: National Center for Health Statistics.

Olin, J.T., Katz, I.R., Meyers, B.S., Schneider, L.S., and Lebowitz, B.D. (2002b). Provisional diagnostic criteria for depression of Alzheimer disease: Rationale and background. *Am J Geriatr Psychiatry* 10:129–141.

Olin, J.T., Schneider, L.S., Katz, I.R., Meyers, B.S., Alexopoulos, G.S., Breitner, J.C., Bruce, M.L., Caine, E.D., Cummings, J.L., Devanand, D.P., Krishnan, K.R., Lyketsos, C.G., Lyness, J.M., Rabins, P.V., Reynolds, C.F., 3rd, Rovner, B.W., Steffens, D.C., Tariot, P.N., and Lebowitz, B.D. (2002a) Provisional diagnostic criteria for depression of Alzheimer disease. *Am J Geriatr Psychiatry* 10:125–128.

Oslin, D.W., Streim, J.E., Katz, I.R., et al. (2000) Heuristic comparison of sertraline with nortriptyline for the treatment of depression in frail elderly patients. *Am J Geriatr Psychiatry* 8:141–149.

Oslin, D.W., TenHave, T.R., Streim, J.E., Datto, C.J., Weintraub, D., DiFilippo, S., and Katz, I.R. (2003) Probing the safety of medications in the frail elderly: Evidence from a randomized clinical trial of sertraline and venlafaxine in depressed nursing home residents. *J Clin Psychiatry*. 64:875–882.

Parmelee, P.A., Katz, I.R., and Lawton, M.P. (1989a) Depression among institutionalized aged: Assessment and prevalence estimation. *J Gerontol* 44:M22–M29.

Parmelee, P.A., Katz, I.R., and Lawton, M.P. (1991a) The relation of pain to depression among institutionalized aged. *J Gerontol [Psychol Sci]* 46:P15–P21.

Parmelee, P.A., Katz, I.R., and Lawton, M.P. (1992a) Incidence of depression in long term care settings. *J Gerontol [Med Sci]* 47:M189–M196.

Parmelee, P.A., Katz, I.R., and Lawton, M.P. (1992b) Depression and mortality among institutionalized aged. *J Gerontol [Psychol Sci]* 47:P3–P10.

Parmelee, P.A., Kleban, M.H., Lawton, M.P., and Katz, I.R. (1991b) Depression and cognitive change among institutionalized aged. *Psychol Aging* 6:504–511.

Parmelee, P., Lawton, M.P., and Katz, I.R. (1989b) Psychometric properties of the Geriatric Depression Scale among the institutionalized aged. *Psychol Assess J Consult Clin Psychol* 1:331–338.

Ray, W.A., Federspiel, C.F., and Schaffner, W. (1980) A study of antipsychotic drug use in nursing homes: Epidemiologic evidence suggesting misuse. *Am J Public Health* 70:485–491.

Rhoades, J., and Krauss, N. (1999) Nursing Home Trends, 1987 and 1996 (MEPS Chart Book No. 3, AHCPR Pub. No. 99-0032). Rockville, MD: Agency for Health Care Policy and Research.

Rosen, J., Mulsant, B.H., and Pollock, B.G. (2000) Sertraline in the treatment of minor depression in nursing home residents: A pilot study. *Int J Geriatr Psychiatry* 15:177–180.

Rovner, B.W., German, P.S., Brant, L.J., et al. (1991) Depression and mortality in nursing homes. *JAMA* 265:993–996.

Rovner, B.W., German, P.S., Broadhead, J., Morriss, R.K., Brant, L.J., Blaustein, J., and Folstein, M.F. (1990) The prevalence and management of dementia and other psychiatric disorders in nursing homes. *Int Psychogeriatr* 2:13–24.

Rovner, B.W., and Katz, I.R. (1993) Psychiatric disorders in the nursing home: A selective review of studies related to clinical care. *Int J Geriatr Psychiatry* 8:75–87.

Samuels, S.C., Katz, I.R., Parmelee, P.A., Boyce, A.A., and DiFilippo, S. (1996) Use of the Hamilton and Montgomery Asberg Depression Scales in institutionalized elderly patients. *Am J Geriatr Psychiatry* 4:237–246.

Strahan, G.W. (1997) An overview of nursing homes and their current residents. Data from the 1995 National Nursing Home Survey. Centers for Disease Control and Prevention. National Center for Health Statistics. Advance Data No. 280, January 27. Available at www.cdc.gov/nchs/products/pubs/pubd/ad/280-271/ad.280.

Streim, J.E., and Katz, I.R. (1996) Clinical psychiatry in the nursing home. In: Busse, E.W., and Blazer, D.G., eds. *Geriatric Psychiatry*, 2nd ed. Washington, DC: American Psychiatric Press, pp. 413–432.

Streim, J.E., Oslin, D.W., Katz, I.R., et al. (2000) Drug treatment of depression in frail elderly nursing home residents. *Am J Geriatr Psychiatry* 8:150–159.

Thapa, P.B., Gideon, P., Cost, T.W., Milam, A.B., and Ray, W.A. (1998) Antidepressants and the risk of falls among nursing home residents. *N Engl J Med* 339:875–882.

Trappler, B., and Cohen, C.I. (1996) Using fluoxetine in "very old" depressed nursing home residents. *Am J Geriatr Psychiatry* 4:258–262.

Trappler, B., and Cohen, C.I. (1998) Use of SSRIs in "very old" depressed nursing home residents. *Am J Geriatr Psychiatry* 6:83–89.

# V | DEPRESSION CO-MORBID WITH OTHER ILLNESSES

Perhaps no other issue has received so much attention and been the focus of so much excellent research in the past decade as the complex relationships between depression and other illnesses. There are many types of co-morbid relationships. Probably most familiar to the clinician is *clinical co-morbidity*, defined as one disorder influencing the course, outcome, or treatment response of a second disorder when they occur concurrently. This effect has been documented when depression is co-morbid with ischemic heart disease. Patients with ischemic heart disease who are depressed have higher cardiac mortality than comparably medically ill patients who are not depressed.

However, there are other types of co-morbid relationships that are also important. *Familial co-morbidity* is defined as the situation in which family members of a patient with a disorder are more likely to have a second disorder than individuals in a family without either disorder. Members of a family often have many things in common, and familial co-morbidity may result from linked genes for the two disorders or shared environmental risk factors. The evolving story of the co-morbid relationship between depression and vascular disease has brought into focus *epidemiological co-morbidity*, defined in this circumstance as the increased likelihood that a patient with one disease will become depressed compared to a patient without that disease. In studies of epidemiological co-morbidity, it is critical to study the population throughout the risk period for both disorders since the illnesses may occur in the same patient at different times. Furthermore, the sequence of the presentation of the two disorders—that is, whether their onset is concurrent or whether one condition most often precedes the other—is particularly important because it may suggest a causal link between the two disorders. For example, if depression occurs before ischemic disease, then depression may be a risk factor for ischemic disease.

There is also a not uncommon clinical circumstance that can be erroneously misinterpreted as representing a co-morbid relationship: when different manifestations of the same disorder are mistaken for two distinct disorders. An example of this is the apparent co-morbidity of depression and dementia; these two disorders are frequently concurrent, and they complicate both assessment and treatment. However, new evidence suggests that in many patients there may not be two distinct disorders; rather, cognitive impairment or affective symptoms may simply be different first presentations of the same degenerative process.

# 25 | Depression co-morbid with ischemic heart disease

S T E V E N   P .   R O O S E   A N D   A L E X A N D E R   H .   G L A S S M A N

Over the past two decades, a number of rigorous epidemiological studies and clinical trials have illuminated the complex relationship between depression and ischemic heart disease (IHD). This relationship has many dimensions, including the following: (1) patients with depression have a higher rate of sudden cardiovascular death than age-matched controls, (2) depression early in life is associated with an increased rate of symptomatic and fatal IHD, (3) depression co-morbid with IHD is associated with an increased rate of cardiovascular mortality, and (4) treatment of depression in patients with IHD may reduce the cardiovascular risk. Although the relationship between depression and heart disease may begin at a young age, this topic belongs in a volume on late-life depression because both disorders are prevalent in the elderly and it is in this age group that the clinical implications of co-morbidity are most significant.

In order to understand the layered relationship between depression and IHD, it must first be appreciated that there are different types of co-morbidity. The two most relevant to this topic are clinical and epidemiological co-morbidity. *Clinical co-morbidity* is defined as one disorder influencing the course, outcome, or treatment response to a second disorder when they occur concurrently. *Epidemiological co-morbidity* means that patients with one disease are more likely to become depressed than those without the disease. In determining co-morbidity between depression and medical disorders, it is critical to know if the disorders occur in the same patient at different times and the sequence of the presentation of the two disorders, that is, whether their onset is concurrent or whether one condition generally precedes the other. The sequencing issue is particularly important to the degree that it may suggest a mechanistic link between the two disorders. For example, if heart disease tends to occur before depression, then heart disease may be a risk factor for depression.

The decision of whether symptoms can be considered as resulting from depression strongly influences the diagnosis of depression in the medically ill population. Some symptoms (e.g., anorexia, fatigue, sleep disturbance) that fulfill the diagnostic criteria for depression in DSM-IV are also nonspecific symptoms of serious medical conditions. Consequently, there is a long-standing debate about whether, in the setting of medical illness, it is more accurate to take the *inclusive* or *exclusive* approach to counting symptoms with respect to the diagnosis of depression. In the exclusive approach, a symptom is not counted for the diagnosis of depression if it can reasonably be attributed to an underlying medical condition or medication side effect. In the inclusive approach, all symptoms are counted for the diagnosis of depression without consideration of this presumed etiology. The inclusive approach is currently favored because of evidence that it has greater sensitivity for the diagnosis of depression without significantly sacrificing specificity (Koenig et al., 1988, 1997).

## DEPRESSION IN PATIENTS WITH CARDIAC DISEASE

Depression has long been associated with heart disease, and a number of studies have documented the prevalence of major depressive disorder and subsyndromal depression in patients with cardiac disease. The rate of depression in patients following myocardial infarction (MI) is approximately 20%, and an additional 20%–25% have significant depressive symptoms, as indicated by high scores on the Beck Depression Inventory (BDI) (Carney et al., 1987; Forrester et al., 1992; Frasure-Smith et al., 1993; Schleifer et al., 1989). It has long been assumed that the depression follows the cardiac event. However, studies reporting that 20% of patients are depressed at the time of cardiac catheterization before an MI (Carney et al., 1987; Gonzalez et al., 1996; Hance et al., 1995) raise the question of whether the MI is a precipitant of the depression or the depression contributes to the precipitation of the ischemic event. The latter possibility is supported by studies documenting that depression tends to follow a chronic course during the first year after MI and may not be a brief reaction to a life-threatening event (Schleifer et al., 1989; Stern et al., 1977; Travella et al., 1994).

## DEPRESSION AND DEVELOPMENT OF CORONARY ARTERY DISEASE

Although strongly associated with the post-MI period, there is now convincing evidence that depression early in life before the development of IHD is actually a risk factor for the development of coronary artery disease (CAD). Table 25.1 summarizes the results of 10 longitudinal studies establishing the relationship between depression and CAD. A prototypic example of these studies is the one by Ford et al. (1998) that followed all male medical students who entered. In an unadjusted analysis, clinical depression was associated with an almost twofold higher risk of later CAD. This association remained after adjustment for established risk factors for IHD such as hyperlipidemia requiring treatment, hypertension, and diabetes. The relative risk ratio for the development of CAD among men with versus without clinical depression was 2.12. Of special interest with respect to the sequence of the presentations of illness was that the median time from the first episode of clinical depression to the first CAD event was 15 years. The evidence that depression is a risk factor for the development of IHD does not just apply to men. Hallstrom et al. (1986) reported on a sample of Swedish women, aged 38–54, followed for 12 years after a comprehensive medical and psychiatric assessment at baseline. Subjects with depressive disorder at baseline had a significantly higher risk of developing symptomatic IHD.

In summary, it is a reasonable conclusion that depression plays a significant role in the development of CAD, independent of conventional risk factors, and that its adverse influence endures over time. The impact of depression on the risk of MI is probably comparable to that of smoking. Longitudinal studies suggest that depression occurs before the onset of clinically significant CAD; however, atherosclerosis begins at very young ages.

## THE EFFECT OF DEPRESSION ON CARDIAC OUTCOMES IN PATIENTS WITH ISCHEMIC HEART DISEASE

Depression is associated with an increased risk of cardiac morbidity and mortality across a wide range of patients with cardiac disease including patients following cardiac catheterization (Barefoot et al., 1996; Carney et al., 1988), patients with unstable angina (Lespérance et al., 2000), patients post MI, and patients post heart transplant (Dew et al., 1999).

TABLE 25.1. *Studies of the Relation Between Depression and Prognosis in CAD in People without Existing CAD*

| Study | Follow-up (yrs) | Events (n) | Types of Events | Relative Risk* |
|---|---|---|---|---|
| Hallstrom et al. (1986) | 12 | 75 | Nonfatal MI, angina, ischemic ECG change | Severity of depression, predicted angina only |
| Appels et al. (2000) | 4.5 | 59 | MI (fatal = 21; nonfatal = 38) | 2.28 for nonfatal MI; no association with fatal MI |
| Anda et al. (1993) | 12.4 | 189 | Fatal MI | 1.5, depression affect |
| Aromaa et al. (1994) | 6.6 | 91 | Fatal CAD | 3.36 |
| Wassertheil-Smoller et al. (1996) | 4.5 | A. 355 B. 321 C. 126 | A. All deaths B. MI or stroke C. MI | A. 1.26 B. 1.18 C. 1.14 but not significant* |
| Barefoot et al. (1996) | 24 | A. 290 B. 122 | A. All deaths B. MI | A. 1.59 B. 1.71 |
| Pratt et al. (1996) | 13 | 64 | MI, self reported | 4.54, major depressive episode 2.07, dysphoria |
| Ford et al. (1998) | 37 | A. 103 B. 163 | A. MI B. CAD | A and B: 2.12† |
| Mendes de Leon et al. (1998) | 9 | A. 255 B. 391 | A. CAD death B. nonfatal MI, cardiac death | A and B: 1.03‡ |

*Adjusted for multiple factors (various across studies, in general age, conventional cardiovascular risk factors such as smoking, cholesterol, weight or body mass index, and physical conditions at entry of the study).

†Per 5-unit increase in CES-D score during follow-up versus baseline.

‡Per unit increase in CES-D score.

CAD, coronary artery disease; CES-D, Center for Epidemiologic Studies Depression; DSM-III, *Diagnostic and Statistical Manual*, 3rd ed.; ECG, electrocardiogram; GHQ, General Health Questionnaire; MI, myocardial infarction; MMPI, Minnesota Multiphasic Personality Inventory; PSE, Psychiatric State Examination.

In a seminal study, Frasure-Smith et al. (1993) reported on a cohort of 222 patients with electrocardiogram (ECG)- and enzyme-confirmed acute MI, who were classified as having major depression by DSM criteria, having depressive symptoms but not meeting criteria for major depression as indicated by BDI scores of 10 or greater, or no depression. Patients were followed for 18 months, and after controlling for other variables already established as predictors of outcome post-MI (e.g., previous MI or Killip class), major depression emerged as a significant independent predictor of an adverse outcome (adjusted hazard ratio = 4.29; 95% CI, 3.14–5.44; $p$ = .013). Most intriguingly, at the 18-month evaluation point, the mortality rate for post-MI patients with only BDI scores above 10 was comparable to that of patients with major depression (Frasure-Smith et al., 1995). Table 25.2 lists studies of the relationship between depression and prognosis in patients with CAD.

Depression also significantly impacts behaviors that can influence cardiac outcomes. Depressed post-MI patients take longer to return to work than patients without depression, and are more likely to drop out of exercise and cardiac rehabilitation programs or to be noncompliant with medical regimens (Blumenthal and Emery, 1988). For example, depressed patients with CAD are less likely to comply with low-dose aspirin therapy, and depressed smokers are 40% less likely to stop smoking than nondepressed smokers (Glassman and Shapiro, 1998).

## PHYSIOLOGICAL MECHANISMS UNDERLYING THE RELATIONSHIP BETWEEN VASCULAR DISEASE AND DEPRESSION

Studies of platelet function and heart rate variability in normal controls, patients with depression, and patients with depression and IHD provide intriguing data suggesting possible physiological mechanisms underlying the association between depression, IHD, and sudden cardiac death. When injury to blood vessel endothelium occurs, such as in patients with atherosclerosis, both platelets and circulating leukocytes attach to exposed subendothelial layers. This begins a cascade of events that includes conversion of platelet membrane GPIIB/IIIa complexes into receptors for fibrinogen and release from storage granules of chemotactic factors such as platelet factor 4 (PF4), beta-thyroglobulin (BTG), and serotonin that stimulate other platelets and thereby induce the process of platelet aggregation. Mechanical obstruction secondary to platelet aggregation can play a central role in the development of acute coronary ischemia in patients with atherosclerosis (Musselman et al., 2000).

Platelet activity in depressed patients with and without cardiac disease has been studied by a number of investigators using different methodologies (Musselman et al., 1998). Musselman et al., demonstrated that young depressed patients without vascular disease have increased platelet activation and responsiveness compared to age- and gender-matched normal controls (Musselman, 1996). Pollock et al. (2000) compared indices of platelet activity, PF4 and BTG, in normal controls, depressed and nondepressed patients with IHD. Despite being on aspirin therapy, patients with IHD and depression had statistically significant increases in PF4 and BTG compared to both nondepressed IHD patients and normal controls. When the patients with depression and IHD were treated with paroxetine, there were significant reductions in platelet-active factors such that this patient group was no longer different from nondepressed patients or normal controls with respect to measures of platelet activity. The *anti-platelet* effect of the selective serotonin reuptake inhibitor (SSRI) was not dependent on the response to depression; normalization of platelet activity occurred in both responders and nonresponders to paroxetine. Furthermore, the anti-platelet effect was specific to the SSRI. Patients with IHD and depression treated with a tricyclic antidepressant, nortriptyline, did not have normalization of platelet activation despite the robust antidepressant effect of the medication.

The increased platelet activity in depressed patients may result from sympatho-adrenal hyperactivity

TABLE 25.2. *Studies of the Relation Between Depression and Prognosis in CAD, in People with Existing CAD*

| Study | $n$ | Follow-up (mo) | RR* |
|---|---|---|---|
| Stern et al. (1977) | 68 | 12 | 7.5 (OR) |
| Schleifer et al. (1989) | 282 | 6 | 3.1 |
| Ahern et al. (1990) | 265 | 12 | NA ($p < .05$) |
| Ladwig et al. (1991) | 552 | 6 | 4.9 2.8 |
| Frasure-Smith et al. (1993) | 222 | 6 | 3.1 |
| Frasure-Smith et al. (1995) | 218 | 18 | 6.64 |
| Denollet and Brutsaert (1998) | 87 | 7.9 yr | 4.3 |
| Lespérance et al. (2000) | 896 | 12 | 3.66 |
| Kaufman et al. (1983) | 361 | 12 | 2.33 |

*Adjusted relative risk ratio for mortality after myocardial infarction with versus without depression.

CAD, coronary artery disease; OR, odds ratio.

thought to be secondary to hypothalamic-pituitary-adrenal (HPA) hyperactivity (Musselman et al., 1996, 1998). Elevated levels of plasma cortisol may contribute to vascular damage by inducing hypercholesterolemia and hypertension (Troxler et al., 1977). Direct effects of catecholamine on the heart and blood vessels also promote vascular injury. There may also be a connection between catecholamine and platelet function; human platelets contain adrenergic and serotonergic receptors. Thus, either increased circulating levels of catecholamine or increased platelet 5-HT$_2$ binding sites may lead to increased platelet activation.

Hypothalamic-pituitary-adrenal hyperactivity may also contribute to the development of insulin resistance (Gold and Chrousos, 1999). Elevated plasma cortisol can cause hyperglycemia, which leads to insulin resistance. Furthermore, increased plasma cortisol, as well as other hormone abnormalities associated with depression, such as decreased secretion of growth hormone and sex steroids, can result in increased visceral fat, which can further contribute to insulin resistance (Troxler et al., 1977). The development of insulin resistance may explain, in part, the mechanism by which depression is a risk factor for the development of vascular disease. Insulin resistance promotes hypertension through multiple mechanisms including (1) increased renal tubular reabsorption of sodium, (2) increased sympathetic activity, and (3) proliferation of vascular smooth muscle. Furthermore, independent of its role in the development of insulin resistance, visceral fat promotes vascular damage by activating hepatic secretion of tumor necrosis factor. This initiates a cascade of events that ultimately results in an inflammatory process now recognized as a critical component in the pathogenesis of atherosclerosis. Recently, a number of studies have reported that indices of inflammatory process are elevated in patients with depression (Appels et al., 2000).

## DEPRESSION AND SUDDEN CARDIOVASCULAR DEATH

The first observation that suggested a link between depression and cardiovascular disease was that depressed patients have an increased risk of sudden cardiovascular death (Malzberg, 1937). Though HPA hyperactivity and increased catecholamine activity may explain why depression is a risk factor for the development of vascular disease, these processes cannot explain why depression is associated with an increased frequency of sudden cardiac death in patients with IHD or in patients free of cardiac disease. The increased risk of sudden cardiovascular death in depressed patients with and without IHD is primarily the result of ventricular fibrillation. Ventricular fibrillation occurs when the heart receives an electrical stimulus during a brief vulnerable period of the cardiac cycle (repolarization) that is significantly greater than the threshold required to cause electrical instability of the myocardium. Activity in the central nervous system can significantly affect electrophysiological properties of the heart so as to decrease or increase the threshold for ventricular fibrillation, an effect that is presumably mediated through the autonomic nervous system. The threshold for ventricular fibrillation is lowered by increased sympathe-tic neuronal input to the heart, whereas increased parasympathetic tone raises the threshold and therefore reduces the risk of ventricular fibrillation.

Heart-rate variability is the standard deviation of successive R-to-R intervals in normal sinus rhythm, and reflects the interplay and balance between sympathetic and parasympathetic input on the cardiac pacemaker. Sudden cardiac death is presumed to result from ventricular arrhythmias; parasympathetic tone is protective with respect to the generation of arrhythmias, whereas sympathetic tone increases the vulnerability to arrhythmia. A noninvasive method of assessing the state of sympathetic and parasympathetic tone as they relate to cardiac function and the vulnerability to arrhythmia is the measurement of heart-rate variability. Heart-rate variability results from the moment-to-moment interplay between sympathetic and parasympathetic input on the cardiac pacemaker. Power spectral analysis separates heart-rate variability into high-, low-, and ultra-low-frequency domains that are of specific interest because high-frequency variability reflects parasympathetic tone, whereas the lower frequencies are indicators of sympathetic input (Akselrod et al., 1981; Pomeranz et al., 1985). In a patient free of cardiac disease, there is maximum interplay between parasympathetic and sympathetic input, resulting in the full range of heart-rate variability. Restricted heart-rate variability, resulting primarily from increased sympathetic or decreased parasympathetic input, is present in many forms of cardiac disease and generally is a predictor of a poor prognosis (Kleiger et al., 1987).

Measurements of heart-rate variability in depressed patients show abnormalities that are interpreted to reflect an increased vulnerability to fatal arrhythmias. Studies of depressed patients without cardiac disease have consistently reported reduced variability, and some, though not all, studies have specifically reported reduced high-frequency variability indicating decreased parasympathetic tone (Roose et al., 1991b; Yeragani, 2000; Yeragani et al., 1991, 2000). In depressed patients with IHD, a study of post-MI patients reported that depressed patients had significantly deceased heart-rate variability compared to nondepressed patients (Carney et al., 2001).

Whereas sympathetic tone decreases heart-rate variability, it increases QT interval variability (Murakawa et al., 1992). Increased variability in the QT interval is also an indicator of vulnerability to arrhythmia, presumably because of an increased risk of R-on-T phenomena (Elming et al., 1998; Molnar et al., 1997), and is a strong predictor of mortality in cardiac patients (Bonnemeier et al., 2001; Vrtovec et al., 2000). Consistent with this finding is a recent report that depressed post-MI patients have increased QT variability compared to nondepressed post-MI patients (Carney et al., 2001).

In summary, the preponderance of data suggests that patients with depression have changes in autonomic nervous system balance, reflecting increased sympathetic tone and/or decreased parasympathetic tone, which may predispose them to a fatal arrhythmia, especially in the context of an ischemic event.

## TREATMENT OF DEPRESSION IN PATIENTS WITH ISCHEMIC HEART DISEASE

With respect to treatment, there are a number of questions relevant to both clinicians and researchers: (1) Does treatment of depression reduce the risk of developing IHD? (2) Are there safe and effective treatments for depression in patients with IHD? (3) Does treatment of depression in patients with IHD reduce cardiac morbidity and/or mortality? Not surprisingly, given the nature of the long-term prospective studies necessary, there are currently no systematic data available to address question 1. However, there are an increasing number of studies to address question 2, and results are just now becoming available from studies designed to answer question 3. Interpretation of data relevant to this question may be especially complex.

Treatment may increase or decrease the cardiac risk as a consequence of the physiological changes associated with resolution of a depressive episode or as a consequence of a direct or indirect medication effect independent of an antidepressant effect. If a reduction in cardiac mortality were a direct result of the treatment of depression, then it would be observed only in treatment responders. In contrast, if a treatment effect, either positive or negative, on cardiac status were not dependent on the antidepressant effect, then it would be observed equally in responders and nonresponders.

## THE CARDIOVASCULAR EFFECTS OF TRICYCLIC ANTIDEPRESSANTS

The cardiovascular effects of a therapeutic plasma level of a tricyclic antidepressant (TCA) have been extensively studied in depressed patients both with and without cardiovascular disease (Roose and Glassman, 1989). Most of the cardiovascular effects of the TCAs

are not problematic in a younger and healthy population. However, these same effects may cause significant adverse events in older and/or medically ill patients. In patients over age 60, TCAs routinely increase the heart rate by 11%; induce symptomatic orthostatic hypotension in 20%, which can result in falls and serious injuries; and slow cardiac conduction, which can result in two-to-one atrioventricular block in patients with preexisting bundle branch block. Tricyclics do not routinely have an adverse effect on ventricular function even in patients with severe left ventricular impairment. The electrophysiological profile of the TCAs, specifically an effect on the initial inward sodium current of the Purkinje fiber and a reduction of intraventricular conduction velocity, is similar to that of type 1A antiarrhythmic compounds such as quinidine and moricizine. It is this action that accounts for the antiarrhythmic effect of the TCAs at normal plasma levels. However, in an overdose, this activity results in a high rate of mortality secondary to ventricular arrhythmias and heart block.

Some of the cardiovascular effects of TCAs are mediated by actions thought to be unrelated to the therapeutic mechanism of action. For example, the increased heart rate caused by TCAs results primarily from the anticholinergic effect and is observed equally in responders and nonresponders. Though TCA-induced tachycardia is frequently symptomatic, an 11% increase in heart rate (e.g., from 72 to 80) will neither be experienced by the patient nor cause the clinician alarm in the course of an acute (6- to 8-week) antidepressant trial. Consequently, the potential for this effect to result in long-term adverse events has been overlooked. Depressed patients require antidepressant medications for a minimum of 6 months to treat a single depressive episode, and patients with recurrent illness must be treated indefinitely. After years of TCA treatment, the increased cardiac work associated with an 11% increase in heart rate may result in significant adverse events, especially in patients with IHD. There may be such a great separation in time from the occurrence of these adverse events to the initiation of antidepressant therapy that a cause-and-effect relationship can easily be missed.

## THE ANTIARRHYTHMIC EFFECT OF TRICYCLIC ANTIDEPRESSANTS: CARDIAC RISK RECONSIDERED

Given the robust therapeutic effectiveness of the TCAs, the awareness of their adverse cardiac events that forewarn the clinician, and the belief that treatment of depression would reduce the associated increase in cardiac mortality, it is not surprising that for a period of time, it was believed that in most circumstances there is a favorable risk-benefit ratio to TCA treatment in depressed patients with heart disease. However, results from the CAST (Cardiac Arrhythmia Suppression Trial) studies illuminated adverse cardiovascular effects of the TCAs not previously appreciated and led to a reconsideration of their safety in patients with IHD. The CAST trials tested the hypothesis that suppression of post-MI ventricular irritability would result in decreased mortality. The first study, CAST I, was prematurely discontinued by the data safety monitoring board because treatment with two of the three antiarrhythmics being tested, encainide and flecainide, was associated with a significant excess of deaths compared to placebo-treated controls (CAST, 1989). Encainide and flecainide are both type 1C antiarrhythmics, and it was not clear that the increase in mortality was associated with the third drug in the trial, moricizine, a drug with type 1A antiarrhythmic action. However, a second study, CAST II, which compared moricizine to placebo, also was prematurely discontinued when it became apparent that moricizine also induced an increase in mortality comparable to that of encainide and flecainide (CAST II, 1992).

Subsequent studies indicate that antiarrhythmic drugs may carry a risk of increased mortality not only in patients with ventricular arrhythmias post-MI but also in patients with a broader range of ischemic disease (Coplen et al., 1990; Falk 1989; Selzer and Wray, 1964). The current belief is that there is an interaction between the antiarrhythmic drug and ischemic myocardium, which results in an increased probability of ventricular fibrillation (Bigger 1990; Echt et al., 1991; Greenberg et al., 1995). If correct, this would imply that the risk of using a type 1 antiarrhythmic medication increases proportionately with the severity of IHD. The relevance of this information with respect to the treatment of depression is that TCAs are type 1A antiarrhythmics similar to moricizine. Therefore, it would be prudent to assume that TCAs carry a similar risk of increased mortality if given to depressed patients with IHD. Consequently, the treatment of depression with TCAs in patients with even mild IHD must be carefully considered, and TCA treatment may be relatively contraindicated in patients with severe ischemic disease (Glassman et al. 1993).

## TRICYCLIC ANTIDEPRESSANTS, HEART-RATE VARIABILITY, AND CARDIAC DEATH

Studies of TCAs in depressed patients with IHD indicate that these drugs decrease all heart-rate variability components including high-frequency variability, which reflects parasympathetic tone (Roose et al., 1991b; Yeragani et al., 1991, 2000). In a study comparing nortriptyline to paroxetine in depressed patients with IHD,

both heart-rate variability and high-frequency variability were significantly decreased in the nortriptyline-treated patients, but there was no effect on these measures in the paroxetine-treated patients (Roose et al., 1998b). Nortriptyline also significantly increased QT variability in patients with panic disorder, whereas paroxetine has no effect on any measure of heart-rate variability in this patient population (Yeragani et al., 2000). To date, multiple studies have consistently demonstrated that TCAs decrease all component measures of heart-rate variability and increase QT variability, whereas SSRIs, including paroxetine, fluoxetine, and sertraline, have shown no effect on heart-rate variability.

## THE CARDIOVASCULAR EFFECTS OF THE SELECTIVE SEROTONIN REUPTAKE INHIBITORS

Given the presumed risk of increased mortality associated with TCA use in patients with IHD, the obvious question is whether other classes of antidepressant medication offer a safe and effective alternative. Only the SSRIs have been extensively and systematically studied in patients with heart disease. Given the contribution of platelet aggregation to thrombus formation that results in ischemia, the SSRIs might be expected to decrease mortality because of their significant antiplatelet effect. There is some evidence to support this hypothesis. A study comparing the rate of MI in patients treated with an SSRI or with no antidepressant reported that the SSRI-treated patients had a significantly lower rate of MI than the non-SSRI-treated patients (Sauer et al., 2001). This result can be more directly attributed to the administration of the SSRI or the resolution of depression rather than to a nonspecific reduction of psychiatric symptoms because, in the same study, a comparison of patients treated with an anxiolytic versus no anxiolytic failed to show a similar reduction in the rate of MI in the medication-treated group.

In studies of depressed patients without heart disease, SSRIs neither slowed cardiac conduction nor induced orthostatic hypotension. Heart rate was slightly decreased (1–3 bpm); whether this effect may be greater in patients with sinus node dysfunction is not known. In contrast to the TCAs, the SSRIs are rarely lethal in overdosage (Barbey and Roose, 1998). Whereas TCAs decrease all components of heart-rate variability and increase QT variability, studies of paroxetine, fluoxetine, and sertraline report no effect on heart-rate variability or QT-variability measures.

Because of their efficacy, relatively benign side effect profile, and absence of adverse events in patients without cardiac disease, the SSRIs have been studied to determine their efficacy and safety in depressed patients with IHD.

## Fluoxetine

An open-label study was conducted to determine the cardiovascular effects of fluoxetine in depressed patients with cardiac disease (Roose et al., 1998a). Patients with major depression and at least one of the following conditions—an ejection fraction of ≤50%, 10 or more ventricular premature depolarizations per hour, and/or a QRS interval of at least 0.10 second—were started on 20 mg/day of fluoxetine, which was increased to 40 mg/day after 2 weeks and to 60 mg/day for 4 additional weeks if necessary. Cardiac testing, including radionuclide angiography and 24-hour ECG recordings, was conducted at baseline and after 7 weeks of treatment.

The study included 27 patients, mean age 73, 26% female; 44% had a history of MI, 52% of left ventricular impairment, and 63% of conduction defects. After 2 weeks of 20 mg/day fluoxetine, supine systolic blood pressure increased from 128 to 131 mmHg ($p = .02$), heart rate decreased from 78 to 73 bpm ($p = .0002$), and ejection fraction increased from 35% to 37.5% ($p = .05$). Fluoxetine did not prolong the PR, QRS, or QTc interval or have any effect on ventricular arrhythmias. Eight patients (30%) discontinued medication, including one patient with arrhythmia at baseline who developed increasing arrhythmia during the trial that continued to increase after drug discontinuation and was considered to be unrelated to the fluoxetine treatment.

Thus, in this relatively small sample of elderly depressed patients with cardiac disease, fluoxetine was relatively safe with respect to cardiovascular adverse events. An important caveat is that this study was not designed to test for drug–drug interactions. Fluoxetine and other SSRIs inhibit cytochrome P450 isoenzymes. The possibility of drug–drug interactions may be especially important in cardiac patients who are often taking multiple medications, many of which have a relatively narrow therapeutic range.

## Paroxetine

The one study of paroxetine in patients with cardiac disease is a multicenter, double-blind trial comparing the safety and efficacy of paroxetine to nortriptyline in depressed patients with IHD (Roose et al., 1998b). The inclusion criteria were a diagnosis of major depression and IHD, as evidenced by previous MI, a coronary artery bypass graft, angioplasty, a positive stress test, or angiographic findings of coronary luminal occlusion. After a 1-week single-blind, placebo treatment, patients were randomly assigned to 6 weeks of treatment with either paroxetine (20–30 mg/day) or nortriptyline (with the dose adjusted to achieve a plasma concentration of

80–120 ng/ml). Cardiac assessments, including 12-lead ECGs and 24-hour continuous ECG readings, were performed at baseline, after 2 weeks of treatment, and at the end point or week 6. Supine and standing blood pressures were measured weekly.

The mean age of the sample was 58 years, and there were no significant differences in baseline characteristics between the paroxetine and nortriptyline groups. With respect to the antidepressant effect, 61% of the paroxetine group and 55% of the nortriptyline group met remission criteria, defined as a final Hamilton Rating Scale of Depression (HRSD) score of <8. At end point, nortriptyline caused an 11% increase in heart rate but paroxetine had no effect. Neither drug caused clinically significant changes in blood pressure or cardiac conduction intervals. Heart-rate variability was significantly decreased at week 6 in the nortriptyline- but not the paroxetine-treated patients. Most important, the discontinuation rate due to cardiac adverse events was significantly greater in the nortriptyline group (7 of 40 [18%]) compared with the paroxetine group (1 of 41 [2%]; $p < .03$).

## Sertraline

Sertraline was the first antidepressant to be systematically studied in post-MI depressed patients (Shapiro et al., 1999). Patients with major depression, an MI within the past 30 days, and an ejection fraction ≥35% were treated openly with sertraline, 50 to 200 mg/day, for 16 weeks. Twenty-six patients, 58% male and with a mean age of 58, began medication treatment. There was no medication effect on heart rate, standing or supine blood pressure, or conduction intervals. No patient had a significant cardiac adverse event that required medication discontinuation.

The open trial of sertraline was followed up by the recently completed SADHART study (Sertraline Antidepressant Heart Attack Randomized Trial), which is the largest, and to date the most influential and important, study of antidepressant treatment in patients with IHD (Glassman et al., 2002). This double-blind, randomized, placebo-controlled trial was conducted in North America, Europe, and Australia. Patients with major depression and hospitalized for MI or unstable angina received 2 weeks of single-blind placebo followed by randomization to sertraline (flexible dose of 50 to 200 mg/day) or placebo for 24 weeks. A total of 369 patients were randomized, 74% were post-MI, and 26% had unstable angina; the sample was 64% male, with a mean age 57. The treatment effect was assessed using a continuous measure, the change in HRSD, and a dichotomous classification, responder/nonresponder, with a responder defined as a subject with a final global clinical impression score of 1 or 2 (very much improved: 85%–100%; much improved: 60%–85%). The treatment effect was evaluated in three groups of patients: (1) all randomized patients, (2) patients with recurrent depression, and (3) patients with at least two prior depressive episodes and a baseline HRSD score ≥18. For all three groups, sertraline had a significantly higher response rate than placebo: group 1—67% versus 53%, $p < .01$; group 2—72% versus 51%, $p < .003$; group 3—78% versus 45%, $p < .004$. The change in HRSD was significantly greater for sertraline only in groups 2 and 3: group 1—8.4 versus 7.6, $p = .14$; group 2—9.8 versus 7.6, $p < .009$; group 3—12.3 versus 8.9, $p < .001$.

Sertraline had no significant effect on heart rate, blood pressure, cardiac conduction, left ventricular function, ventricular ectopy, or any component of heart-rate variability. In a comparison of sertraline and placebo, there were no significant differences on any cardiovascular parameter assessed. An intriguing result of the study was that the incidence of severe cardiovascular adverse events (death, MI, congestive heart failure, angina, and stroke) was numerically, but not significantly, greater in the placebo group (22.4%) than in the sertraline group (14.5%). The published data to date do not report the frequency of severe cardiovascular adverse events in the depression responder versus nonresponder groups treated with medication and placebo. Therefore, whether the apparent improvement in cardiac morbidity and mortality in the sertraline group was associated with the resolution of depression or with the antiplatelet effect of the SSRIs cannot be determined. The results of this study extend the relative safety of the SSRIs, and of sertraline in particular, to treatment of depressed patients with unstable angina or immediately post-MI.

## OTHER ANTIDEPRESSANTS

### Bupropion

There is one study of bupropion treatment in depressed patients with congestive heart failure, conduction disturbances, or ventricular arrhythmias (Roose et al., 1991a). Thirty-six patients were treated openly with a starting dose of 150 mg/day that was raised to 450 mg/day over 1 week. Cardiovascular assessments, including radionuclide angiography and 24-hour continuous ECGs, were recorded at baseline and after 3 weeks of treatment. Lying and standing systolic and diastolic blood pressure was measured three times per day. After 3 weeks of bupropion treatment, there was a 5 mmHg increase in supine systolic ($p < .01$), a 3 mmHg increase in supine diastolic blood pressure ($p < .005$), and an 82% suppression of ventricular premature depolarization ($p < .005$). There was no significant effect on heart rate, ejection fraction, or cardiac conduction. Four patients experienced an adverse cardiac event: ex-

acerbation of hypertension (two patients), orthostatic drop resulting in a fall (one patient), and worsening of angina (one patient).

### Venlafaxine and Mirtazapine

Other antidepressant medications, particularly venlafaxine and mirtazapine, have not been systematically studied in depressed patients with IHD. Venlafaxine can induce sustained hypertension, and this effect is dose-related. The rate of sustained hypertension is reported as 3%–7% at a dose range of 100–300 mg/day, increasing to 13% at doses greater than 300 mg/day. The effect on blood pressure may reflect increased norepinephrine activity that is consistent with the dose effect. Increased noradrenergic activity results in sympathetic tone that is associated with increased QT variability. Therefore, there are theoretical reasons to wonder whether medications such as venlafaxine or mirtazapine may have long-term insidious negative cardiac effects that will not be detected without systematic study.

The concern about increased sympathetic tone, increased QT variability, and the risk of ventricular fibrillation also extends to another class of medications: stimulants that are frequently prescribed in older patients with medical illness and minor or major depression. In older medically ill and nursing home residents, the baseline prevalence rate of sudden cardiovascular death is high. Thus, even if stimulant medication were associated with a significant increase in QT variability and resultant sudden cardiac death, without systematic study this effect may go undetected in the clinical setting.

## PSYCHOTHERAPY

Although there have been a number of studies of psychosocial interventions in post-MI patients, to date only one large study has tested a psychotherapy treatment in a depressed post-MI sample. The Enhancing Recovery in Coronary Heart Disease Patients Randomized Trial (ENRICHD) included 2481 post-MI patients, 56% male, with a mean age of 61 (Writing Committee for the ENRICHD, 2003). Patients were entered if they met criteria for major or minor depression, dysthymia, or low perceived social support. Patients were randomized to treatment with cognitive-behavioral therapy for up to 6 months or treatment as usual. A major complicating feature of the study design was that all patients in the intervention group with a baseline HRSD score >24, or without at least a 50% reduction in BDI scores after 5 weeks of therapy, were started on antidepressant medication, primarily sertraline. At the 6-month evaluation point there was a statistically significant ($p < .001$), but modest and of questionable clinical significance (1.7 HRSD points), difference in the change in

HRSD in the intervention group compared to the treatment-as-usual group. After an average follow-up of 29 months, there was no significant difference in cardiac event–free survival between the intervention and comparator groups, 75.8% and 75.9%, respectively. However, medication treatment was associated with a lower risk of nonfatal MI and death in both the intervention and treatment-as-usual patients. The intervention treatment had no benefit on cardiac outcomes in patients who did not receive medication. Thus, the ENRICHD study further suggests that antidepressant treatment may produce lower cardiac morbidity and mortality rates in depressed post-MI patients, but it does not help clarify whether the outcome results from resolution of depression or the antiplatelet effects of the SSRIs.

## CONCLUSION

There is a growing body of evidence that depression significantly and adversely affects cardiovascular health. Depression is a risk factor for the development of IHD and is associated with increased cardiac morbidity and mortality in a wide range of patients with IHD, most notably post-MI patients. Treatment with SSRIs appears to be relatively safe in depressed patients with IHD and may improve the cardiac outcomes. However, by virtue of age and cardiac illness, many of these patients are taking multiple medications before the initiation of antidepressant therapy, so special attention must be paid to the potential for drug–drug interactions.

REFERENCES

Ahern, D.K., Gorkin, L., Anderson, J.L., Tierney, C., Ewart, C., Capone, R.J., et al. (1990) Biobehavioral variables and mortality or Cardiac Arrhythmia Pilot Study (CAPS). *Am J Cardiol* 66:59–62.

Akselrod, S., Gordon, D., Ubel, F.A., Shannon, D.C., Barger, A.C., and Cohen, R.J. (1981) Power spectrum analysis of heart rate fluctuation: a quantitative probe of beat-to-beat cardiovascular control. *Science* 213:220–222.

Anda, R., Williamson, D., Jones, D., et al. (1993) Depressed affect, hopelessness, and the risk of ischemic heart disease in a cohort of U.S. adults [comment]. *Epidemiol* 4:285–294.

Appels, A.D., Barr, F.W., Bar, J., Bruggeman, C., and DeBaets, M. (2000) Inflammation, depressive symptomatology, and coronary artery disease. *Psychosom Med* 62:601–605.

Aromaa, A., Raitasalo, R., Reunanen, A., Impivaara, O., Heliovaara, M., Knekt, P.K., et al. (1994) Depression and cardiovascular diseases. *Acta Psychiatr Scand* 377(S):77–82.

Barbey, J.T., and Roose, S.P. (1998) SSRI safety in overdose. *J Clin Psychiatry* 59(suppl 15):42–48.

Barefoot, J.C., Helms, M.J., Mark, D.B., Blumenthal, J.A., Califf, R.M., Haney, T.L., et al. (1996) Depression and long-term mortality risk in patients with coronary artery disease. *Am J Cardiol* 78:613–617.

Bigger, J.T., Jr. (1990) Implications of the cardiac arrhythmia suppression trial for antiarrhythmic drug treatment. *Am J Cardiol* 65:3D–10D.

Blumenthal, J.A., and Emery, C.F. (1988) Rehabilitation of patients following myocardial infarction. *J Consult Clin Psychol* 56:374–381.

Bonnemeier, H., Hartmann, F., Wiegand, U.K., Bode, F., Katus, H.A., and Richard, G. (2001) Course and prognostic implications of QT interval and QT interval variability after primary coronary angioplasty in acute myocardial infarction. *J Am Coll Cardiol* 37:44–50.

Cardiac Arrhythmia Suppression Trial (CAST) Investigators. (1989) Preliminary report: Effect of encainide and flecainide on mortality in a randomized trial of arrhythmia suppression after myocardial infarction. *N Engl J Med* 321:406–412.

Cardiac Arrhythmia Suppression Trial II Investigators. (1992) Effect of the antiarrhythmic agent moricizine on survival after myocardial infarction. *N Engl J Med* 327:227–233.

Carney, R.M., Berkman, L.F., Blumenthal, J.A., et al, (2001) Heart rate variability and depression in patients with a recent acute myocardial infarction (abstract). *Psychosom Med* 63:102.

Carney, R.M., Rich, M.W., Freedland, K.E., teVelde, A.J., Saini, J., Simeone, C., et al. (1988) Major depressive disorder predicts cardiac events in patients with coronary artery disease. *Psychosom Med* 50:627–633.

Carney, R.M., Rich, M.W., teVelde, A.J., Freedland, K.E., Saini, J., Simeone, C., et al. (1987) Major depressive disorders in coronary artery disease. *Am J Cardiol* 60:1273–1275.

Coplen, S.E., Antman, E.M., Berlin, J.A., Hewitt, P., and Chalmers, T.C. (1990) Efficacy and safety of quinidine therapy for maintenance of sinus rhythm after cardioversion: A meta-analysis of randomized control trials. *Circulation* 82:1106–1116.

Denollet, J., and Brutsaert, D.L. (1998) Personality, disease severity, and the risk of long term cardiac events in patients with a decreased ejection fraction after myocardial infarction {comment}. *Circulation* 97:167–173.

Dew, M.A., Kormos, R.L., Roth, L.H., Murali, S., DiMartini, A.F., and Griffith, B.P. (1999) Early post-transplant medical compliance and mental health predict physical morbidity and mortality one to three years after heart transplantation. *J Heart Lung Transplant* 18:549–562.

Echt, D.S., Liebson, P.R., Mitchell, L.B., et al. (1991) Mortality and morbidity in patients receiving encainide, flecainide, or placebo. The Cardiac Arrhythmia Suppression Trial. *N Engl J Med* 324:781–788.

Elming, H., Holm, E., Jun, L., Torp-Pedersen, C., Kober, L., Kirschoff, M., Malik, M., and Camm, J. (1998) The prognostic value of the QT interval and QT interval dispersion in all cause and cardiac mortality and morbidity in a population of Danish citizens. *Eur Heart J* 19:1391–1400.

Falk, R.H. (1989) Flecainide-induced ventricular tachycardia and fibrillation in patients treated for atrial fibrillation. *Ann Intern Med* 111:107–111.

Ford, D.E., Mead, L.A., Change, P.P., Cooper-Patrick, L., Wang, N.Y., and Klag, M.J. (1998) Depression is a risk factor for coronary artery disease in men. *Arch Intern Med* 158:1422–1426.

Forrester, A.W., Lipsey, J.R., Teitelbaum, M.L., DePaulo, J.R., Andrzejewski, P.L., and Robinson, R.G. (1992) Depression following myocardial infarction. *Int J Psychiatry Med* 22:33–46.

Frasure-Smith, N., Lespérance, F., and Talajic, M. (1993) Depression following myocardial infarction: Impact on 6 month survival. *JAMA* 270:1819–1825.

Frasure-Smith, N., Lespérance, F., and Talajic, M. (1995) Depression and 18 month prognosis after myocardial infarction. *Circulation* 91:999–1005.

Glassman, A.H., O'Connor, C.M., Califf, R.M., Swedberg, K., Schwartz, P., Bigger, J.T., Jr., Krishnan, K.R.R., vanZyl, L.T., Swenson, J.R., et al. (2002) Sertraline treatment of major depression in patients with acute MI or unstable angina. *JAMA* 288:701–709.

Glassman, A.H., Roose, S.P., and Bigger, J.T., Jr. (1993) The safety of tricyclic antidepressants in cardiac patients. Risk/benefit reconsidered. *JAMA* 269:2673–2675.

Glassman, A.H., and Shapiro, P.A. (1998) Depression and the course of coronary artery disease. *Am J Psychiatry* 155:4–11.

Gold, P.W., and Chrousos, G.P. (1999) The endocrinology of melancholic and atypical depression: Relation to neurocircuitry and somatic consequences. *Proc Assoc Am Physicians* 111(1):22–34.

Gonzalez, M.B., Snyderman, T.B., Colket, J.T., Arias, R.M., Jiang, J.W., O'Connor, C.M., et al. (1996) Depression in patients with coronary artery disease. *Depression* 4:57–62.

Greenberg, H.M., Dwyer, E.M., Jr., Hochman, J.S., Steinberg, J.S., Echt, D.S., and Peters, R.W. (1995) Interaction of ischemia and encainide/flecainide treatment: A proposed mechanism for the increased mortality in CAST I. *Br Heart J* 74:631–635.

Hallstrom, T., Lapidus, L., Bengtsson, C., et al. (1986) Psychosocial factors and risk of ischaemic heart disease and death in women: A twelve-year follow-up of participants in the population study of women in Gothenburg, Sweden. *J Psychosom Res* 30:451–459.

Hance, M., Carney, R.M., Freedland, K.E., and Skala, J. (1995) Depression in patients with coronary heart disease: A twelve month follow-up. *Gen Hosp Psychiatry* 18:61–65.

Kleiger, R.E., Miller, J.P., Bigger, J.T., and Moss, A.J. (1987) Decreased heart rate variability and its association with increased mortality after acute myocardial infarction. *Am J Cardiol* 59:256–262.

Kaufman, D.W., Helmrich, S.P., Rosenberg, L., Miettinen, O.S., and Shapiro, S. (1983) Nicotine and carbon monoxide content of cigarette smoke and the risk of myocardial infarction in young men. *N Engl J Med* 308:409–413.

Koenig, H.G., George, L.K., Peterson, B.L., and Pieper, C.F. (1997) Depression in medically ill hospitalized older adults: Prevalence, characteristics, and course of symptoms according to six diagnostic schemes. *Am J Psychiatry* 154:1376–1383.

Koenig, H.G., Meador, K.G., Cohen, H.J., and Blazer, D.G. (1988) Detection and treatment of major depression in older medically ill hospitalized patients. *Int J Psychiatry Med* 18:17–31.

Ladwig, K.H., Kieser, M., Konig, J., Breithardt, G., and Borggrefe, M. (1991) Affective disorders and survival after acute myocardial infarction. *Eur Heart J* 12:959–964.

Lespérance, F., Frasure-Smith, N., Juneau, M., and Théroux, P. (2000) Depression and 1-year prognosis in unstable angina. *Arch Intern Med* 160:1354–1360.

Malzberg, B. (1937) Mortality among patients with involution melancholia. *Am J Psychiatry* 93:1231–1238.

Mendes de Leon, C.F., Krumholz, H.M., Seeman, T.S., et al. (1998) Depression and risk of coronary heart disease in elderly men and women: New Haven EPESE, 1982–1991. Established Populations for the Epidemiologic Studies of the Elderly. *Arch Intern Med* 158:2341–2348.

Molnar, J., Rosenthal, J.E., Weiss, J.S., and Somberg, J.C. (1997) QT interval dispersion in healthy subjects and survivors of sudden cardiac death: Circadian variation in a twenty-four-hour assessment. *Am J Cardiol* 79:1190–1193.

Murakawa, Y., Inoue, H., Nozaki, A., and Sugimoto, T. (1992) Role of sympathovagal interaction in diurnal variation of QT interval. *Am J Cardiol* 69:339–343.

Musselman, D.L., Evans, D.L., and Nemeroff, C.B. (1998) The relationship of depression to cardiovascular disease: Epidemiology, biology, and treatment. *Arch Gen Psychiatry* 55:580–592.

Musselman, D.L., Marzec, U.M., Manatunga, A., et al. (2000) Platelet reactivity in depressed patients treated with paroxetine: Preliminary findings. *Arch Gen Psychiatry* 57:875–882.

Musselman, D.L., Tomer, A., Manatunga, A.K., Knight, B.T., Porter, M.R., Kasey, S., et al. (1996) Exaggerated platelet reactivity in major depression. *Am J Psychiatry* 153:1212–1217.

Pollock, B.G., Laghrissi-Thode, F., and Wagner, W.R. (2000) Evaluation of platelet activation in depressed patients with ischemic heart disease after paroxetine or nortriptyline treatment. *J Clin Psychopharmacol* 20:137–140.

Pomeranz, B., Macaulay, R.J., Caudill, M.A., Kutz, I., Adam, D., Gordon, D., Kilborn, K.M., Barger, A.C., Shannon, D.C., Cohen, R.J., and Benson, H. (1985) Assessment of autonomic function in humans by heart rate spectral analysis. *Am J Physiol* 248(1, Pt 2):H151–H153.

Pratt, L.A., Ford, D.E., Crum, R.M., et al. (1996) Depression, psychotropic medication, and risk of myocardial infarction: Prospective data from the Baltimore ECA follow-up. *Circulation* 94:3123–3129.

Roose, S.P., Dalack, G.W., Glassman, A.H., Woodring, S., Walsh, B.T., and Giardina, E.G.V. (1991a) Cardiovascular effects of bupropion in depressed patients with heart disease. *Am J Psychiatry* 148:512–516.

Roose, S.P., Dalack, G.W., and Woodring, S. (1991b) Death, depression, and heart disease. *J Clin Psychiatry* Suppl 52:34–39.

Roose, S.P., and Glassman, A.H. (1989) Cardiovascular effects of TCAs in depressed patients with and without heart disease. *J Clin Psychiatry Monograph* 7(2):1–19.

Roose, S.P., Glassman, A.H., Attia, E., Woodring, S., Giardina, E.G.V., and Bigger, J.T., Jr. (1998a) Cardiovascular effects of fluoxetine in depressed patients with heart disease. *Am J Psychiatry* 155(5):660–665.

Roose, S.P., Laghrissi-Thode, F., Kennedy, J.S., Nelson, J.C., Bigger, J.T. Jr., Pollock, B.G., et al. (1998b) Comparison of paroxetine and nortriptyline in depressed patients with ischemic heart disease. *JAMA* 279(4):287–291.

Sauer, W.H., Berlin, J.A., and Kimmel, S.E. (2001) Selective serotonin reuptake inhibitors and myocardial infarction. *Circulation* 104:1894–1898.

Schleifer, S.J., Macari-Hinson, M.M., Coyle, D.A., Slater, W.R., Kahn, M., Gorlin, R., et al. (1989) The nature and course of depression following myocardial infarction. *Arch Intern Med* 149:1785–1789.

Selzer, A., and Wray, H.W. (1964) Quinidine syncope: Paroxysmal ventricular fibrillation occurring during treatment of chronic atrial arrhythmias. *Circulation* 10:17–26.

Shapiro, P.A., Lespérance, F., Frasure-Smith, N., et al., for the Sertraline Anti-Depressant Heart Attack Trial. (1999) An open-label preliminary trial of sertraline for treatment of major depression after acute myocardial infarction (the SADHAT Trial). *Am Heart J* 137:1100–1106.

Stern, J.J., Pascale, L., and Ackerman, A. (1977) Life adjustment post myocardial infarction: Determining predictive variables. *Arch Intern Med* 137:1680–1685.

Travella, J.I., Forrester, A.W., Schultz, S.K., and Robinson, R.G. (1994) Depression following myocardial infarction: A one year longitudinal study. *Int J Psychiatry Med* 24(4):357–369.

Troxler, R.G., Sprague, E.A., Albanese, R.A., Fuchs, R., and Thompson, A.J. (1977) The association of elevated plasma cortisol and early atherosclerosis as demonstrated by coronary angiography. *Atherosclerosis* 26:151–162.

Vrtovec, B., Starc, V., and Starc, R. (2000) Beat-to-beat QT interval variability in coronary patients. *J Electrocardiol* 33:119–125.

Wassertheil-Smoller, S., Applegate, W.B., Berge, K., et al. (1996) Change in depresssion as a precursor of cardiovascular events. SHEP Cooperative Research Group (Systolic Hypertension in the Elderly Project). *Arch Intern Med* 156:553–561.

Writing Committee for the ENRICHD Investigators. (2003) Effects of treating depression and low perceived social support on clinical events after nyocardial infarction. *JAMA* 289(23):3106–3116.

Yeragani, V.K. (2000) Major depression and long-term heart period variability. *Depression Anxiety* 12:51–52.

Yeragani, V.K., Pohl, R., Balon, R., Ramesh, C., Glitz, D., Jung, I., and Sherwood, P. (1991) Heart rate variability in patients with major depression. *Psychiatry Res* 37:35–46.

Yeragani, V.K., Pohl, R., Jampala, V.C., Balon, R., Ramesh, C., and Srinivasan, K. (2000) Increased QT variability in patients with panic disorder and depression. *Psychiatry Res* 93:225–235.

# 26 | Vascular disease and late-life depression: stroke

ROBERT G. ROBINSON

Cerebrovascular disease is the third leading cause of mortality in the elderly and therefore represents a major public health problem in all industrialized countries (American Heart Association, 1996). Cerebrovascular disease includes a wide range of disorders from atherosclerotic narrowing of cerebral blood vessels leading to transitory ischemia, to permanent brain infarction due to an intramural thrombus or an embolic infarction caused by the breakup of thrombi within the heart or large arterial vessels that travel to the brain, to hemorrhagic phenomena caused by weakness of the vascular wall. Stroke is defined as a sudden loss of the blood supply to the brain leading to permanent tissue damage. This chapter will focus on depression associated with stroke caused by thrombotic, embolic, or hemorrhagic events.

Stroke is the most common serious neurological disorder in the world and accounts for half of all the acute hospitalizations for neurological disease (Hachinski and Norris, 1985). The age-specific incidence of stroke varies dramatically over the life course. The annual incidence in developed countries around the world among persons aged 55 to 64 ranges from 10 to 20 per 10,000, while among those over age 85 the incidence is almost 200 per 10,000 (Bonita, 1992).

The association of depression with cerebrovascular disease has been recognized by clinicians for almost 100 years, but it is only within the past 30 years that systematic studies of depression following stroke have been conducted.

## HISTORICAL PERSPECTIVE

Early reports of depression after brain damage (usually caused by cerebrovascular disease) were made by neurologists and psychiatrists in case descriptions. Meyer (1904) warned that new discoveries of cerebral localization in the early 1900s, such as language function, led to an overly hasty identification of centers and functions of the brain. He identified several disorders such as delirium, dementia, and aphasia that were the direct

result of brain injury. In keeping with his view of biopsychosocial causes of most mental "reactions," however, he saw manic-depressive illness and paranoiac conditions as arising from a combination of brain injury (specifically citing left frontal lobe and cortical convexities) and a family history of psychiatric disorder and premorbid personal psychiatric disorders to produce the specific mental reaction. Bleuler (1951, p. 230) noted that after stroke, "melancholic moods lasting for months and sometimes longer appear frequently." Kraepelin (1921, p. 271) recognized an association between manic-depressive insanity and cerebrovascular disease. He stated that "the diagnosis of states of depression may offer difficulties, especially when arteriosclerosis is involved." Kraepelin concluded that cerebrovascular disorder may be a phenomenon accompanying manic-depressive disease or may itself produce depressive disorder.

Despite the assertions by Kraepelin (1921) and others that emotional disorder may be produced directly by focal brain injury, many investigators have adopted *psychological* explanations for poststroke depression. Studies in which the emotional symptoms specifically associated with cerebrovascular disease were examined began to appear in the early 1960s. Ullman and Gruen (1960) reported that stroke was a particularly severe stress to the patient, as Goldstein (1942) had suggested, because the organ governing the emotional response to injury had itself been damaged. Fisher (1961, p. 379) described depression associated with cerebrovascular disease as reactive and understandable because "the brain is the most cherished organ of humanity." Thus, depression was viewed as a natural emotional response to a decrease in self-esteem from a life-threatening injury and the resulting disability and dependence.

Systematic studies, however, led other investigators, impressed by the frequency of the association between depression and brain injury, to hypothesize more direct causal links. In a study of 100 elderly patients with affective disorder, Post (1962) stated that the high frequency of brain ischemia associated with first episodes of depressive disorder suggested that the causes for atherosclerosis and depression may be linked. Folstein et al. (1977) compared 20 stroke patients with 10 orthopedic patients and found that, although the functional disability in both groups was comparable, more of the stroke patients were depressed. These authors concluded that "mood disorder was a more specific complication of stroke than simply a response to motor disability" (p. 1018).

Thus, poststroke depression has been viewed historically either as an understandable psychological reaction to the associated impairment or as the direct result of injury to specific structures within neuronal circuits mediating depression.

## DIAGNOSIS OF POSTSTROKE DEPRESSION

Although strict diagnostic criteria have not been used in some studies of depression associated with cerebrovascular disease (Andersen et al., 1993), most studies have used structured interviews and diagnostic criteria defined by DSM-III-R (American Psychiatric Association, 1987, 1994) or Research Diagnostic Criteria (Eastwood et al., 1989; Morris et al., 1990; Robinson et al., 1983a; Spitzer et al., 1978). Poststroke major depression is now categorized in DSM-IV-TR, (American Psychiatric Association, 2000) as "mood disorder due to stroke with major depressive-like episode" (p. 404). For patients with less severe forms of depression, there are "research criteria" in DSM-IV for minor depression (i.e., subsyndromal major depression characterized by depression or anhedonia with at least one but fewer than four additional symptoms of major depression) or, alternatively, a DSM-IV diagnosis of "mood disorder due to stroke with depressive features."

Investigators of depression associated with physical illness have debated the most appropriate method for the diagnosis of depression when some symptoms (e.g., sleep or appetite disturbance) can result from the physical illness. Cohen-Cole and Stoudemire (1987) re-

ported that four approaches have been used to assess depression in the physically ill. These are the *inclusive approach*, in which depressive diagnostic symptoms are counted regardless of whether they may be related to physical illness (Rifkin et al., 1985); the *etiological approach*, in which a symptom is counted only if the diagnostician feels that it is not caused by the physical illness (Rapp and Vrana, 1989); the *substitutive approach*, in which other psychological symptoms of depression replace the vegetative symptoms (Endicott, 1984); and the *exclusive approach*, in which symptoms are removed from the diagnostic criteria if they are not found to be more frequent in depressed than nondepressed patients. (Bukberg et al., 1984)

Paradiso et al. (1997) have examined the utility of these methods in the diagnosis of poststroke depression (PSD) during the first 2 years following stroke. Among 205 patients with acute stroke, 142 patients were followed up for examination at 3, 6, 12, or 24 months following stroke. The patients who were not included in the follow-up had either died, could not be located, or refused to attend follow-up evaluations. Of 142 patients with follow-up, 60 (42%) reported having a depressed mood (depressed group) while they were in the hospital and the remaining 82 patients were nondepressed. There were no significant differences in the background characteristics of the depressed and nondepressed groups except that the depressed group was significantly younger ($p = .006$) and had a significantly more frequent personal history of psychiatric disorder ($p = .04$).

The frequency of vegetative symptoms in the hospital and at each of the follow-up visits is shown in Table 26.1. Throughout the 2-year follow-up period, the depressed patients demonstrated both vegetative and psychological symptoms more frequently than the nondepressed patients. The only symptoms that were not more frequent in the depressed patients were weight loss and early awakening at the initial evaluation; weight loss and early morning awakening at 6 months;

TABLE 26.1. *Number of Patients with Vegetative Depressive Symptoms at Each Post-Stroke Evaluation*

| | Initial Evaluation | | 3-Month Follow-Up | | 6-Month Follow-Up | | 1-Year Follow-Up | | 2-Year Follow-Up | |
|---|---|---|---|---|---|---|---|---|---|---|
| | Dep Mood | Non-Dep Mood | Dep Mood | Non-Dep Mood | Dep Mood | Non-Dep Mood | Dep Mood | Non-Dep Mood | Dep Mood | Non-Dep Mood |
| Autonomic anxiety | 23 (39) | 4 (5)* | 15 (52) | 5 (11)* | 18 (58) | 7 (15)* | 9 (45) | 6 (12)* | 16 (64) | 8 (20)* |
| Anxious foreboding | 21 (36) | 8 (10)* | 13 (46) | 3 (6)* | 9 (29) | 7 (15) | 4 (20) | 4 (8) | 11 (44) | 2 (5)* |
| Morning depression | 38 (63) | 4 (5)* | 17 (67) | 2 (4)* | 20 (65) | 2 (4)* | 11 (55) | 2 (4)* | 17 (68) | 0 (0)* |
| Weight loss | 20 (34) | 16 (20) | 6 (22) | 3 (6) | 10 (32) | 11 (24) | 4 (20) | 2 (4) | 7 (28) | 6 (15) |
| Delayed sleep | 24 (40) | 12 (15)* | 10 (36) | 9 (19) | 15 (48) | 7 (15)* | 8 (40) | 5 (10)* | 11 (44) | 2 (5)* |
| Subjective anergia | 35 (58) | 16 (20)* | 17 (61) | 12 (28)* | 19 (61) | 10 (22)* | 10 (50) | 8 (16)* | 15 (60) | 10 (24)* |
| Early awakening | 16 (27) | 13 (16) | 9 (32) | 8 (17) | 4 (13) | 7 (15) | 3 (15) | 3 (6) | 11 (44) | 5 (12)* |
| Loss of libido | 16 (27) | 7 (9)* | 12 (46) | 11 (12)* | 12 (39) | 6 (14)* | 5 (25) | 7 (14) | 11 (44) | 10 (24) |

*Significant at the .05 level.

weight loss, early morning awakening, anxious foreboding, and loss of libido at 1 year; and weight loss and loss of libido at 2 years. The depressed patients had a higher frequency of most psychological symptoms throughout the 2-year follow-up period. The only psychological symptoms that were not significantly more frequent in the depressed than in the nondepressed group were suicide plans, simple ideas of reference, and pathological guilt at 3 months; pathological guilt at 6 months; pathological guilt, suicide plans, guilty ideas of reference, and irritability at 1 year; and pathological guilt and self-depreciation at 2 years.

The effect of using each of the proposed alternative diagnostic methods for poststroke depression using DSM-IV criteria was examined. The symptoms were obtained using the inclusive approach (i.e., symptoms that the patients acknowledged were included as positive even if there was some suspicion that the symptoms may have been related to the physical illness). Thus, the initial diagnoses were based on the inclusive criteria. During the in-hospital evaluation, 26 of 142 patients (18%) met DSM-IV diagnostic criteria for major depression. Using the exclusive approach, diagnostic criteria required five or more specific symptoms (i.e., we excluded weight loss and early morning awakening from DSM-IV diagnostic criteria because they were not significantly more frequent in the depressed than the nondepressed patients). Of 27 patients with major depression, 3 were excluded. Compared to diagnoses based solely on the existence of five or more specific symptoms for the diagnosis of DSM-IV major depression, diagnoses based on unmodified symptoms (i.e., early awakening and weight loss included) had a specificity of 98% and a sensitivity of 100%.

The exclusive diagnostic criteria were then used to examine the substitutive approach (i.e., all vegetative symptoms were eliminated, and the presence of four psychological symptoms plus depressed mood was required for the diagnosis of major depression). Using this approach, none of the original 27 patients with major depression was excluded. In addition, four patients presented with four or more specific symptoms of major depression but denied having a depressed mood. These cases may represent *masked* depression.

Similar results were found at 3, 6, 12, and 24 months of follow-up. The unmodified DSM-IV criteria consistently showed a sensitivity of 100% and a specificity that ranged from 95% to 98% compared to criteria using only specific symptoms. Thus, one could reasonably conclude that modifying DSM-IV criteria because of the existence of an acute medical illness is probably unnecessary.

These findings also suggest that the nature of PSD may change over time. Since the symptoms specific to depression changed over time, this may reflect an alteration in the underlying etiology of PSD associated with early-onset depression compared to the late or chronic poststroke period.

Gainotti et al. (1999) examined the phenomenology of PSD using their own Poststroke Depression Rating Scale (PSDRS). The scale includes 10 items: depressed mood, guilt feelings, thoughts of death or suicide, vegetative symptoms, apathy and loss of interest, anxiety, catastrophic reactions, hyperemotionalism, anhedonia, and diurnal mood variations. The last section on diurnal mood variations is scored between +2 and −2. A score of +2 indicates a motivated depression associated with situational stresses, handicaps, or disabilities. A score of −2 indicates that a lack of motivation associated with depression is more prominent in the early morning.

Gainotti et al. (1999) compared patients with major depression who were less than 2 months (n = 58), 2–4 months (n = 52), and more than 4 months (n = 43) post-stroke, using this scale and compared them to 30 patients admitted to a psychiatric hospital with a diagnosis of endogenous major depression. Although statistical adjustments controlling for the large number of comparisons were not made, the data indicated that patients with endogenous depression (i.e., no associated brain injury) had higher scores on suicide and anhedonia, while patients with PSD had higher scores on catastrophic reactions, hyperemotionalism, and diurnal mood variation. These findings were construed to support an association of depression with disability.

Gainotti et al. (1999) asserted that failure to assess these aspects of depression (included in the PSDRS) indicates methodological errors in the assessment of depression by Robinson et al. (1984a). There are, however, clearly established criteria for the diagnosis of major depression, as validated by numerous studies supporting DSM-IV-TR (American Psychiatric Association, 2000). Catastrophic reactions, hyperemotionalism, and diurnal variations (which are scored on the basis of the patients' attribution of their depression to life stressors and disability) are clearly idiosyncratic criteria for the diagnosis of depression arbitrarily added to the diagnostic criteria to show differences from primary depression. Both catastrophic reactions and hyperemotionalism, however, occur in patients without depression indicating the co-morbid nature of these conditions and not symptoms which are integral to the diagnosis of depression (Robinson et al., 1993; Starkstein et al., 1993). The addition of symptoms to the widely accepted criteria for depression must be validated as defining a specific population of patients with a unique PSD disorder. Validation of this new form of depressive disorder should include demonstration of the predictable duration of the disorder, specific associated clinical and pathological correlates, and responses to treatment that are not found when standard criteria are used. The only evidence available in the studies that compared primary depression and PSD using standard criteria indicated a close correspondence between these two forms of depression in the elderly (Lipsey et al., 1986).

## PREVALENCE OF DEPRESSION

Over the past 10 years, a large number of studies throughout the world have examined the prevalence of PSD. These studies indicate an increasing interest among clinicians caring for patients with stroke in the frequency and effect of depression on the long-term outcome. The results of these studies are shown in Table 26.2. In general, these studies found similar rates of major and minor depression among patients hospitalized for acute stroke, in rehabilitation hospitals, and in outpatient clinics. Based on pooled data, the mean prevalence of major depression among patients in acute and rehabilitation hospitals was 22% for major depression and 17% for minor depression. Among patients studied in community settings, however, the mean prevalence of major depression was 13% and that of minor depression was 10%. Thus, PSD is common both among patients receiving treatment for stroke as well as among community samples. The higher rate of depression among patients receiving treatment for stroke is probably related to the greater severity of stroke seen in treatment settings compared to community settings. Reports using community samples have included many patients with no physical or intellectual impairment and only a clinical history of stroke.

## DURATION OF DEPRESSION

A consecutive series of 103 acute stroke patients were prospectively studied in a 2-year longitudinal study of PSD (Robinson et al., 1987). At the time of the initial in-hospital evaluation, 26% of the patients had the symptom cluster of major depression and 20% had the symptom cluster of minor depression. Although both major and minor depressive disorders were still present in 86% of patients with in-hospital major or minor depression at the 6-month follow-up evaluation, only one of five patients with major depression continued to have major depression at 1-year follow-up (two patients had minor depression). Patients with minor depression had a less favorable prognosis; only 40% had no depression at 1-year follow-up, and only 30% had no depression at 2-year follow-up. In addition, about 30% of patients who were not depressed in the hospital became depressed after discharge. Thus, the natural duration of major depression appeared to be between 6 months and 1 year. The duration of minor depression was more variable, and in many cases the patients appeared to be chronically depressed.

Morris et al. (1990) found that among a group of 99 patients in a stroke rehabilitation hospital in Australia, those with major depression had a duration of 40 weeks, whereas those with adjustment disorders (minor depression) had a duration of depression of only 12 weeks. These findings confirm that major depression has a duration of approximately 9 months to 1 year but suggest that less severe depressive disorders may be more variable in their duration. Astrom et al. (1993) found that among 80 patients with acute stroke, 27 developed major depression in the hospital or at 3-month follow-up. Of those patients with major depression, 15 (60%) had recovered by 1-year follow-up, but by 3-year follow-up, only 1 more patient had recovered. This finding indicates that there may be a minority of patients with either major or minor depression who develop prolonged PSD. Thus, although all studies found that the majority of depressions were less than 1 year in duration, the mean frequency of major depression that persisted beyond 1 year was 26%.

## RELATIONSHIP TO LESION VARIABLES

The relationship between depressive disorder and lesion location is perhaps the most controversial area of research in the field of poststroke mood disorder. Although elucidating the association between specific clinical symptomatology and lesion location is one of the fundamental goals of clinical practice in neurology, this has rarely been the case with psychiatric disorders. Cognitive functions, speech impairment, and the extent and severity of motor or sensory impairment are all symptoms of stroke that are commonly used by clinicians to localize lesions to particular brain regions. There is, however, no known neuropathology consistently associated with primary mood disorders (i.e., mood disorders without known brain injury) or secondary mood disorders (i.e., mood disorders associated with a physical illness). The idea that there may be a neuropathology associated with the development of major depression has caused both surprise and skepticism.

The first study to report a significant clinical–pathological correlation in PSD was an investigation by Robinson and Szetela (1981) of 29 patients with left hemisphere brain injury secondary to stroke ($n = 18$) or to traumatic brain injury ($n = 11$). Based on localization of the lesion by computed tomography (CT) scan, there was a significant inverse correlation between the severity of depression and the distance of the anterior border of the lesion from the frontal pole ($r = .76$). This surprising finding led to a number of subsequent examinations of this phenomenon in other populations. Herrmann et al. (1993) found a significant correlation in 20 patients with acute left hemisphere stroke and aphasia who were in an acute or rehabilitation hospital and had no prior history of psy-

TABLE 26.2. *Prevalence Studies of Poststroke Depression*

| Study | Patient Population | N | Criteria | % Major Dep. | % Minor Dep. | Total % |
|---|---|---|---|---|---|---|
| Wade et al. (1987) | Community | 379 | Cutoff score | | | 30 |
| House et al. (1991) | Community | 89 | PSE-DSM-III | 11 | 12 | 23 |
| Burvill et al. (1995) | Community | 294 | PSE-DSM-III | 15 | 8 | 23 |
| Kotila et al. (1998) | Community | 321 | Cutoff score | | | 44 |
| Pooled data means for community study | | | | 14.1 | 9.1 | 31.8 |
| Robinson et al. (1983b) | Acute hosp | 103 | PSE-DSM-III | 27 | 20 | 47 |
| Ebrahim et al. (1987) | Acute hosp | 149 | Cutoff score | | | 23 |
| Fedoroff et al. (1991) | Acute hosp | 205 | PSE-DSM-III | 22 | 19 | 41 |
| Castillo et al. (1995) | Acute hosp | 291 | PSE-DSM-III | 20 | 18 | 38 |
| Starkstein et al. (1992) | Acute hosp | 80 | PSE-DSM-III | 16 | 13 | 29 |
| Astrom et al. (1993) | Acute hosp | 80 | DSM-III | 25 | NR | 25* |
| Herrmann et al. (1993) | Acute hosp | 21 | RDC | 24 | 14 | 38 |
| Singh et al. (2000) | Acute hosp | 81 | Cutoff score | | | 36 |
| Andersen et al. (1994b) | Acute hosp or outpatient | 285 | HDRS cutoff | 10 | 11 | 21 |
| Gainotti et al. (1999) | Acute or rehab hosp | 153 | PSDRS | | | 31 |
| | <2 mo | 27% | | | | |
| | 2–4 mo | 27% | | | | |
| | >4 mo | 40% | | | | |
| Folstein et al. (1977) | Rehab hosp | 20 | PSE and items | | | 45 |
| Finklestein et al. (1982) | Rehab hosp | 25 | Cutoff score | | | 48 |
| Sinyor et al. (1986) | Rehab hosp | 35 | Cutoff score | | | 36 |
| Finset et al. (1989) | Rehab hosp | 42 | Cutoff score | | | 36 |
| Eastwood et al. (1989) | Rehab hosp | 87 | SADS-RDC | 10 | 40 | 50 |
| Morris et al. (1990) | Rehab hosp | 99 | CIDI-DSM-III | 14 | 21 | 35 |
| Schubert et al. (1992) | Rehab hosp | 18 | DSM-III-R | 28 | 44 | 72 |
| Schwartz et al. (1993) | Rehab hosp | 91 | DSM-III | 40 | | 40* |
| Pooled data for all acute and rehab hospital studies | | | | 19.3 | 18.5 | 35.5* |
| Pohjasvaara et al. (1998) | Outpatient | 277 | PSE-DSM-III-R | 26 | 14 | 40 |
| Feibel and Springer (1982) | Outpatient (6 mo) | 91 | Nursing eval | | | 26 |
| Robinson and Price (1982) | Outpatient (6 mo–10 yr) | 103 | Cutoff score | | | 29 |
| Herrmann et al. (1998) | Outpatient (3 mo) | 150 | Cutoff score | | | 27 |
| | (1 yr) | 136 | Cutoff score | | | 22 |
| Vataja et al. (2001) | Outpatient (3 mo) | 275 | PSE-DSM-III-R | 26 | 14 | 40 |
| Collin et al. (1987) | Outpatient | 111 | Cutoff score | | | 42 |
| Astrom et al. (1993) | Outpatient (3 mo) | 77 | DSM-III | 31 | NR | 31* |
| | (1 yr) | 73 | DSM-III | 16 | NR | 16* |
| | (2 yr) | 57 | DSM-III | 19 | NR | 19* |
| | (3 yr) | 49 | DSM-III | 29 | NR | 29* |
| Castillo et al. (1995) | Outpatient (3 mo) | 77 | PSE-DSM-III | 20 | 13 | 33 |
| | (6 mo) | 80 | PSE-DSM-III | 21 | 21 | 42 |
| | (1 yr) | 70 | PSE-DSM-III | 11 | 16 | 27 |
| | (2 yr) | 67 | PSE-DSM-III | 18 | 17 | 35 |
| Pooled data for outpatient studies | | | | 23.3 | 15.0 | 32.9* |

*Because minor depression was not included, these values may be low.

CIDI, Composite International Diagnostic Interview; HDRS, Hamilton Depression Rating Scale; NR, not reported; PSDRS, Poststroke Depression Rating Scale; PSE, Present State Examination; RDC, Research Diagnostic Criteria; SADS, Schedule for Affective Disorders and Schizophrenia.

chiatric disorder. A meta-analysis by Narushima et al. (2003) found a significant inverse correlation between severity of depression and distance of the left hemisphere lesion from the frontal pole $Z = -7.04$, $p < .001$ using the fixed model and $Z = 4.68$, $p < .001$ using the random model pooled correlates $-.53$ or $-.59$ for 163 patients in eight studies. Among 106 patients with right hemisphere lesions, the meta-analysis using fixed or random models found no significant relationship correlation between severity of depression and distance of the lesion from the frontal pole (i.e., pooled correlation below $-0.15$ fixed and $-0.17$ random). The correlation in the left hemisphere was significantly greater than the right hemisphere ($Z$ fixed = 3.43, $p < .001$, 2 random = 2.63, $p < .008$). Thus, the location of the lesion along the anterior-posterior dimension appears to be an important variable in the severity of depression after stroke.

In addition, however, lesion location also influences the frequency of depression. In a study of 45 patients with single lesions restricted to either cortical or subcortical structures in the left or right hemisphere, Starkstein et al. (1987) found that 44% of patients with left cortical lesions were depressed, whereas 39% of patients with left subcortical lesions, 11% of patients with right cortical lesions, and 14% of patients with right subcortical lesions were depressed. Thus, patients with lesions in the left hemisphere had significantly higher rates of depression than did those with lesions in the right hemisphere, regardless of the cortical or subcortical location of the lesion, supporting the hypothesis that depressive disorders after stroke are more frequent among patients with acute left hemisphere lesions compared with right hemisphere lesions ($p < .05$).

When patients were further divided into those with anterior and those with posterior lesions, 5 of 5 patients with left cortical lesions involving the frontal lobe had depression compared with 2 of 11 patients with left cortical posterior lesions ($p < .05$). Moreover, four of the six patients with left subcortical anterior lesions had depression compared with one of seven patients with left subcortical posterior lesions ($p < .05$). Finally, correlations between depression scores and the distance of the lesion from the frontal pole were significant for patients with left cortical lesions and patients with left subcortical lesions. These relationships were not significant for patients with right hemisphere lesions.

In a subsequent study, Starkstein et al. (1988a) examined the relationship between lesions of specific subcortical nuclei and depression. Basal ganglia (caudate and/or putamen) lesions produced major PSD in 7 of 8 patients with left-sided lesions compared with only 1 of 7 patients with right-sided lesions and 0 of 10 with thalamic lesions ($p < .001$).

Astrom et al. (1993) similarly found that among patients with acute stroke, 12 of 14 with left anterior lesions had major depression compared with only 2 of 7 patients with left posterior lesions ($p = .017$) and 2 of 23 with right hemisphere lesions ($p < .001$). Herrmann et al. (1993), however, found major depression in 7 of 10 patients with nonfluent aphasia and left anterior lesions compared with 0 of 7 patients with fluent aphasia and left posterior lesions ($p = .0014$), but only during the acute poststroke period.

Numerous studies, however, have failed to replicate these findings. For example, Gainotti et al. (1999) examined lesion location in 53 patients using magnetic resonance (MR) or CT scans. Among patients with left anterior lesions who were less than 2 months poststroke, only one of nine patients had major depression, while three of seven patients with right anterior lesions had major depression. Among patients 2–4 months poststroke, two of six patients with left anterior lesions had major depression compared with three of seven with right anterior lesions. Among patients who were more than 4 months poststroke, five of nine patients with left anterior lesions had major depression compared to two of three with right anterior lesions.

Carson et al. (2000) reported on a meta-analysis of all studies of PSD that examined the association of depression with lesion location. The authors concluded that "this systemic review offered no support for the hypothesis that the risk of depression after stroke is affected by the location of the brain lesion" (p. 122). The Robinson (1998) hypothesis, however, was that patients with lesions involving the left frontal basal ganglia circuit would have a significantly greater frequency of major depression than patients with comparable lesions of the right hemisphere or posterior left hemisphere, but only during the first one or two months following stroke. The Carson et al. (2000) analysis of studies conducted within 1 month poststroke included 10 studies, but only 2 studies examined the hypothesis regarding left frontal and left basal ganglia lesions (Morris et al., 1996b; Robinson et al. (1983a). Both of these studies found a significantly greater frequency of major depression following left compared with right anterior lesions. Carson et al., however, omitted other relevant studies that appeared to have met their criteria (e.g., Astrom et al., 1993; Robinson et al., 1985a). A meta-analysis of all the relevant studies (Astrom et al., 1993; Gainotti et al., 1999; Herrmann et al., 1995; House et al., 1990b; Morris et al., 1996a; Robinson et al., 1984b, 1986b) examined the relative risk of poststroke major depression following left anterior versus right anterior lesions (relative risk-fixed combined (N = 112) = 2.18, CI = 1.4–3.3, p = .000; random combined = 2.16, CI = 1.3–3.6, p = .004) and following left anterior versus left posterior lesions (relative risk-fixed combined (N = 128) = 2.29, CI = 1.6–3.4 p = .000; random combined = 2.29, CI 1.5–3.4, p = .000) (Robinson, 2003). Thus, in spite of some investigators' failure to replicate these findings, the data support the conclusion that within the first 2 months poststroke, lesions involving the left frontal or left basal ganglia are associated with a significantly greater frequency of major depression than comparable lesions of the right hemisphere or posterior lesions of the left hemisphere.

This reanalysis also suggests that the failure of other investigators to replicate the association of left anterior lesion location with increased frequency of depression, in most cases, is probably related to the time since the stroke. The lateralized effect of left anterior lesions on both major and minor depression is a phenomenon of the acute poststroke period (when the patients are less than 1–2 months following stroke). In a longitudinal study by Shimoda and Robinson (1999), at short-term follow-up (3–6 months), patients with right hemisphere lesions, as well as patients with left hemisphere lesions, showed a significant correlation between severity of depression and proximity of the lesion to the frontal pole.

At long-term follow-up (12–24 months), there was no significant correlation between severity of depression, as measured by the Hamilton Depression Rating Scale (HDRS) or the Present State Examination (PSE), and proximity of the lesion to the frontal pole among patients with left hemisphere lesions ($n = 25$). Among patients with right hemisphere stroke ($n = 21$), however, severity of depression was significantly correlated with proximity of the lesion to the occipital pole (i.e., lesions farther from the frontal pole were associated with more severe depression).

Although it is uncertain why this temporal dynamic occurs in the relationship between the existence and severity of depression and lesion location, it suggests that if physiological changes such as depletion of biogenic amines occur in patients with left anterior lesions, leading to depression, these changes are hemisphere specific for only a few weeks. By 2–3 months following stroke (i.e., short-term follow-up), similar or alternative mechanisms occur in patients with right frontal lesions that lead to correlations of depression severity with proximity of the lesion to the frontal pole in both the right and left hemisphere.

## PREMORBID RISK FACTORS

The studies just reviewed indicate that although a significant proportion of patients with left anterior lesions developed PSD, not every patient with a lesion in these locations developed a major depression. This observation raises the questions of why clinical variability occurs and why some but not all patients with lesions in these locations develop depression.

Starkstein (1988b) examined this issue by comparing 13 patients with major PSD with 13 stroke patients without depression, all of whom had lesions of the same size and location. Eleven pairs of patients had left hemisphere

lesions, and two pairs had right hemisphere lesions. Damage was cortical in 10 pairs and subcortical in 3 pairs. The groups did not differ on important demographic variables such as age, sex, socioeconomic status, or education. They also did not differ on family or personal history of psychiatric disorders or neurological deficits. Patients with major PSD, however, had significantly more subcortical atrophy ($p < .05$), as measured both by the ratio of third ventricle to brain (i.e., the area of the third ventricle divided by the area of the brain at the same level) and by the ratio of lateral ventricle to brain (i.e., the area of the body of the lateral ventricle contralateral to the brain lesion divided by the brain area at the same level). It is likely that the subcortical atrophy preceded the stroke because acute stroke would probably not increase the ventricular size in patients with depression but not identical strokes in patients without depression. Thus, a mild degree of subcortical atrophy may be a premorbid risk factor that increases the risk of developing major depression following a stroke.

Among patients with right hemisphere lesions, Starkstein et al. (1989) found that patients who developed major depression after a right hemisphere lesion had a significantly more frequent family history of psychiatric disorders than did either nondepressed patients with right hemisphere lesions or patients with major depression following left hemisphere lesions. This finding suggests that a genetic predisposition to depression may play an important role after the occurrence of right hemisphere lesions. Eastwood et al. (1989) and Morris et al. (1990) also reported that depressed patients were more likely than nondepressed patients to have either a personal or a family history of psychiatric disorders.

In summary, lesion location is not the only factor that influences the development of PSD. Subcortical atrophy that probably precedes the stroke and a family or personal history of affective disorders also seem to play an important role.

## POSTSTROKE DEPRESSION AND ACTIVITIES OF DAILY LIVING

### Relationship with Depression

Examining the association between PSD and activities of daily living (ADL) is a complicated task because there are so many variables that may influence this association. Robinson et al. (1983b) reported that the severity of depressive symptoms, as measured by the Zung Self-Rating Depression Scale (SDS) (Zung, 1965), the HDRS Hamilton, 1960), or the PSE (Wing et al., 1974), was significantly correlated with severity of impairment in ADL, including the patients' ability to dress and feed themselves, walk, find their way around, express needs, read and write, and keep their room in order (Robinson et al., 1983b). Numerous other investigators have also reported that severity of poststroke depression was associated with severity of impairment in ADL (Feibel and Springer, 1982; Herrmann et al., 1998; Ingles et al., 1999; Kauhanen et al., 1999; Kotila et al., 1984; Morris et al., 1994; Parikh et al., 1987; Pohjasvaara et al., 1998; Ramasubbu, 1994; Sinyor et al., 1986; Wade et al., 1987).

In the acute stroke period, Sinyor et al. (1986) studied 64 stroke patients within weeks of their stroke and reported that patients with PSD, defined as those with an SDS score ≥50, had lower functional status scores (i.e., the Patient Evaluation Conference System) (Harvey and Jellinek, 1981) than nondepressed patients (Sinyor et al., 1986). Similar findings were reported by Pohjaasvara et al. (1998) at short-term follow-up (i.e., at 3 months poststroke). Patients with depression were more severely physically handicapped, as measured by the Barthel Index (BI)(Mahoney and Barthel, 1965); had more physically disabling strokes, as measured by the Scandinavian Stroke Scale (SSS)(Scandinavian Stroke Study Group, 1985); and were more often dependent than nondepressed patients (Pohjasvaara et al., 1998). Ingels et al. (1999) also reported that fatigue, commonly reported as a symptom of PSD, caused more functional limitation after stroke, and the impact of fatigue on functional ability was strongly influenced by depression. Parikh et al. (1987) compared 25 patients with major or minor depression following an acute stroke to 38 patients who were never depressed during 2 years of poststroke follow-up. Although both groups had similar impairment in ADL in the hospital, the depressed patients had significantly less improvement (the group by time interaction was significant, $p < .05$) than the nondepressed patients. This finding held true even after controlling for important variables such as the type and extent of rehabilitation, the size and location of the lesion, patient demographic characteristics, nature of the stroke, and concurrent medical illness or recurrent stroke. Paradiso and Robinson (1998) examined the gender differences in PSD and found that poststroke major depression was significantly associated with greater impairment of ADL in male patients but not female patients.

Although the association between physical impairment and PSD appears to be bidirectional (i.e., greater physical impairment leads to depression and depression leads to greater physical impairment), most investigations have found that patients with PSD have greater impairment in ADL than patients without PSD.

### Effect of Poststroke Depression on Recovery of Activities of Daily Living

Dove et al. (1984) reported that baseline neurological deficits, early intervention, the presence of a specialized stroke unit, type of infarct, and the use of physiotherapy influenced patients' recovery. The effects of depression on recovery in ADL cannot be evaluated unless all of these factors, as well as others, are either comparable across groups or controlled.

Several investigators have studied the effect of poststroke depression on recovery in ADL (Paolucci et al., 1999; Parikh et al., 1990; Robinson et al., 1986b). A multiple regression analysis of ADL scores at 2-year follow-up in 63 patients studied by Parikh (1990), examining the effects of in-hospital depression scores, 2-year depression scores, in-hospital ADL scores, intellectual impairment scores in the hospital and at 2 years, social functioning in the hospital and at follow-up, and distance of the lesion from the frontal pole, found that in-hospital depression scores were independently and positively correlated with ADL scores at 2 years. The only other significant correlate was in-hospital ADL scores. Interestingly, in-hospital ADL scores did not correlate significantly with depression scores at 2-year follow-up (Parikh et al., 1988; Robinson et al., 1985b). Schubert et al. (1992) examined 21 patients with PSD and reported that the severity of depression, as measured by the Beck Depression Inventory (BDI) (Beck et al., 1961), was associated with the severity of ADL, as measured by the BI (Mahoney and Barthel, 1965), and that patients with PSD recovered their ADL more slowly than nondepressed patients. These findings suggest that in-hospital depression is one of the strongest predictors of recovery of ADL over 2 years and that the initial ADL impairment has no significant effect on depression 2 years poststroke.

### Effect of Treatment on Activities of Daily Living

If PSD impairs recovery in ADL, recovery from PSD would be expected to improve recovery in ADL. Starkstein et al. (1988c) reported that patients who recovered from PSD had significantly lower Johns Hopkins Functioning Inventory (JHFI) scores (i.e. less impaired ADL) than patients who did not recover from PSD.

Several studies have reported that antidepressant treatment improved poststroke patients' ADL (Gainotti et al., 2001; Gonzalez-Torrecillas et al., 1995; Reding et al., 1986). Reding et al. studied 27 patients with stroke and found that those with abnormal dexamethasone suppression test (DST) results showed significantly greater improvement on the BI if they were given trazodone over 4 to 5 weeks compared with placebo. Similar results were reported by Gonzales-Torrecillas et al. (1995) in 37 patients with PSD receiving open-label antidepressants (26 fluoxetine, 11 nortriptyline) compared to 11 patients with PSD who remained untreated. Both nortriptyline and fluoxetine improved depression, as measured by the HDRS; ADL, as measured by the BI; and neurological function, as assessed by the Orgogozo scale. These differences between treated and nontreated patients were statistically significant from week 3 to the end of the 6-week treatment trial.

Chemerinski et al. (2001a, 2001b) reported similar findings. Twenty-one depressed patients, whose mood improved spontaneously between in-hospital evaluation and 3 or 6 months after stroke, had significantly greater recovery in ADL at follow-up than did 34 patients whose mood did not improve (Fig. 26.1) (Chemerinski et al., 2001b). Interestingly, patients with either major or minor depression showed the same amount of recovery in ADL. This finding that major and minor depression did not differ in their relationship to recovery in ADL suggests that the effect may not be mediated by biological or physiological mechanisms, but rather by psychological mechanisms such as poor motivation or social withdrawal.

Chemerinski et al. (2001a, 2001b) also conducted a merged analysis of patients who were treated in one of two double-blind trials with nortriptyline versus placebo for the treatment of PSD. There were 10 patients whose depression responded to treatment and who were matched in severity of initial ADL impairment to another 10 patients who failed to respond to treatment. At a dose of 100 mg/day, the patients who responded to treatment had significantly lower ADL scores (i.e., were less impaired) at 6 or 9 weeks of treatment than the 10 patients who failed to respond at the same time and dose (Chemerinski et al., 2001a).

In summary, PSD has been associated with greater impairment in ADL both in the hospital and at follow-up. Furthermore, not only poststroke major depression but also poststroke minor depression had a negative impact on recovery in ADL. Effective treatment of PSD, on the other hand, increased recovery in ADL.

## POSTSTROKE DEPRESSION AND COGNITIVE IMPAIRMENT

### Relationship to Depression

Numerous investigators have reported that elderly patients with functional major depression have intellectual deficits that improve with treatment of depression (Wells, 1979). This issue was first examined in patients with PSD by Robinson et al. (1986a). Patients with major depression after a left hemisphere infarct were found to have significantly lower scores (i.e., more impairment) on the Mini-Mental State Exam (MMSE) (Folstein et al., 1975) than did a comparable group of nondepressed patients. Using a multiple regression analysis, both the size of the patients' lesions and their depression scores correlated independently with severity of cognitive impairment.

In a second study discussed in the section "Premorbid Risk Factors" (Starkstein et al., 1988b), stroke patients with and without major depression were matched for lesion location and volume. Of 13 patients with major PSD, 10 had an MMSE score lower than that of their matched control subjects, 2 had the same score, and only 1 patient had a higher score (i.e., less impairment) ($p < .001$). Thus, even when patients were matched for lesion size and location, depressed patients were more cognitively impaired. This finding demonstrated that there is a cognitive impairment in patients with poststroke major depression that is due to depression and not simply to the lesion's location.

In another study, Bolla-Wilson et al. (1989) administered a comprehensive neuropsychological battery and found that patients with major depression and left hemisphere lesions had significantly greater cognitive impairment than did nondepressed patients with com-

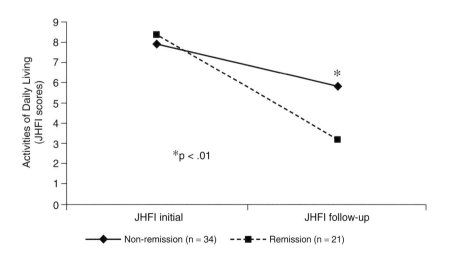

FIGURE 26.1 Poststroke patients with remission of depression showed significantly greater recovery in activities of daily living than nonremitted patients at 3- or 6-month follow-up ($F = 6.37$; $df = 1$; 53, $p = .015$) as measured by the Johns Hopkins Functioning Inventory (JHFI). (From Chemerinski et al., 2001b, reprinted with permission)

parable left hemisphere lesions ($p < .05$). These cognitive deficits involved tasks of temporal orientation, language, and executive motor and frontal lobe functions. On the other hand, among patients with right hemisphere lesions, those with major depression did not differ from nondepressed patients on any of the measures of cognitive impairment. This finding indicated that the dementia of poststroke major depression was related to mechanisms induced by left hemisphere injury and that right hemisphere injury leading to depression did not provoke the same mechanisms.

The association of PSD with cognitive impairment has also been demonstrated by other investigators (House et al., 1990a; Kauhanen et al., 1999). Kauhanen et al. examined 106 patients with stroke using not only the MMSE but also other neuropsychological examinations (i.e., two subtests of the Wechsler Memory Scale (Wechsler, 1997) and the visual recognition memory task (Cronholm and Ottosson, 1963; Kauhanen et al., 1999). In this study, PSD was associated with impairments in memory, nonverbal problem solving, attention, and psychomotor speed. The association between PSD and cognitive impairment has been reported in the acute stroke period (House et al., 1990a), at short-term follow-up (Bolla-Wilson et al., 1989; House et al., 1990a; Kauhanen et al., 1999) and at long-term follow-up (Kauhanen et al., 1999; Starkstein et al., 1988c).

## Effect of Poststroke Depression on Recovery from Cognitive Impairment

The effect of PSD on recovery from cognitive impairment has been examined in several studies (Downhill and Robinson, 1994; Kahn et al., 1960; Robinson et al., 1985b, 1986a, 1986b). Downhill and Robinson (1994) conducted a 2-year follow-up study of 140 patients after the occurrence of stroke. They found that major depression was associated with a greater degree of cognitive impairment, as measured by the MMSE, than minor depression or no depression for 1 year after a stroke. The intellectual deficit, however, was most prominent among patients with major depression after a left hemisphere lesion. Patients who had major depression following a right hemisphere stroke, patients with minor depression, and patients in whom stroke had occurred 2 years previously did not show an effect of major depression on cognitive impairment. This study demonstrated that the dementia produced by left hemisphere stroke and major depression lasts for 1 year, which is the usual course of major depression.

## Effect of Antidepressant Treatment on Cognitive Function

Since PSD has a negative effect on recovery of cognitive function and is a treatable disorder, it is expected that treatment of PSD would lead to improved cog-

nitive function. Several studies using double-blind methodology, however, failed to show an improvement in cognitive function among patients given nortriptyline or citalopram for PSD even though they showed a significant reduction in HDRS scores (Andersen et al., 1996; Lipsey et al., 1984; Robinson et al., 2000).

Using a merged analysis of prior treatment studies, Kimura et al. (2000) examined 47 patients with PSD (major = 33, minor = 14), divided into those who responded (i.e. had a greater than 50% reduction in the HDRS score) ($n = 24$, major = 15, minor = 9) and those who failed to respond ($n = 23$, major = 18, minor = 5). The responder group included 16 patients treated with nortriptyline and 9 with placebo. The nonresponder group included 5 patients treated with nortriptyline and 18 with placebo. Although there was no significant difference between the responder and nonresponder groups in their baseline HDRS scores, repeated-measures analysis of variance (ANOVA) of the MMSE scores demonstrated a significant time-by-group interaction (i.e., MMSE scores in the responder group improved more over the course of double-blind treatment than MMSE scores in the nonresponder group) (Fig. 26.2).

Planned post hoc comparisons demonstrated that the responders had significantly higher MMSE scores than the nonresponders at nortriptyline doses of 75 mg/day ($p = .0360$) and 100 mg/day ($p = .024$). If only nortriptyline-treated patients (responders) were compared with only placebo-treated patients (nonresponders), there was still a significant group-by-time interaction ($p = .036$). This indicates that the failure to show sig-

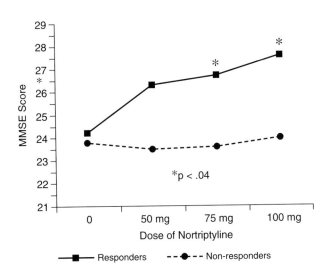

FIGURE 26.2 Change in Mini-Mental State Examination scores in patients with poststroke major depression during the treatment study. Treatment responders ($n = 13$) showed significantly greater improvement in cognitive function than nonresponders ($n = 18$) (group-by-time interaction F = 4.98; df = 3,126, $p = .002$; at 75 mg/day, group diff $p = .036$; at 100 mg/day, group diff $p = .024$). Error bars represent standard errors on the mean (SE). (From Kimura et al., 2000. Reprinted with permission)

nificant improvement in prior studies was not the result of nortriptyline drug effects such as impaired attention due to anticholinergic effects or sedation.

Prior treatment studies did not show a significant effect of treatment of depression on cognitive function as a result of effect size. When patients treated with nortriptyline (i.e., both responders and nonresponders) were compared with placebo-treated patients (i.e., both responders and nonresponders), the effect size was only 0.16. When patients were divided into those who responded and those who did not respond, the effect size increased to .96, thus allowing a significant difference to be demonstrated with a much smaller group size.

## POSTSTROKE DEPRESSION AND MORTALITY

Mortality is the most important outcome following stroke. Increased mortality associated with primary depression (i.e., no known brain lesion) has been demonstrated by numerous investigators. Avery and Winokur (1976), for example, examined 519 depressed patients and demonstrated that there was a significantly increased death rate among patients who had been inadequately treated with antidepressants or electroconvulsive therapy compared to patients who had been adequately treated for depression. Although mortality was also influenced by the effects of age, gender, social class, and medical co-morbid illnesses, depression has been shown to be an independent factor in mortality among older patients (Murphy et al., 1988).

Wade et al. (1987) studied 976 patients with stroke. They found that patients with depression, assessed at 3 weeks poststroke using the Wakefield self-assessment depression inventory (Snaith et al., 1971), had 50% higher mortality at 1 year than nondepressed patients and concluded that early depression correlated with early death. Morris et al. (1993) examined this association among 103 acute stroke patients followed for 10 years. Although the in-hospital background characteristics were not significantly different between depressed and nondepressed patients, major or minor depression during in-hospital evaluation was significantly associated with an increased mortality rate over the next 6 to 7 years. The mortality rate among patients with acute in-hospital major or minor depression was 71% and 70%, respectively, over the next 10 years. This rate was significantly higher than that of patients without in-hospital depression, whose 10-year mortality rate was only 41%. The relative risk of depression on mortality rate was 3.4 (CI = 1.4–8.4, $p = .007$). A logistic regression analysis to assess the contribution of depression, social function, co-morbid medical illness, age, sex, social class, physical and cognitive impairment, and size and location of stroke found that depression remained an independent factor for mortality with an odds ratio of 3.7 (CI = 1.1–12.2, $p = .03$).

Morris et al. (1993) also found this association of mortality and depression among another group of patients in an Australian rehabilitation hospital followed up at 15 months after stroke. The death rate among 99 stroke patients initially seen at 2–3 months poststroke was 23% for patients with major depression, 10% for those with minor depression, and 2% for patients with no mood disorder (odds ratio 8.1, CI = 0.9–72.9, $p = .06$). Astrom et al. (1993), however, failed to find an increased mortality rate among patients with major poststroke depression compared with nondepressed patients during their 3-year evaluation. Mortality in this study was associated with older age, disorientation in the hospital, greater impairment in ADL, and increased cortical atrophy. Recently, House et al. (2001) reported that among 448 patients evaluated at 1 month poststroke, scoring in the highest quartile of the General Health Questionnaire was associated with increased mortality at 1 year (odds ratio 3.1, CI = 1.1–8.8) and at 24 months (odds ratio 2.2, CI = 1.0–4.8). The score on the Depression subscale of the General Health Questionnaire was the only significant predictor of mortality using a logistic regression to control for other variables.

Findings from a 9-year follow-up of the PSD treatment study (Jorge et al., 2003) found that active treatment with nortriptyline or fluoxetine ($N = 69$) versus placebo ($N = 35$) over 12 weeks increased the probability of survival at the 6-year follow-up (Kaplan Meier log rank $\chi^2 = 7.3$, $df = 1$, $p = .006$). The survival rate among patients given antidepressants was 61%, while the survival rate among patients given placebo was 34%. A logistic regression analysis of the effects of age, diabetes, relapsing depression, and antidepressant use found that antidepressant use was independently associated with increased survival (Jorge et al., 2003).

In summary, several studies have found that depression following stroke is associated with increased mortality as early as 1 year and as late as 10 years poststroke. Although the mechanism remains uncertain, the majority of patients died from cardiac (46%) or cerebrovascular disease (24%). The finding that the risk of increased mortality remains elevated even after most depressions have remitted suggests that the mechanisms leading to death are not linked to the pathophysiology of depression but may involve long-lasting changes in heart rate variability, coagulation states, or immune system function. Preliminary findings from a controlled treatment trial suggest that treatment of depression may significantly reduce the mortality associated with PSD.

## MECHANISM OF POSTSTROKE DEPRESSION

Although the cause of PSD remains unknown, one of the mechanisms that has been hypothesized to play an etiological role is dysfunction of the biogenic amine system. The noradrenergic and serotonergic cell bodies are located in the brain stem and send ascending projections through the median forebrain bundle to the frontal cortex. The ascending axons then arc posteriorly and run longitudinally through the deep layers of the cortex, arborizing and sending terminal projections into the superficial cortical layers (Morrison et al., 1979). Lesions that disrupt these pathways in the frontal cortex or the basal ganglia may affect many downstream fibers. Based on these neuroanatomical facts and the clinical finding that the severity of depression correlates with the proximity of the lesion to the frontal pole, Robinson et al. (1984a) suggested that acute PSD in some patients may be related to depletion of norepinephrine and/or serotonin produced by lesions in the left lateral frontal lobe or left basal ganglia.

In support of this hypothesis, laboratory investigations in rats have demonstrated that the biochemical response to ischemic lesions is lateralized. Right hemisphere lesions produce depletion of norepinephrine and spontaneous hyperactivity, whereas comparable lesions of the left hemisphere do not (Robinson, 1979). A similar lateralized biochemical response to ischemia in human subjects was also reported by Mayberg et al. (1988). Patients with stroke lesions in the right hemisphere had significantly higher ratios of ipsilateral to contralateral spiperone binding (presumably 5-hydroxytryptamine [5-HT] type 2 receptor binding) in noninjured temporal and parietal cortex than comparable patients with left hemisphere strokes. Patients with left hemisphere lesions, on the other hand, showed a significant inverse correlation between the amount of spiperone binding in the left temporal cortex and depression scores (i.e., higher depression scores were associated with less serotonin receptor binding).

Thus, a greater depletion of biogenic amines in patients with right hemisphere compared with left hemisphere lesions could lead to a compensatory up-regulation of receptors that might protect against depression. On the other hand, patients with left hemisphere lesions may have moderate depletions of biogenic amines but without a compensatory up-regulation of 5-HT receptors and, therefore, a dysfunction of biogenic amine systems in the left hemisphere.

This dysfunction must also be related to the growing consensus about the anatomical circuits that seem to play a dynamic role in the mechanism of both primary (i.e., no brain lesion) and secondary (i.e., known structural abnormality) depression. The work of Alexander et al. (1986) has demonstrated the existence of at least five cortical basal ganglia circuits that play an important role in movement disorders. Soares and Mann (1997) reviewed all the functional imaging studies of patients with mood disorders. Decreased prefrontal cortex blood flow and metabolism in depressed unipolar and bipolar patients was the most consistently replicated finding, and the degree of hypometabolism correlated with the severity of illness. Basal ganglia abnormalities have also been found in depressed unipolar and bipolar patients (Greenwald et al., 1998). In addition, temporal lobe abnormalities are present in bipolar and perhaps unipolar patients. In addition to these functional imaging findings, changes in the anatomical volume of the subgenual cortex, hippocampus, and amygdala have been reported in unipolar depressive disorder (Drevets et al., 1992).

Robinson (1998) has hypothesized that PSD may involve dysfunction of the lateral limbic circuit (i.e., orbital frontal cortex, basal ganglia, basal temporal cortex, amygdala, dorsal medial thalamus). Frontal dysfunction or temporal dysfunction may be produced by biogenic amine depletions, leading to abnormal function throughout the limbic circuit. Alternatively, direct injury or diaschisis (distant effects of injury) affecting some of these structures may also change the limbic balance and ultimately lead to dysphoria or depression.

## TREATMENT OF POSTSTROKE DEPRESSION

At present, there are five placebo-controlled, randomized, double-blind treatment studies on the efficacy of single antidepressant treatment of PSD. In the first study, Lipsey et al. (1984) examined 14 patients treated with nortriptyline and 20 patients given placebo. The 11 patients treated with nortriptyline who completed the 6-week study showed significantly greater improvement in their HDRS scores (Hamilton, 1960) than did 15 placebo-treated patients ($p < .01$). Successfully treated patients had serum nortriptyline levels of 50–150 ng/ml. Three patients experienced side effects (including delirium, confusion, drowsiness, and agitation) that were severe enough to require the discontinuation of nortriptyline therapy.

Reding et al. (1986) reported that 27 patients who were about 6 weeks poststroke and were enrolled in a stroke rehabilitation program were randomly assigned to trazodone (50–200 mg/day) or placebo. When the analysis was restricted to 16 patients with abnormal DST test results, 7 patients receiving trazodone had greater improvement in BI ADL scores (Granger et al., 1979) than did 9 placebo-treated control subjects during 4 to 5 weeks of treatment ($p < .05$).

Another double-blind, placebo-controlled trial compared 33 patients with HDRS scores >13 given citalopram (20 mg/day for patients below 66 years of age and 10 mg/day for older patients) compared to 33 similar patients given placebo. The patients were 2 to 4 months after acute stroke. Among the study completers, HDRS scores were significantly more improved over 6 weeks in patients receiving active treatment ($n = 27$)

than placebo ($n = 32$) (Andersen et al., 1994a). At both 3 and 6 weeks, the group receiving active treatment had significantly lower HRDS scores than did the group receiving placebo. The response rate to citalopram was 59%, and to placebo it was 28% ($p < .05$). This study established for the first time the efficacy of a selective serotonin reuptake inhibitor in the treatment of PSD. Side effects included nausea, vomiting, and fatigue.

Lauritzen et al. (1994) compared combined treatment with imipramine (mean dose 75 mg/day) plus mianserin (25 mg/day) ($n = 10$) to treatment with desipramine (mean dose 66 mg/day) plus mianserin (27 mg/day) ($n = 10$). The melancholia scale (MES) showed a greater change in the imipramine group than in the desipramine group. No differences were found when the HDRS was used.

The most recent treatment study was conducted by Robinson et al. (2000). This study compared depressed patients treated with fluoxetine ($n = 23$), nortriptyline ($n = 16$), or placebo ($n = 17$) in a double-blind, randomized treatment design. Patients were enrolled if they had a diagnosis of either major or minor PSD and had no contraindication to the use of fluoxetine or nortriptyline such as intracerebral hemorrhage (fluoxetine) or cardiac induction abnormalities (nortriptyline). Patients were treated with 10 mg/day doses of fluoxetine for the first 3 weeks, 20 mg/day for weeks 4–6, 30 mg/day for weeks 7–9, and 40 mg/day for weeks 10–12 (the last 3 weeks). The nortriptyline-treated patients were given 25 mg/day for the first week, 50 mg/day for weeks 2 and 3, 75 mg/day for weeks 4–6, and 100 mg/day for weeks 7–12. Patients treated with placebo were given identical capsules of the same number used for the actively treated patients. Intention-to-treat analysis demonstrated significant time-by-treatment interaction, with nortriptyline-treated patients showing a significantly greater decline in HDRS scores than either the placebo- or fluoxetine-treated patients at 12 weeks. There were no significant differences between the fluoxetine and placebo groups.

Nortriptyline treatment led to a significantly higher response rate (response is defined as more than a 50% drop in HRDS score and the patient no longer meeting diagnostic criteria for major or minor depression) (10 of 16, 62%) than either fluoxetine (2 of 23, 9%) or placebo (4 of 17, 24%) (Fisher exact $p = .001$). In addition, fluoxetine treatment was associated with a mean weight loss of 15.1 pounds, or 8.5% of initial body weight from the beginning to the end of the 12-week treatment trial, which was not seen among patients treated with placebo or nortriptyline. Of the 12 patients treated with fluoxetine, 10 lost 10 or more pounds; only 2 of 13 nortriptyline-treated patients and 1 of 11 placebo-treated patients lost this amount of weight (Fisher exact $p = .004$).

Based on the available data, if there are no con-

traindications to nortriptyline, such as heart block, cardiac arrhythmia, narrow angle glaucoma, sedation, or orthostatic hypotension, nortriptyline remains the first-line treatment for PSD. Doses of nortriptyline should be increased slowly and blood levels should be monitored, with the goal of achieving serum concentrations between 50 and 150 ng/ml. If there are contraindications to the use of nortriptyline, citalopram (20 mg/day for patients under age 66, 10 mg/day for those aged 66 and over) would be the next choice.

Electroconvulsive therapy has also been reported to be effective for treating PSD (Murray et al., 1987). It causes few side effects and no neurological deterioration. Psychostimulants have also been reported in open-label trials to be effective for the treatment of PSD. Finally, psychological treatment, including cognitive-behavioral therapy (Hibbard et al., 1990), group therapy, and family therapy, have also been reported to be useful (Oradei and Waite, 1974; Watzlawick and Coyne, 1980). However, controlled studies for these treatment modalities have not been conducted.

REFERENCES

Alexander, G.E., DeLong, M.R., and Strick, P.L. (1986) Parallel organization of functionally segregated circuits linking basal ganglia and cortex. *Annu Rev Neurosci* 9:357–381.

American Heart Association. (1996) *American Heart Association: Heart and Stroke Facts. 1996 Statistical Supplement*. Dallas: American Heart Association.

American Psychiatric Association. (1987) *Diagnostic and Statistical Manual of Mental Disorders*, 3rd rev. ed. Washington, DC: American Psychiatric Press.

American Psychiatric Association. (1994) *Diagnostic and Statistical Manual of Mental Disorders*, 4th ed. Washington, DC: American Psychiatric Press.

Andersen, G., Vestergaard, K., and Lauritzen, L. (1994a) Effective treatment of poststroke depression with the selective serotonin reuptake inhibitor citalopram. *Stroke* 25:1099–1104.

Andersen, G., Vestergaard, K., and Riis, J. (1993) Citalopram for post-stroke pathological crying. *Lancet* 342(8875):837–839.

Andersen, G., Vestergaard, K., Riis, J.O., and Ingeman-Nielsen, M. (1996) Dementia of depression or depression of dementia in stroke? *Acta Psychiatr Scand* 94:272–278.

Andersen, G., Vestergaard, K., Riis, J.O., and Lauritzen, L. (1994b) Incidence of post-stroke depression during the first year in a large unselected stroke population determined using a valid standardized rating scale. *Acta Psychiatr Scand* 90:190–195.

Astrom, M., Adolfsson, R., and Asplund, K. (1993) Major depression in stroke patients: A 3-year longitudinal study. *Stroke* 24:976–982.

Avery, D., and Winokur, G. (1976) Mortality in depressed patients treated with electroconvulsive therapy and antidepressants. *Arch Gen Psychiatry* 33:1029–1037.

Beck, A.T., Ward, C.H., Mendelson, M., Mock, J., and Erbaugh, J. (1961) An inventory for measuring depression. *Arch Gen Psychiatry* 4:551–571.

Bleuler, E.P. (1951) *Textbook of Psychiatry*. New York: Macmillan, pp. 131–197.

Bolla-Wilson, K., Robinson, R.G., Starkstein, S.E., Boston, J., and Price, T.R. (1989) Lateralization of dementia of depression in stroke patients. *Am J Psychiatry* 146:627–634.

Bonita, R. (1992) Epidemiology of stroke. *Lancet* 339:342–344.

Bukberg, J., Penman, D., and Holland, J.C. (1984) Depression in hospitalized cancer patients. *Psychosom Med* 46:199–212.

Burvill, P.W., Johnson, G.A., Jamrozik, K.D., Anderson, C.S., Stewart-Wynne, E.G., and Chakera, T.M.H. (1995) Prevalence of depression after stroke: The Perth Community Stroke Study. *Br J Psychiatry* 166:320–327.

Carson, A.J., MacHale, S., Allen, K., Lawrie, S.M., Dennis, M., House, A., and Sharpe, M. (2000) Depression after stroke and lesion location: A systematic review. *Lancet* 356:122–126.

Castillo, C.S., Schultz, S.K., and Robinson, R.G. (1995) Clinical correlates of early-onset and late-onset poststroke generalized anxiety. *Am J Psychiatry* 152:1174–1179.

Chemerinski, E., Robinson, R.G., Arndt, S., and Kosier, J.T. (2001a) The effect of remission of poststroke depression on activities of daily living in a double-blind randomized treatment study. *J Nerv Ment Dis* 189:421–425.

Chemerinski, E., Robinson, R.G., and Kosier, J.T. (2001b) Improved recovery in activities of daily living associated with remission of post-stroke depression. *Stroke* 32:113–117.

Cohen-Cole, S.A., and Stoudemire, A. (1987) Major depression and physical illness: Special considerations in diagnosis and biologic treatment. *Psychiatr Clin North Am* 10:1–17.

Collin, S.J., Tinson, D., and Lincoln, N.B. (1987) Depression after stroke. *Clin Rehabil* 1:27–32.

Cronholm, B., and Ottosson, J.O. (1963) Reliability and validity of a memory test battery. *Acta Psychiatr Scand* 39:218–234.

Dove, H.G., Schneider, K.C., and Wallace, J.D. (1984) Evaluating and predicting outcome of acute cerebral vascular accident. *Stroke* 15:858–864.

Downhill, J.E., Jr., and Robinson, R.G. (1994) Longitudinal assessment of depression and cognitive impairment following stroke. *J Nerv Ment Dis* 182:425–431.

Drevets, W.C., Videen, T.O., Price, J.L., Preskorn, S.H., Carmichael, S.T., and Raichle, M.D. (1992) A functional anatomical study of unipolar depression. *J Neurosci* 12:3628–3641.

Eastwood, M.R., Rifat, S.L., Nobbs, H., and Ruderman, J. (1989) Mood disorder following cerebrovascular accident. *Br J Psychiatry* 154:195–200.

Ebrahim, S., Barer, D., and Nouri, F. (1987) Affective illness after stroke. *Br J Psychiatry* 151:52–56.

Endicott, J. (1984) Measurement of depression in patients with cancer. *Cancer* 53(suppl):2243–2248.

Fedoroff, J.P., Starkstein, S.E., Parikh, R.M., Price, T.R., and Robinson, R.G. (1991) Are depressive symptoms nonspecific in patients with acute stroke? *Am J Psychiatry* 148:1172–1176.

Feibel, J.H., and Springer, C.J. (1982) Depression and failure to resume social activities after stroke. *Arch Phys Med Rehabil* 63:276–278.

Finklestein, S., Benowitz, L.I., Baldessarini, R.J., Arana, G.W., Levine, D., Woo, E., Bear, D., Moya, K., and Stoll, A.L. (1982) Mood, vegetative disturbance, and dexamethasone suppression test after stroke. *Ann Neurol* 12:463–468.

Finset, A., Goffeng, L., Landro, N.I., and Haakonsen, M. (1989) Depressed mood and intra-hemispheric location of lesion in right hemisphere stroke patients. *Scand J Rehabil Med* 21:1–6.

Fisher, S.H. (1961) Psychiatric considerations of cerebral vascular disease. *Am J Cardiol* 7:379–385.

Folstein, M.F., Folstein, S.E., and McHugh, P.R. (1975) Mini-Mental State: A practical method for grading the cognitive state of patients for the clinician. *J Psychiatr Res* 12:189–198.

Folstein, M.F., Maiberger, R., and McHugh, P.R. (1977) Mood disorder as a specific complication of stroke. *J Neurol Neurosurg Psychiatry* 40:1018–1020.

Gainotti, G., Antonucci, G., Marra, C., and Paolucci, S. (2001) Relation between depression after stroke, antidepressant therapy, and functional recovery. *J Neurol Neurosurg Psychiatry* 71:258–261.

Gainotti, G., Azzoni, A., and Marra, C. (1999) Frequency, phenomenology and anatomical-clinical correlates of major post-stroke depression. *Br J Psychiatry* 175:163–167.

Goldstein, K. (1942) *After Effects of Brain Injuries in War.* New York: Grune and Stratton.

Gonzalez-Torrecillas, J.L., Mendlewicz, J., and Lobo, A. (1995) Effects of early treatment of poststroke depression on neuropsychological rehabilitation. *Int Psychogeriatr* 7:547–560.

Granger, C.V., Denis, L.S., Peters, N.C., Sherwood, C.C., and Barrett, J.E. (1979) Stroke rehabilitation: Analysis of repeated Barthel Index measures. *Arch Phys Med Rehabil* 60:14–17.

Greenwald, B.S., Kramer-Ginsberg, E., Krishnan, R.R., Ashtari, M., Auerbach, C., and Patel, M. (1998) Neuroanatomic localization of magnetic resonance imaging signal hyperintensities in geriatric depression. *Stroke* 29:613–617.

Hachinski, V., and Norris, J.W. (1985) *The Acute Stroke.* Philadelphia: F.A. Davis.

Hamilton, M.A. (1960) A rating scale for depression. *J Neurol Neurosurg Psychiatry* 23:56–62.

Harvey, R.F., and Jellinek, H.M. (1981) Functional performance assessment: A program approach. *Arch Phys Med Rehabil* 62:456–460.

Herrmann, M., Bartels, C., Schumacher, M., and Wallesch, C.-W. (1995) Poststroke depression: Is there a pathoanatomic correlate for depression in the postacute stage of stroke? *Stroke* 26:850–856.

Herrmann, M., Bartles, C., and Wallesch, C.-W. (1993) Depression in acute and chronic aphasia: Symptoms, pathoanatomical-clinical correlations and functional implications. *J Neurol Neurosurg Psychiatry* 56:672–678.

Herrmann, N., Black, S.E., Lawrence, J., Szekely, C., and Szalai, J.P. (1998) The Sunnybrook stroke study. A prospective study of depressive symptoms and functional outcome. *Stroke* 29:618–624.

Hibbard, M.R., Grober, S.E., Gordon, W.A., and Aletta, E.G. (1990) Modification of cognitive psychotherapy for the treatment of post-stroke depression. *Behav Therapist* 13:15–17.

House, A., Dennis, M., Mogridge, L., Warlow, C., Hawton, K., and Jones, L. (1991) Mood disorders in the year after first stroke. *Br J Psychiatry* 158:83–92.

House, A., Dennis, M., Warlow, C., Hawton, K., and Molyneaux, A. (1990a) The relationship between intellectual impairment and mood disorder in the first year after stroke. *Psychol Med* 20:805–814.

House, A., Dennis, M., Warlow, C., Hawton, K., and Molyneux, K. (1990b) Mood disorders after stroke and their relation to lesion location. A CT scan study. *Brain* 113:1113–1130.

House, A., Knapp, P., Bamford, J., and Vail, A. (2001) Mortality at 12 and 24 months after stroke may be associated with depressive symptoms at 1 month. *Stroke* 32:696–701.

Ingles, J.L., Eskes, G.A., and Phillips, S.J. (1999) Fatigue after stroke. *Arch Phys Med Rehabil* 80:173–178.

Jorge, R.E., Robinson, R.G., Arndt, S., and Starkstein, S.E. (2003) Mortality and post-stroke depression: a placebo controlled trial of antidepressants. *Am J Psychiatry* 160:1823–1829.

Kahn, R.L., RGoldfarb, A.I., Pollack, M., and Peck, A. (1960) Brief objective measures for the determination of mental status in the aged. *Am J Psychiatry* 117:326–328.

Kauhanen, M., Korpelainen, J.T., Hiltunen, P., Brusin, E., Mononen, H., Maatta, R., Nieminen, P., Sotaniemi, K.A., and Myllyla, V.V. (1999) Poststroke depression correlates with cognitive impairment and neurological deficits. *Stroke* 30:1875–1880.

Kimura, M., Robinson, R.G., and Kosier, T. (2000) Treatment of cognitive impairment after poststroke depression. *Stroke* 31:1482–1486.

Kotila, M., Numminen, H., Waltimo, O., and Kaste, M. (1998) Depression after stroke. Results of the FINNSTROKE study. *Stroke* 29:368–372.

Kotila, M., Waltimo, O., Niemim, L., Laaksonen, R., and Lempinen, M. (1984) The profile of recovery from stroke in factors influencing outcome. *Stroke* 15:1039–1044.

Kraepelin, E. (1921) *Manic Depressive Insanity and Paranoia*. Edinburgh: E&S Livingstone.

Lauritzen, L., Bendsen, B.B., Vilmar, T., Bendsen, E.B., Lunde, M., and Bech, P. (1994) Post-stroke depression: Combined treatment with imipramine or desipramine and mianserin: A controlled clinical study. *Psychopharmacology* 114:119–122.

Lipsey, J.R., Robinson, R.G., Pearlson, G.D., Rao, K., and Price, T.R. (1984) Nortriptyline treatment of post-stroke depression: A double-blind study. *Lancet* i:297–300.

Lipsey, J.R., Spencer, W.C., Rabins, P.V., and Robinson, R.G. (1986) Phenomenological comparison of functional and post-stroke depression. *Am J Psychiatry* 143:527–529.

Mahoney, F.I., and Barthel, D.W. (1965) Functional evaluation: Barthel index. *Md Med J* 14:61–65.

Mayberg, H.S., Robinson, R.G., Wong, D.F., Parikh, R.M., Bolduc, P., Starkstein, S.E., Price, T.R., Dannals, R.F., Links, J.M., Wilson, A.A., Ravert, H.T., and Wagner, H.N., Jr. (1988) PET imaging of cortical $S_2$-serotonin receptors after stroke: Lateralized changes and relationship to depression. *Am J Psychiatry* 145:937–943.

Meyer, A. (1904) The anatomical facts and clinical varieties of traumatic insanity. *Am J Insanity* 60:373–441.

Morris, P.L.P., Robinson, R.G., Andrezejewski, P., Samuels, J., and Price, T.R. (1993) Association of depression with 10-year post-stroke mortality. *Am J Psychiatry* 150:124–129.

Morris, P.L.P., Robinson, R.G., Carvalho, M.L., Albert, P., Wells, J.C., Eden-Fetzer, D., and Price, T.R. (1996a) Lesion characteristics and depressed mood in the stroke data bank study. *J Neuropsychiatry Clin Neurosci* 8:153–159.

Morris, P.L.P., Robinson, R.G., and Raphael, B. (1990) Prevalence and course of depressive disorders in hospitalized stroke patients. *Int J Psychiatr Med* 20:349–364.

Morris, P.L.P., Robinson, R.G., Raphael, B., and Hopwood, M.J. (1996b) Lesion location and post-stroke depression. *J Neuropsychiatry Clin Neurosci* 8:399–403.

Morris, P.L.P., Shields, R.B., Hopwood, M.J., Robinson, R.G., and Raphael, B. (1994) Are there two depressive syndromes after stroke? *J Nerv Ment Dis* 182:230–234.

Morrison, J.H., Molliver, M.E., and Grzanna, R. (1979) Noradrenergic innervation of the cerebral cortex: Widespread effects of local cortical lesions. *Science* 205:313–316.

Murphy, E., Smith, R., Lindesay, J., and Slattery, J. (1988) Increased mortality rates in late-life depression. *Br J Psychiatry* 152:347–353.

Murray, G.B., Shea, V., and Conn, D.R. (1987) Electroconvulsive therapy for post-stroke depression. *J Clin Psychiatry* 47:458–360.

Narushima, K., Kosier, J.T., and Robinson, R.G. (2003) A reappraisal of post-stroke depression, intra and inter-hemispheric lesion location using meta-analysis. *J Neuropsychiatry Clin Neurosci* 15:422–430.

Oradei, D.M., and Waite, N.S. (1974) Group psychotherapy with stroke patients during the immediate recovery phase. *Am J Orthopsychiatry* 44:386–395.

Paolucci, S., Antonucci, G., Pratesi, L., Traballesi, M., Grasso, M.G., and Lubich, S. (1999) Poststroke depression and its role in rehabilitation of inpatients. *Arch Phys Med Rehabil* 80:985–990.

Paradiso, S., Ohkubo, T., and Robinson, R.G. (1997) Vegetative and psychological symptoms associated with depressed mood over the first two years after stroke. *Int J Psychiatr Med* 27:137–157.

Paradiso, S., and Robinson, R.G. (1998) Gender differences in post-stroke depression. *J Neuropsychiatry Clin Neurosci* 10:41–47.

Parikh, R.M., Eden, D.T., Price, T.R., and Robinson, R.G. (1988) The sensitivity and specificity of the Center for Epidemiologic Studies depression scale as a screening instrument for post-stroke depression. *Int J Psychiatr Med* 18:169–181.

Parikh, R.M., Lipsey, J.R., Robinson, R.G., and Price, T.R. (1987) Two-year longitudinal study of post-stroke mood disorders: dynamic changes in correlates of depression at one and two years. *Stroke* 18:579–584.

Parikh, R.M., Robinson, R.G., Lipsey, J.R., Starkstein, S.E., Fedoroff, J.P., and Price, T.R. (1990) The impact of post-stroke depression on recovery in activities of daily living over two year follow-up. *Arch Neurol* 47:785–789.

Pohjasvaara, T., Leppavuori, A., Siira, I., Vataja, R., Kaste, M., and Erkinjuntti, T. (1998) Frequency and clinical determinants of poststroke depression. *Stroke* 29:2311–2317.

Post, F. (1962) *The Significance of Affective Symptoms in Old Age*. London: Oxford University Press.

Ramasubbu, R. (1994) Denial of illness and depression in stroke. *Stroke* 25:226–227.

Rapp, S.R., and Vrana, S. (1989) Substituting nonsomatic for somatic symptoms in the diagnosis of depression in elderly male medical patients. *Am J Psychiatry* 146:1197–1200.

Reding, M.J., Orto, L.A., Winter, S.W., Fortuna, I.M., DiPonte, P., and McDowell, F.H. (1986) Antidepressant therapy after stroke: A double-blind trial. *Arch Neurol* 43:763–765.

Rifkin, A., Reardon, G., Siris, S., Karagji, B., Kim, Y.S., Hackstaff, L., and Endicott, N. (1985) Trimipramine in physical illness with depression. *J Clin Psychiatry* 46:4–8.

Robinson, R.G. (2003) The controversy over post-stroke depression and lesion location. *Psychiatric Times* 20:39–40.

Robinson, R.G. (1979) Differential behavioral and biochemical effects of right and left hemispheric cerebral infarction in the rat. *Science* 105:707–710.

Robinson, R.G., Bolduc, P., and Price, T.R. (1987) A two year longitudinal study of post-stroke depression: Diagnosis and outcome at one and two year follow-up. *Stroke* 18:837–843.

Robinson, R.G., Bolla-Wilson, K., Kaplan, E., Lipsey, J.R., and Price, T.R. (1986a) Depression influences intellectual impairment in stroke patients. *Br J Psychiatry* 148:541–547.

Robinson, R.G., Kubos, K.L., Starr, L.B., Rao, K., and Price, T.R. (1983a) Mood changes in stroke patients: Relationship to lesion location. *Compr Psychiatry* 24:555–566.

Robinson, R.G., Kubos, K.L., Starr, L.B., Rao, K., and Price, T.R. (1984a) Mood disorders in stroke patients: Importance of location of lesion. *Brain* 107:81–93.

Robinson, R.G., Lipsey, J.R., Bolla-Wilson, K., Bolduc, P.L., Pearlson, G.D., Rao, K., and Price, T.R. (1985a) Mood disorders in left handed stroke patients. *Am J Psychiatry* 142:1424–1429.

Robinson, R.G., Lipsey, J.R., Rao, K., and Price, T.R. (1986b) Two-year longitudinal study of post-stroke mood disorders: Comparison of acute-onset with delayed-onset depression. *Am J Psychiatry* 143:1238–1244.

Robinson, R.G., Parikh, R.M., Lipsey, J.R., Starkstein, S.E., and Price, T.R. (1993) Pathological laughing and crying following stroke: validation of measurement scale and double-blind treatment study. *Am J Psychiatry* 150:286–293.

Robinson, R.G., and Price, T.R. (1982) Post-stroke depressive disorders: A follow-up study of 103 outpatients. *Stroke* 13:635–641.

Robinson, R.G., Schultz, S.K., Castillo, C., Kopel, T., and Kosier, T. (2000) Nortriptyline versus fluoxetine in the treatment of depression and in short term recovery after stroke: A placebo controlled, double-blind study. *Am J Psychiatry* 157:351–359.

Robinson, R.G., Starr, L.B., Kubos, K.L., and Price, T.R. (1983b) A two year longitudinal study of post-stroke mood disorders: Findings during the initial evaluation. *Stroke* 14:736–744.

Robinson, R.G., Starr, L.B., Lipsey, J.R., Rao, K., and Price, T.R. (1985b) A two year longitudinal study of post-stroke mood disorders: In-hospital prognostic factors associated with six month outcome. *J Nerv Ment Dis* 173:221–226.

Robinson, R.G., Starr, L.B., and Price, T.R. (1984b) A two-year longitudinal study of post-stroke mood disorders: Dynamic changes in associated variables over the first six months of follow-up. *Stroke* 15:510–517.

Robinson, R.G., and Szetela, B. (1981) Mood change following left hemispheric brain injury. *Ann Neurol* 9:447–453.

Scandinavian Stroke Study Group. (1985) Multicenter trial of hemodilution in ischemic stroke—background and study protocol. *Stroke* 16:885–890.

Schubert, D.S.P., Taylor, C., Lee, S., Mentari, A., and Tamaklo, W. (1992) Physical consequences of depression in the stroke patient. *Gen Hosp Psychiatry* 14:69–76.

Schwartz, J.A., Speed, N.M., Brunberg, J.A., Brewer, T.L., Brown, M., and Greden, J.F. (1993) Depression in stroke rehabilitation. *Biol Psychiatry* 33:694–699.

Shimoda, K., and Robinson, R.G. (1999) The relationship between post-stroke depression and lesion location in long-term follow-up. *Biol Psychiatry* 45:187–192.

Singh A.B., Herrmann, S.E.N., Leibovitch, F.S., Ebert, P.L., Lawrence, J., and Szalai, J.P. (2000) Functional and neuroanatomic correlations in poststroke depression: the Sunnybrook Stroke Study. *Stroke* 31:637–644.

Sinyor, D., Amato, P., and Kaloupek, P. (1986) Post-stroke depression: Relationship to functional impairment, coping strategies, and rehabilitation outcome. *Stroke* 17:112–117.

Snaith, R.P., Ahmed, S.N., Mehta, S., and Hamilton, M. (1971) Assessment of the severity of primary depressive illness. Wakefield self-assessment depression inventory. *Psychol Med* 1:143–149.

Soares, J.C., and Mann. J.J. (1997) The anatomy of mood disorders—review of structural neuroimaging studies. *Biol Psychiatry* 41:86–106.

Spitzer, R.L., Endicott, J., and Robins, E. (1978) Research diagnostic criteria: Rationale and reliability. *Arch Gen Psychiatry* 35:773–782.

Starkstein, S.E., Boston, J.D., and Robinson, R.G. (1988a) Mechanisms of mania after brain injury: 12 case reports and review of the literature. *J Nerv Ment Dis* 176:87–100.

Starkstein, S.E., Fedoroff, J.P., Price, T.R., Leiguarda, R., and Robinson, R.G. (1992) Anosognosia in patients with cerebrovascular lesions. A study of causative factors. *Stroke* 23:1446–1453.

Starkstein, S.E., Fedoroff, Price, T.R., Leiguarda, R., and Robinson, R.G. (1993) Catastrophic reaction after cerebrovascular lesions: Frequency, correlates, and validation of a scale. *J Neurol Neurosurg Psychiatry* 5:189–194.

Starkstein, S.E., Robinson, R.G., Honig, M.A., Parikh, R.M., Joselyn, P., and Price, T.R. (1989) Mood changes after right hemisphere lesion. *Br J Psychiatry* 155:79–85.

Starkstein, S.E., Robinson, R.G., and Price, T.R. (1987) Comparison of cortical and subcortical lesions in the production of post-stroke mood disorders. *Brain* 110:1045–1059.

Starkstein, S.E., Robinson, R.G., and Price, T.R. (1988b) Comparison of patients with and without post-stroke major depression matched for size and location of lesion. *Arch Gen Psychiatry* 45:247–252.

Starkstein, S.E., Robinson, R.G., and Price, T.R. (1988c) Comparison of spontaneously recovered versus non-recovered patients with post-stroke depression. *Stroke* 19:1491–1496.

Ullman, M., and Gruen, A. (1960) Behavioral changes in patients with stroke. *Am J Psychiatry* 117:1004–1009.

Vataja, R., Pohjasvaara, T., Leppavuori, A., Mantyla, R., Aronen, H.J., Salonen, O., Kaste, M., and Erkinjuntti, T. (2001) Magnetic resonance imaging correlates of depression after ischemic stroke. *Arch Gen Psychiatry* 58:925–931.

Wade, D.T., Legh-Smith, J., and Hewer, R.A. (1987) Depressed mood after stroke, a community study of its frequency. *Br J Psychiatry* 151:200–205.

Watzlawick, P., and Coyne, J.C. (1980) Depression following stroke: Brief, problem-focused family treatment. *Family Process* 19: 13–18.

Wechsler, D. (1997) *Wechsler Memory Scale*, 3rd ed. San Antonio: Harcourt, Brace.

Wells, C.E. (1979) Pseudodementia. *Am J Psychiatry* 136:895–900.

Wing, J.K., Cooper, J.E., and Sartorius, N. (1974) *The Measurement and Classification of Psychiatric Symptoms: An Instructional Manual for the PSE and CATEGO Programs*. New York: Cambridge University Press.

Zung, W.W.K. (1965) A self-rating depression scale. *Arch Gen Psychiatry* 12:377–395.

# 27 | Substance abuse co-morbidity

DAVID W. OSLIN

The impact of late-life addictive disorders is a growing public health concern. Epidemiological studies have demonstrated that the abuse of addictive substances is common among older adults. Moreover, substance abuse in early adulthood can have lasting effects into late life, including an increase in the likelihood of developing other late-life mental health problems. Thus, in measuring the impact of addictions on older adults, one must consider the lifetime use and abuse of these substances. This chapter will focus on the intersection between the use and abuse of addictive substances and the presence and course of depressive disorders. Emphasis will be placed on those substances that are most commonly abused by older adults, namely, alcohol, cigarettes, and benzodiazepines. Only brief attention will be given to other abused drugs.

## DEFINING CO-MORBIDITY

Co-morbidity has been recognized as a significant factor in the effectiveness of various treatments in most areas of medicine. With regard to late-life major depression, co-morbidity with medical problems or with substance abuse is often the rule rather than the exception (Blazer and Koenig, 1993). Because the terms "co-morbidity" and "dual diagnosis" have been used to refer to a variety of different interactions of diseases, these terms can be misleading. Most often, "co-morbidity" is used to describe the co-occurrence of two diseases—for example, alcoholism and depression. At the other end of the spectrum, "co-morbidity" has been used to imply any lifetime correlation between two disorders even when the disorders occur at different times in a person's life—for example, an older adult with current symptoms of a depressive disorder who has a past history of alcohol dependence but does not currently drink. The past history of alcohol dependence may be important in predicting the treatment outcome of the depressive disorder and may influence the choices of treatment. "Co-morbidity" has also been defined more narrowly as two or more disorders that interact to produce an effect not seen by either disorder alone—for example, failure to respond to an antidepressant. This effect may also occur despite years of separation between the acute phases of the disorders. While all of these definitions are valid and acceptable, it is important, when reading literature and communicating with others, to clarify which definition is in use. Although not typically considered co-morbidity, the use of addictive substances like alcohol or benzodiazepines may impact on the treatment of depression when the depressed older adult is using the substance but not to a degree that warrants a diagnosis of abuse or dependence. These interactions will also be considered in this chapter. In an effort to collate information from a variety of research studies, this chapter will include the spectrum of definitions of co-morbidity.

## THE EPIDEMIOLOGY OF LATE-LIFE ADDICTIONS

The health and social costs of alcohol dependence have been well described for middle-aged and younger adults, and the patterns of drinking leading to alcohol dependence have been well documented. Alcohol consumption of older adults differs significantly from that of middle-aged and younger adults. The majority of older adults do not drink, and those who do, drink moderately with few or no apparent consequences due to their drinking. However, the prevalence of alcohol dependence is rising among healthy adults age 65–75 who were raised during a time of greater drug and alcohol use. Current prevalence estimates suggest that 40% of older adults drink and that 10% to 22% of older adults drink daily, with the majority of older adults drinking within recommended drinking limits (Adams et al., 1996; Barry et al., 1998; Douglass et al., 1988; Fillmore, 1987; Goodwin et al., 1987; Herd, 1990; Molgaard et al., 1990).

Rates of alcohol dependence among community-dwelling elderly persons have been estimated in two recent studies. Kandel and colleagues (1997) reported on symptoms of alcohol dependence using the National Household Survey on Drug Abuse. Study participants included 87,915 noninstitutionalized adults over 12 years of age. Among the participants aged 50 and older, both alcohol use and cigarette use were common (54.9% reported alcohol use in the last year, and 22.6% reported cigarette use). However, the prevalence of alcohol dependence was 1.6%, and the prevalence of nicotine dependence was 5.4%. The prevalence of marijuana and cocaine dependence was reported as 0.01% and 0.1%. Black and colleagues (1998) reported on a cohort of 865 elderly adults living in a public housing project in Baltimore. The prevalence of current alcohol-related problems was 4%, with a lifetime prevalence of 22%. Put into perspective, the prevalence of alcohol dependence among elderly men exceeds the prevalence of major depression among elderly men (Liberto et al., 1992).

Other recent studies have examined the epidemiology of substance use disorders among the elderly, focusing on primary care practices, nursing homes, and hospitals. Barry and colleagues (1998) conducted an alcohol screening program in over 12,000 elderly primary care patients. Among those evaluated, 15% screened positive for alcohol problems based upon alcohol consumption, binge drinking, or the presence of alcohol-related problems. A similar project conducted by Callahan and colleagues (1996) found that 10.6% of the older primary care patients had alcohol problems. Patients were considered to have an alcohol-related problem if they reported any drinking in the last year and scored ≥2 on the CAGE questionnaire. Among 140 patients enrolled in a geriatric mental health outpatient clinic, Holroyd and Duryee (1997) reported the prevalence of alcohol dependence (DSM-IV diagnosis) to be 8.6%. The authors also reported that 11.4% of the patients were dependent on benzodiazepines.

Little is known about the epidemiology of substance use disorders other than alcoholism in the elderly. The general belief is that older drug addicts represent only younger addicts grown old, with few older adults initiating drug use in their later years. In addition to the National Household Survey noted above, the Epidemiologic Catchment Area (ECA) study is one of the few community epidemiological surveys that included older adults (Robins and Regier, 1991). Using the Diagnostic Interview Schedule (DIS) to determine prevalence rates for psychiatric diagnoses as defined by DSM-III, the study found the lifetime prevalence rates of drug abuse and dependence to be 0.12% for elderly men and 0.06% for elderly women, respectively. No active cases were reported for either gender. In contrast, a more recent study of an elder-specific drug program in a population of veterans found that one-quarter of patients had either a primary drug problem or a concurrent drug and alcohol problem (Schonfeld et al., 2000).

### Benzodiazepines

A common problem with the elderly is the misuse of prescription and over-the-counter medications. This includes the misuse of substances such as sedative/hypnotics, narcotic and nonnarcotic analgesics, diet aids, decongestants, and a wide variety of other over-the-counter medications. Historically, benzodiazepines have been among the most commonly prescribed medications in the United States. The prevalence of benzodiazepine use increases with age, and the elderly are more likely to take benzodiazepines chronically (Holroyd and Duryee, 1997; Simon et al., 1996). Studies mostly from the 1970s and 1980s suggested that 10%–15% of the elderly were taking a benzodiazepine (Dunbar et al., 1989; Krska and MacLeod, 1995; Wright et al., 1994; Zisselman et al., 1994). However, a more recent study by Blazer and colleagues (2000) suggests that there have been few changes in the use of benzodiazepines over the past decade. Previous research has also shown that benzodiazepines are often inappropriately prescribed for illnesses such as depression, psychosis, and chronic insomnia (Isacson et al., 1993; Rickels et al., 1991; Simon et al., 1996; Straand and Rokstad, 1997; Zisselman et al., 1994).

### Smoking

Smoking is often overlooked as a problem for the elderly, but it contributes significantly to the disability and poor health of some elders. Although smoking rates decrease with age (primarily due to differential mortality among smokers and nonsmokers), one out of every five smokers is age 50 or older (Gourlay and Benowitz, 1996; Orleans et al., 1990). Approximately 15.2% of community-dwelling individuals age 65 to 74 and 8.4% of those aged 75 and older are smokers, with higher rates found among African-American men (22.1% of those between ages 65–74 and 12% of those age 75 or older) (Center for Disease Control and Prevention 1999).

In summary, the use and abuse of alcohol, cigarettes, and benzodiazepines are common in late life. The impact of late-life addictions will continue to grow as the population of older adults increases. Cohort changes may also influence the magnitude of late-life addictions since the baby boom generation, which is now entering late life, grew up during a time when alcohol and drug use was more acceptable compared to earlier periods. This may be even more significant for older women, as evidenced by the increased use of cigarettes and the associated increase in cancer rates over the past several decades. There is strong speculation that similar increases are occurring in alcohol and drug dependence in women and that these rates will continue to increase over the next several decades.

## THE CO-OCCURRENCE OF LATE-LIFE DEPRESSION AND USE OF ADDICTIVE SUBSTANCES

Several studies that have examined the co-occurrence of depression with substance abuse and dependence have included older adults. The National Co-morbidity Study, which was designed to explore the epidemiology of various co-morbid conditions, indicated that alcoholism and depression were the most common co-morbid conditions across the life span (Kessler et al., 1996). Other studies, including the ECA study, have found that alcoholism occurs 1.6 times more often in depressed than nondepressed subjects (Helzer and Pryzbeck 1988; Kessler et al., 1996; Merikangas and Gelernter, 1990). Although less is known about older adults, the few studies that have included the older population indicate that concurrent alcohol use and depression are common, especially among those seeking treatment. For older subjects discharged from a psychiatric hospital, Blixen and colleagues (1997) found that 27 of 74 (37%) elderly subjects with major depression had a concurrent diagnosis of alcoholism. Speer and Bates (1992) also found that 18% of the older patients in an inpatient psychiatric facility had a diagnosis of concurrent major depression and alcoholism. Callahan and associates (1994) also found alcoholism to be common among older subjects with major depression and suggested that alcoholism be used as a clinical factor that should alert a clinician to evaluate a subject for depression.

Studies of subjects with alcoholism also indicate high rates of co-morbidity with major depression. In one of the larger studies of the interaction of alcohol dependence and depression, Blow and colleagues (1992) reviewed the diagnosis of 22,463 veterans presenting for alcohol treatment. The most common co-morbid psychiatric disorder was an affective disorder, which was found in 21% of the subjects. As shown in Figure 27.1, there was an age-related increase in co-morbid major depression across the entire life cycle, indicating that the co-morbidity of depression and alcoholism was a more significant issue for older adults than for younger adults. In addition, those with co-morbid disorders were shown to have greater functional impairment than those with only one of the two problems.

## Smoking and Benzodiazepines

Smoking and depression have also been shown to co-occur at higher rates than would be expected if they were unrelated disorders. For instance, in a study of 526 primary care patients, smoking was one of several factors associated with the presence of significant depressive symptoms (Brown et al., 2000). In one of the largest primary care studies focused on older adults, 26,588 patients were screened. The rate of smoking among those who screened positive for depression was 13.4% compared to 9.9% in those who were not depressed (Kirchner, 2002). The value of benzodiazepines for older depressed patients is debatable because of both the possible risks and benefits associated with benzodiazepine use. This practice remains controversial because few studies have examined the impact of benzodiazepine use in the elderly. Two unpublished reports indicate that the prescription of benzodiazepines is common practice in the management of late-life depression. In a study of over 2500 elderly patients treated for a depressive disorder as inpatients, nearly 40% were taking a benzodiazepine at the time of admission to the geripsychiatric unit, and of those taking a benzodiazepine at the time of admission, 77% continued to take the medication as outpatients (Oslin, 2002). Recent data from a study of randomly selected primary care patients found that 19.5% of those who screened positive for depression were currently taking a benzodiazepine, with the most common medications being alprazolam and lorazepam (Bruce, 2002).

## Consequences of Co-Morbidity

Concurrent alcohol abuse and depressive disorders are not only common in late life, but alcohol use is an important factor in the course and prognosis of the depressive disorder. Among younger patients, Hanna and Grant (1997) demonstrated that symptoms of depression were more severe in subjects with co-morbid conditions than in those with either disorder alone. Depressed adults with alcohol dependence also have a more complicated clinical course of depression, with an increased risk of suicide, more social dysfunction than nondepressed alcohol-dependent adults, and a worse prognosis (Blixen et al., 1997; Conwell, 1991; Cook et al., 1991; Hanna and Grant, 1997; Hasin et al., 1996; Helzer and Pryzbeck, 1988; Schuckit et al., 1997). They

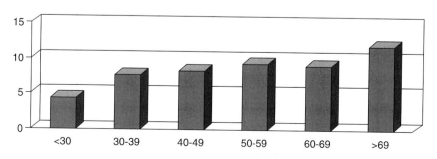

FIGURE 27.1 The prevalence of co-morbid depression among patients seeking treatment for alcoholism.

also seek more treatment and use more health services (Fortney et al., 1999).

However, other studies have not shown that co-morbidity is a significant factor in treatment outcome. Helzer and Pryzbeck (1988) found that relapse rates for those with alcoholism do not appear to be influenced by the presence of depression. Kranzler and colleagues (1996) also found that the presence of depression among those with alcoholism did not influence alcohol-related symptoms or the number of drinking days over the course of 3 years. Most recently, Hodgins et al. (1999) found that although there was synchrony between alcohol relapse and depression relapse, one did not predict the other. One difficulty in interpreting these studies is that the majority of them have focused on patients seeking treatment for alcoholism and have not distinguished substance-induced or secondary depression from a primary depressive disorder.

Few studies have specifically explored the effects of co-morbid substance abuse on late-life depression. Oslin and colleagues (1999) conducted a longitudinal descriptive study of middle-aged and older adults who recently received a charge of driving while intoxicated. The results of the study demonstrated greater self-rated disability among older subjects suffering from concurrent alcoholism and major depression compared to subjects with either alcohol abuse or dependence alone. Moreover, there was no change in drinking behavior or level of depression over the course of 1 year. Among those with current major depression, the 1-year assessment continued to show greater dysfunction in several areas after accounting for the baseline level of disability. These results suggest a low rate of spontaneous recovery and a need for disease-specific interventions among subjects with co-morbid major depression. There was also infrequent use of specialty addiction treatment in the prior 2 months and extremely frequent use of primary care facilities. This pattern concurs with the findings of previous studies demonstrating that older adults are less likely to have addiction treatment services recommended and less likely to undergo addiction treatment than younger adults (Brennan et al., 2001; Curtis et al., 1986).

Alcohol abuse prior to late life has also been shown to influence the treatment of late-life depression. Cook and colleagues (1991) found that a prior history of alcohol abuse predicted a more severe and chronic course of late-life depression, and is a risk factor for suicide in late life (Waern, 2003). Similarly, several studies have shown that alcohol problems earlier in life increase the risk of developing depression or dementia in subsequent years, even after prolonged periods of abstinence from alcohol (Crum et al., 2001; Saunders et al., 1991; Schutte et al., 1997). Finally, alcoholism significantly increases noncompliance with medication regimens and reduces attendance at treatment programs, both of which can substantially impact on treatment outcomes (Burman et al., 1997; Maarbjerg et al., 1988).

Of special interest to mental health service providers are the effects of moderate or at-risk alcohol consumption on other mental health disorders. In a recent study of over 2000 elderly patients, Oslin and colleagues (2000) demonstrated an added benefit of reducing low levels of alcohol use while treating a depressive disorder. Co-morbid alcoholism (self-reported lifetime history of alcohol problems) occurred in 9.4% of the sample. However, 38.8% of the patients reported some drinking within the past 6 months, and 3.5% of them reported drinking nearly every day. In contrast to the study hypothesis, current alcohol use did not predict a poor outcome for treatment; in fact, those patients who were moderate or heavy drinkers had better outcomes on several measures. However, all of the patients stopped drinking while in the hospital, and the majority continued to be abstinent after discharge. Thus, the combination of treatment of depression and elimination of alcohol use was beneficial. It should also be noted that most of these patients were moderate drinkers. Similarly, nondiagnostic levels of depression or distress have been shown to increase the use of alcohol or relapse in older adults being treated for alcoholism (Holahan et al., 2001; Schonfeld and Dupree, 1991; Schutte et al., 1998). These studies underscore the importance of addressing the use of alcohol or mild affective symptoms when treating late-life depression or alcoholism. Treating concurrent nonproblematic substance abuse would not *traditionally* be viewed as co-morbidity or a dual diagnosis but is nonetheless an important aspect of improving treatment outcomes.

## Smoking

Research conducted over the past 50 years, including many large–scale epidemiological studies, has produced overwhelming evidence that smoking is harmful at any age. Cigarette smoking accounts for more than 400,000 deaths annually in the United States and is considered the most significant cause of preventable morbidity and mortality (McGinnis and Foege, 1993). It has been well documented that smoking increases the risk of respiratory and nonrespiratory cancers, cardiovascular disease, cerebrovascular disease, and nonmalignant respiratory disease (e.g., chronic obstructive pulmonary disease), as well as other nonmalignant diseases such as ulcer and osteoporosis (Hays et al., 1998; Samet, 1992).

The effects of smoking on the treatment of late-life depression have been addressed in relatively few studies. Patten and colleagues (2001) compared hospitalized smokers with a primary mood disorder with a matched sample of depressed nonsmokers. Although smoking did not predict overall worse treatment outcomes, it was associated with less improvement in certain symptoms such as fatigue. In another study, the presence of depression did not appear to impact the success of smoking cessation (Keuthen et al., 2000; Vazquez and Becona, 1999). Together these findings suggest that it may be important to address co-morbid smoking in the treatment of depression, although it is clear that more research needs to be conducted in this area.

## Benzodiazepines

Understanding the consequences of using benzodiazepines in the context of depression has evolved over the years from a recognition that benzodiazepines alone are a poor choice for treatment of depression to questions regarding the risks and benefits of benzodiazepine use as an adjunct to antidepressant use. There is clear evidence that benzodiazepines can increase the risk of falls and may impair cognition in older adults (Gales and Menard, 1995; Hemmelgarn et al., 1997; Herings et al., 1995; Newman et al., 1997; Ried et al., 1998). These problems have occurred most consistently with longer-acting benzodiazepines and with higher doses. The risks are also more apparent with chronic use rather than short-term (<3 months) use. A recent review of randomized, controlled trials of depression management, mostly in younger adults, indicates that patients may have greater improvement and less attrition with the use of a benzodiazepine in addition to an antidepressant (Furukawa et al., 2001). The reviewed studies were conducted over short time periods (≤8 weeks) and did not address the long-term risks or benefits of benzodiazepine use. Given that most older adults take benzodiazepines chronically, it is not clear that the short-term studies are an indication of the risks associated with benzodiazepine use.

Overall, the interaction between depression and co-morbid substance abuse is complex. Findings suggest a strong interaction between depression and substance abuse in some patients and a weaker interaction in others. There are suggestions that these interactions can be better understood in the context of primary and secondary disorders. However, these distinctions are very difficult to make reliably, and it is likely that other factors are also important in understanding the interaction, including environmental factors, personality traits, genetic factors, and social supports. Figure 27.2 presents one conceptual model for understanding the reciprocal interaction of these problems. Given the weight of evidence suggesting that these problems do interact to produce greater disability, it is reasonable to conclude that focusing treatment in a way that addresses both problems would be beneficial to patients.

## DIAGNOSTIC CONSIDERATIONS

The epidemiological studies demonstrating higher than expected rates of co-morbid depression and substance abuse are based on the ability to recognize and diagnose distinct disorders. Intoxication and withdrawal cause many behavioral and mood states that mimic other psychiatric illnesses such as depression, psychosis, or cognitive disorders. Thus, the relationship between substance abuse and other psychiatric symptoms is difficult to ascertain with good reliability and validity (Oslin et al., 2001). Ideally, co-morbidity with psychiatric symptoms is best described prospectively while monitoring for the emergence of new symptoms. A retrospective diagnosis has the drawback that the reliability and validity of the information gathered may be suspect. This is a particularly relevant problem among

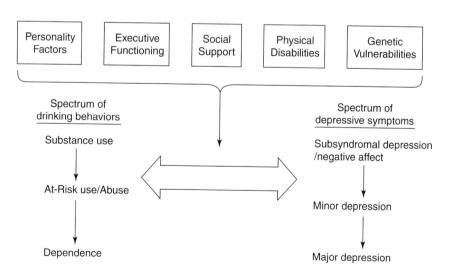

FIGURE 27.2 Complex interactions between substance use and depressive symptoms.

older patients and among alcoholics, who as part of their illness may suffer from cognitive deficits that make reporting of information problematic.

In a seminal paper, Brown and Schuckit (1988) reported that 42% of subjects present to detoxification facilities with significant depressive symptoms but only 6% continue to have significant symptoms at 4 weeks. This work led to the recognition that significant depressive symptoms and alcohol use can interact in a number of ways. Significant depressive symptoms can precede (primary or independent depression), occur simultaneously with (indeterminate depression), or develop as a consequence of (reactive or secondary depression) significant alcohol use. Clinically, a diagnosis of primary depression would lead to treatment plans to address both disorders concurrently, whereas a diagnosis of secondary depression would suggest treating the addiction while watchfully waiting for the resolution of the depressive symptoms. Making a distinction between these diagnoses places an emphasis on the temporal relationship of the symptoms of depression and periods of abstinence. Thus, depression that either precedes the onset of substance use or occurs during a prolonged period of abstinence is considered primary depression or independent depression. Correspondingly, depression that develops as a consequence of substance use is considered reactive or secondary depression.

The distinction between primary and secondary alcoholism has implications for understanding the consequences of the co-morbidity. At least three studies have found that people with primary major depression with co-morbid alcoholism have more severe symptoms, are less likely to show improvement of depressive symptoms, and have a greater chance of suicide than subjects with secondary depression (Hasegawa et al., 1990; Schuckit et al., 1997; Tsuang et al., 1995). Thus, it is entirely possible that the consequences of co-morbid depression, including long-term outcomes, are worse in primary depressed patients compared to patients with secondary depression. The significance of these treatment outcome differences among older adults is unclear. It is speculated that because of the lower prevalence of alcohol dependence and the modest prevalence of depressive disorders in elders, primary depression may be more common in late life.

Several strategies have evolved to address problems related to distinguishing co-morbid psychiatric disorders from symptoms of alcohol intoxication or withdrawal. Methods for distinguishing symptoms of alcohol use from other syndromes have been formalized in many semistructured interviews such as the DIS and the Structured Clinical Interview for DSM-IV (SCID) (First et al., 1981; Robins et al., 1981). These instruments generally rely on interviewer judgment to determine the relationship between alcohol use and symptoms such as depression or psychosis. The interviewer relies on information regarding periods of abstinence and the timing of the onset of both problems. The diagnosis of a primary affective disorder is made if the symptoms occur during a period of abstinence or precede the onset of the second illness. Otherwise, the symptoms are considered related to the alcohol use. This method is useful for categorizing syndromes and has been shown to be reliable. Other, more recent semistructured interviews include criteria embedded for making distinctions between primary and secondary major depression, the Semi-Structured Assessment for the Genetics of Alcoholism (SSAGA) and the Psychiatric Research Interview for Substance and Mental Disorders (PRISM) (Bucholz et al., 1994; Hasin et al., 1996a). However, both of these instruments require a considerably longer time to administer than the SCID.

## TREATMENT ISSUES

There is a limited number of studies that address the treatment of patients who present with co-morbid alcoholism and depression. Rigorous treatment recommendations are few, as many patients with co-morbid substance use are excluded from clinical trials. For example, concurrent alcohol or drug misuse was found to be the most important factor for exclusion (17%) of subjects from antidepressant trials. Other significant exclusions included current use of an antidepressant (15%), concurrent physical disability (14%), and organizational difficulty (16%) (Partonen et al., 1996). Several recent studies have included subjects with co-morbid major depression and alcoholism. In one study, McGrath and colleagues (1996) conducted a 12-week placebo-controlled trial of imipramine in outpatients with co-morbid major depression and alcoholism. The results demonstrated an antidepressant effect of the medication but no overall effect on drinking outcomes, and less than half of the subjects had improvement in both their depression and drinking.

Mason and colleagues (1996) conducted a placebo-controlled study of desipramine in patients with alcoholism with and without major depression. In this study, all of the depressed subjects had a diagnosis of secondary major depression and the sample size was small, with 10 to 15 subjects in each group. Despite this, the drug significantly reduced depressive symptoms in the desipramine-treated group compared to the placebo-treated group. There was no effect on the number of subjects who relapsed, but the drug significantly increased the time to relapse.

In a third study, Cornelius and colleagues (1997) evaluated subjects with primary major depression and co-morbid alcoholism. Patients were randomly assigned to placebo or fluoxetine treatment. Fluoxetine significantly improved depressive symptoms over the

12-week study period. This study also found that flu-oxetine reduced total alcohol consumption, although there was no information regarding the number of subjects who achieved full remission from both illnesses.

In a fourth study, Roy-Byrne and colleagues (2000) examined nefazadone as monotherapy in treating primary depression complicated by alcoholism. This study demonstrated an antidepressant effect but no effect on drinking outcomes.

Published studies combining pharmacological treatments for major depression and alcoholism, such as naltrexone and an antidepressant, are also absent. However, the rationale for treating both disorders is sound and is logically based on the concurrent treatment of any two disorders, such as hypertension and major depression or cognitive disorders and major depression. Results from a recent randomized placebo controlled trial of naltrexone as an adjunct to sertraline and psychosocial support in older adults failed to demonstrate added value of naltrexone (Oslin, submitted for publication). However, there was a robust association with relapse during treatment or frequent drinking during treatment and reduced depression response. This trial underscores the need to treat alcohol dependence concurrently while treating depression.

In the absence of empirical data, specific treatment recommendations for older adults with co-morbid substance abuse are derived from a consensus development process that reviewed existing data to develop treatment guidelines (Blow, 1998). Once significant substance use and any associated problems have been identified, it is important to note that older persons with a substance use problem often present with a variety of treatment needs. It is therefore important to have an array of services available for older adults that can be tailored to these individual needs and have the flexibility to adapt to changing needs over time. The spectrum of alcohol interventions for older adults ranges from minimal advice or brief structured interventions for at-risk or problem drinkers to formalized alcoholism treatment for drinkers who meet criteria for abuse and/or dependence. The array of formalized treatment options available includes various psychotherapeutic options, educational tools, rehabilitative and residential models, and psychopharmacological treatments. An example of why this tailoring of needs is important is the contrast between the at-risk drinker or benzodiazepine user and the severely dependent patient. It is unlikely that the at-risk user will need the intensity of services required by the severely dependent patient. Indeed, requiring the at-risk drinker to receive a mandatory set of services may be more detrimental to the outcome than helpful. The use of brief interventions and individual therapy focused on alcohol use can also easily be incorporated into the treatment

of depression without necessitating a referral to a specialty addiction service.

The assessment of any substance abuser starts with a thorough history, physical examination, and laboratory tests. In addition to quantifying the frequency and quantity of use, assessing the presence of substance-specific problems should be considered part of routine practice. For older adults who drink, instruments such as the Short Geriatric Michigan Alcohol Screening Test (S-GMAST), the Alcohol Use Disorders Test (AUDIT), or the Alcohol Related Problems Survey can be helpful in documenting problems (Blow, 1993; Moore et al., 2000; Saunders et al., 1993). The S-GMAST (Table 27.1) was developed specifically for older adults and is useful both as a screening tool and to track progress in treatment. Included in the initial assessment is the patient's potential to suffer acute withdrawal symptoms. Severe symptoms of withdrawal, such as those from alcohol use, can be life-threatening and warrant careful attention. Patients with severe symptoms of dependency or withdrawal potential and patients with significant medical or psychiatric co-morbidity may require inpatient hospitalization for acute stabilization prior to implementing an outpatient management strategy.

TABLE 27.1. *Short Geriatric Michigan Alcoholism Screening Test (S-GMAST)*

| In the past year: | YES | NO |
|---|---|---|
| 1. When talking with others, do you ever underestimate how much you actually drink? | (1) | (0) |
| 2. After a few drinks, have you sometimes not eaten or been able to skip a meal because you didn't feel hungry? | (1) | (0) |
| 3. Does having a few drinks help decrease your shakiness or tremors? | (1) | (0) |
| 4. Does alcohol sometimes make it hard for you to remember parts of the day or night? | (1) | (0) |
| 5. Do you usually take a drink to relax or calm your nerves? | (1) | (0) |
| In the past year: | | |
| 6. Do you drink to take your mind off your problems? | (1) | (0) |
| 7. Have you ever increased your drinking after experiencing a loss in your life? | (1) | (0) |
| 8. Has a doctor or nurse ever said they were worried or concerned about your drinking? | (1) | (0) |
| 9. Have you ever made rules to manage your drinking? | (1) | (0) |
| 10. When you feel lonely, does having a drink help? | (1) | (0) |

TOTAL SMAST-G SCORE (0–10) _____

A score of greater than 2 is indicative of alcohol problems.

*Source:* Reprinted with permission of the University of Michigan Alcohol Research Center. © The Regents of the University of Michigan, 1991

344    DEPRESSION CO-MORBID WITH OTHER ILLNESSES

Traditionally, outpatient substance abuse treatment has been reserved for specialized clinics focused only on substance abuse. It is becoming increasingly apparent that this model is inadequate in addressing the broader public health demand and that there is a need to involve a variety of clinicians and clinical settings in delivering substance abuse treatment. This is particularly important in older adults with concurrent depression who rarely seek specialized addiction services. The traditional addiction clinic is focused on supportive group psychotherapy and encouragement to attend regular self-help group meetings such as those of Alcoholics Anonymous (AA), Alcoholics Victorious, Rational Recovery, or Narcotics Anonymous. For older adults, peer-specific group activities are considered superior to mixed-age group activities. Individual psychosocial support is also very effective in the treatment of late-life alcoholism (Oslin et al., 2002).

Outpatient rehabilitation, in addition to focusing on active addiction issues, usually needs to address issues of time management. Abstinence reduces the time spent in maintaining the substance use disorder. The management of this time, which is often the greater part of a patient's day, is critical to the prognosis of treatment. Use of resources such as day programs and senior centers can be beneficial, especially in cognitively impaired patients. Social services such as financial support are often needed to stabilize the patient in early recovery. Supervised living arrangements such as halfway houses, group homes, nursing homes, and residing with relatives should also be considered.

Low-intensity, brief interventions have been suggested as cost-effective and practical techniques that can be used as an initial approach to at-risk and problem drinkers in primary care settings or for those patients with low levels of drinking followed in a mental health clinic. Treatment manuals for at-risk drinkers specifically designed for older adults have been published (Barry et al., 2001). Brief intervention studies have been conducted in a wide range of health-care settings, ranging from hospitals and primary health care locations to mental health clinics. To date, there have been two brief alcohol intervention trials with older adults (Barry et al., 1998; Fleming et al., 1999). Both studies were designed as randomized, clinical, brief intervention trials to reduce hazardous drinking in older adults, using advice protocols in primary care settings. These studies showed that older adults can be engaged in brief intervention protocols, that the protocols are acceptable to this population, and that there is a substantial reduction in drinking among at-risk drinkers receiving the interventions compared to a control group.

The use of medications to support abstinence may be of benefit but has not been well studied. No research to date has addressed the pharmacological treatment of older alcoholics, although studies are underway using naltrexone, as well as various antidepressants including the selective serotonin reuptake inhibitors (SSRIs). Some of the general principles used in treating younger patients should be applied to older drinkers as well. For example, benzodiazepines are important in the treatment of alcohol detoxification but have no clinical use in maintaining long-term abstinence because of their abuse potential and the potential for fostering further alcohol or benzodiazepine abuse. Disulfiram may benefit some well-motivated patients, but cardiac and hepatic disease limits the use of this agent in the older alcoholic.

## Benzodiazepines

Addressing inappropriate use and misuse of medications relies on physicians and pharmacists to monitor medication use carefully, avoiding dangerous combinations of drugs, medications with a high potential for side effects, and ineffective or unnecessary medications. A practical approach to monitoring psychoactive medication use would be to reevaluate its use every 3 to 6 months. Only patients with a documented response to the treatment should continue on to maintenance treatment. Patients without a response or with a partial response should be reevaluated to consider the appropriate diagnosis and further care. In this situation, consultation with a specialty geriatric mental health provider could be advantageous.

While withdrawal from benzodiazepines may be considered difficult, Rickels and colleagues demonstrated that the elderly can successfully be withdrawn from chronic benzodiazepine use (Rickels et al., 1991; Schweizer et al., 1989). However, they also demonstrated that the elderly are more likely to return to benzodiazepine use within 3 years of discontinuation. Given that the negative effects of benzodiazepines, such as increased risks of falls and cognitive effects, are dose dependent and occur more often with longer-acting medications, a practical approach to managing long-term use would be to decrease the medication to the lowest possible dose and avoid long-acting medications.

## Smoking

Although the 1990 Surgeon General's Report concluded that smoking cessation is beneficial at any age, its application and significance to older adults continues to be underused and underappreciated (Morgan et al., 1996; U.S. Department of Health and Human Services, 1990). Nevertheless, the health benefits of smoking cessation for older adults are unequivocal and often quite dramatic. The most profound effects for older adults are on the cardiovascular system; quitting smoking almost immediately reduces the risk of heart disease and stroke (Hermanson et al., 1988; Howard et al., 1987). Benefits to the respiratory system accrue gradually, but even moderately symptomatic patients show improvement in lung function following smoking cessation (Pathak et al., 1986). Other benefits for older adults who quit smoking include significant and rapid improvements in circulation and pulmonary perfusion, increased mobility, improved physical function, and reduced osteoporosis and hip fracture (LaCroix et al., 1993; Rimer et al., 1994; Seeman et al., 1983). Thus, there is now substantial evidence that smoking cessation, by preventing or reducing acute and chronic illnesses, improves both the length and quality of life for older adults (Rimer et al., 1990). The impact of smoking cessation, particularly in conjunction with other lifestyle improvements, can be enormous.

## SUMMARY

Substance use and abuse in late life are growing public health issues. As older adults live longer and as generational changes occur, more older adults are abusing alcohol and other substance than ever before. As a complicating factor in the treatment of depression, it is also clear that alcohol, cigarettes, and possibly benzodiazepines significantly decrease the chance of positive treatment outcomes. Thus, it seems imperative that mental health providers be able to recognize these issues and make the management of substance use problems a part of the treatment plan for depression.

Because few older adults with substance abuse problems seek help from addiction services, it can also be argued that the identification and initial management of addiction problems in late life should be addressed by mental health professionals. All too often, older adults find the maze of insurance, paperwork, and referrals to be complex. These logistical issues may severely limit patients' access to formal care. This is particularly true of older adults with addiction problems, who must cope with these logistical barriers as well as with the personal barriers of shame and stigma. It is also not clear that there are benefits to dividing up care among multiple providers such as a depression specialist and an addiction specialist. As older patients with co-morbid depression and substance use are more likely to seek help for their depression, mental health professionals may be particularly poised to manage older patients with co-morbid substance abuse, although all behavioral health providers should be trained in the management of depression and substance abuse.

ACKNOWLEDGMENTS
This work was supported in part by Grant 1K08MH 01599 from the National Institute of Mental Health.

REFERENCES

Adams, W.L., Fleming, M., et al. (1996) Screening for problem drinking in older primary care patients. *JAMA* 276:1964–1967.

Barry, K.L., Blow, F.C., et al. (1998) Elder-specific brief alcohol intervention: 3-month outcomes. *Alcoholism: Clin Exp Res* 22:32A.

Barry, K.L., Oslin, D.W., et al. (2001) *Prevention and Management of Alcohol Problems in Older Adults*. New York: Springer.

Black, B.S., Rabins, P.V., et al. (1998) Alcohol use disorder is a risk factor for mortality among older public housing residents. *Int Psychogeriatr* 10:309–327.

Blazer, D., Hybels, C., et al. (2000) Sedative, hypnotic, and antianxiety medication use in an aging cohort over ten years: A racial comparison. *J Am Geriatr Soc* 48(9):1073–1079.

Blazer, D.G., and Koenig, H.G. (1993) Mood Disorders. In: Busse, E.W., and Blazer, D.G., eds. *The American Psychiatric Association Textbook of Geriatric Psychiatry*. Washington, DC: APA Press, pp. 235–263.

Blixen, C.E., McDougall, G.J., et al. (1997) Dual diagnosis in elders discharged from a psychiatric hospital. *Int J Geriatr Psychiatry* 12:307–313.

Blow, F. (1993) *A Geriatric Version of the MAST*. New Orleans: American Association of Geriatric Psychiatry.

Blow, F. (1998) Substance abuse among older Americans. *Treatment Improvement Protocol*. Washington, DC: U.S. Government Printing Office.

Blow, F., Cook, C.L., et al. (1992) Age-related psychiatric co-morbidities and level of functioning in alcoholic veterans seeking outpatient treatment. *Hosp Commun Psychiatry* 43:990–995.

Brennan, P.L., Kagay, C.R., et al. (2001) Predictors and outcomes of outpatient mental health care: a 4-year prospective study of elderly Medicare patients with substance use disorders. *Med Care* 39(1):39–49.

Brown, C., Madden, P.A., et al. (2000) The association between depressive symptoms and cigarette smoking in an urban primary care sample. *Int J Psychiatry Med* 30(1):15–26.

Brown, S.A., and Schuckit, M.A. (1988) Changes in depression among abstinent alcoholics. *J Studies Alcohol* 49:412–417.

Bruce, M. (2002) The use of benzodiazepines among primary care patients with depression (personal communication)

Bucholz, K.K., Cadoret, R., et al. (1994) A new, semi-structured psychiatric interview for use in genetic linkage studies: A report on the reliability of the SSAGA. *J Studies Alcohol* 55:149–158.

Burman, W.J., Cohn, D.L., et al. (1997) Noncompliance with directly observed therapy for tuberculosis. Epidemiology and effect on the outcome of treatment. *Chest* 111:1168–1173.

Callahan, C., Hendrie, H., et al. (1996) The recognition and treatment of late-life depression: A vew from primary care. *Int J Psychiatry Med* 26:155–171.

Callahan, C.M., Hendrie, H.C., et al. (1994) Depression in late life: The use of clinical characteristics to focus screening efforts. *J Gerontol* 49:M9–M14.

Centers for Disease Control and Prevention. (1999) Surveillance for five health risks among older adults—United States, 1993–1997. *Morbid Mort Week Rep* 48:89–130.

Conwell, Y. (1991) Suicide in elderly patients. In: Schneider, L.S., Reynolds, C.F., Lebowitz, B.D., and Friedhoff, A.J., eds. *Diagnosis and Treatment of Depression in Late Life*. Washington, DC: American Psychiatric Press, pp. 397–418.

Cook, B., Winokur, G., et al. (1991) Depression and previous alcoholism in the elderly. *Br J Psychiatry* 158:72–75.

Cornelius, J.R., Salloum, I.M., et al. (1997) Fluoxetine in depressed alcoholics: A double-blind, placebo-controlled trial. *Arch Gen Psychiatry* 54:700–705.

Crum, R.M., Brown, C., et al. (2001) The association of depression and problem drinking: Analyses from the Baltimore ECA follow-up study. Epidemiologic Catchment Area. *Addict Behav* 26(5):765–773.

Curtis, J., Millman, E., et al. (1986) Prevalence rates for alcoholism, associated depression and dementia on the Harlem hospital medicine and surgery services. *Adv Alcohol Substance Abuse* 6:45–65.

Douglass, R.L., Schuster, E.O., et al. (1988) Drinking patterns and abstinence among the elderly. *Int J Addict* 23:399–415.

Dunbar, G.C., Perera, M.H., et al. (1989) Patterns of benzodiazepine use in Great Britain as Measured by a general population survey. *Br J Psychiatry* 155:836–841.

Fillmore, K. (1987) Prevalence, incidence and chronicity of drinking patterns and problems among men as a function of age: A longitudinal and cohort analysis. *J Addict* 82:77–83.

First, M.B., Spitzer, R.L., et al. (2002) *Structured Clinical Interview for DSM IV Axis I Disorders—Patient Edition (SCID-I/P*, New York: New York State Psychiatric Institute, Biometrics Research Department.

Fleming, M., Manwell, L., et al. (1999) Brief physician advice for alcohol problems in older adults: A randomized community-based trial. *J Family Pract* 48:378–384.

Fortney, J.C., Booth, B.M., et al. (1999) Do patients with alcohol dependence use more services? a comparative analysis with other chronic disorders. *Alcoholism: Clin Exp Res* 23:127–133.

Furukawa, T.A., Streiner, D.L., et al. (2001) Is antidepressant-benzodiazepine combination therapy clinically more useful? A meta-analytic study. *J Affect Disord* 65(2):173–177.

Gales, B.J., and Menard, S.M. (1995) Relationship between the administration of selected medications and falls in hospitalized elderly patients. *Ann Pharmacother* 29(4):354–358.

Goodwin, J.S., Sanchex, C.J., et al. (1987) Alcohol intake in a healthy elderly population. *Am J Public Health* 77:173–177.

Gourlay, S., and Benowitz, N. (1996) The benefits of stopping smoking and the role of nicotine replacement therapy in older patients. *Drugs Aging* 9:8–23.

Hanna, E.Z., and Grant, B.F. (1997) Gender differences in DSM-IV alcohol use disorders and major depression as distributed in the general population: Clinical implications. *Compr Psychiatry* 38:202–212.

Hasegawa, K., Mukasa, H., et al. (1990) Primary and secondary depression in alcoholism—clinical features and family history. *Drug Alcohol Depend* 27:275–281.

Hasin, D.S., Trautman, K.D., et al. (1996a) Psychiatric Research Interview for Substance and Mental Disorders (PRISM): Reliability for substance abusers. *Am J Psychiatry* 153:1195–1201.

Hasin, D.S., Tsai, W.-Y., et al. (1996b) Five-year course of major depression: Effects of co-morbid alcoholism. *J Affect Disord* 41:63–70.

Hays, J., Dale, L., et al. (1998) Trends in smoking-related diseases: Why smoking cessation is still the best medicine. *Postgrad Med* 104:56–71.

Helzer, J.E., and Pryzbeck, T.R. (1988) The co-occurrence of alcoholism with other psychiatric disorders in the general population and its impact on treatment. *J Studies Alcohol* 49:219–224.

Hemmelgarn, B., Suissa, S., et al. (1997) Benzodiazepine use and the risk of motor vehicle crash in the elderly [see comments]. *JAMA* 278(1):27–31.

Herd, D. (1990) Subgroup differences in drinking patterns among black and white men: Results from a national survey. *J Studies Alcohol* 51:221–232.

Herings, R.M.C., Stricker, B.H.C., et al. (1995) Benzodiazepines and the risk of falling leading to femur fractures. *Arch Intern Med* 155:1801–1807.

Hermanson, B., Omenn, G., et al. (1988) Beneficial six-year outcome of smoking cessation in older men and women with coronary artery disease. *N Engl J Med* 319:1365–1369.

Hodgins, D.C., el-Guebaly, N., et al. (1999) Implications of depression on outcome from alcohol dependence: A 3-year prospective follow-up. *Alcoholism: Clin Exp Res* 23:151–157.

Holahan, C.J., Moos, R.H., et al. (2001) Drinking to cope, emotional distress and alcohol use and abuse: A ten-year model. *J Studies Alcohol* 62(2):190–198.

Holroyd, S., and Duryee, J. (1997) Substance use disorders in a geriatric psychiatry outpatient clinic: Prevalence and epidemiologic characteristics. *J Nerv Ment Dis* 185(10):627–632.

Howard, G., Toole, J., et al. (1987) Factors influencing the survival of 451 transient ischemic attack patients. *Stroke* 18:552–557.

Isacson, D., Bingefors, K., et al. (1993) Factors associated with high-quantity prescriptions of benzodiazepines in Sweden. *Soc Sci Med* 36(3):343–351.

Kandel, D., Chen, K., et al. (1997) Prevalence and demographic correlates of symptoms of last year dependence on alcohol, nicotine, marijuana and cocaine in the U.S. population. *Drug Alcohol Depend* 44(1):11–29.

Kessler, R.C., Nelson, C.B., et al. (1996) Co-morbidity of DSM-III-R major depressive disorder in the general population: Results from the US national co-morbidity survey. *Br J Psychiatry* 168(suppl 30):17–30.

Keuthen, N.J., Niaura, R.S., et al. (2000) Co-morbidity, smoking behavior and treatment outcome. *Psychother Psychosom* 69(5):244–250.

Kirchner, J. (2002) The co-occurance of depressive symptoms and smoking among the elderly (Personal communication).

Kranzler, H.R., DelBoca, F.K., et al. (1996) Co-morbid psychiatric diagnosis predicts three-year outcomes in alcoholics: A posttreatment natural history study. *J Studies Alcohol* 57:619–626.

Krska, J., and MacLeod, T.N., (1995) Sleep quality and the use of benzodiazepine hypnotics in general practice. *J Clin Pharm Ther* 20(2):91–96.

LaCroix, A.Z., Guralnik, J.M., et al. (1993) Maintaining mobility in late life. *J Epidemiol* 137:858–869.

Liberto, J.G., Oslin, D.W., et al. (1992) Alcoholism in older persons: A review of the literature. [Review] [70 refs]. *Hosp Commun Psychiatry* 43(10):975–984.

Maarbjerg, K., Aagaard, J., et al. (1988) Adherence to lithium prophylaxis: I. clinical predictors and patient's reasons for nonadherence. *Pharmacopsychiatry* 21:121–125.

Mason, B.J., Kocsis, J.H., et al. (1996) A double-blind, placebo-controlled trial of desipramine for primary alcohol dependence stratified on the presence or absence of major depression. *JAMA* 275:761–767.

McGinnis, J.M., and Foege, W.H. (1993) Actual causes of death in the United States. *JAMA* 270:2207–2212.

McGrath, P.J., Nunes, E.V., et al. (1996) Imipramine treatment of alcoholics with primary depression a placebo-controlled clinical trial. *Arch Gen Psychiatry* 53:232–240.

Merikangas, K., and Gelernter, C.S. (1990) Co-morbidity for alcoholism and depression. *Psychiatr Clin North Am* 13:613–632.

Molgaard, C.A., Nakaamura, C.M., et al. (1990) Prevalence of alcohol consumption among older persons. *J Commun Health* 15:239–251.

Moore, A.A., Hays, R.D., et al. (2000) Using a criterion standard to validate the Alcohol-Related Problems Survey (ARPS): A screening measure to identify harmful and hazardous drinking in older persons. *Aging (Milano)* 12(3):221–227.

Morgan, G.D., Noll, E.L., et al. (1996) Reaching midlife and older smokers: Tailored interventions for routine medical care. *Prev Med* 25:346–354.

Newman, A., Enright, P., et al. (1997) Sleep disturbances, psyhcosocial correlates, and cardiovascular disease in 5201 older adults: The cardiovasular health study. *J Am Geriatr Soc* 45:1–7.

Orleans, C., Rimer, B., et al. (1990) Psychological and behavioral consequences and correlates of smoking cessation. In: *The Health Benefits of Smoking Cessation—A Report of the Surgeon General*. Rockville, MD: U.S. Government Printing Office, pp. 521–578.

Oslin, D.W. The Treatment of Late Life Depression Complicated by Alcohol Dependence. *Am J Geriatr Psychiatry*, submitted.

Oslin, D., Katz, I., et al. (2000) The effects of alcohol consumption on the treatment of depression among the elderly. *Am J Geriatr Psychiatry* 8:215–220.

Oslin, D.W. (2002) *Benzodiazepine Use in Hospitalized Depressed Older Adults*. Philadelphia (Personal communication).

Oslin, D.W., O'Brien, C.P., et al. (1999) The disabling nature of co-morbid depression among older DUI recipients. *Am J Addict* 8(2):128–135.

Oslin, D.W., Pettinati, H.M., et al. (2002) Alcoholism treatment adherence: Older age predicts better adherence and drinking outcomes. *Am J Geriatr Psychiatry* 10(6):740–747.

Oslin, D.W., H.R., et al. (2001) *Failure to Validate Primary and Secondary Depression Diagnoses*. Denver, CO: Research Society on Alcoholism.

Partonen, R., Sihvo, S., et al. (1996) Patients excluded from an antidepressant efficacy trial. *J Clin Psychiatry* 57:572–575.

Pathak, D., Samet, J., et al. (1986) Determinants of lung cancer risk in cigarette smokers in New Mexico. *J Natl Cancer Inst* 76:597–604.

Patten, C.A., Gillin, J.C., et al. (2001) Relationship of mood disturbance to cigarette smoking status among 252 patients with a current mood disorder. *J Clin Psychiatry* 62(5):319–324.

Rickels, K., Case, W., et al. (1991) Long-term benzodiazepine users 3 years after participation in a discontinuation program. *Am J Psychiatry* 148:757–761.

Ried, L.D., Lohnson, R.E., et al. (1998) Benzodiazepine exposure and functional status in older people. *J Am Geriatr Soc* 46:71–76.

Robins, L.N., Helzer, J.E., et al. (1981) National Institute of Mental Health Diagnostic Interview Schedule: Its history, characteristics, and validity. *Arch Gen Psychiatry* 38:381–389.

Rimer, B.K., Orleans, C.T., et al. (1990) The older smoker: Status, challenges and opportunities for intervention. *Chest* 97:547–553.

Rimer, B.K., Orleans, C.T., et al. (1994) Does tailoring matter? The impact of a tailored guide on ratings and short-term smoking-related outcomes for older smokers. *Health Ed Res* 9:69–84.

Robins, L.N., and Regier, D.A., eds. (1991) *Psychiatric Disorders in America: The Epidemiologic Catchment Area Study*. New York: Free Press.

Roy-Byrne, P.P., Pages, K.P., et al. (2000) Nefazodone treatment of major depression in alcohol-dependent patients: A double-blind, placebo-controlled trial. *J Clin Psychopharmacol* 20(2):129–136.

Samet, J. (1992) The health benefits of smoking cessation. *Med Clin North Am* 76:399–414.

Saunders, J.B., Asland, O.G., et al. (1993) Development of the alcohol-use disorders identification test (AUDIT)—WHO collaborative project on early detection of persons with harmful alcohol-consumption. *Addiction* 88:791–804.

Saunders, P.A., Copeland, J.R., et al. (1991) Heavy drinking as a risk

factor for depression and dementia in elderly men. *Br J Psychiatry* 159:213–216.

Schonfeld, L., and Dupree, L.W. (1991) Antecedents of drinking for early- and late-onset elderly alcohol abusers. *J Studies Alcohol* 52:587–592.

Schonfeld, L., Dupree, L.W., et al. (2000) Cognitive-behavioral treatment of older veterans with substance abuse problems. *J Geriatr Psychiatry Neurol.* 13:124–129.

Schuckit, M.A., Tipp, J.E., et al. (1997) Comparison of induced and independent major depressive disorders in 2,945 alcoholics. *Am J Psychiatry* 154:948–957.

Schutte, K.K., Brennan, P.L., et al. (1998) Predicting the development of late-life late-onset drinking problems: A 7-year prospective study. *Alcoholism: Clin Exp Res* 22(6):1349–1358.

Schutte, K.K., Hearst, J., et al. (1997) Gender differences in the relations between depressive symptoms and drinking behavior among problem drinkers: A three-wave study. *J Consult Clin Psychol* 65(3):392–404.

Schweizer, E., Case, W.G., et al. (1989) Benzodiazepine dependence and withdrawal in elderly patients. *Am J Psychiatry* 146(4):529–531.

Seeman, E., Melton, L.J., III, et al. (1983) Risk factors for spinal osteoporosis in men. *Am J Med* 75:977–983.

Simon, G., VonKorff, M., et al. (1996) Predictors of chronic benzodiazepine use in a health maintenance organization sample. *J Clin Epidemiol* 49:1067–1073.

Speer, D., and Bates, K. (1992) Co-morbid mental and substance disorders among older psychiatric patients. *J Am Geriatr Soc* 40:886–890.

Straand, J., and Rokstad, K. (1997) General practitioners' prescribing patterns of benzodiazepine hypnotics: Are elderly patients at particular risk for overprescribing? A report from the More and Romsdal Prescription Study [see comments]. *Scand J Primary Health Care* 15(1):16–21.

Tsuang, D., Cowley, D., et al. (1995) The effects of substance use disorder on the clinical presentation of anxiety and depression in an outpatient psychiatric clinic. *J Clin Psychiatry* 56:549–555.

U.S. Department of Health and Human Services. (1990) *The Health Benefits of Smoking Cessation*. Washington, DC: U.S. Government Printing Office.

Vazquez, F.L., and Becona, E. (1999) Depression and smoking in a smoking cessation programme. *J Affect Disord* 55(2–3):125–132.

Waern, M. (2003) Alcohol dependence and misuse in elderly suicides. *Alcohol Alcohol* 38(3):249–254.

Wright, N., Caplan, R., et al. (1994) Community survey of long term daytime use of benzodiazepines [see comments]. *BMJ* 309(6946):27–28.

Zisselman, M.H., Rovner, B.W., et al. (1994) Benzodiazepine utilization in a university hospital. *Am J Med Quality* 9(3):138–141.

# 28 | Basal ganglia disease and depression

### ANJAN CHATTERJEE AND KAREN MARDER

## INTRODUCTION TO BASAL GANGLIA DISEASE

Diseases of the basal ganglia are quintessential neuropsychiatric disorders, characterized by abnormal movements, cognitive impairment, and psychiatric symptoms and signs. Depression is common in these illnesses and may occur at presentation or during the course of the illness. Individuals may present to the psychiatrist before seeing a neurologist. Depression is an important target for research, as it affords a unique perspective on the pathophysiology of basal ganglia diseases as well as an alternative method of understanding the biology of mood disorders. Traditionally, basal ganglia diseases are diagnosed and treated by neurologists, who define their onset by specific motor manifestations. Psychiatric symptomatology has been considered peripheral to the understanding of the motor disorders that define basal ganglia diseases. There is growing evidence for the contrary view that mood and affect are integrally related to the evolution of these diseases. For example, in diseases such as Huntington's disease or Wilson's disease, where the genetic mutation has been identified, it is possible to identify presymptomatic individuals, prior to the development of motor signs, who are unaware of their genetic status, and determine whether cognitive or psychiatric manifestations occur more often in gene-positive than in gene-negative individuals. Another way to examine the role of psychiatric impairment is to study individuals in the general population who have undergone psychiatric assessments and to determine if individuals with a history of affective disorder are more likely to develop specific basal ganglia diseases (e.g., Parkinson's disease) than individuals without mood disorders. This chapter includes a review of the epidemiology, prevalence, and correlates of depression in basal ganglia diseases and their treatment.

## ANATOMY AND CONNECTIONS OF THE BASAL GANGLIA

Research over the past two decades has led to a better understanding of the structure and function of the basal ganglia in terms of their connections among basal gan-

glia nuclei as well as with the overlying cortex. Circuit models for these structures have become progressively more refined and, although still a simplification, are very useful in guiding new research as well as surgical and pharmacological treatments for these disorders.

The basal ganglia are subcortical structures that include the corpus striatum, which consists of the caudate nucleus and the putamen, the globus pallidus with its internal (Gpi) and external portions (Gpe) (together, the paleostriatum), the subthalamic nucleus of Luys (STN), and the substantia nigra, made up of the pars compacta (SNc) and pars reticulata (SNr) (Parent, 1996). These nuclei are a part of larger segregated circuits that involve the cortex and the thalamus. The circuits are thought to begin in the cortex, travel through various basal ganglia structures, and then continue on to the thalamus for further processing before being projected back to the original cortices. Ideas regarding the circuit connectivity of the basal ganglia have been influenced by theories of parallel circuits linking cortical association areas through the basal ganglia and thalamus back to the cortex (Kultas-Ilinsky and Ilinsky, 2001). The first circuit described was the motor circuit that arises in the pre- and postcentral sensorimotor fields and projects to the putamen.

Subsequently Alexander et al. (1986) described evidence for other circuits (two of which, when dysfunctional, can have depressive symptoms as a feature) that were segregated from one another and projected to specific and restricted areas of the frontal lobe. This idea of complete segregation of each of these circuits has been called into question, and studies in primates indicate that these motor, cognitive, and behavioral systems probably interact within the basal ganglia and that the segregation is not as complete as was initially thought (Parent and Cicchetti, 1998). The circuits included the oculomotor circuit (which goes to the frontal eye fields), the dorsolateral prefrontal circuit, the lateral orbitofrontal circuit, and the anterior cingulate circuit.

The dorsolateral prefrontal circuit subserves executive function (Cummings, 1993). Damage to the dorsolateral prefrontal lobe, the basal ganglia circuits, or the intervening white matter can cause deficits in executive function. Reduced verbal and design fluency is seen, as well as poor organizational strategies in learning tasks and impaired sequential motor tasks (Cummings, 1985). Neuropsychiatric disturbances include depression and anxiety with dorsolateral prefrontal strokes and with caudate dysfunction (Starkstein et al., 1990). The orbitofrontal circuit has two major subdivisions: a lateral division and a medial division (Carmichael and Price, 1995). The medial portion of the orbitofrontal circuit mediates mood and neurovegetative function (Price, 1999). Hypofunctioning of the medial division (as demonstrated by positron emission tomography [PET]) is associated with depressive symptoms in patients with Parkinson's disease that normalizes when the mood disorder is treated with fluoxetine (Mayberg, 1995). The anterior cingulate circuit mediates motivated behavior, and apathy is the behavior associated with dysfunction in this circuit. Akinetic mutism occurs with bilateral lesions of the anterior cingulate. There is poverty of spontaneous speech, almost no movement, and incontinence, and basic behaviors such as eating and drinking are not initiated (Fesenmeier et al., 1990).

The above discussion underscores the fact that these circuits are involved in normal neuropsychiatric function, and damage to portions of the circuits can cause one or more abnormalities in behavior and cognition. What is also apparent from this discussion is that diseases or lesions of subcortical basal ganglia structures and circuits, specifically the medial orbitofrontal and dorsolateral prefrontal circuits, may be associated with depression.

## THE NEUROANATOMY OF DEPRESSION

Major depressive disorder (MDD) can occur without concomitant neurological disease. Research into the anatomical and biochemical pathways and structures involved in the pathogenesis of MDD is an area of intense scrutiny. Anatomical studies of depression have shown normal brain structure and volume but have been less useful in understanding the pathogenesis of this illness. One exception has been a study that showed subgenual frontal volume loss in depressed patients (Drevets, 1997). In contrast, PET and single photon emission computer tomography (SPECT) studies in major depression have shown frontal and cingulate abnormalities (which correlate more closely with patterns in patients with neurological disease and depression) and, less commonly, temporal and parietal abnormalities in metabolism (Mayberg, 2001).

The most frequently replicated finding is decreased frontal lobe function, though the changes sometimes involved the dorsolateral-prefrontal cortex as well as the ventral-prefrontal and orbitofrontal cortex (Baxter et al.,

1989; Buchsbaum et al., 1986; Lesser et al., 1994; Mayberg, 1997). Most of these studies report bilateral cortical involvement, although there are asymmetries. Changes in the amygdala (Drevets et al., 1992) as well as in the anterior temporal lobe and the cingulate (Bench et al., 1992; Drevets, 1997; Ebert and Ebmeier, 1996; Mayberg et al., 1994; Wu et al., 1992), have also been reported. Finally, there have been reports involving the basal ganglia and thalamus but less consistently so (Buchsbaum et al., 1986; Drevets et al., 1992). There is thus a paucity of evidence linking basal ganglia structures to MDD, although cortical areas intimately connected to them have been repeatedly shown to be involved.

Baxter and colleagues have gone further to show normalization of frontal hypometabolism upon drug treatment of depression (Baxter et al., 1989; Buchsbaum et al., 1997).

Neurochemical studies show involvement of neurotransmitters that have also been implicated in motor disorders of the basal ganglia. They have added to the anatomical data from imaging and have implicated serotonergic and adrenergic mechanisms. These are believed to be involved in the pathogenesis of MDD because of the therapeutic effects of antidepressants that alter these systems in vivo (Ballenger, 1988). Dietary restriction of tryptophan, resulting in an acute reduction in brain serotonin, as well as restriction of catecholamines (the alpha-methyl paratyrosine challenge), resulted in abrupt relapse in remitted depressed patients, further indicating that these systems are intimately involved in the disease process (Delgado et al., 1990). Each of these neurotransmitters is involved in the pathology of basal ganglia disorders as well and may be one common pathway linking depression to these illnesses.

## PARKINSON'S DISEASE

### Epidemiology and Neurology of Parkinson's Disease

Idiopathic Parkinson's disease (PD) is a neurodegenerative disorder of middle or late life and was first described by James Parkinson in his "Essay on the Shaking Palsy" (Parkinson, 1817). Parkinson's disease affects approximately 107 per 100,000 persons across all age groups, and the prevalence increases with increasing age (Mayeux et al., 1995). There is a slight male preponderance. In all populations, PD is rare below the age of 50. The prevalence of PD over the age of 65 is 1.6% (de Rijk et al., 1997).

Parkinson's disease is diagnosed clinically and is defined by the triad of tremor, bradykinesia, and rigidity. Research criteria have been proposed, and include asymmetrical onset and a response to levodopa (Gelb et al., 1999).

Pathologically, PD is characterized by the loss of pigmented neurons in the substantia nigra and other pigmented brain stem nuclei as well as the presence, in the remaining nigral cells, of the intracytoplasmic lewy bodies (Jellinger, 2001; Takahashi and Wakabayashi, 2001). Lewy bodies are the sine qua non of PD; their role in the pathogenesis of the disease is unknown. Cortical Lewy bodies in small numbers have also been consistently described (Hughes et al., 1993; Sugiyama et al., 1994). The cause of PD is unknown. Current hypotheses favor the possibility of excitotoxic injury and environmental toxins, as well as genetic factors in a significant minority of patients. Three genes (*Parkin, alpha-synuclein,* and *UCH-L1*) and five genetic loci have been identified in a minority of patients with early-onset PD (Mouradian, 2002).

Parkinson's disease is treated with the exogenous administration of dopamine (DA) or a DA agonist. Dopamine is given as a combination of levodopa and carbidopa to enhance the central nervous system availability of DA and also to reduce the side effects of DA caused by excessive peripheral decarboxylation of levodopa. Dopamine agonists have also been successfully used in the treatment of PD and form an important part of the armamentarium for this disorder.

## Epidemiology of Depression in Parkinson's Disease

The prevalence of depression in PD is reported as varying from 4% to 70% (Cummings, 1992), depending on the sampling, diagnostic criteria, and instruments employed. Cummings (1992) noted dysphoria, pessimism, irritability, sadness, and suicidal ideation as the most reliable indicators of depression in PD. Although PD patients experience suicidal ideation, rates of suicide are not higher in the PD population than in the general population. Stenager et al. (1994) looked at case records of 458 PD patients at a Danish university hospital and then evaluated the cause of death in the 254 patients who died over the 17 years of follow-up. They did not find an increased rate of suicide in the PD group (2 of the 254) compared to the general population.

Is depression in PD reactive or endogenous to the illness? There is an ongoing debate about the etiology of depression in PD and whether it represents an endogenous or reactive illness. The mechanism of depression in patients with PD is poorly understood, and it is unclear why some patients develop depression and others do not. Prior to the availability of levodopa treatment for PD, depression was believed to be related to lack of DA and the presence of the motor disorder. After the introduction of levodopa, investigators found that PD patients continued to report depressive symptoms. Mindham (1970) demonstrated the first successful treatment of these symptoms (in a double-blind study) with antidepressants. Evidence for the reactive hypothesis includes a recent paper by Schrag (2001) that looked at factors contributing to depression in PD in 97 patients and concluded that depression was related to advancing disease severity, recent deterioration due to disease, and occurrence of falls. This study also suggested that depression in PD was related to the patients' perceptions of the extent of their disability. Other studies have also suggested that depression is a reaction to the disability on the basis of correlations between motor disability and depression severity (Gotham et al., 1986; Huber et al., 1988). Disease severity, however, may merely be a marker of the extent of damage to the basal ganglia and as such is not clear evidence of the reactive hypothesis. Studies looking at depression in PD patients and physically disabled controls have concluded that depression was more common in PD patients, a result that contradicts the reactive hypothesis (Horn, 1974; Warburton, 1967).

Another argument against the reactive hypothesis is evidence suggesting that depressive symptoms can precede development of the motor symptoms, implying that depression itself is an early nonmotor symptom of PD in these patients (Mayeux et al., 1981; Sano et al., 1989; Santamaria et al., 1986). A recent retrospective cohort study reported the outcome of patients who were diagnosed with depression and then followed for 15 years to assess the hazard ratio for the depressed versus the nondepressed patients to develop PD (Schuurman et al., 2002). The authors found that among depressed patients, 1.4% (Hazard ratio 3.13; 95% CI = (1.95–5.01)) developed PD versus 0.4% in the nondepressed group. The authors sought to explain this finding by stating that reduced DA in patients with PD would cause a feedback reduction in serotonin since serotonin has an inhibitory effect on DA transmission (Kapur and Remington, 1996). This may predispose a patient who has lowered DA as part of the diathesis for PD to have depression as a result of the altered serotonin levels, which are compensatory.

## Anatomy of Depression in Parkinson's Disease

Anatomical and neurochemical evidence also suggests that depression represents an endogenous feature of the disease. The diverse motor and nonmotor symptoms of PD have been related to dysfunction in cortical–basal ganglionic–thalamic loops (Alexander et al., 1986). Studies have demonstrated that depressed patients with PD have increased neuronal loss in the dorsal raphe compared to patients with psychosis who had no specific neuropathological features (Paulus and Jellinger, 1991). Further studies have discovered a relative hypometabolism in the caudate and inferior orbital-frontal regions and in the medial frontal lobes in PET studies that compared depressed PD patients to nondepressed PD patients and controls matched by age, disease duration, and stage of illness (Mayberg et al., 1990; Ring et al., 1994).

A case report by Bejjani et al. (1999) illustrates further the intricate relationship between cortical and subcortical structures in the pathophysiology of depression in basal ganglia disease. The authors described a 65-year-old woman with PD who received bilateral deep-brain stimulation for treatment of the PD symptoms. Electrode 0 on the left side was placed too deep in the substantia nigra within both pars compacta and reticulata. Stimulation of this electrode produced intense dysphoria with crying, suicidal ideation, and hopelessness. Cessation of this stimulation normalized the patient's mood in 90 seconds. This experiment was repeated, and concomitant PET scanning revealed increased blood flow to the right parietal lobe, left orbitofrontal cortex, left globus pallidus, left amygdala, and anterior thalamus during the period of left-sided nigral stimulation, possibly implicating these cortical and subcortical areas in this patient's acute dysphoria.

## Neurochemistry of Depression in Parkinson's Disease

Neurotransmitters such as serotonin, norepinephrine (NE), and DA, all of which have been implicated in depression, have also been implicated in the pathogenesis of depression in PD. Evidence has accumulated for all three, but it is still not clear which, if any, is the primary neurotransmitter to be affected.

Dopamine deficiency has been suspected by some to be the primary neurotransmitter associated with depression in PD since the serotonergic neuronal damage is less pervasive and loss of neurons in the locus ceruleus is not consistently correlated with depression in PD patients (Sandyk and Fisher, 1989). Degeneration of DA neurons in the ventral tegmental area (VTA) (Taylor and Saint-Cyr, 1990) has been postulated to predispose PD patients to depression. Further, decreased tyrosine hydroxylase activity in the VTA (caused by degeneration of DA neurons) implies decreased dopaminergic output to cingulate, entorhinal, and frontal cortices, areas of the brain that have been linked to depression (Javoy-Agid and Agid, 1980). However, there have been no correlations between homovanillic acid (HVA), a DA metabolite and depression in PD (Mayeux et al., 1984, 1988; Wolfe et al., 1990).

There is also evidence for reduced peripheral and central metabolites of serotonin (5-HT) (Mayeux et al., 1984; Sano et al., 1989). Mayeux et al. (1988) showed that 5-HT reduces depression. Other evidence in favor of serotonin as the causative neurotransmitter includes the finding of low levels of 5-hydroxyindoleacetic acid (5-HIAA) in the cerebrospinal fluid (CSF) of PD patients with depression, although there is no correlation between 5-HIAA level and the severity of depression (Mayeux et al., 1984, 1986, 1988). There are also reports of degeneration of 5-HT neurons of the dorsal raphe (Sano et al., 1990), and abnormal binding at 5-HT uptake sites has been demonstrated (Cash et al., 1985). Also, transcranial sonography reveals greater disruption of brain stem dorsal raphe echogenicity in depressed PD patients than in nondepressed patients (Becker et al., 1997).

Decreased platelet–imipramine binding has also been described in depressed PD patients (Langer et al., 1987; Raisman et al., 1986), possibly implicating intrinsic neurochemical defects in NE as being related to the pathogenesis of depressive symptoms in this disease. Degeneration of NE-contaning neurons of the locus ceruleus (Chan-Palay, 1993; Chan-Palay and Asan, 1989; Sandyk, 1990) may also predispose PD patients to depression.

## Treatment of Depression in Parkinson's Disease

Evaluating depression in the context of a motor disorder such as PD may be difficult because of the overlap of somatic symptoms of depression and the motor deficits of PD such as bradykinesia and flat affect. Some authors have suggested that the Montgomery-Asburg Depression Rating Scale (MADRS) is more useful in neurological disease because it has less focus on the motor/vegetative symptoms than the Hamilton Depression Rating Scale (HAM-D) (Hammond, 1996; Leentjens et al., 2000).

Another issue is the fact that both of these scales, as well as the Beck Depression Inventory (BDI), were not designed to be diagnostic and are commonly used as such in the investigation of neurological disease. However, authors have addressed this issue in the PD population and have concluded that they are valid when certain cutoffs are used (16/17 for the HAM-D and 17/18 for the MADRS) (Leentjens et al., 2000). It is possible that patients with PD may score high on these scales and not have depression, and authors have suggested that they be used only if the patient scores on the depression items on these scales (Mayeux et al., 1981). Williams (2001) and others have also commented on the fact that there are several different versions of the scales, such as the HAM-D, and frequently published literature fails to cite the correct version of the scale used, increasing confusion. Efforts are underway to develop a "Grid" HAM-D that will score the intensity and severity of a symptom first, and thereby clarify the exact nature of the symptom endorsed and go a long way toward reducing the confusion and uncertainty in the interpretation of the results.

There are few double-blind, placebo-controlled clinical trials assessing the effects of antidepressants specifically in the context of mood changes in PD (Poewe and Seppi, 2001). Four double-blind, randomized, controlled trials were conducted using tricyclic antidepressants and one using bupropion (Laitinen, 1969; Strang, 1965; Anderson et al., 1980; Goetz et al., 1984). No randomized, blind, controlled trials are available on the use of serotonin reuptake inhibitors (Klaassen et al., 1995) (see Table 28.1). A recent survey of 49 investigators from the Parkinson's Study Group (PSG) to assess physician preferences for treatment found that 51% of physicians use selective serotonin reuptake inhibitors (SSRIs) first, 41% use tricyclic antidepressants (TCAs) first, and 8% use other drugs first to treat depression in PD (Richard and Kurlan, 1997). Although TCAs or SSRIs are widely used in clinical practice, there continues to be a need for controlled clinical trials proving the efficacy of SSRIs, specifically in PD. Studies using monoamine oxidase inhibitors (MAOIs) are even rarer (Greenberg and Meyers, 1985; Hargrave and Ashford, 1992). Steur and Ballering (1997) treated 10 patients (6 women) with PD of varying duration and depression (diagnosed according to DSM criteria) with a combination of a MAOI-A and a MAOI-B (moclobemide and selegiline). All these patients were on levodopa, and six were on a dopaminergic agonist. Moclobemide, 600 mg in two divided doses, with or without selegiline, 10 mg daily, was administered during a 6-week study period. At the end of this period, improvement in depression (measured by change on the HAM-D scale) was present in both groups but was significantly less in the moclobemide-only group as compared to the moclobemide-plus-selegiline group. Since

selegiline at doses of 10 mg/day does not have an antidepressant effect, and since doses of 30 mg/day or more have been shown to be associated with a greater drop in HAM-D scores than doses less than 30 mg/day (Mann et al., 1989), Steur and Ballering explained the difference in the responses of the two groups on the basis of simultaneous inhibition of two isoforms of MAO or, alternatively, by the fact that having both types of MAOIs caused inhibition of serotonin and/or NE as well as DA and thus increased the overall antidepressant response.

Dopamine agonists are commonly used to treat the symptoms of PD. Since dopaminergic abnormalities have been proposed to be involved in the pathophysiology of depression in PD, some investigators have looked at the use of DA in the treatment of depression in PD. It is sometimes unclear whether improvement in symptoms is related to motor improvement or is the direct result of the drug on depression, since the symptoms may overlap. Bromocriptine is one agonist that has been used to improve depressive symptoms in 10 PD patients (Jouvent et al., 1983), with dosages ranging from 85 to 220 mg/day. The small sample size and open study design make this hard to interpret. Rektorova and colleagues (2001) have reported an 8-month randomized, open-label trial of the antidepressant effects of pramipexole and pergolide in 38 PD patients with motor complications. Significant decreases in the Zung Self-Rating Depression Scale (SDS) scores were

TABLE 28.1. *Treatment Studies of Depression in Parkinson Disease*

| Number | Year | Author | Type of Study | Drug | Dose | No. of Patients | Response |
|---|---|---|---|---|---|---|---|
| 1 | 1965 | Strang | Double blind | Imipramine | 150–200 mg | 20 | 60% responders |
| 2 | 1969 | Laitinen | Double blind | Desipramine | 100 mg | 39 | 50% responders |
| 3 | 1980 | Anderson | Double blind | Nortryptiline | 150 mg | 22 | All improved |
| 4 | 1983 | Jouvent | Open label | Bromocriptine | 85–220 mg | 10 | Improved |
| 5 | 1984 | Goetz | Double blind | Bupropion | 450 mg | 20 | 42% improved |
| 6 | 1988 | Mayeux | Open label | 5-Hydroxy-tryptophan | | 7 | Improved |
| 7 | 1994 | Waters | Chart review | Fluoxetine and selegiline | 20–40 mg of fluoxetine 5–10 mg of selegiline | 23 | 6 were better |
| 8 | 1996 | Rabey | Open label | Amytriptiline vs. fluvoxamine | Fluvoxamine 78 mg (mean) and amytriptiline 69 mg (mean) | 47 | 55% of amitryptiline and 60% of fluvoxamine patients got better |
| 9 | 1997 | Hauser | Open label | Sertraline | 50 mg | 15 | All improved |
| 10 | 1999 | Steur | Open label | Moclobemide and selegiline | Moclobemide 600 mg with or without selegiline 10 mg | 10 | All improved and Moclobemide plus selegiline group improved more than moclobemide only |
| 11 | 2001 | Slaughter | Open label | Sertraline | 25–50 mg | 10 | 9 of 10 reported moderate to complete resolution and the 10th patient had increased anxiety |
| 12 | 2001 | Rektorova | Open label | Pramipexole (21) and pergolide (17) | no dosage mentioned | 38 | Both groups improved |

noted in both DA agonist groups, while the improvement in the MADRS rating reached statistical significance only in the pramipexole group.

Electroconvulsive therapy (ECT), another extremely useful treatment for MDD, has proven efficacy as antidepressant therapy in patients with PD (Burke et al., 1988). Treatment with ECT may cause loss of short-term memory and may by itself improve symptoms of PD, thereby necessitating a temporary reduction in the dosage of antiparkinsonian medications.

Transcranial magnetic stimulation (TMS) has provided temporary relief of depression under experimental conditions (George et al., 1996; Mally and Stone, 1999; Tom and Cummings, 1998). George and colleagues have described a temporary improvement in mood using TMS to the right prefrontal cortices, the mechanism for which is unclear but may be mediated by the pineal gland (Sandyk and Derpapas, 1993). There are no studies of TMS in the treatment of depression in PD, although it does appear to help the motor symptoms in some cases (Mally and Stone, 1999).

When drug therapy is chosen for the treatment of depression, careful consideration must be given to potential drug–drug interactions, as adverse effects of polypharmacy in the attempted treatment of depression in patients with PD are common in the elderly. There is a concern that SSRIs may actually worsen the motor symptoms of PD (Richard and Kurlan, 1997). A *serotonin syndrome* was described in the coadministration of selegiline with SSRIs (Richard et al., 1997), but others have been able to coadminister these drugs safely (Waters, 1994). The frequency of the serotonin syndrome has been estimated to be 0.24%, with 0.04% of patients experiencing symptoms considered to be serious, but this was a survey and not a population-based sample, and thus may have underestimated the true prevalence of this phenomenon (Richard et al., 1997). The use of TCAs for depression may affect memory because of the anticholinergic effects of these drugs. Other anticholinergic effects that must be watched for include urinary hesitancy and blurry vision. These drugs may also cause orthostasis in elderly patients, and blood pressure should be monitored.

Depression itself may affect the evaluation for surgery (deep brain stimulation) in PD patients, with severe persistent depression being a relative contraindication to surgery (Saint-Cyr and Trepanier, 2000). The authors have suggested using the BDI, the Geriatric Depression Scale, the HAM-D, or the MADRS to screen patients who are candidates for surgery. This would be done as part of a much larger neuropsychological evaluation.

Fluctuations in the severity of depression may be seen with the fluctuations of motor symptoms in PD (Friedenberg and Cummings, 1989). Treatment of the motor symptoms may sometimes improve the depression as

well (Maricle et al., 1995). The pathophysiology of this on-off state may be related to catecholaminergic systems, and the use of catechol-o-methyltransferase (COMT) inhibitors may have beneficial effects on mood instability (Sandyk, 1989). Our understanding of the etiology and treatment of depression in PD is far from clear, and further research is needed to clarify these several issues.

## HUNTINGTON'S DISEASE

### Epidemiology of Huntington's Disease

Huntington's disease (HD) is an autosomal dominant, neurodegenerative disease characterized by a triad of symptoms and signs, including a movement disorder, cognitive impairment, and psychiatric syndromes. These conditions may occur alone or in combination, and any one may predominate in an individual. Huntington's disease occurs worldwide, with a prevalence of 4.1–7.5 per 100,000 (Folstein et al., 1987). Up to half of all individuals in a retrospective study of families and patients with HD (110 patients) presented with purely psychiatric symptoms before onset of the movement disorder (Shiwach, 1994).

Huntington's disease is caused by an abnormal expansion of trinucleotide (cytosine-adenine-guanine, [CAG]) repeats, which code for glutamine at the N terminus of a protein called *huntingtin* (IT15 at 4p16.3) (Huntington's Disease Collaborative Research Group, 1993). The function of normal huntingtin is unknown. Current thinking favors the idea that mutant huntingtin causes HD via a toxic gain of function. An expanded IT15 CAG repeat of 37 or more is 100% specific and 98.8% sensitive for HD (Kremer et al., 1994). In the United States, the mean age of onset of HD is approximately 40, but onset as early as age 2 and as late as age 80 has been reported (Folstein, 1989). An inverse relationship between CAG repeat length and age of onset has also been demonstrated, such that higher CAG repeat numbers are associated with earlier age of onset (Andrew et al., 1993).

The pathological change in HD is a decline in the number of striatal medium spiny $\gamma$-aminobutyric (GABA) neurons, which is most marked in the caudate and also in the globus pallidus (Vonsattel and DiFiglia, 1998).

Neurological deficits in HD include abnormal involuntary movements (chorea, dystonia, tremor), rigidity, and impairment of normal voluntary movements (gait disturbance, impairment of saccades and smooth pursuit, speech and swallowing difficulties). The impairment of eye movements may be one of the earliest signs of HD (Beenen et al., 1986; Kirkwood et al., 2000). Some patients have juvenile onset of HD (age less than 20 years, approximately 6% of patients), and have little chorea and a clinical picture that is more consistent with PD. They may have seizures and myoclonus, and school failure is commonly reported.

## Epidemiology of Depression in Huntington's Disease

There is no population-based estimate of depression in HD that uses research criteria such as the Structured Clinical Interview for DSM (SCID). Slaughter et al. (2001) reviewed the depression literature in HD and identified 16 HD depression studies. There were 461 patients who were reported to have depressive symptoms, the large majority (301) by clinical impression and the rest by DSM criteria (160). This was out of a total of 1558 patients, and the authors concluded that the overall prevalence of depression was 30% in HD patients. They noted that 5.6% of patients met DSM-III or DSM-III-R criteria for dysthymia in the six studies using those criteria. Depression in HD frequently coexists with other nonmotor symptoms such as apathy. Levy and colleagues (1998) evaluated the significance of apathy in HD and its relationship to depression, and found that in a sample of 34 HD outpatients, depression did not significantly correlate with apathy. They recommended that despite considerable overlap in the frontal and subcortical regions implicated in both conditions, the two conditions should be evaluated separately. Depression was significantly correlated, however, with anxiety and with agitation.

As with other psychiatric symptoms, onset of depression may occur several years prior to neurological abnormalities, which is evidence against depression being a purely reactive phenomenon. In fact, Folstein et al. (1983) observed that depression may occur up to 5 years prior to the onset of movement abnormalities. In a sample of 110 patients with HD, 40% had a lifetime prevalence of depression. One-third of the patients displayed mood symptoms prior to the onset of motor abnormalities (Shiwach, 1994). However, the population was carefully selected as a group of families that were being followed by a regional genetic center, and therefore the data are most likely not generalizable. A case registry study by Jensen et al. (1993) from Denmark found that HD patients had significantly more psychiatric admissions and diagnoses than their unaffected relatives.

Patients with HD have a high rate of suicide compared to that seen in the general population, perhaps due to their reported poor impulse control (Cummings, 1995) or irritability (Paulsen et al., 2001). Reported suicide rates in HD vary from 3.0% to 7.3% of patients (Di Maio et al., 1993; Lipe et al., 1993). Farrer (1986) looked at rates of suicide among 452 deceased patients with HD out of 831 HD patients in the National Huntington's Disease Research Roster. They found that 5.7% of the deaths were attributable to sui-

cide and reported a 27.6% rate of attempted suicide in HD patients. The proportion of deaths due to suicide is almost four times that of the general population. Given the nature of the data collected in this study, the results are probably valid and an accurate reflection of the increased risk incurred by patients with HD. Lipe and colleagues (1993) found that risk factors for suicide in HD patients were similar to those seen in the general population. Suicide was more likely in patients who lived alone and were childless, unmarried, and depressed.

## Anatomy of Depression in Huntington's Disease

Several neurobiological explanations have been suggested for the increased rate of depression in HD patients. Functional imaging studies in depressed HD patients indicate that disruption of frontal-striatal circuitry may be involved in the pathology of depression (Mayberg et al., 1992). Krishnan et al. (1992) reported decreased caudate volume in depressed individuals without HD compared with normal controls, and since damage to the caudate is related to depression in lesion studies (Bhatia and Marsden, 1994), this by itself is not surprising. The striatum receives input from the limbic system, disruption of which could lead to changes in mood. The dorsomedial caudate, a primary target for limbic projection, is one of the earliest regions to show neuronal loss in HD (Vonsattel and DiFiglia, 1998), and this early pathology may explain why mood disorders are seen early in some HD patients.

## Neurochemistry of Depression in Huntington's Disease

Serotonin is elevated in the caudate and putamen but normal in the substantia nigra and the nucleus accumbens, implicating its involvement in HD (Peyser and Folstein, 1990). Since serotonin is an important neurotransmitter in mood disorders, Kurlan and colleagues (1988) investigated 5-HIAA levels in the CSF of depressed versus nondepressed HD patients. They were unable to find any differences.

Other neurotransmitters implicated in the pathology of HD include GABA and glutamic acid decarboxylase (GAD) (Lloyd et al., 1989). These have been shown to be reduced in HD (Bird and Iversen, 1974; Bird et al., 1979; Spokes, 1980), but they have not been systematically evaluated in depressed patients with HD.

## Treatment of Depression in Huntington's Disease

There are no controlled clinical trials of treatment of depression in HD. Small open trials and case reports suggest that standard medications, including SSRIs and TCAs, as well as ECT, are all useful (see Table 28.2) (Caine and Shouldson, 1983; Como et al., 1997; Fol-

TABLE 28.2. *Treatment Studies of Depression in Huntington Disease*

| Number | Year | Author | Type of Study | Drug | Number of Patients | Response |
|---|---|---|---|---|---|---|
| 1 | 1971 | Heathfield | Case report | ECT | 1 (agitated depression) | Improvement |
| 2 | 1979 | Folstein | Open trial | Amytriptiline or chlorpromazine | 4 (3 given amitryptiline) | Improvement |
| 3 | 1981 | Shoulson | Open trial | TCA | 10 | 7 had improvement some patients given neuroleptics concomitantly |
| 4 | 1983 | Caine | Open trial | TCA | 6 | 5/6 improved in neurovegetative sxs |
| 5 | 1983 | Folstein | Retrospective case report | ECT | 2 | Improvement |
| 6 | 1984 | Moldawsky | Case report | Amoxapine | 1 | Improvement |
| 7 | 1986 | Ford | Case series | Phenelzine and isocarboxazid | 3 | Improvement in mood in 2 of 3 with concomitant psychosis |
| 8 | 1991 | Knowling | Case report | Sulpiride | 1 | Improvement |
| 9 | 1991 | Sajatovic | Case report | Clozapine | 1 (psychotic depression) | Improvement |
| 10 | 1994 | Ranen | Retrospective case reports | ECT | 6 (5 depressed, 1 bipolar depressed) | Improvement in 4 of the depressed and the bipolar depressed pt |
| 11 | 1996 | Patel | Case report | Fluoxetine and deprenyl | 1 | Improvement |
| 12 | 1997 | Como | Open label trial | Fluoxetine | 8 | Improvement in mood |
| 13 | 2001 | Slaughter | Case series | Sertraline | 7 | Marked improvement in 5, moderate in 2 |

stein et al., 1979; Ford, 1986; Heathfield and MacKenzie, 1971; Moldawsky, 1984; Patel et al., 1996; Ranen et al., 1994; Sajatovic et al., 1991; Shoulson, 1981; Slaughter et al., 2001).

## WILSON'S DISEASE

### Epidemiology and Neurology of Wilson's Disease

Wilson's disease (WD) is an autosomal recessive disease that results in the deposition of excess copper in the body, especially in the liver and the brain. The gene responsible (*ATP7B*) lies on chromosome 13q14.3 (Petrukhin et al., 1993; Tanzi et al., 1993). Inevitably fatal when first described, this is now a treatable illness. Wilson's disease is largely a disorder of children and young adults, although occurrences have been reported as early as 3 years and as late as the seventh decade. Hepatic, neurological, and psychiatric symptoms are common and may be seen alone or in combination (Brewer, 2000). The classic ocular finding in WD is the Kayser-Fleischer (K-F) ring. These rings are due to the deposition of copper in Descemet's membrane and are best seen with the help of a slit lamp exam. Neurological manifestations without the K-F ring are exceedingly rare. Neurological manifestations of WD are most commonly a movement disorder and

include tremor, dystonia, and parkinsonism. Dysarthria and drooling are common. The tremor has been described as wing beating in character, but postural and mixed tremors may be more common. The illness may be asymmetrical and may wax and wane, and because of this variability it is sometimes misdiagnosed as psychogenic. Psychiatric manifestations include psychosis, depression, and cognitive abnormalities, as well as personality changes (irritability, etc.) (Dening and Berrios, 1989).

Studies have indicated that WD presents with hepatic disease in up to a third of patients and that another third present with neurological dysfunction (Akil and Brewer, 1995; Brewer, 2000). It has an estimated prevalence of 1 case per 40,000, and the carrier rate is 1 per 90 persons (Olivarez et al., 2001). Wilson's disease is autosomal recessive and heterozygotes do not have symptoms, although they may exhibit mild abnormalities of copper metabolism (Reilly et al., 1993). The gene has been linked to chromosome 13q14.3 and is a copper-transporting P-type adenosine triphosphatase (ATPase) gene (Cuthbert, 1995).

Pathologically, copper accumulates in the lenticular nucleus in the brain as well as in the liver (hence hepatolenticular degeneration), and serum ceruloplasmin levels are low. Caudate and putaminal cavitary necrosis is seen with neuronal loss, axonal degeneration, and astrocytosis (Saatci et al., 1997). The serum copper level is also low, and there is increased urinary free copper excretion. Diagnosis is made in the presence of relevant clinical findings by measuring serum ceruloplasmin and copper and, if necessary, quantifying 24-hour urinay copper.

## Epidemiology of Depression in Wilson's Disease

Depression has been reported in WD in 20% to 30% of cases (Akil et al., 1991). Dening and Berrios, (1989) looked at a series of 195 patients with WD retrospectively and found that depression was a common psychiatric manifestation in patients with WD. However, this retrospective study was based on the series of Walshe (the so-called Cambridge series), and the study reported only the index admission of these patients and thus was the point prevalence of a selected sample of patients with WD. No lifetime prevalence numbers are available, and these are considered to be underestimates of the true prevalence of the phenomenon (Akil and Brewer, 1995). Akil et al. (1991) postulate that depression is the second most common psychiatric manifestation of WD after personality changes, which include irritability and aggressiveness. In their series of 124 patients, 4 had depression severe enough to have suicidal ideation and 2 actually attempted suicide. Some authors have argued that depression in WD is reactive, and although this is hard to refute, it does not explain the onset of these symptoms in patients before their motor symptoms are manifest (Xu et al., 1981).

## Treatment of Depression in Wilson's Disease

Controlled trials of antidepressant treatment in WD have not been done. A few case reports exist (Keller et al., 1999; Walter and Lyndon, 1997).

## PARKINSON-PLUS SYNDROMES AND THE TAUOPATHIES

Multiple system atrophy (MSA) is a Parkinson-plus syndrome that also involves the basal ganglia, as do progressive supranuclear palsy (PSP) and cortical basal ganglionic degeneration (CBGD), which are tauopathies (i.e., their pathology involves deposition of tau protein in the brain).

Each of these illnesses is associated with depression, but estimates of their prevalence is sparse (Aarsland et al., 2001; Fetoni et al., 1999; Gill et al., 1999; Goto et al., 2000; Litvan et al., 1996, 1998; Menza et al., 1995; Pilo et al., 1996; Stefanova et al., 2000). Treatment studies of depression are virtually nonexistent, with most reports in the literature being case reports and

small series (Fetoni et al., 1999; Roane et al., 2000; Tamai and Almeida, 1997). There are no controlled clinical trials of medications for depression in these illnesses.

## Lesion Studies of the Basal Ganglia

Lesion studies looking at behavioral effects of damage to the basal ganglia have found that depression correlates with caudate nucleus damage (Bhatia and Marsden, 1994). Poststroke depression studies have also implicated the caudate as well as the frontal lobes as regions more often involved (Mendez et al., 1989). These findings underscore the close relationship of these structures to the pathophysiology of depression.

## CONCLUSIONS

This chapter describes the epidemiology, pathology, and clinical characteristics of depression in patients with basal ganglia disease. These illnesses share commonalities including prominent subcortical pathology as well as cortical-subcortical pathway dysfunction. Depression is among the most common psychiatric disorders, and although etiopathogenic factors related to it are still under intense scrutiny, theories implicating selective dysfunction of known neural pathways have been postulated (Drevets, 2001). Abnormalities of frontal lobe metabolism as well as limbic and basal ganglia dysfunction have been proposed in imaging studies of endogenous depression (MDD) (Drevets, 2000), and the reversal of this hypometabolism is evidence in favor of these regions being involved in the anatomy of melancholia (Baxter et al., 1989).

This review has demonstrated that anatomico-physiological correlates of depression in basal ganglia disease involve structures similar to those in MDD, including the caudate in lesion studies (Bhatia and Marsden, 1994), frontal lobes in stroke studies (Starkstein et al., 1987), basal ganglia in stroke studies (Mendez et al., 1989), and hypometabolism of the caudate and inferior and medial frontal lobes in depressed patients with PD (Mayberg et al., 1990). Additionally, cellular damage to the caudate occurs in HD and WD patients and may explain the origin of depression in these disorders. Treatment of depression in PD (as in MDD) results in reversal of the PET changes seen in depressed patients with PD, strongly implicating these regions in the pathogenesis of the mood disorder in PD (Mayberg, 2001). Further, neurotransmitters implicated in the pathogenesis of MDD have been implicated in PD depression (Chan-Palay, 1993; Javoy-Agid and Agid, 1980; Mayeux, 1990; Sandyk and Fisher, 1989) and are probably involved in the depression seen in other basal ganglia diseases. Summating this collective data set, the evidence appears to implicate depression as a syndrome with multifactorial causation and dysfunction along separate but functionally linked pathways that involve not only subcortical but also cortical sites, as well as multiple neurotransmitter systems (Heilman, 1997). This has several important implications both for our understanding of these illnesses and for directions for future research. Research aimed at understanding the cerebral correlates of depression might focus on individuals who have well-defined neurological disease as an alternative to MDD in an effort to subscribe to a more uniform population of depressed patients, resulting in a novel way of investigating the neural underpinnings of mood.

Since the *motor* illnesses of the basal ganglia and depression share common structural localizations, it is therefore intuitive that depression would be enmeshed in the syndromic picture. The segregated circuits described earlier in this chapter all pass through the basal ganglia, and the motor and nonmotor circuits have interconnections. Damage to one or more circuits can understandably cause repercussions in other functionally segregated circuits and explains why all basal ganglia motor disorders have been associated with affective disorders. So far, neurologists have defined these illnesses on the basis of their motor manifestations. Our argument would be that this is less than adequate, as psychiatric symptomatology such as depression may be an integral and even an initial derangement in these diseases and not simply a reactive component to the disease burden, as was argued in the past. The question remains whether depression in these diseases is a risk factor for the motor disorder, a marker of a variant pathology of the disease, or an integral component of the pathophysiological process. If depression predates the motor disorder and is integral to the disease process, then our understanding of the processes involved would lead to a better identification of presymptomatic or early symptomatic phases of these devastating diseases. This would, in turn, allow us to plan and investigate neuroprotective strategies that may be more effective than those available at present. Further research in these areas is clearly indicated to clarify these issues.

## REFERENCES

Aarsland, D., Litvan, I., and Larsen, J.P. (2001) Neuropsychiatric symptoms of patients with progressive supranuclear palsy and Parkinson's disease. *J Neuropsychiatry Clin Neurosci* 13:42–49.

Akil, M., and Brewer, G.J. (1995) Psychiatric and behavioral abnormalities in Wilson's disease. *Adv Neurol* 65:171–178.

Akil, M., Schwartz, J.A., Dutchak, D., Yuzbasiyan-Gurkan, V., and Brewer, G.J. (1991) The psychiatric presentations of Wilson's disease. *J Neuropsychiatry Clin Neurosci* 3:377–382.

Alexander, G.E., DeLong, M.R., and Strick, P.L. (1986) Parallel organization of functionally segregated circuits linking basal ganglia and cortex. *Annu Rev Neurosci* 9:357–381.

Anderson, G., Aabro, E., Gulamann, N., Hjelmsted, A., and Peder-

sen, H.E. (1980) Antidepressant treatment in Parkinson's disease: A controlled trial of the effect of nortryptiline in patients with Parkinson's disease treated with L-dopa. *Acta Neurol Scand* 62:210–219.

Andrew, S.E., Goldberg, Y.P., Kremer, B., Telenius, H., Theilmann, J., Adam, S., et al. (1993) The relationship between trinucleotide (CAG) repeat length and clinical features of Huntington's disease. *Nat Genet* 4:398–403.

Ballenger, J.C. (1988) Biological aspects of depression: Implications for clinical practice. In: Frances, A.J., and Hales, R.E., eds. *Review of Psychiatry*, vol. 7. Washington, DC: American Psychiatric Press, pp. 169–187.

Baxter, L.R., Jr., Schwartz, J.M., Phelps, M.E., Mazziotta, J.C., Guze, B.H., Selin, C.E., et al. (1989) Reduction of prefrontal cortex glucose metabolism common to three types of depression. *Arch Gen Psychiatry* 46:243–250.

Becker, T., Becker, G., Seufert, J., Hofmann, E., Lange, K.W., Naumann, M., et al. (1997) Parkinson's disease and depression: Evidence for an alteration of the basal limbic system detected by transcranial sonography. *J Neurol Neurosurg Psychiatry* 63:590–596.

Beenen, N., Buttner, U., and Lange, H.W. (1986) The diagnostic value of eye movement recordings in patients with Huntington's disease and their offspring. *Electroencephalogr Clin Neurophysiol* 63:119–127.

Bejjani, B.P., Damier, P., Arnulf, I., Thivard, L., Bonnet, A.M., Dormont, D., Cornu, P., Pidoux, B., Samson, Y., and Agid, Y. (1999) Transient acute depression induced by high-frequency deep-brain stimulation. *N Engl J Med* 340:1476–1480.

Bench, C.J., Friston, K.J., Brown, R.G., Scott, L.C., Frackowiak, R.S., and Dolan, R.J. (1992) The anatomy of melancholia—focal abnormalities of cerebral blood flow in major depression. *Psychol Med* 22:607–615.

Bhatia, K.P., and Marsden, C.D. (1994) The behavioural and motor consequences of focal lesions of the basal ganglia in man. *Brain* 117:859–876.

Bird, E.D., and Iversen, L.L. (1974) Huntington's chorea. Post-mortem measurement of glutamic acid decarboxylase, choline acetyltransferase and dopamine in basal ganglia. *Brain* 97:457–472.

Bird, E.D., Spokes, E.G., and Iversen, L.L. (1979) Increased dopamine concentration in limbic areas of brain from patients dying with schizophrenia. *Brain* 102:347–360.

Brewer, G.J. (2000) Recognition, diagnosis, and management of Wilson's disease. *Proc Soc Exp Biol Med* 223:39–46.

Buchsbaum, M.S., Wu, J., DeLisi, L.E., Holcomb, H., Kessler, R., Johnson, J., et al. (1986) Frontal cortex and basal ganglia metabolic rates assessed by positron emission tomography with [18F]2-deoxyglucose in affective illness. *J Affect Disord* 10:137–152.

Buchsbaum, M.S., Wu, J., Siegel, B.V., Hackett, E., Trenary, M., Abel, L., et al. (1997) Effect of sertraline on regional metabolic rate in patients with affective disorder. *Biol Psychiatry* 41:15–22.

Burke, W.J., Peterson, J., and Rubin, E.H. (1988) Electroconvulsive therapy in the treatment of combined depression and Parkinson's disease. *Psychosomatics* 29:341–346.

Caine, E.D., and Shoulson, I. (1983) Psychiatric syndromes in Huntington's disease. *Am J Psychiatry* 140:728–733.

Carmichael, S.T., and Price, J.L. (1995) Limbic connections of the orbital and medial prefrontal cortex in macaque monkeys. *J Comp Neurol* 363:615–641.

Cash, R., Raisman, R., Ploska, A., and Agid, Y. (1985) High and low affinity [3H]imipramine binding sites in control and parkinsonian brains. *Eur J Pharmacol* 117:71–80.

Chan-Palay, V. (1993) Depression and dementia in Parkinson's disease. Catecholamine changes in the locus ceruleus, a basis for therapy. *Adv Neurol* 60:438–446.

Chan-Palay, V., and Asan, E. (1989) Alterations in catecholamine neurons of the locus coeruleus in senile dementia of the Alzheimer type and in Parkinson's disease with and without dementia and depression. *J Comp Neurol* 287:373–392.

Como, P.G., Rubin, A.J., O'Brien, C.F., Lawler, K., Hickey, C., Rubin, A.E., et al. (1997) A controlled trial of fluoxetine in nondepressed patients with Huntington's disease. *Mov Disord* 12:397–401.

Cummings, J.L. (1985) *Clinical Neuropsychiatry*. New York: Grune & Stratton.

Cummings, J.L. (1992) Depression and Parkinson's disease: A review. *Am J Psychiatry* 149:443–454.

Cummings, J.L. (1993) Frontal-subcortical circuits and human behavior. *Arch Neurol* 50:873–880.

Cummings, J.L. (1995) Behavioral and psychiatric symptoms associated with Huntington's disease. *Adv Neurol* 65:179–186.

Cuthbert, J.A. (1995) Wilson's disease: a new gene and an animal model for an old disease. *J Invest Med* 43:323–336.

de Rijk, M.C., Tzourio, C., Breteler, M.M., Dartigues, J.F., Amaducci, L., Lopez-Pousa, S., Manubens-Bertran, J.M., Alperovitch, A., and Rocca, W.A. (1997) Prevalence of parkinsonism and parkinson's disease in Europe: The EUROPARKINSON Collaborative Study. European Community Concerted Action on the Epidemiology of Parkinson's disease. *J Neurol Neurosurg Psychiatry* 62:10–15.

Delgado, P.L., Charney, D.S., Price, L.H., Aghajanian, G.K., Landis, H., and Heninger, G.R. (1990) Serotonin function and the mechanism of antidepressant action. Reversal of antidepressant-induced remission by rapid depletion of plasma tryptophan. *Arch Gen Psychiatry* 47:411–418.

Dening, T.R., and Berrios, G.E. (1989) Wilson's disease. Psychiatric symptoms in 195 cases. *Arch Gen Psychiatry* 46:1126–1134.

Di Maio, L., Squitieri, F., Napolitano, G., Campanella, G., Trofatter, J.A., and Conneally, P.M. (1993) Onset symptoms in 510 patients with Huntington's disease. *J Med Genet* 30:289–292.

Drevets, W.C. (2000) Neuroimaging studies of mood disorders. *Biol Psychiatry* 48:813–829.

Drevets, W.C. (2001) Neuroimaging and neuropathological studies of depression: Implications for the cognitive-emotional features of mood disorders. *Curr Opin Neurobiol* 11:240–249.

Drevets, W.C., Price, J.L., Simpson, J.R., Jr., Todd, R.D., Reich, T., Vannier, M., and Raichle, M.E. (1997) Subgenual prefrontal cortex abnormalities in mood disorders. *Nature* 386(6627):824–827.

Drevets, W.C., Videen, T.O., Price, J.L., Preskorn, S.H., Carmichael, S.T., and Raichle, M.E. (1992) A functional anatomical study of unipolar depression. *J Neurosci* 12:3628–3641.

Ebert, D., and Ebmeier, K.P. (1996) The role of the cingulate gyrus in depression: From functional anatomy to neurochemistry. *Biol Psychiatry* 39:1044–1050.

Farrer, L.A. (1986) Suicide and attempted suicide in Huntington disease: Implications for preclinical testing of persons at risk. *Am J Med Genet* 24:305–311.

Fesenmeier, J.T., Kuzniecky, R., and Garcia, J.H. (1990) Akinetic mutism caused by bilateral anterior cerebral tuberculous obliterative arteritis. *Neurology* 40:1005–1006.

Fetoni, V., Soliveri, P., Monza, D., Testa, D., and Girotti, F. (1999) Affective symptoms in multiple system atrophy and Parkinson's disease: Response to levodopa therapy. *J Neurol Neurosurg Psychiatry* 66:541–544.

Folstein, S.E. (1989) *Huntington's Disease. A Disorder of Families.* Baltimore: Johns Hopkins University Press.

Folstein, S.E., Abbott, M.H., Chase, G.A., Jensen, B.A., and Folstein, M.F. (1983) The association of affective disorder with Huntington's disease in a case series and in families. *Psychol Med* 13:537–542.

Folstein, S.E., Chase, G.A., Wahl, W.E., McDonnell, A.M., and Folstein, M.F. (1987) Huntington disease in Maryland: Clinical aspects of racial variation. *Am J Hum Genet* 41:168–179.

Folstein, S.E., Folstein, M.F., and McHugh, P.R. (1979) Psychiatric syndromes in Huntington's disease. *Adv Neurol* 23:281–289.

Ford, M.F. (1986) Treatment of depression in Huntington's disease with monoamine oxidase inhibitors. *Br J Psychiatry* 149:654–656.

Friedenberg, D.L., and Cummings, J.L. (1989) Parkinson's disease, depression, and the on-off phenomenon. *Psychosomatics* 30:94–99.

Gelb, D.J., Oliver, E., and Gilman, S. (1999) Diagnostic criteria for Parkinson disease. *Arch Neurol* 56:33–39.

George, M.S., Wassermann, E.M., and Post, R.M. (1996) Transcranial magnetic stimulation: A neuropsychiatric tool for the 21st century. *J Neuropsychiatry Clin Neurosci* 8:373–382.

Gill, C.E., Khurana, R.K., and Hibler, R.J. (1999) Occurrence of depressive symptoms in Shy-Drager syndrome. *Clin Auton Res* 9:1–4.

Goetz, C.G., Tanner, C.M., and Klawans, H.L. (1984) Bupropion in Parkinson's disease. *Neurology* 34:1092–1094.

Gotham, A.M., Brown, R.G., and Marsden, C.D. (1986) Depression in Parkinson's disease: A quantitative and qualitative analysis. *J Neurol Neurosurg Psychiatry* 49:381–389.

Goto, K., Ueki, A., Shimode, H., Shinjo, H., Miwa, C., and Morita, Y. (2000) Depression in multiple system atrophy: A case report. *Psychiatry Clin Neurosci* 54:507–511.

Greenberg, R., and Meyers, B.S. (1985) Treatment of major depression and Parkinson's disease with combined phenelzine and amantadine. *Am J Psychiatry* 142:273–274.

Hammond, M.F. (1996) Rating depression severity in the elderly physically ill patient: Reliability and factor structure of the Hamilton and Montgomery-Asberg Depression Rating Scales. *Int J Geriatr Psychiatry* 13:257–261.

Hargrave, R., and Ashford, J.W. (1992) Phenelzine treatment of depression in Parkinson's disease. *Am J Psychiatry* 149:1751–1752.

Heathfield, K.W.G., and Mackenzie, I.C.K. (1971) Huntington's chorea in Bedfordshire, England. *Guys Hosp Rep* 120:295–309.

Heilman, K.M. (1997) The neurobiology of emotional experience. *J Neuropsychiatry Clin Neurosci* 9:439–448.

Horn, S. (1974) Some psychological factors in parkinsonism. *J Neurol Neurosurg Psychiatry* 37:27–31.

Huber, S.J., Paulson, G.W., and Shuttleworth, E.C. (1988) Relationship of motor symptoms, intellectual impairment, and depression in Parkinson's disease. *J Neurol Neurosurg Psychiatry* 51:855–858.

Hughes, A.J., Daniel, S.E., Blankson, S., and Lees, A.J. (1993) A clinicopathologic study of 100 cases of Parkinson's disease. *Arch Neurol* 50:140–148.

The Huntington's Disease Collaborative Research Group. (1993) A novel gene containing a trinucleotide repeat that is expanded and unstable on Huntington's disease chromosomes. *Cell* 72(6):971–983.

Javoy-Agid, F., and Agid, Y. (1980) Is the mesocortical dopaminergic system involved in Parkinson disease? *Neurology* 30:1326–1330.

Jellinger, K.A. (2001) The pathology of Parkinson's disease. *Adv Neurol* 86:55–72.

Jensen, P., Sorensen, S.A., Fenger, K., and Bolwig, T.G. (1993) A study of psychiatric morbidity in patients with Huntington's disease, their relatives, and controls. Admissions to psychiatric hospitals in Denmark from 1969 to 1991. *Br J Psychiatry* 163:790–797.

Jouvent, R., Abensour, P., Bonnet, A.M., Widlocher, D., Agid, Y., and Lhermitte, F. (1983) Antiparkinsonian and antidepressant effects of high doses of bromocriptine. An independent comparison. *J Affect Disord* 5:141–145.

Kapur, S., and Remington, G. (1996) Serotonin–dopamine interaction and its relevance to schizophrenia. *Am J Psychiatry* 153:466–476.

Keller, R., Torta, R., Lagget, M., Crasto, S., and Bergamasco, B. (1999) Psychiatric symptoms as late onset of Wilson's disease: Neuroradiological findings, clinical features and treatment. *Ital J Neurol Sci* 20:49–54.

Kirkwood, S.C., Siemers, E., Bond, C., Conneally, P.M., Christian, J.C., and Foroud, T. (2000) Confirmation of subtle motor changes among presymptomatic carriers of the Huntington disease gene. *Arch Neurol* 57:1040–1044.

Klaassen, T., Verhey, F.R., Sneijders, G.H., Rozendaal, N., de Vet, H.C., and van Praag, H.M. (1995) Treatment of depression in Parkinson's disease: A meta-analysis. *J Neuropsychiatry Clin Neurosci* 7:281–286.

Kremer, B., Goldberg, P., Andrew, S.E., Theilmann, J., Telenius, H., Zeisler, J., et al. (1994) A worldwide study of the Huntington's disease mutation. The sensitivity and specificity of measuring CAG repeats. *N Engl J Med* 330:1401–1406.

Krishnan, K.R., McDonald, W.M., Escalona, P.R., Doraiswamy, P.M., Na, C., Husain, M.M., et al. (1992) Magnetic resonance imaging of the caudate nuclei in depression. Preliminary observations. *Arch Gen Psychiatry* 49:553–557.

Kultas-Ilinsky, K., and Ilinsky, I.A. (2001) *Basal Ganglia and Thalamus in Health and Movement Disorders.* New York: Kluwer Academic/Plenum.

Kurlan, R., Caine, E., Rubin, A., Nemeroff, C.B., Bissette, G., Zaczek, R., et al. (1988) Cerebrospinal fluid correlates of depression in Huntington's disease. *Arch Neurol* 45:881–883.

Laitinen, L. (1969) Desipramine in the treatment of Parkinson's disease. *Acta Neurol Scand* 45:109–113.

Langer, S.Z., Galzin, A.M., Poirier, M.F., Loo, H., Sechter, D., and Zarifian, E. (1987) Association of [3H]-imipramine and [3H]-paroxetine binding with the 5HT transporter in brain and platelets: Relevance to studies in depression. *J Recept Res* 7:499–521.

Leentjens, A.F., Verhey, F.R., Lousberg, R., Spitsbergen, H., and Wilmink, F.W. (2000) The validity of the Hamilton and Montgomery-Asberg depression rating scales as screening and diagnostic tools for depression in Parkinson's disease. *Int J Geriatr Psychiatry* 15:644–649.

Lesser, I.M., Mena, I., Boone, K.B., Miller, B.L., Mehringer, C.M., and Wohl, M. (1994) Reduction of cerebral blood flow in older depressed patients. *Arch Gen Psychiatry* 51:677–686.

Levy, M.L., Cummings, J.L., Fairbanks, L.A., Masterman, D., Miller, B.L., Craig, A.H., et al. (1998) Apathy is not depression. *J Neuropsychiatry Clin Neurosci* 10:314–319.

Lipe, H., Schultz, A., and Bird, T.D. (1993) Risk factors for suicide in Huntington's disease: A retrospective case controlled study. *Am J Med Genet* 48:231–233.

Litvan, I., Mega, M.S., Cummings, J.L., and Fairbanks, L. (1996) Neuropsychiatric aspects of progressive supranuclear palsy. *Neurology* 47:1184–1189.

Litvan, I., Paulsen, J.S., Mega, M.S., and Cummings, J.L. (1998) Neuropsychiatric assessment of patients with hyperkinetic and hypokinetic movement disorders. *Arch Neurol* 55:1313–1319.

Lloyd, K.G., Zivkovic, B., Scatton, B., Morselli, P.L., and Bartholini, G. (1989) The gabaergic hypothesis of depression. *Prog Neuropsychopharmacol Biol Psychiatry* 13:341–351.

Mally, J., and Stone, T.W. (1999) Improvement in parkinsonian symptoms after repetitive transcranial magnetic stimulation. *J Neurol Sci* 162:179–184.

Mann, J.J., Aarons, S.F., Wilner, P.J., Keilp, J.G., Sweeney, J.A., Pearlstein, T., et al. (1989) A controlled study of the antidepressant efficacy and side effects of (−)-deprenyl. A selective monoamine oxidase inhibitor. *Arch Gen Psychiatry* 46:45–50.

Maricle, R.A., Nutt, J.G., Valentine, R.J., and Carter, J.H. (1995) Dose-response relationship of levodopa with mood and anxiety in fluctuating Parkinson's disease: A double-blind, placebo-controlled study. *Neurology* 45:1757–1760.

Mayberg, H.S. (1997) Limbic-cortical dysregulation: A proposed model of depression. *J Neuropsychiatry Clin Neurosci* 9:471–481.

Mayberg, H.S. (2001) Depression: Focus on prefrontal–limbic interactions. In: Lichter, D.G., and Cummings, J.L., eds. *Frontal-Subcortical Circuits in Psychiatric and Neurological Disorders.* New York: Guilford Press, pp. 177–207.

Mayberg, H.S., Lewis, P.J., Regenold, W., and Wagner, H.N., Jr. (1994) Paralimbic hypoperfusion in unipolar depression. *J Nucl Med* 35:929–934.

Mayberg, H.S., Mahurin, R.K., and Brannan, S.K. (1995) Parkinson's depression: Discrimination of mood sensitive and mood insensitive cognitive deficits using fluoxetine and FDG PET. *Neurology* 45(suppl 4):A166.

Mayberg, H.S., Starkstein, S.E., Peyser, C.E., Brandt, J., Dannals, R.F., and Folstein, S.E. (1992) Paralimbic frontal lobe hypometabolism in depression associated with Huntington's disease. *Neurology* 42:1791–1797.

Mayberg, H.S., Starkstein, S.E., Sadzot, B., Preziosi, T., Andrezejewski, P.L., Dannals, R.F., et al. (1990) Selective hypometabolism in the inferior frontal lobe in depressed patients with Parkinson's disease. *Ann Neurol* 28:57–64.

Mayeux, R. (1990) The "serotonin hypothesis" for depression in Parkinson's disease. *Adv Neurol* 53:163–166.

Mayeux, R., Marder, K., Cote, L.J., Denaro, J., Hemenegildo, N., Mejia, H., et al. (1995) The frequency of idiopathic Parkinson's disease by age, ethnic group, and sex in northern Manhattan, 1988–1993. *Am J Epidemiol* 142:820–827.

Mayeux, R., Stern, Y., Cote, L., and Williams, J.B. (1984) Altered serotonin metabolism in depressed patients with parkinson's disease. *Neurology* 34:642–646.

Mayeux, R., Stern, Y., Rosen, J., and Leventhal, J. (1981) Depression, intellectual impairment, and Parkinson disease. *Neurology* 31:645–650.

Mayeux, R., Stern, Y., Sano, M., Williams, J.B., and Cote, L.J. (1988) The relationship of serotonin to depression in Parkinson's disease. *Mov Disord* 3:237–244.

Mayeux, R., Stern, Y., Williams, J.B., Cote, L., Frantz, A., and Dyrenfurth, I. (1986) Clinical and biochemical features of depression in Parkinson's disease. *Am J Psychiatry* 143:756–759.

Mendez, M.F., Adams, N.L., and Lewandowski, K.S. (1989) Neurobehavioral changes associated with caudate lesions. *Neurology* 39:349–354.

Menza, M.A., Cocchiola, J., and Golbe, L.I. (1995) Psychiatric symptoms in progressive supranuclear palsy. *Psychosomatics* 36:550–554.

Mindham, R.H. (1970) Psychiatric symptoms in parkinsonism. *J Neurol Neurosurg Psychiatry* 33:188–191.

Moldawsky, R.J. (1984) Effect of amoxapine on speech in a patient with Huntington disease. *Am J Psychiatry* 141:150.

Mouradian, M.M. (2002) Recent advances in the genetics and pathogenesis of Parkinson disease. *Neurology* 58:179–185.

Olivarez, L., Caggana, M., Pass, K.A., Ferguson, P., and Brewer, G.J. (2001) Estimate of the frequency of Wilson's disease in the U.S. Caucasian population: A mutation analysis approach. *Ann Hum Genet* 65:459–463.

Parent, A. (1996) *Carpenter's Human Neuroanatomy.* Baltimore: Williams & Wilkins.

Parent, A., and Cicchetti, F. (1998) The current model of basal ganglia organisation under scrutiny. *Mov Disord* 13:199–202.

Parkinson, J. (1817) *An Essay on the Shaking Palsy.* London: Whittingham & Rowland.

Patel, S.V., Tariot, P.N., and Asnis, J. (1996) L-Deprenyl augmentation of fluoxetine in a patient with Huntington's disease. *Ann Clin Psychiatry* 8:23–26.

Paulsen, J.S., Ready, R.E., Hamilton, J.M., Mega, M.S., and Cummings, J.L. (2001) Neuropsychiatric aspects of Huntington's disease. *J Neurol Neurosurg Psychiatry* 71:310–314.

Paulus, W., and Jellinger, K. (1991) The neuropathologic basis of different clinical subgroups of Parkinson's disease. *J Neuropathol Exp Neurol* 50:743–755.

Petrukhin, K., Fischer, S.G., Pirastu, M., Tanzi, R.E., Chernov, I., Devoto, M., et al. (1993) Mapping, cloning and genetic characterization of the region containing the Wilson disease gene. *Nat Genet* 5:338–343.

Peyser, C.E., and Folstein, S.E. (1990) Huntington's disease as a model for mood disorders. Clues from neuropathology and neurochemistry. *Mol Chem Neuropathol* 12:99–119.

Pilo, L., Ring, H., Quinn, N., and Trimble, M. (1996) Depression in multiple system atrophy and in idiopathic Parkinson's disease: A pilot comparative study. *Biol Psychiatry* 39:803–807.

Poewe, W., and Seppi, K. (2001) Treatment options for depression and psychosis in Parkinson's disease. *J Neurol* 248(suppl 3):III12–21.

Price, J.L. (1999) Prefrontal cortical networks related to visceral function and mood. *Ann NY Acad Sci* 877:383–396.

Raisman, R., Cash, R., and Agid, Y. (1986) Parkinson's disease: Decreased density of 3H-imipramine and 3H-paroxetine binding sites in putamen. *Neurology* 36:556–560.

Ranen, N.G., Peyser, C.E., and Folstein, S.E. (1994) ECT as a treatment for depression in Huntington's disease. *J Neuropsychiatry Clin Neurosci* 6:154–159.

Reilly, M., Daly, L., and Hutchinson, M. (1993) An epidemiological study of Wilson's disease in the Republic of Ireland. *J Neurol Neurosurg Psychiatry* 56:298–300.

Rektorova, I., Rektor, I., and Hortova, H. (2001) Depression in Parkinson's disease: An eight month randomised, open-label, national, multi-centre comparative study of pramipexole and pergolide. *Parkinsonism Rel Disord* 7:S68.

Richard, I.H., and Kurlan, R. (1997) A survey of antidepressant drug use in Parkinson's disease. Parkinson Study Group. *Neurology* 49:1168–1170.

Richard, I.H., Kurlan, R., Tanner, C., Factor, S., Hubble, J., Suchowersky, O., et al. (1997) Serotonin syndrome and the combined use of deprenyl and an antidepressant in Parkinson's disease. Parkinson Study Group. *Neurology* 48:1070–1077.

Ring, H.A., Bench, C.J., Trimble, M.R., Brooks, D.J., Frackowiak, R.S., and Dolan, R.J. (1994) Depression in Parkinson's disease. A positron emission study. *Br J Psychiatry* 165:333–339.

Roane, D.M., Rogers, J.D., Helew, L., and Zarate, J. (2000) Electroconvulsive therapy for elderly patients with multiple system atrophy: A case series. *Am J Geriatr Psychiatry* 8:171–174.

Saatci, I., Topcu, M., Baltaoglu, F.F., Kose, G., Yalaz, K., Renda, Y., et al. (1997) Cranial MR findings in Wilson's disease. *Acta Radiol* 38:250–258.

Saint-Cyr, J.A., and Trepanier, L.L. (2000) Neuropsychologic assessment of patients for movement disorder surgery. *Mov Disord* 15:771–783.

Sajatovic, M., Verbanac, P., Ramirez, L.F., and Meltzer, H.Y. (1991) Clozapine treatment of psychiatric symptoms resistant to neuroleptic treatment in patients with Huntington's chorea. *Neurology* 41:156.

Sandyk, R. (1989) Locus coeruleus–pineal melatonin interactions in the pathogenesis of the "on-off" phenomenon associated with mood changes and sensory symptoms in Parkinson's disease. *Int J Neurosci* 49:95–101.

Sandyk, R. (1990) Pineal melatonin functions and the depression of Parkinson's disease: A hypothesis. *Int J Neurosci* 51:73–77.

Sandyk, R., and Derpapas, K. (1993) The effects of external pico-Tesla range magnetic fields on the EEG in Parkinson's disease. *Int J Neurosci* 70:85–96.

Sandyk, R., and Fisher, H. (1989) The relationship of serotonin metabolism and melatonin secretion to the pathophysiology of tardive dyskinesia. *Int J Neurosci* 48:133–136.

Sano, M., Stern, Y., Cote, L., Williams, J.B., and Mayeux, R. (1990) Depression in Parkinson's disease: A biochemical model. *J Neuropsychiatry Clin Neurosci* 2:88–92.

Sano, M., Stern, Y., Williams, J., Cote, L., Rosenstein, R., and Mayeux, R. (1989) Coexisting dementia and depression in Parkinson's disease. *Arch Neurol* 46:1284–1286.

Santamaria, J., Tolosa, E., and Valles, A. (1986) Parkinson's disease with depression: A possible subgroup of idiopathic parkinsonism. *Neurology* 36:1130–1133.

Schrag, A., Jahanshahi, M., and Quinn, N.P. (2001) What contributes to depression in Parkinson's disease? *Psychol Med* 31:65–73.

Schuurman, A.G., Van Den Akker, M., Ensinck, K.T., Metsemakers, J.F., Knottnerus, J.A., Leentjens, A.F., et al. (2002) Increased risk of Parkinson's disease after depression: A retrospective cohort study. *Neurology* 58:1501–1504.

Shiwach, R. (1994) Psychopathology in Huntington's disease patients. *Acta Psychiatr Scand* 90:241–246.

Shoulson, I. (1981) Huntington disease: Functional capacities in patients treated with neuroleptic and antidepressant drugs. *Neurology* 31:1333–1335.

Slaughter, J.R., Martens, M.P., and Slaughter, K.A. (2001) Depression and Huntington's disease: Prevalence, clinical manifestations, etiology, and treatment. *CNS Spectrums* 6:306–326.

Spokes, E.G. (1980) Neurochemical alterations in Huntington's chorea: A study of post-mortem brain tissue. *Brain* 103:179–210.

Starkstein, S.E., Cohen, B.S., Fedoroff, P., Parikh, R.M., Price, T.R., and Robinson, R.G. (1990) Relationship between anxiety disorders and depressive disorders in patients with cerebrovascular injury. *Arch Gen Psychiatry* 47:246–251.

Starkstein, S.E., Robinson, R.G., and Price, T.R. (1987) Comparison of cortical and subcortical lesions in the production of poststroke mood disorders. *Brain* 110:1045–1059.

Stefanova, N., Seppi, K., Scherfler, C., Puschban, Z., and Wenning, G.K. (2000) Depression in alpha-synucleinopathies: Prevalence, pathophysiology and treatment. *J Neural Transm Suppl* 60:335–343.

Stenager, E.N., Wermuth, L., Stenager, E., and Boldsen, J. (1994) Suicide in patients with Parkinson's disease. An epidemiological study. *Acta Psychiatr Scand* 90:70–72.

Steur, E.N., and Ballering, L.A. (1997) Moclobemide and selegeline in the treatment of depression in Parkinson's disease. *J Neurol Neurosurg Psychiatry* 63:547.

Strang, R.R. (1965) Imipramine in the treatment of parkinsonism. *Br Med J* 2:33–34.

Sugiyama, H., Hainfellner, J.A., Yoshimura, M., and Budka, H. (1994) Neocortical changes in Parkinson's disease, revisited. *Clin Neuropathol* 13:55–59.

Takahashi, H., and Wakabayashi, K. (2001) The cellular pathology of Parkinson's disease. *Neuropathology* 21:315–322.

Tamai, S., and Almeida, O.P. (1997) Nortriptyline for the treatment of depression in progressive supranuclear palsy. *J Am Geriatr Soc* 45:1033–1034.

Tanzi, R.E., Petrukhin, K., Chernov, I., Pellequer, J.L., Wasco, W., Ross, B., et al. (1993) The Wilson disease gene is a copper transporting ATPase with homology to the Menkes disease gene. *Nat Genet* 5:344–350.

Taylor, A.E., and Saint-Cyr, J.A. (1990) Depression in Parkinson's disease: Reconciling physiological and psychological perspectives. *J Neuropsychiatry Clin Neurosci* 2:92–98.

Tom, T., and Cummings, J.L. (1998) Depression in Parkinson's disease. Pharmacological characteristics and treatment. *Drugs Aging* 12:55–74.

Vonsattel, J.P., and DiFiglia, M. (1998) Huntington disease. *J Neuropathol Exp Neurol* 57:369–384.

Walter, G., and Lyndon, B. (1997) Depression in hepatolenticular degeneration (Wilson's disease). *Aust NZJ Psychiatry* 31:880–882.

Warburton, J.W. (1967) Depressive symptoms in Parkinson patients referred for thalamotomy. *J Neurol Neurosurg Psychiatry* 30:368–370.

Waters, C.H. (1994) Fluoxetine and selegiline—Lack of significant interaction. *Can J Neurol Sci* 21:259–261.

Williams, J.B. (2001) Standardizing the Hamilton Depression Rating Scale: Past, present, and future. *Eur Arch Psychiatry Clin Neurosci* 251:II6–12.

Wolfe, N., Katz, D.I., Albert, M.L., Almozlino, A., Durso, R., Smith, M.C., et al. (1990) Neuropsychological profile linked to low dopamine: In Alzheimer's disease, major depression, and Parkinson's disease. *J Neurol Neurosurg Psychiatry* 53:915–917.

Wu, J.C., Gillin, J.C., Buchsbaum, M.S., Hershey, T., Johnson, J.C., and Bunney, W.E., Jr. (1992) Effect of sleep deprivation on brain metabolism of depressed patients. *Am J Psychiatry* 149:538–543.

Xu, X.H., Yang, B.X., and Feng, Y.K. (1981) Wilson's disease (hepatolenticular degeneration): Clinical analysis of 80 cases. *Chin Med J (Engl)* 94:673–678.

# 29 | Major depressive disorder in Alzheimer's disease

GEORGE S. ZUBENKO

Clinically significant depression is a common and important complication of Alzheimer's disease (AD) that increases the suffering of patients and their families, produces excess disability, promotes institutionalization, and hastens death (Olin et al., 2002; U.S. DHHS, 1999). Estimates of the prevalence of depressive symptoms among patients with AD have been as high as 86% (Merriam et al., 1988). Most cross-sectional estimates of the coexistence of syndromal major depressive disorder (MDD) in elderly outpatients with probable AD range from about 15% to 25% (for reviews, see Mulsant and Zubenko, 1994; Olin et al., 2002; Teri and Reifler, 1987; Wragg and Jeste, 1989). The recurrent nature of this behavioral complication of AD suggests that an even larger proportion of patients eventually experience a major depressive episode (MDE) before death (Zubenko, 1992; Zubenko et al., 2003).

In a recent collaborative study that employed a common, reliable methodology for the assessment and diagnosis of MDEs in demented patients, the prevalence of MDD in the aggregate sample of 243 patients who met clinical consensus criteria for probable AD was 35%, and reached nearly 50% among the most demented individuals (Zubenko et al., 2003). Since current population estimates indicate that AD affects 8% to 15% of Americans over the age of 65, these findings suggest that the major depressive syndrome of AD may be among the most common mood disorders of late life. Furthermore, the high rate of MDEs that occurred at or after the onset of cognitive impairment among patients with AD (the majority of whom had no premorbid history of MDD), their common emergence in the early stages of dementia when symptoms of cognitive impairment are least likely to contribute to the syndromal diagnosis of MDD, and differences in the clinical presentations of the MDEs of AD patients and nondemented elderly controls all supported the validity of the major depressive syndrome of AD. These observations and the current lack of an effective means of preventing or controlling the pathophysiological events that lead to dementia in late life have stimulated efforts to understand and treat MDD and

other behavioral complications of AD, efforts that may also provide insight into the clinical biology of major mood disorders more generally among older adults.

Emerging clinicopathological studies of MDD in AD suggest that the development of this behavioral syndrome is associated with degeneration of the major brain stem aminergic nuclei (locus ceruleus [LC], substantia nigra [SN], dorsal raphe [DR]) and the relative preservation of the cholinergic basal nucleus of Meynert (bnM) (Chan-Palay, 1990; Forstl et al., 1992; Zubenko and Moossy, 1988; Zweig et al., 1988). Reported changes in the levels of monoaminergic neurotransmitters/metabolites and choline acetyltransferase (ChAT) in the projection areas of these nuclei have been largely consistent with the histopathological findings (Zubenko et al., 1990). The neuropathological and neurochemical correlates of MDD in AD appear to be relatively specific for this behavioral complication, and may explain aspects of the course and treatment responsiveness of MDD when it emerges in AD (Zubenko, 1992, 1997, 2000b; Zubenko et al., 1990; Zubenko et al., 1991).

## NEUROPATHOLOGICAL AND NEUROCHEMICAL CORRELATES OF MAJOR DEPRESSIVE DISORDER IN ALZHEIMER'S DISEASE

The original catecholamine hypothesis of affective disorders focused largely on the role of the noradrenergic components of the central nervous system (CNS) in the etiology of depression and mania (Bunney and Davis, 1965; Schildkraut, 1965). Additional evidence from clinical, pharmacological, and physiological studies has emerged since the original hypothesis was proposed and is generally supportive of the view that clinically significant depression may result from a dysfunction of CNS mechanisms employing the catecholamine neurotransmitters, norepinephrine (NE) and dopamine (DA) (Jimerson, 1987; Siever, 1987). Neurochemical studies of serotonin (5-HT) receptors and 5-hydroxyindoleacetic acid (5-HIAA) in spinal fluid or brain tissue have also suggested an alteration in serotonergic components of the CNS in both idiopathic MDD and suicide (Brikmayer and Riederer, 1975; Mendlewicz et al., 1981; Crow et al., 1984; Lloyd et al., 1974; Stanley and Mann, 1983). In contrast to these hypotheses, which suggest that depression may result from the decreased function of one or more central aminergic systems, the cholinergic hypothesis of affective disorders (Janowsky and Risch, 1987) predicts that idiopathic depression may be associated with the hyperfunctioning of cholinergic systems. This last prediction is especially interesting in the context of AD, since the progression of the central cholinergic deficit that occurs in this disorder may interact with the pathophysiology of depression to limit the prevalence of MDD in late stages of this disorder.

The pigmented nuclei of the brain stem contain the cell bodies of the majority of the catecholaminergic neurons in the brain. The LC and the SN are the largest of these nuclei, and project noradrenergic afferents to the forebrain and dopaminergic afferents to the striatum, thalamus, and amygdala (Carpenter, 1985; Foote and Morrison, 1987). Studies in primates and humans indicate that the brain stem raphe nuclei contain predominantly serotonergic cell bodies that likewise project to the forebrain and subcortical structures (Felten and Sladek, 1983; Foote and Morrison, 1987). Finally, the bnM is an important source of the cholinergic innervation of the cortex (Whitehouse et al., 1982). Since AD is often associated with degenerative changes in these nuclei (Boller et al., 1980; Bondareff and Mountjoy, 1986; Huber et al., 1986; Mayeux et al., 1981;

Whitehouse et al., 1982) as well as concurrent depression, we have presented evidence supporting the hypothesis that degeneration of one or more of these nuclei is associated with the occurrence of MDD in patients with this multifocal brain disease.

Five published postmortem studies have addressed the neuropathological and neurochemical correlates of MDD in AD. A comparison of the study designs and methods is presented in Table 29.1. Sample sizes of AD cases have ranged from 3 to 52 (50 with complete data). All studies employed prospective behavioral assessments of demented patients who were enrolled in longitudinal studies of AD and related dementias, as well as neuropathologically determined diagnoses of dementia. Our initial studies included 81% with AD, 19% with Parkinson's disease, and 14% with multiple infarctions. The remaining studies included patients with autopsy-confirmed AD, although it is uncertain whether patients with the Lewy body variant of AD (ADLBV) or concurrent brain diseases were excluded.

In all studies, patients with concurrent diagnoses of AD "with depression" fulfilled the DSM-III or DSM-III-R symptom criteria for an MDE. In the context of dementia, depressed mood was required to be one of these symptoms. According to these criteria, 27% to 39% of patients developed an episode of MDD during their follow-up assessments. This proportion is higher than expected based on the reported 15% to 25% estimates of the co-morbidity of MDD and AD among individuals who present for evaluation and treatment at geriatric outpatient clinics. This observation has suggested that MDD may be a risk factor for mortality

TABLE 29.1. *Methodological Comparison of Four Neuropathological Studies of Major Depressive Disorder in Alzheimer's Disease*

| | Zubenko et al. (1988, 1990) | Zweig et al. (1988) | Chan-Palay (1990) | Forstl et al. (1992) |
|---|---|---|---|---|
| Sample size (N) | 37 | 21–25 | 3 | 50–52 |
| Prospective behavioral assessments | Yes | Yes | Unknown | Yes |
| Neuropathological diagnoses of dementia | 81% AD, 20% PD, 14% infarcts | 100% AD (+?) | 100% AD | 100% AD (+?) |
| Symptom criteria for depression | DSM-III Major depressive episode | DSM-III Major depressive episode | DSM-III-R Major depressive episode | DSM-III-R Major depressive episode |
| Depressed; N (%) | 14 (39%) | 8 (38%) | 1 (33%) | 14 (27%) |
| FHx assessment of MDD | Yes | No | No | No |
| Analyses blind to clinical information | Yes | Yes | Unknown | Yes |
| Characterization of aminergic nuclei | Five cyto/histopathological features | Cell loss | Cell loss | Cell loss |
| Measurements of neurotransmitters/ChAT | Yes | No | No | No |
| Multivariate statistics | Yes | No | No | Yes |

AD, Alzheimer's disease; ChAT, choline acetyltransferase; FHx, family history; PD, Parkinson's disease.
*Source:* Modified from Zubenko et al. (2000b).

among patients with AD. In a recently completed prospective study of 196 patients with clinically diagnosed AD, the severity of depressive symptoms as measured by the 17-item Hamilton Depression Rating Scale score was an independent predictor of mortality (Zubenko et al., unpublished). Our results in this regard are consistent with those of Hoch and coworkers (1989), who found that survivorship in a 2-year study of patients with AD and concurrent depression was predicted by abnormalities of rapid eye movement (REM) latency and the presence of sleep-disordered breathing, functions whose anatomical substrates are also thought to reside in the brain stem.

In three of the studies, neuropathological and neurochemical assessments were reported to have been performed by investigators who were blind to demographic and clinical information. Neuropathological evaluations of the aminergic nuclei in our studies included five indices of neurodegeneration; in the remaining studies, neuron counts served as the sole index of neurodegeneration. In our published neurochemical study, the levels of aminergic neurotransmitters, their metabolites, and ChAT specific activity were measured in eight regions (four cortical, four subcorti-

cal) to which these aminergic nuclei project. In only two studies were the samples of sufficient size to support multivariate statistical approaches that minimize the number of comparisons needed to test a hypothesis and to control for the effects of potentially confounding variables.

A summary and comparison of the major findings of these studies is presented in Table 29.2. Neither age at onset nor duration of dementia differentiated AD patients with or without MDD in any of these studies. In our initial study, 43% of demented patients with MDD had a family history of MDD, while the corresponding value for demented patients without depression was 9% (exact $p = .02$, one-tailed). These results are consistent with those previously reported by Pearlson and coworkers (1990).

All of the existing neuropathological studies have reported increased degeneration of the LC associated with the emergence of MDD in AD. This has been a robust finding considering that these studies involved four geographically disparate populations of AD patients with differing mean durations of illness at the time of autopsy and varying laboratory methods. Consistent with these observations, demented patients with this behav-

TABLE 29.2. *Clinical, Neuropathological, and Neurochemical Correlates of Major Depressive Disorder in Alzheimer's Disease*

|  | Zubenko et al. (1988, 1990) | Zweig et al. (1988) | Chan-Palay (1990) | Forstl et al. (1992) |
|---|---|---|---|---|
| *Clinical features* | | | | |
| Age at onset of dementia | No effect | No effect | — | No effect |
| Duration of Dementia | No effect | No effect | — | No effect |
| FHx of MDD | ↑ | — | — | — |
| *Neuropathological features* | | | | |
| LC | ↑ Degeneration | ↑ Degeneration | ↑ Degeneration | ↑ Degeneration |
| SN | ↑ Degeneration | — | — | No effect |
| DR | — | ↑ Degeneration | — | — |
| bnM | — | — | — | Preservation |
| Cortical SP | No effect | — | — | No effect |
| Cortical NFT | No effect | — | — | — |
| *Neurochemical features* | | | | |
| NE | ↓ esp. in cortex | — | — | — |
| DA | No consistent effect | — | — | — |
| 5-HT/5-HIAA | Modest ↓ all regions | — | — | — |
| ChAT | Preservation, esp. in subcortical regions | — | — | — |

Associations not addressed in a study are indicated by a dash.

bnM, basal nucleus of Meynert (cholinergic); ChAT, choline acetyltransferase; DA, dopamine; DR, dorsal raphe (serotonergic); FHx, family history; 5-HIAA, 5-hydroxyindoleacetic acid (serotonin metabolite); 5-HT, serotonin; LC, locus ceruleus (noradrenergic); MDD, major depressive disorder; NE, norepinephrine; NFT, neurofibrillary tangles; SN, substantia nigra (dopaminergic); SP, senile plaques.

*Source:* Modified from Zubenko (2000b).

ioral complication have been reported to manifest substantial reductions of NE levels in the cortex.

Demented patients with MDD in our initial study also exhibited increased degeneration of the SN, a result that was not found in the study of Forstl and colleagues (1992). This difference may be attributable to the inclusion of patients with Parkinson's disease or ADLBV in our study population and highlights the importance of diagnostic homogeneity in investigations of biological correlates of behavioral complications of dementia. Corresponding neurochemical measurements revealed an increased DA level in the entorhinal cortex that did not reach statistical significance after correction for multiple comparisons and no consistent pattern of change in the levels of this neurotransmitter in the remaining seven brain regions.

Increased degeneration of the serotonergic raphe nuclei were associated with MDD in the study reported by Zweig and coworkers (1988), a finding that has not yet been reexamined. However, this association is supported by several additional lines of evidence. The development of MDD in primary dementia was accompanied by consistent modest reductions in both 5-HT and 5-HIAA in eight projection areas of the DR (Zubenko et al., 1990). In addition, the highly selective 5-HT reuptake blocker citalopram has been demonstrated to significantly outperform placebo in the treatment of depression in a double-blind, placebo-controlled study of 98 patients with Alzheimer-type or vascular dementia (Gottfries et al., 1992).

In our study of primary dementia, ChAT specific activity was measured as a proxy for degeneration of the bnM, whose anatomical boundaries make reproducible morphometric analyses difficult. In this neurochemical study, MDD was associated with the relative preservation of ChAT activity, especially in subcortical areas. Consistent results from the study of Forstl and coworkers (1992) indicate that MDD in AD is likewise accompanied by the preservation of the bnM.

The relative preservation of bnM and ChAT activity in depressed, demented patients suggests that there is a threshold for central cholinergic function below which the clinical expression of depression is not possible. Since primary degenerative dementia is associated with a progressive loss of cholinergic function in the CNS (Davies and Maloney, 1976; Perry and Perry, 1980; Zubenko et al., 1989), this interpretation suggests that the prevalence of MDD in primary dementia may decrease as dementia progresses. Several groups of investigators have observed such a clinical relationship among patients with primary degenerative dementia of the Alzheimer type (Fischer et al., 1990; Forsell et al., 1993; Reifler et al., 1982; 1989; Zubenko et al., 1992). Interestingly, this relationship may have some specificity for AD, since it was not observed in patients with vascular dementia (Fischer et al., 1990).

The existence of such a threshold might also explain the high rate of induction of depression (five of seven cases) during the treatment of patients with AD with oxotremorine, a potent cholinergic agonist (Davis et al., 1987).

## MECHANISM(S) OF NEURONAL DEATH IN ALZHEIMER'S DISEASE

Neuronal death in the brains of patients with AD appears to occur by mechanisms of both necrosis and apoptosis. While these pathways may overlap to some extent, they are typically triggered by different events, are manifested by distinguishable cytological and biochemical features, and have somewhat different outcomes (Kerr et al., 1972). Necrosis usually results from physical injury, is not genetically controlled, is typified by the destruction of organelles and the plasma membrane, and results in the release of cellular debris that often stimulates a local inflammatory response. In contrast, apoptosis or programmed cell death represents a genetically controlled response to specific developmental or environmental stimuli. Cells undergoing apoptosis manifest shrinkage, membrane blebbing, chromatin condensation, and DNA fragmentation. The last two characteristics have commonly been used to identify apoptotic cells in formalin-fixed, paraffin-embedded sections of brain tissue. Apoptotic cells and their fragments undergo phagocytosis by microglia and do not stimulate an inflammatory response.

Several lines of evidence have implicated apoptosis in the loss of neurons from vulnerable brain areas in AD. Increased oxidative damage, disturbances of calcium homeostasis, reductions in neurotrophic factors, deposition of $\beta$-amyloid aggregates, and reduced energy metabolism are all characteristic of the central neurodegeneration that occurs in AD (Zubenko, 1997), and all of these conditions induce or stimulate apoptosis in cultured neuronal cell lines (for review, see Cotman and Su, 1996). DNA fragmentation labeling techniques have been used to identify substantial numbers of cells in vulnerable cortical regions (frontal, temporal, hippocampus) that appear to have initiated the apoptosis pathway in AD patients, a process that occurs to a far lesser extent in normal aging (Dragunow et al., 1995; Lassmann et al., 1995; Smale et al., 1995; Su et al., 1994; Thomas et al., 1995). These observations do not appear to result from DNA damage that occurs during the postmortem period or to be due to agonal factors (Anderson et al., 1996; Cotman and Su, 1996) and are consistent with evolving research on one of the regulatory functions of the presenilin genes (Vita et al., 1996; Wolozin et al., 1996). Our data also implicate apoptotic events in cell loss from the brain stem aminergic nuclei in AD (Color Fig. 29.1 in separate color insert) and invite an exploration of the role of apoptosis in the increased degeneration of these nuclei associated with the emergence of MDD.

## DISCUSSION

In the context of AD, these studies suggest that the diagnosis of MDD describes a clinically and pathologically distinct subgroup of patients who have degenerative changes in the brain stem aminergic nuclei (especially the LC) that are disproportionate to those that occur in the cerebral cortex, as well as relative preservation of the bnM. Whether there are important pathogenetic differences between these patients and those who do not develop MDD or whether they represent merely extremes of the distributions of degenerative changes in these structures that occur in all patients with AD cannot be determined from available data. Furthermore, these results do not exclude the potential importance of degenerative changes other than those measured or psychosocial factors that were not assessed in the pathogenesis of MDD in patients with AD.

Our existing published studies provide considerable evidence that the neuropathological and neurochemical correlates of MDD in primary dementia have specificity. Demented patients with or without MDD included in our studies and that of Forstl and colleagues (1992) did not differ with respect to mean age at onset, age at death, duration of illness, or brain weight, or in the mean densities of senile plaques (SP) or neurofibrillary tangles (NFT) in the cortex. Therefore, the emergence of MDD did not appear to result from greater global brain degeneration. Furthermore, the profile of neurochemical changes associated with MDD differed qualitatively from that for dementia (Zubenko et al., 1990, 1991). The relative preservation of cholinergic neurons in the bnM and of ChAT activity in its projection areas in demented patients with MDD was the most dramatic example of this. Finally, two reports failed to find an association of increased LC degeneration with psychosis (delusions or hallucinations) in AD (Bierer et al., 1990; Zweig et al., 1988), and the profiles of neurochemical changes associated with MDD and psychosis appear to be qualitatively and topographically distinct (Zubenko et al., 1990, 1991). This evidence further suggests that the observed neuropathological and neurochemical correlates of MDD are not nonspecifically related to all behavioral complications of AD.

The demented patients with or without MDD in our previous study were similar with respect to a variety of potentially important covariates including sex ratio, age at onset, age at death, duration of illness, postmortem interval, and medication history at or near the time of death, supporting the specificity of the observed neu-

rochemical correlates of MDD in dementia. These medications were grouped into one of eight classes: antibiotics, anticonvulsants, antidepressants, antiparkinson medications, cardiovascular medications, pain medications, steroids, and other. After corrections for multiple comparisons were made, none of these classes of medications was found to be associated with significant or consistent effects on any of the neurochemical measurements made. Similar negative results have been reported by investigators at the Mt. Sinai Alzheimer's Disease Research Center (Bierer et al., 1990, and personal communication) and may reflect (1) the true inability of some medications to modulate the neurochemical variables studied, (2) compensatory mechanisms that blunt acute effects of medications over time, (3) the reduced responsiveness of these neurochemical measures to medication effects in the context of neurodegeneration, or (4) a combination of these.

The pathophysiology of MDD may not be identical in dementias of differing etiology. The importance of achieving diagnostic homogeneity in studies of the biological correlates of MDD in AD was illustrated in the previous section. For this reason, patients with AD and ADLBV should be analyzed separately in future clinicopathological studies. While the nomenclature of ADLBV has been somewhat inconsistent and controversial, the distinguishing features of this subgroup of AD patients is the presence of Lewy bodies (LBs) in addition to an age-specific increase in the density of SPs in the neocortex (Hansen et al., 1990). Historically, this subtype of AD has been underrecognized due to the difficulty of visualizing neocortical LBs, which require immunolabeling with anti-ubiquitin or anti-$\alpha$-synuclein antibodies for reliable detection. Pathologically, ADLBV is associated with fewer cortical NFTs (Hansen et al., 1990, 1993; Lippa et al., 1994) and greater degeneration of the brain stem aminergic nuclei than AD alone (Hansen et al., 1990; Langlais et al., 1993). Retrospective clinical-correlative studies suggest that, as a group, patients with ADLBV are more likely to develop clinically significant depression, psychotic symptoms, fluctuations in cognitive impairment, extrapyramidal symptoms, and increased sensitivity to neuroleptic medications compared to patients with AD alone (Hansen et al., 1990; McKeith et al., 1992). Estimates of the proportion of AD cases that have cortical LBs have ranged widely (Hansen et al., 1990, 1993; Joachim et al., 1988; Kazee and Han, 1995; Victoroff et al., 1995). The LB variant of AD may be associated with both greater degeneration of the brain stem aminergic nuclei and a higher prevalence of MDD than patients with AD alone. Such a finding would provide additional support for an etiological relationship between degeneration of these nuclei and MDD in AD.

The etiopathogenesis of MDD seems likely to be heterogeneous across the age spectrum as well as within particular age strata. The results described in the preceding sections are largely consistent with preexisting neurochemical hypotheses of MDD that emerged from studies of young and middle-aged adults. However, these individuals are likely to develop depression through dysfunctions of one or more of these systems by mechanisms that are more subtle than neuronal loss. In contrast, normal aging is accompanied by progressive neuronal loss in the brain stem aminergic nuclei (Mann et al., 1983; McGeer et al., 1977; Vijayashankar and Brody, 1977), a process that may have relevance to the pathogenesis of late-onset depression among elders with normal cognition.

Several characteristics of depressed AD patients appear to distinguish them as a group from elderly depressed patients with normal cognition. Most estimates of the prevalence of MDD among outpatients with AD have been in the range of 15% to 25%, and recent prevalence estimates resulting from the use of a common, reliable method for the assessment and diagnosis of MDEs among AD patients are even higher (Zubenko et al., 2003). These prevalence estimates substantially exceed the 1.4% figure reported by the Epidemiologic Catchment Area study of community-dwelling nondemented elders (Weissman et al., 1991). Furthermore, the clinical presentations of MDEs among AD patients have been reported to differ in meaningful ways from those experienced by nondemented elders (Zubenko et al., 2003).

In addition, Pearlson and coworkers (1990) reported that a family history of MDD was more common among first-degree relatives of AD patients with MDD than among those who did not develop this behavioral complication, and our preliminary data support this finding. This latter result suggests that the development of MDD in AD may rely upon an interaction of specific degenerative events with one or more familial (possibly inherited) factors that confer a constitutional vulnerability to the development of this mood disorder.

This observation also distinguishes MDD in AD from late-onset MDD in older patients with normal cognition, a disorder that is rarely familial (for review, see Greenwald and Kramer-Ginsberg, 1988). If confirmed, these results suggest that the pathophysiological events that lead to MDD in these two contexts may overlap but are not identical.

Considerable evidence implicates elements of the programmed cell death pathway in the loss of neurons from the neocortex, hippocampus, and brain stem aminergic nuclei in AD. However, the process that affects mature neurons in the CNS during normal aging and AD appears to differ in important ways from most examples of apoptosis. The time course from the initiation of apoptosis until cell death (and resumption in vivo) is typically measured in hours (Wyllie, 1992). In AD, neurons that manifest chromatic condensation and DNA fragmentation appear to be in a state of dynamic and extended competition between progression toward cell death and compensatory (potentially restorative) processes that include the up-regulation of the anti-apoptotic Bcl-2 and p21 (also called waf1) proteins and the DNA repair enzyme Ref-1 (Anderson et al., 1996; Cotman and Su, 1996; Engidawork et al., 2001; Satou et al., 1995; Su et al., 1996). Moreover, the association of Bcl-2 up-regulation with greater disease severity in AD (Satou et al., 1995) suggests that postmortem studies provide an appropriate time window within which to study this phenomenon.

The apparent bimodality in the frequency distributions of LC neurons in AD with or without MDD suggests that the loss of neurons from this nucleus does not result from a stochastic process. Instead, it suggests that the subset of AD patients who develop MDD have increased susceptibility to neuronal loss from the LC (and possibly from the DR and SN). At least some of the variability in the susceptibility of aminergic neurons to degeneration in AD may be attributable to ge-

TABLE 29.3. *Phenotypic Characterization of Six Susceptibility Alleles in 50 Autopsied Cases of Alzheimer's Disease*

| Allele | Clinical Features | | Histopathological Features | | Neurochemical Features* | |
|---|---|---|---|---|---|---|
| | AAO | AAD | SP | NFT | NE | DA |
| APOE E4 | 0 | 0 | + | + | 0 | 0 |
| D12S1045 91bp | − | − | 0 | + | 0 | − |
| D10S1423 234bp | 0 | 0 | 0 | 0 | + | − |
| DXS1047 202bp | 0 | 0 | 0 | 0 | + | −tr |
| D1S518 195bp | 0 | 0 | 0 | −tr | 0 | 0 |
| D1S547 286bp | 0 | 0 | 0 | 0 | 0 | 0 |

*None of the alleles manifested an association with cortical choline acetyltransferase activities or serotonin levels.

(+) Positive association; (−) negative association; (−tr) negative trend; (0) no association; AAD, age at death; AAO, age at onset; DA, dopamine levels; NE, norepinephrine levels; NFT, neurofibrillary tangle density; SP, senile plaque density.

*Source:* Modified from Zubenko (2000a).

netic heterogeneity in the pathophysiology of this disorder. We have recently reported the results of a genome survey that identified five novel AD susceptibility loci in addition to the apolipoprotein E (APOE) locus (Zubenko et al., 1998). Alleles at three of these loci—D10S1423, D12S1045, and DXS1047—appear to modulate the cortical levels of both NE and DA (Zubenko et al., 1999a–1999c) in patients with AD (Table 29.3). Specifically, the D10S1423 234bp allele, the D12S1045 91bp allele, and the DXS1047 202 bp allele were associated with greater loss of cortical DA levels and relative preservation of cortical NE levels among 50 autopsy-confirmed AD cases. These three alleles did not modulate cortical levels of 5-HT or ChAT, and none of the remaining AD risk alleles detected by our genomic survey (D1S518 195bp, D1S547 286 bp, APOE $\varepsilon$4) affected any of these neurochemical indices. Whether these alleles influence the emergence of depression, other behavioral symptoms/syndromes, or parkinsonian features among AD patients remains to be determined. Genetic loci that affect susceptibility to the development of MDD earlier in adulthood may also contribute to the development of MDD in AD (Jorm, 2000; Zubenko, 2000a; Zubenko et al., 2001, 2002).

The potential clinical significance of this integrative, translational research approach is noteworthy. Systematic studies of the morphological and neurochemical correlates of MDD in AD, cellular mechanism(s) that affect the vulnerability of aminergic nuclei in AD, and the further evaluation of the potential role of susceptibility genes in the pathogenesis of MDD in AD may provide important new information that leads to improved treatment of this behavioral complication and of AD more generally. Such an intergrated approach may provide new opportunities for drug development and disease prevention, as well as insights into the biology of mood and other normal brain functions (Zubenko, 1997, 2000a).

## ACKNOWLEDGMENTS

This work was supported by research grants MH43261 and MH/AG47346 and by Independent Scientist Award MH00540 from the National Institute of Mental Health and the National Institute on Aging. Copyrighted materials were reprinted with permission of the International Psychogeriatric Association (2000b).

## REFERENCES

Anderson, A.J., Su, J.H., and Cotman, C.W. (1996) DNA damage and apoptosis in Alzheimer's disease: Colocalization with c-Jun immunoreactivity, relationship to brain area, and effect of postmortem delay. J Neurosci 16:1710–1719.

Bierer, L.M., Haroutunian, V., Perl, D., Knott, P.J., Kanof, P.D., Schmeidler, J., Mohs, R.C., and Davis, K.L. (1990) Relationship of non-cognitive behavioral disturbances to neuropathologic and neurochemical indices in brain specimens of patients with Alzheimer's disease, December 1990. Presented at the 29th annual meeting of the American College of Neuropsychopharmacology, San Juan, Puerto Rico.

Boller, F., Mizutani, T., Roessmann, U., and Gambetti, P. (1980) Parkinson's disease, dementia, and Alzheimer's disease: Clinicopathological correlations. Ann Neurol 7:329–335.

Bondareff, W., and Mountjoy, C.Q. (1986) Number of neurons in nucleus locus ceruleus in demented and non-demented patients: Rapid estimation and correlated parameters. Neurobiol Aging 7:297–300.

Brikmayer, W., and Riederer, P. (1975) Biochemical postmortem findings in depressed patients. J Neural Transm 37:95–109.

Bunney, W.E., and Davis, J. (1965) Norepinephrine in depressive reactions: A review of supporting evidence. Arch Gen Psychiatry 13:483–497.

Carpenter, M.B. (1985) Core Text of Neuroanatomy, 3rd ed. Baltimore: Williams & Wilkins.

Chan-Palay, V. (1990) Depression and senile dementia of the Alzheimer type: Catecholamine changes in the locus coeruleus—basis for therapy. Dementia 1:253–261.

Cotman, C.W., and Su, J.H. (1996) Mechanisms of neuronal death in Alzheimer's disease. Brain Pathol 6:493–506.

Crow, T.J., Cross, A.J., Cooper, S.J., Deakin, J.F., Ferrier, I.N., Johnson, J.A., Joseph, M.H., Owen, F., Poulter, M., Lofthouse, R., Corsellis, J.A.N., Chambers, D.R., Blessed, G., Perry, E.K., Perry, R.H., and Tomlinson, B.E. (1984) Neurotransmitter receptors and monoamine metabolites in the brains of patients with Alzheimer-type dementia and depression, and suicides. Neuropharmacology 23:1561–1569.

Davies, P., and Maloney, A.J. (1976) Selective loss of cholinergic neurons in Alzheimer's disease. Lancet 2:1403.

Davis, K.L., Hollander, E., Davidson, M., Davis, B.M., Mohs, R.C., and Horvath, T.B. (1987) Induction of depression with oxotremorine in patients with Alzheimer's disease. Am J Psychiatry 144:468–471.

Dragunow, M., Fauli, R.L.M., Lawlor, P., Beiharz, E.J., Singleton, K., Walker, E.B., and Mee, E. (1995) In situ evidence for DNA fragmentation in Huntington's disease striatum and Alzheimer's disease temporal lobes. NeuroReport 6:1053–1057.

Engidawork, E., Gulessarian, T., Seidl, R., Cairns, N., and Lubec, G. (2001) Expression of apoptosis related proteins in brains of patients with Alzheimer's disease. Neurosci Lett 303(2):79–82.

Felten, D.L., and Sladek, J.R. (1983) Monoamine distribution in primary brain vs. monoaminergic nuclei: Anatomy, pathways and local organization. Brain Res Bull 10:171–284.

Fischer, P., Simanyi, M., and Danielczyk, W. (1990) Depression in dementia of the Alzheimer type and in multi-infarct dementia. Am J Psychiatry 147:1484–1487.

Foote, S.L., and Morrison, J.H. (1987) Curr Top Dev Biol. 21:391–423, 1987.

Forsell, Y., Jorm, A.F., Fratiglioni, L., Grut, M., and Winblad, B. (1993) Application of DSM-III-R criteria for major depressive episode to elderly subjects with and without dementia. Am J Psychiatry 150:1199–1202.

Forstl, H., Burns, A., Luthert, P., Cairns, N., Lantos, P., and Levy, R. (1992) Clinical and neuropathological correlates of depression in Alzheimer's disease. Psychol Med 22:877–884.

Gottfries, C.G., Karlsson, I., and Nyth, A. (1992) Treatment of depression in elderly patients with and without dementia disorders. Int J Clin Psychopharmacol 5:55–64.

Greenwald, B.S., and Kramer-Ginsberg, E. (1988) Age at onset of geriatric depression: Relationship to clinical variables. J Affect Disord 15:61–68.

Hansen, L.A., Masliah, E., Galasko, D., and Terry, R.D. (1993) Plaque-only Alzheimer's disease is usually the Lewy body variant, and vice versa. J Neuropathol Exp Neurol 52:648–654.

Hansen, L., Salmon, D., Galasko, D., Masliah, E., Katzman, R., DeTeresa, R., Thal, L., Pay, M.M., Hofstetter, R., Klauber, M., Rice,

V., Butters, N., and Alford, M. (1990) The Lewy body variant of Alzheimer's disease: A clinical and pathologic entity. *Neurology* 40:1–8.

Hoch, C.C., Reynolds, C.F., Houck, P.R., Hall, F., Berman, S.R., Buysse, D.J., Dahl, R., and Kupfer, D.J. (1989) REM latency and apnea-hypopnea index predict two-year mortality in mixed depressed-demented patients. *J Neuropsychiatry Clin Neurol* 1: 366–371.

Huber, S.J., Shuttleworth, E.C., and Paulson, G.W. (1986) Dementia in Parkinson's disease. *Arch Neurol* 43:987–995.

Janowsky, D.S., and Risch, S.C. (1987) Role of acetylcholine mechanisms in the affective disorders. In: Meltzer, H.Y., ed. *Psychopharmacology: The Third Generation of Progress*. New York: Raven Press, pp. 527–533.

Jimerson, D.C. (1987) Role of dopamine mechanisms in the affective disorders. In: Meltzer, H.Y., ed. *Psychopharmacology: The Third Generation of Progress*. New York: Raven Press, pp. 505–511.

Joachim, C.L., Morris, J.H., and Selkoe, D.J. (1988) Clinically diagnosed Alzheimer's disease: Autopsy results in 150 cases. *Ann Neurol* 24:50–56.

Jorm, A.F. (2000) Is depression a risk factor for dementia or cognitive decline? *Gerontology* 46(4):219–227.

Kazee, A.M., and Han, L.Y. (1995) Cortical Lewy bodies in Alzheimer's disease. *Arch Pathol Lab Med* 119:448–453.

Kerr, J.F., Wylie, A.H., and Currie, A.R. (1972) Apoptosis: A basic biolgoical phenomenon with wide-ranging implications in tissue kinetics. *Br J Cancer* 26:239–257.

Langlais, P.J., Thal, L., Hansen, L., Galasko, D., Alford, M., and Masliah, E. (1993) Neurotransmitters in basal ganglia and cortex of Alzheimer's disease with and without Lewy bodies. *Neurology* 43:1927–1934.

Lassmann, H., Bancher, C., Breitschopf, H., Wegiel, J., Bobinski, M., Jellinger, K., and Wisniewski, H.M. (1995) Cell death in Alzheimer's disease evaluated by DNA fragmentation in situ. *Acta Neuropathol* 89:35–41.

Lippa, C.F., Smith, T.W., and Swearer, J.M. (1994) Alzheimer's disease and Lewy body disease: A comparative clinicopathological study. *Ann Neurol* 35:81–88.

Lloyd, K.J., Farley, I.J., Deck, J.H.N., and Hornykiewicz, O. (1974) Serotonin and 5-hydroxyindoleacetic acid in discrete areas of brainstem of suicide victims and control patients. *Adv Biochem Psychopharmacol* 11:387–397.

Mann, D.M.A., Yates, P.O., and Hawkes, J. (1983) The pathology of the human locus ceruleus. *Clin Neuropathol* 2:1–7.

Mayeux, R., Stern, Y., Rosen, J., and Leventhal, J. (1981) Depression, intellectual impairment, and Parkinson disease. *Neurology* 31:645–650.

McGeer, P.L., McGeer, E.G., and Suzuki, J.S. (1977) Aging and extapyramidal function. *Arch Neurol* 34:33–35.

McKeith, I.G., Perry, R.H., Fairbairn, A.F., Jabeen, S., and Perry, E.K. (1992) Operational criteria for senile dementia of Lewy body type (SDLT). *Psychol Med* 22:911–922.

Mendlewicz, J., Vanderheyden, J.E., and Noel, G. (1981) Serotonin and dopamine in patients with unipolar depression and parkinsonism. *Adv Exp Med Biol* 133:753–767.

Merriam, A.E., Aronson, M.K., Gaston, P., Wey, S.-L., and Katz, I. (1988) The psychiatric symptoms of Alzheimer's disease. *JAGS* 36:7–12.

Mulsant, B.H., and Zubenko, G.S. (1994) Clinical, neuropathologic, and neurochemical correlates of depression and psychosis in primary dementia. In: Emery, V.O.B., and Oxman, T.E., eds. *Dementia: Presentations, Differential Diagnosis, and Nosology*. Baltimore: Johns Hopkins University Press, pp. 336–352.

Olin, J.T., Katz, I.R., Meyers, B.S., Schneider, L.S., and Lebowitz, B. (2002) Provisional diagnostic criteria for depression of Alzheimer

disease. Rationale and background. *Am J Geriatr Psychiatry* 10:129–141.

Pearlson, G.D., Ross, C.A., Lohr, W.D., Rovner, B.W., Chase, G.A., and Folstein, M.F. (1990) Association between family history of affective disorder and the depressive syndrome of Alzheimer's disease. *Am J Psychiatry* 147:452–456.

Perry, E.K., and Perry, R.H. (1980) The cholinergic system in Alzheimer's disease. In: Roberts, P.J., ed. *Biochemistry of Dementia*. New York: Wiley, pp. 135–183.

Reifler, B.V., Larson, E., and Hanley, R. (1982) Coexistence of cognitive impairment and depression in geriatric outpatients. *Am J Psychiatry* 139:623–626.

Reifler, B.V., Teri, L., Raskind, M., Veith, R., Barnes, R., White, E., and McLean, P. (1989) Double-blind trial of imipramine in Alzheimer's disease patients with and without depression. *Am J Psychiatry* 146:45–49.

Satou, T., Cummings, B.J., and Cotman, C.W. (1995) Immunoreactivity for Bcl-2 protein within neurons in the Alzheimer's disease brain increases with disease severity. *Brain Res* 697:35–43.

Schildkraut, J.J. (1965) The catecholamine hypothesis of affective disorders: A review of supporting evidence. *Am J Psychiatry* 122:509–522.

Siever, L.J. (1987) Role of noradreneric mechanisms in the etiology of the affective disorders. In: Meltzer, H.Y., ed. *Psychopharmacology: The Third Generation of Progress*. New York: Raven Press, pp. 493–504.

Smale, G., Nichols, N.R., Brady, D.R., Finch, C.E., and Horton, W.E. (1995) Evidence for apoptotic cell death in Alzheimer's disease. *Exp Neurol* 133:225–230.

Stanley, M., and Mann, J.J. (1983) Increased serotonin-2 binding sites in frontal cortex of suicide victims. *Lancet* 1:214–216.

Su, J.H., Anderson, A.J., Cummings, B.J., and Cotman, C.W. (1994) Immunohistochemical evidence for apoptosis in Alzheimer's disease. *NeuroReport* 5:2529–2533.

Su, J.H., Satou, T., Anderon, A.J., and Cotman, C.W. (1996) Upregulation of Bcl-2 is associated with neuronal DNA damage in Alzheimer's disease. *NeuroReport* 7:437–440.

Teri, L., and Reifler, B.V. (1987) Depression and dementia. In: Carstensen, L., and Edelstein, B., eds. *Handbook of Clinical Gerontology*. New York: Pergamon Press, pp. 112–119.

Thomas, L.B., Gates, D.J., Richfield, E.K., O'Brian, T.F., Schweitzer, J.B., and Steindler, D.A. (1995) DNA end labeling (TUNEL) in Huntington's disease and other neuropathological conditions. *Exp Neurol* 133:265–272.

U.S. Department of Health and Human Services (1999) Mental Health: A Report of the Surgeon General. Chapter 5, Older Adults and Mental Health. Barry Lebowitz, Section Editor. Rockville, MD: U.S. Department of Health and Human Services, Substance Abuse and Mental Health Services Administration, Center for Mental Health Services, National Institutes of Health, National Institute of Mental Health.

Victoroff, J., Mack, W.J., Lyness, S.A., and Chui, H.C. (1995) Multicenter clinicopathological correlation in dementia. *Am J Psychiatry* 152:1476–1484.

Vijayashankar, N., and Brody, H. (1977) Aging in the human brain stem: A study of the nucleus of the trochlear nerve. *Acta Anat* 99:169–172.

Vita, P., Lacana, E., and D'Adamio, L. (1996) Interfering with apoptosis: $Ca^{2+}$-binding protein ALG-2 and Alzheimer's disease gene ALG-3. *Science* 271:521–525.

Weissman, M.M., Bruce, M.L., Leaf, P.J., Florio, L.P., and Holzer, C. (1991) Affective disorders. In: Robins, L.N., and Regier, D.A., eds. *Psychiatric Disorders in America. The Epidemiologic Catchment Area Study*. New York: Free Press, pp. 53–80.

Whitehouse, P.J., Price, D.L., Struble, R.G., Clark, A.W., Coyle, J.T., and DeLong, M.R. (1982) Alzheimer's disease and senile dementia: Loss of neurons in the basal forebrain. *Science* 215:1237–1239.

Wolozin, B., Iwasaki, K., Vito, P., Ganjei, J.K., Lacana, E., Sunderland, T., Zhao, B., Kusiak, J.W., Wasco, W., and D'Adamio, L. (1996) Participation of presenilin 2 in apoptosis: Enhanced basal activity conferred by an Alzheimer mutation. *Science* 274:1710–1713.

Wragg, R.E., and Jeste, D.V. (1989) Overview of depression and psychosis in Alzheimer's disease. *Am J Psychiatry* 146:577–587.

Wyllie, A.H. (1992) Apoptosis and the regulation of cell numbers in normal and neoplastic tissues: An overview. *Cancer Met Rev* 11:95–103.

Zubenko, G.S. (1992) Biological correlates of clinical heterogeneity in primary dementia. *Neuropsychopharmacology* 6:77–93.

Zubenko, G.S. (1997) Molecular neurobiology of Alzheimer's disease (syndrome?) *Harv Rev Psychiatry* 5:1–37.

Zubenko, G.S. (2000a) Do susceptibility loci contribute to the expression of more than one mental disorder? A view from the genetics of Alzheimer's disease. *Mol Psychiatry* 5(2):131–136.

Zubenko, G.S. (2000b) Neurobiology of major depression in Alzheimer's disease. *Intl Psychogeriatr* 12:217–230.

Zubenko, G.S., Hughes, H.B., III, Maher, B.H., Stiffler, J.S., Zubenko, W.N., and Marazita, M.L. (2002) Genetic linkage of region containing the *CREB1* gene to depressive disorders in women from families with recurrent, early-onset major depression. *Am J Med Genet (Neuropsychiatr Genet)* 114:980–987.

Zubenko, G.S., Hughes, H.B., and Stiffler, J.S. (1999a) Clinical and neurobiological correlates of D10S1423 genotype in Alzheimer's disease. *Biol Psychiatry* 46:740–749.

Zubenko, G.S., Hughes, H.B., and Stiffler, J.S. (1999b) Clinical and neurobiological correlates of DXS1047 genotype in Alzheimer's disease. *Biol Psychiatry* 46:173–181.

Zubenko, G.S., Hughes, H.B., and Stiffler, J.S. (1999c) Neurobio-

logical correlates of a putative risk allele for Alzheimer's disease on chromosome 12q. *Neurology* 52:725–732.

Zubenko, G.S., and Moossy, J. (1988) Major depression in primary dementia: Clinical and neuropathologic correlates. *Arch Neurol* 45:1182–1186.

Zubenko, G.S., Moossy, J., and Kopp, U. (1990) Neurochemical correlates of major depression in primary dementia. *Arch Neurol* 47:209–214.

Zubenko, G.S., Moossy, J., Martinez, A.J., Rao, G.R., Claassen, D., Rosen, J., and Kopp, U. (1991) Neuropathological and neurochemical correlates of psychosis in primary dementia. *Arch Neurol* 48:619–624.

Zubenko, G.S., Moossy, J., Martinez, A.J., Rao, G.R., Kopp, U., and Hanin, I. (1989) A brain regional analysis of morphologic and cholinergic abnormalities in Alzheimer's disease. *Arch Neurol* 46:634–638.

Zubenko, G.S., Rosen, J., Sweet, R.A., Mulsant, B.H., and Rifai, A.H. (1992) Impact of psychiatric hospitalization on behavioral complications of Alzheimer's disease. *Am J Psychiatry* 149:1484–1491.

Zubenko, G.S., Zubenko, W.N., McPherson, S., Spoor, E., Marin, D.B., Farlow, M.R., Smith, G.E., Geda, Y.E., Cummings, J.L., Petersen, R.C., and Sunderland, T. (2003) A collaborative study of the emergence and clinical features of the major depressive syndrome of Alzheimer's disease. *Am J Psychiatry* 160:857–866.

Zubenko, G.S., Zubenko, W.N., Spiker, D.G., Giles, D.E., and Kaplan, B.B. (2001) The malignancy of recurrent, early-onset major depression: A family study. *Am J Med Genet (Neuropsychiatr Genet)* 105(8):690–699.

Zweig, R.M., Ross, C.A., Hedreen, J.C., Steele, C., Cardillo, J.E., Whitehouse, P.J., Folstein, M.F., and Price, D.L. (1988) The neuropathology of aminergic nuclei in Alzheimer's disease. *Ann Neurol* 24:233–242.

# Epilogue

After 29 chapters, can we say that late-life depression is an entity (or entities) meaningfully distinct from depression in younger adults, or is late-life depression simply the same illness afflicting older people? This question can be addressed in terms of nosology, inquiring whether some form of depression in the elderly should be classified as a separate illness based on consistent differences from depression in younger populations in epidemiology, phenomenology, psychobiology, treatment response, or course of illness. The question can also be answered practically, that is, by determining whether patients with late-life depression present distinct clinical challenges regarding assessment, treatment optimization, frequency and management of side effects, interactions with co-morbid conditions, disposition, and so on.

## DOES LATE-LIFE DEPRESSION PRESENT DISTINCT PRACTICAL DEMANDS?

In practical terms, the answer to the question is affirmative. In multiple dimensions, the care of the patient with late-life depression must address different issues and needs than those encountered in treating younger adults. The detection of a depressive syndrome in older patients is often obfuscated because they may present with a distinct symptom pattern, and diagnosis is further complicated since somatic symptoms of depression are similar to the symptoms of the medical conditions frequent among the elderly. The information regarding the efficacy of antidepressant interventions is far more limited in the elderly, and the presence of cognitive impairment and co-morbid medical conditions presents safety issues that occur infrequently in younger adults. In short, the clinical evaluation and care of the older depressed patient are sufficiently distinct that providers require special training that emphasizes an understanding of the effects of the normal aging process and diseases of aging.

## SHOULD LATE-LIFE DEPRESSION BE CONSIDERED A DISTINCT DIAGNOSTIC ENTITY?

The answer to this question is still uncertain. Perhaps the strongest case for differentiation as a distinct entity can be made for late-onset major depression. This condition has been associated with magnetic resonance im-

aging (MRI) abnormalities, low rate of a family history of mood disorder, cognitive dysfunction, poor treatment outcome, and a deteriorating long-term clinical course. The poor treatment outcome and the deteriorating clinical course, if true, are especially striking observations, since patients with early onset of neuropsychiatric disorders are usually more likely to have greater treatment resistance and cognitive and functional impairment by the time they reach late life relative to patients with late onset of the same disorder (e.g., Alzheimer's disease). In other words, early disease onset is usually associated with a more virulent and treatment-resistant course.

However, what is at issue is the quality of the evidence when considering the possibility of distinct subtypes within late-life depression. The studies comparing late-onset and early-onset depression have reported inconsistent findings, and the methods used to define early- and late-onset groups, as well as comparison groups, have been highly variable.

## TREATMENT

Independent of these theoretical concerns, late-life depression is prevalent and patients require treatment. One of most striking and distressing aspects of late-life depression is that the treatments currently available have either limited efficacy or problematic side effects. The selective serotonin reuptake inhibitors (SSRIs) are the most widely used antidepressant medications in younger adults, and for this age group they are reasonably effective, well tolerated (though not without some problematic side effects), and safe. The SSRIs are also widely prescribed for the elderly and appear to be well tolerated and safe, although medication-induced sexual side effects, inappropriate antidiuretic hormone secretion, and drug–drug interactions are problems.

Beyond safety issues, it is a remarkable fact that that data on the efficacy of SSRIs in the treatment of late-life depression are limited and not impressive. In the more rigorous studies, the margin of benefit of SSRIs relative to placebo has been none to slight. In contrast, tricyclic antidepressants (TCAs) are effective, but their anticholinergic and cardiovascular effects make them problematic or contraindicated for many older patients. Electroconvulsive therapy (ECT) is arguably the most effective acute treatment for depression, and its cognitive side effects can be attenuated by use of the right unilateral electrode placement, an efficient electrical waveform (e.g., ultrabrief stimulation), and an electrical dosing strategy individualized for the patient. However, the clinical challenge presented by ECT typically is not achieving remission but sustaining it. Remission following ECT is rarely maintained without adequate continuation therapy, but even with intensive continuation treatment, relapse is frequent.

Other classes of medication, such as atypical antipsychotics, mood stabilizers, and stimulants, as well as psychotherapy, have not been studied sufficiently to claim effectiveness and safety in late-life depression. Thus, there is little or no systematically collected information about many of the treatments widely used in this condition. Despite the sparse evidence regarding the efficacy of interventions, there has been a shift at the National Institutes of Health and elsewhere to promote effectiveness trials. These trials assess the treatment response in diverse clinical settings, examining relatively unselected patient populations. When a treatment has established efficacy by virtue of consistent findings in placebo-controlled trials, effectiveness studies are the logical next step and provide a better measure of the utility of the intervention in the real world of patients and doctors. However, to shift the focus to effectiveness before efficacy is established runs the risk of promoting treatments of unproven value.

## THE RESEARCH AGENDA: TREATMENT

One of the advances in the treatment of major depression across the life span has been the introduction of new pharmacological agents based on a deliberate plan to achieve a specific neurochemical action. Prior to the advent of the SSRIs, the therapeutic action of all antidepressants in major depression was discovered by accident. In contrast, the SSRIs were developed with the mechanistic goal of blocking serotonin reuptake and thereby exerting antidepressant effects. Similarly, the dual-action agents, such as venlafaxine, mirtazapine, and duloxetine, were developed to be antidepressants from the outset with the view that enhancement of both serotonergic and noradrenergic transmission would have a broader spectrum of therapeutic effect.

The success of the approach of applying basic knowledge of the neurochemical mediators to the design of new antidpressant agents has been astounding. However, for the most part, these newer agents appear to be less effective in patients with late-life depression than in younger depressed patients. It could be concluded that patients with late-life depression are constrained by their biology and/or psychology to have a limited antidepressant response compared to younger individuals, regardless of the intervention. In this respect, the

findings with ECT are especially critical. It is well established that age has positive predictive value for the outcome of ECT, with attainment of acute remission more likely in older than younger patients. Independent of the factors responsibile for this association, this fact demonstrates that age per se is not a barrier to achieving marked symptom reduction.

A likely contributor to the poor track record in the pharmacological treatment of late-life depression is the failure to account for the changes in brain signaling systems that occur with aging. While medications have been designed with specific neurochemical targets in mind, little consideration has been given to how these target systems are transformed over the life span. For example, there is increasing evidence that by the age of 60 years, the serotonin system is markedly depleted, with a sharp reduction in the production of this neurotransmitter. Thus, if the first required step for a medication to exert antidepressant effects is the blockade of serotonin reuptake, there may be insufficient substrate available for reuptake blockade to be effective.

Consider Parkinson's disease (PD) for a similar circumstance. The symptoms of PD are not evident until at least 80% of the cells in the substantia nigra are lost, resulting in a marked reduction of the brain's capacity to produce dopamine. Agents that rely on endogenous dopamine by promoting vesicle release (e.g., stimulants), blocking its reuptake, or preventing its catabolism once released (e.g., monoamine oxidase inhibitiors) at most are only adjunctive treatments for PD. In contrast, primary and widely effective treatments for PD act directly at dopamine receptors (dopamine agonists) or attempt to compensate for the deficit dopamine levels (L-dopa/carbidopa). Thus, distinct treatments may need to be designed for patients with late-life depression that do not assume continuity of the neurochemical substrate available in younger patients, but instead compensate for age-related deficiencies.

Normal aging effects on brain signaling systems are known to account for differences among age groups in the incidence of some side effects. The anticholinergic effects of TCAs, impacting on vagally mediated parasympathetic function, are responsible for the treatment-associated increase in heart rate and the decrease in the high-frequency component of heart rate variability. Cholinergic tone decreases with age. Consequently, because of a floor effect in the elderly, the anticholinergic effect of TCAs on these parasympathetic indices is proportionately greater in younger patients; that is, younger patients show both a greater increase in heart rate and a decrease in high-frequency variability. In contrast, anticholingeric agents show greater adverse cognitive effects in older versus younger patients. In this case, the higher cholinergic tone in younger patients may have a protective effect, while the already depleted cholinergic tone in older patients makes them especially vulnerable. Thus, the effects of aging on neurotransmitter and peptide availability and signaling mechanisms may have a larger role in the response to antidepressant medication than has heretofore been appreciated.

## THE RESEARCH AGENDA: CLINICAL TRIAL METHODOLOGY

New methods are also needed to evaluate the efficacy of antidepressant treatments in late life. The clinical trials' designs and methods used to test efficacy in late-life depression have been imported from studies in younger adults. The same procedures are used for sample selection, diagnosis, randomization and masking, treatment delivery, outcome assessment, and so on. Ironically, the most common exception made to this wholesale importation is the use of longer trial durations in elderly patients. While it is believed that 6–8 weeks provide sufficient exposure to determine antidepressant effects in younger adults, controlled trials in the elderly have increasingly adopted 12 weeks as the standard trial duration. This exception is based on the unsubstantiated belief that elderly patients require long exposure to medication to respond. In fact, only one study has compared patients with mid-life and late-life depression in the duration needed to achieve clinical end points (reponse or remission) or in the earliest time-point during treatment when the final outcome can be reliably predicted. No differences were observed between the age groups. Thus, the designs currently used in controlled trials, sometimes involving placebo, require that elderly patients have especially prolonged exposure to ineffective treatment. An unfortunate and unintended consequence is that the potential burden of study participation is greater for the elderly.

More generally, differences between elderly and younger depressed patients have been documented in several dimensions. These include the signs and symptoms of depression, the physiological changes due to aging and co-morbid medical illnesses that modulate behavior independent of the psychiatric condition (e.g., changes in sleep, appetite, and libido), the contribution of cognitive alterations to presentation and assessment, and so on. To date, industry and academia have endorsed the *inclusive* approach to diagnosis, which ignores the source or modulators of symptoms counted toward the diagnosis of a depressive disorder. Furthermore, there are no agreed-upon scoring conventions to account for presumed age-related effects when the most commonly used instruments are employed to quantify depression severity and define treatment outcome. For example, middle insomnia occurs in the majority of individuals over the age of 70 years independent of a psychiatric condition. At this point, it not known whether adjusting assessment tools and methods for age-related effects will increase validity.

## THE RESEARCH AGENDA: PATHOPHYSIOLOGY

The concept of vascular depression typifies the notion that the elderly may present with distinct disease entities that require special diagnostic instruments and treatment interventions. Vascular depression, an illness characterized by late onset, is associated with significant MRI lesions consistent with subclinical ischemic disease and has a comparatively poor response to medication. The key evidence supporting the concept that vascular depression is a distinct entity comes from studies reporting that patients with late-onset illness have greater prevalence and severity of MRI lesions than early-onset patients.

A major methodological issue in pathophysiological studies in late-life depression concerns identification of the correct control group. Older patients often have a variety of risk factors for ischemic disease; moreover, vascular risk factors may be overrepresented in major depression. In studies of pathophysiology, it is common to require that the control group be comprised of healthy volunteers without major psychiatric or neurological illness and free of medication. Consequently, risk factors for vascular disease are likely to be underrepresented in the control sample, even in relation to age-appropriate norms. Thus, the excess of structural brain abnormalities in late-life or late-onset major depression may be a function of underrepresentation of risk factors in the control or comparison groups.

To clarify the source of the excess of MRI ischemic lesions, it is necessary to compare patients with late-life or specifically late-onset depression to nondepressed controls matched for age and the frequency and profile of risk factors. To date there has been only one study of MRI abnormalities in late-onset depression that has used this more rigorous approach to defining control groups (see Chapter 11), and the results suggest that MRI lesions are comparable in frequency and severity in patients with late-onset depression and normal controls when matched for vascular risk factors. This result should not be unexpected. Patients who develop major depression have an excess of frank vascular illness before the first symptomatic manifestation of the mood disorder. It may be that vascular risk factors are overrepresented in late-late or, specifically, late-onset depression, and not that patients with this disorder are more likely to manifest structural brain abnormalities with the same level of risk factors as elderly individuals who do not develop major depression. Thus, the key issue may be epidemiological. Is there an overrepresentation of these risk factors in individuals who, later in life, show excessive MRI hyperintensities, poor treatment response, deteriorating course, and so on?

A reputed feature of late-onset depression accompanied by MRI abnormalities is the observation that this syndrome is associated with a poor response to antidepressant medication. However, this conclusion is based on nonsystematic studies. In contrast, a recent randomized, controlled trial in the old-old, whose participants had an average age of 80 years, compared citalopram to placebo in depressed patients. In this study, patients with late-onset depression did not differ from patients with early-onset depression in clinical outcome. The presence and extent of MRI hyperintensities were unrelated to the clinical outcome with either medication or placebo.

The point of this discussion is not to dismiss the importance of ischemic disease in the etiology of late-onset depression. The vascular hypothesis is intriguing, and the nature of the supporting evidence makes further study not only necessary but compelling. Rather, the point is that we need to be certain that we do not prematurely transform a hypothesis into a fact. Vascular depression serves the field best as a conceptual model and a stimulus for hypothesis testing. It does not constitute either an *established* diagnostic entity or a *proven* etiology.

Another feature of late-life depression that has been advanced as a possible explanation for the relatively poor response to antidepressants is a pattern of cognitive impairment that has been labeled *executive dysfunction*. In fact, it is suggested that late-onset illness, executive dysfunction, and MRI lesion burden constitute a triad of factors associated with a poor treatment outcome. However, though the data have only established that these features are associated with each other, there has been a tendency to transform a pattern of association into a hierarchy in which one variable is considered the cause of an associated finding (e.g., MRI lesions cause depression and/or executive dysfunction). This is a common error that leads to unsupported, and possibly flawed, conclusions about etiology. Furthermore, as indicated, MRI hyperintensities are common in older individuals, especially those with significant vascular risk factors, and not just in older individuals with a mood disorder. In the study of late-life depression, one is always faced with the recurrent problem of distinguishing the phenomenology and psychobiology of depression from those of aging.

Despite the limited evidence supporting some of the newer theoretical models of late-life depression, the theories focusing on vascular depression and executive dysfunction have heuristic importance and stimulate exciting investigation. The importance of theoretical models does not rest solely, or even significantly, on their validity; rather, these models serve to expand the field of investigation in a meaningful way. This was certainly the case for the catecholamine hypothesis of affective disorder, and it may prove to be the case for current theories of late-life depression.

Other potentially fruitful paths of investigation focus on how depression affects multiple organ systems, including the brain. Depression is associated with increased hypothalamic-pituitary-adrenal axis activity, insulin resistance, and other pathophysiological dysfunctions that promote vascular disease and hippocampal atrophy. Both the ischemic brain changes due to vascular disease and the hippocampal degeneration resulting form neuroendocrine dysregulation are hypothesized to have an etiological role in the genesis of depression. Both are also thought to be exacerbated by or to be a consequence of the state of major depression. Thus, with some forms of major depression in the elderly, these positive feedback loops are hypothesized to consist of a perpetuating, circular disease system that promotes both future episodes of depression (recurrence) and further damage to the brain.

There is preliminary, although controversial, evidence that the length of time a patient is in the phenomenological state of depression is positively correlated with the extent of damage to the brain. Furthermore, there are recent data suggesting that treatment of depression can protect against such changes. This type of evidence would strongly support the belief that maintenance treatment for patients with recurrent depression should be started as soon as the illness is identified. One of the most effective ways to prevent late-life depression may be to treat early-onset depression. Perhaps the most definitive study to help clarify the role played by the natural aging processes of the brain, the impact of recurrent episodes of depression, and the role of ischemic disease would be a longitudinal study of a cohort of people as they enter late life that follows the course of the next 25 years with imaging studies, neurocognitive evaluation, assessment of affective symptoms, social status, medical health, and so on. The availability of the brains for postmortem examination would also be critical. Such a longitudinal project would be formidable to organize and finance. It would likely be frustrating to many of the authors of this volume since the findings would not be available to them in this lifetime, but only in the next. However, we are at the stage of knowledge in late-life depressive disorders where we have identified key factors that contribute to or result from the manifestation of these disorders. In the long run, a large-scale longitudinal study is likely the most efficient method for determining which factors have etiological precedence, which factors have clinical predictive values, and which factors are epiphenomena. We suspect that such an investigation will be invaluable to the next generation of researchers and clinicians studying and treating patients with late-life depression.

# Index

Page numbers followed by f and t refer to figures and tables, respectively.

depression and
consequences, 341
prevalence, 339
treatment issues, 344
epidemiology, 338
during electroconvulsive therapy, 265
Bereavement, 107–13
after unexpected death, 111
anxiety disorders after, 111
complicated or traumatic, 111–12
course, 107–9, 108t–109t
depressive symptoms, 68, 107–9,
108t–109t
depressive syndrome after, 111, 112–13
mania after, 111
medical treatment after, 109
mortality, 110–11
pathological outcomes
predictors, 112
treatment, 112–13
physical symptoms, 109–10, 110t
remarriage and, 110
stages, 107
substance abuse after, 109–10
Beta blockers, prophylactic, in
electroconvulsive therapy, 255–56
Biogenic amine system dysfunction, in
poststroke depression, 331–32
Biological markers. See also Neurobiology
depression in dementia, 83–84
Bipolar disorder, 34–45
age-at-onset, 211
antidepressants for, 44
caregiver burden, 41
cerebrovascular disease and, 37, 44
chronicity, 40–41
cognitive impairment in
age and, 39–40
age-at-onset and, 40
nonaffective outcomes and, 43
treatment outcomes and, 43
comorbidity
medical disorders, 37–38, 41
neurological disorders, 37, 41, 211
psychiatric disorders, 35, 41
treatment outcome and, 44
depression in, 34–45
diagnosis, 34–35
disability and, 40, 41, 43
epidemiology, 35–36
familial/genetic factors, 38
historical perspective, 34
versus major depressive disorder, 211,
212t
mania in. See Mania
mixed states, 38–39
mood stabilizers for, 211–19
carbamazepine, 218–19, 219t
difficulties in conducting studies,
212–13
divalproex, 215–16
lamotrigone, 216–18
lithium, 213–15, 213t
mortality, 42, 211
negative life events and, 38
neuroimaging abnormalities, 37
nonaffective outcomes, 42–43

pathophysiology and etiology, 36–38
psychiatric service use, 41
psychopathology and assessment, 38–39
psychosis in, 35, 39
psychotic depression in, 252
relapse and recurrence, 41
in maintenance treatment, 44
social support level and, 41
suicide and, 41
treatment outcome modifiers, 43–44
type I, 35
type II, 35
ventricular enlargement in, 137
Bipolar-type schizoaffective disorders, 35
Black Americans
electroconvulsive therapy, 241
suicide rates, 96, 97f
Blood pressure abnormalities. See
Hypertension; Hypotension
Body weight. See Weight alterations
Bradycardia, carbamazepine-induced, 219
Brain abnormalities. See also
Neuroimaging studies;
Neuropathology
in aging, 18, xxiii
in late-life depression, xxii
functional, 139–44, 332
structural
development of concepts, 148
MRI hyperintensities, 129–36. See
also Encephalomalacia; Magnetic
resonance imaging,
hyperintensities
volumetric, 136–39
in mania, 36–37
in poststroke depression, 324, 326–27
Brain stem aminergic nuclei, apoptosis, in
Alzheimer's disease, 364–65, 366,
Color Figure 29.1
Brief alcohol intervention trials, 344
Brief dynamic therapy, for late-life
depression, 288–89
Bromocriptine, for depression in
Parkinson's disease, 352
Bupropion
for bereavement-related depression, 113
clinical trials, 198
in Parkinson's disease, 352
pharmacokinetics in elderly persons, 188t
side effects
anticholinergic, 205
cardiovascular, 206, 318
Burden of illness, late-life depression,
12–14

Calcium metabolism, age-related changes,
168
California Verbal Learning Test, 121
Carbamazepine
for bipolar disorder, 218–19, 219t
drug interactions, 219, 219t
plus lamotrigone, 217
side effects, 219
usage guidelines, 218–19
Carbidopa, for Parkinson's disease, 350
Carbohydrate metabolism, age-related
changes, 168

Cardiac Arrhythmia Suppression Trial
(CAST), 316
Cardiac disease
depression in patients with, 311–12
electroconvulsive therapy in patients
with, 255–56
and insulin resistance in depression, 314
ischemic. See Coronary artery disease
Cardiac risk, HPA axis hyperactivity and,
162–63
Cardiovascular death, sudden, depression
and, 314–15
Cardiovascular effects
antidepressants, 206–7, 315–18
antipsychotics, 236
electroconvulsive therapy, 255–56
lithium, 215
selective serotonin reuptake inhibitors,
206–7, 316–18
stimulants, 228, 318
tricyclic antidepressants, 196, 206, 207,
315–16
Caregiver burden, bipolar disorder, 41
Case identification, late-life depression,
3–4
Case management model, for suicide
prevention, 103
CAST (Cardiac Arrhythmia Suppression
Trial), 316
Catecholamines
in affective disorders, 361–62
age-related changes, 168
in depression, 162–63
in dysthymic disorder, 55
platelet activity and, 314
Caudate, 348
lesions, in depression, 356
neuronal loss, in Huntington's disease, 354
Cell death, programmed, in brain stem
aminergic nuclei, in Alzheimer's
disease, 364–65, 366, Color
Figure 29.1
Center for Elder Suicide Prevention, 101–2
Center for Epidemiologic Studies
Depression Scale (CES-D), 4, 25
Central nervous system
mechanisms of hormonal action, 167–68
stimulant effects on, 228
Cerebral atrophy, in late-life major
depression, 56
Cerebral blood flow
in encephalomalacia, 135–36
in late-life major depressive disorder
baseline deficits, 139–41, 140f, 142f
treatment and recovery effects,
141–44, Color Figures 11.5 to
11.7
in vascular depression, 144
Cerebral blood volume, in
encephalomalacia, 135–36
Cerebral infarction, silent, in late-onset
major depression, 132, 133
Cerebral metabolic rate
in encephalomalacia, 135
in late-life major depressive disorder,
140f, 141, 142, 143–44, Color
Figures 11.6 to 11.7